histology

The National Medical Series for Independent Study

histology

Ray C. Henrikson, Ph.D.
*Professor of Pathology and Laboratory Medicine
and Coordinator of Anatomy Education*

Gordon I. Kaye, Ph.D.
Alden March Professor of Pathology and Laboratory Medicine

Joseph E. Mazurkiewicz, Ph.D.
Professor of Microbiology, Immunology, and Molecular Genetics

*Albany Medical College
Albany, New York*

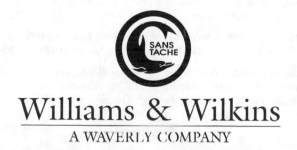

Williams & Wilkins
A WAVERLY COMPANY

BALTIMORE • PHILADELPHIA • LONDON • PARIS • BANGKOK
BUENOS AIRES • HONG KONG • MUNICH • SYDNEY • TOKYO • WROCLAW

Editor: Elizabeth A. Nieginski
Manager, Development Editing: Julie Scardiglia
Managing Editor: Amy G. Dinkel
Marketing Manager: Rebecca Himmelheber
Production Coordinator: Peter J. Carley
Illustration Planner: Peter J. Carley
Cover Designer: Cotter Visual Communications
Typesetter: Maryland Composition Co., Inc.
Printer: Mack Printing Group
Digitized Illustrations: Maryland Components Co., Inc.
Binder: Mack Printing Group

351 West Camden Street
Baltimore, Maryland 21201-2436 USA

Rose Tree Corporate Center
1400 North Providence Road
Building II, Suite 5025
Media, Pennsylvania 19063-2043 USA

Printed in the United States of America

Library of Congress Cataloging-in-Publication Data

Henrikson, Ray C.
    NMS histology / Ray C. Henrikson, Gordon I. Kaye, Joseph E. Mazurkiewicz.—1st ed.
        p. cm.—(The National medical series for independent study)
    Includes index.
    ISBN 0-683-06225-5
    1. Histology—Outlines, syllabi, etc.   2. Histology—Examinations, questions, etc.   I. Kaye, Gordon I.   II. Mazurkiewicz, Joseph E.
III. Title.   IV. Series.
    [DNLM: 1. Histology—outlines.   2. Histology—examination questions.   QS 518.2 H518n 1997]
    QM553.H385   1997
    611'.018'076—dc21
    DNLM/DLC   97-8734
    for Library of Congress   CIP

The publishers have made every effort to trace the copyright holders for borrowed material. If they have inadvertently overlooked any, they will be pleased to make the necessary arrangements at the first opportunity.

To purchase additional copies of this book, call our customer service department at **(800) 638-0672** or fax orders to **(800) 447-8438**. For other book services, including chapter reprints and large quantity sales, ask for the Special Sales department.

Canadian customers should call **(800) 665-1148**, or fax **(800) 665-0103**. For all other calls originating outside of the United States, please call **(410) 528-4223** or fax us at **(410) 528-8550**.

Visit Williams & Wilkins on the Internet: http://www.wwilkins.com or contact our customer service department at **custserv@wwilkins.com**. Williams & Wilkins customer service representatives are available from 8:30 am to 6:00 pm, EST, Monday through Friday, for telephone acces.

                                                98 99 00
                                    2   3   4   5   6   7   8   9   10

Contents

Preface   xiii
Acknowledgments   xv

1   Membrane Structure and Cell Surface   **1**
   I.   Introduction   1
   II. Organization of biological membranes   1
   III. Plasma membrane functions in cell regulation and signaling   4
   IV. Endocytosis: transport of macromolecules and particles   5
   V. Plasma membrane surface structures   8

2   Cytoplasmic Organelles and Inclusions   **13**
   I.   Introduction   13
   II. Endoplasmic reticulum   13
   III. Golgi apparatus   17
   IV. Mitochondria   19
   V. Peroxisomes   21
   VI. Lysosomes   22
   VII. Particles and inclusions   24

3   Cytoskeleton   **25**
   I.   Introduction   25
   II. Actin   25
   III. Microtubules   28
   IV. Intermediate filaments   30

4   Nucleus   **35**
   I.   Introduction   35
   II. Chromosomes   35
   III. Nucleolus   37
   IV. Nuclear envelope   38
   V. Nuclear pores   39
   VI. Nuclear lamina   39
   VII. Nuclear matrix   40
  VIII. Cell cycle   40
   IX. Meiosis   43

5   Epithelium   **47**
    I.   Introduction   47
    II.   General characteristics of epithelia   47
    III.   Functions of epithelia   48
    IV.   Classification of epithelia   48
    V.   Intercellular junctions of epithelial cells   50
    VI.   Epithelial cell mitosis and tissue renewal   58
    VII.   Epithelia–connective tissue interface   58

6   Nerve   **61**
    I.   Introduction   61
    II.   Neurons   61
    III.   Synapses   66
    IV.   Supporting cells of the nervous system   69
    V.   Myelin sheath of the peripheral nervous system   70
    VI.   Myelin sheath of the central nervous system   74
    VII.   Comparison of peripheral myelin and central myelin   75
    VIII.   Unmyelinated nerves in the peripheral and central nervous systems   75
    IX.   Connective tissue sheaths of peripheral nerve   76
    X.   Blood–brain barrier   77
    XI.   Degeneration and regeneration in the nervous system   77
    XII.   Afferent receptors   78

7   Muscle Tissue   **81**
    I.   Introduction   81
    II.   Contractile proteins   81
    III.   Classification of muscle   83
    IV.   Skeletal muscle   83
    V.   Cardiac muscle   93
    VI.   Smooth muscle   94
    VII.   Repair and renewal in muscle tissue   96

8   Connective Tissue   **97**
    I.   Introduction   97
    II.   Fibers of connective tissue   97
    III.   Ground substance of connective tissue   103
    IV.   Cells of connective tissue   106
    V.   Classification of connective tissue   111
    VI.   Histogenesis of connective tissue   113

9   Adipose Tissue   **115**
    I.   Introduction   115
    II.   White adipose tissue   115
    III.   Brown adipose tissue   119

10   Cartilage   **121**
    I.   Introduction   121
    II.   Cartilage cells   121

    III.   Cartilage matrix   122
    IV.   Types of cartilage   124
    V.   Supply of nutrients to chondrocytes   125
    VI.   Cartilage growth   126

11   Bone   127

    I.   Introduction   127
    II.   Bone cells   127
    III.   Bone matrix   129
    IV.   Types of bone   130
    V.   Bone-associated fibrous connective tissue   131
    VI.   Osteogenesis: intramembranous ossification   132
    VII.   Osteogenesis: endochondral ossification   133
    VIII.   Osteons and lamellar bone   136
    IX.   Growth and remodeling of a long bone   139
    X.   Growth and remodeling of a flat bone   139
    XI.   Fracture repair   140
    XII.   Bone and hormonal control of calcium   140

12   Blood   143

    I.   Introduction   143
    II.   Erythrocytes   143
    III.   Neutrophils   145
    IV.   Eosinophils   147
    V.   Basophils   148
    VI.   Lymphocytes   149
    VII.   Monocytes   150
    VIII.   Platelets   151

13   Hematopoiesis   155

    I.   Introduction   155
    II.   Hematopoietic stem cells   155
    III.   Erythropoiesis   158
    IV.   Granulopoiesis   160
    V.   Megakaryocytopoiesis   164
    VI.   Monocytopoiesis   166
    VII.   Microscopic anatomy of the marrow compartment   166

14   Cardiovascular System   169

    I.   Introduction   169
    II.   The heart   169
    III.   General structure of blood vessels   173
    IV.   The arterial vessels   174
    V.   Capillaries   176
    VI.   The venous vessels   180
    VII.   Portal blood vessels   181
    VIII.   Arteriovenous anastomosis (AVA)   182
    IX.   Lymphatic vessels   182

15   Lymphatic Cells and Tissues   185
     I.   Introduction   185
     II.   Lymphocytes   185
     III.   B Lymphocytes and humoral immunity   186
     IV.   T Lymphocytes and cell-mediated immunity   189
     V.   Other features of humoral and cell-mediated immune responses   190
     VI.   Structural framework of lymphatic tissues   191
     VII.   Diffuse lymphatic tissue   191
     VIII.   Lymphatic nodules and germinal centers   192

16   Tonsils, Peyer Patches, and Appendix   195
     I.   Introduction   195
     II.   Tonsils   195
     III.   Peyer patches   196
     IV.   Appendix   197
     V.   M cells   198

17   Lymph Nodes   201
     I.   Introduction   201
     II.   Surface landmarks of lymph nodes   201
     III.   Lymph node compartments: cortex and medulla   201
     IV.   Lymphatic sinuses   204
     V.   Lymph pathway through a lymph node   205
     VI.   Blood pathway through a node and lymphocyte recirculation   205
     VII.   Functions of lymph nodes   206

18   Spleen   209
     I.   Introduction   209
     II.   Histologic landmarks of the spleen   209
     III.   White pulp   209
     IV.   Marginal zone   211
     V.   Red pulp   211
     VI.   Blood vessels of the spleen   213
     VII.   Blood circulation through the red pulp: closed versus open   214

19   Thymus   215
     I.   Introduction   215
     II.   Histologic landmarks of the thymus   215
     III.   Thymic epithelial reticular cells   215
     IV.   Cortex of the thymus   216
     V.   Medulla of the thymus   217
     VI.   Blood-thymus barrier   217
     VII.   Involution of the thymus   218
     VIII.   Role of thymus in immune response   220

20   Skin   221
     I.   Introduction   221
     II.   Epidermis   221

III. Dermis   226
IV. Hair follicles   228
V. Sebaceous glands   230
VI. Eccrine sweat glands   232
VII. Apocrine glands   234
VIII. Nail   235
IX. Skin injury, cutaneous appendages, and wound healing   235

21   General Plan of the Alimentary Tract   **237**
I. Introduction   237
II. Basic plan of the wall of the alimentary canal   237
III. Functions of the alimentary mucosa   240
IV. Functional specializations in the wall of the alimentary canal   243

22   Oral Cavity   **245**
I. Introduction   245
II. Mucosa of the oral cavity   245
III. Tongue   246
IV. Teeth   248
V. Supporting tissues of the teeth   252

23   Exocrine Glands—Salivary Glands   **255**
I. Introduction   255
II. General characteristics of exocrine glands   255
III. Parotid glands   259
IV. Submandibular gland   260
V. Sublingual gland   260
VI. Saliva   260

24   Esophagus and Stomach   **263**
I. Esophagus   263
II. Stomach   265
III. Cells of the gastric glands   269

25   Small intestine and Colon   **273**
I. Small intestine   273
II. Colon   284

26   Liver and Gallbladder   **289**
I. Introduction   289
II. General structure of the liver   289
III. Hepatic circulation   289
IV. Organization of liver parenchyma   292
V. Hepatocytes   293
VI. Perisinusoidal space   298
VII. Biliary system   299
VIII. Bile   300
IX. Gallbladder   302

27   Exocrine Pancreas   **305**
   I.   Introduction   305
   II.   Histologic characteristics   305
   III. Serous acinar cells   305
   IV.   Duct system   307
   V.   Control of pancreatic exocrine secretion   309

28   Respiratory System   **311**
   I.   Introduction   311
   II.   Nasal cavity   311
   III.   Paranasal sinuses and nasopharynx   313
   IV.   Larynx   314
   V.   Trachea   314
   VI.   Bronchi   315
   VII.   Bronchioles   317
   VIII. Alveoli   318
   IX.   Air–blood barrier   320
   X.   Surfactant   321

29   Urinary System   **323**
   I.   Introduction   323
   II.   General characteristics of the kidneys   323
   III.   Organization of the kidney parenchyma   323
   IV.   Interstitium of the kidney   325
   V.   Nephron   325
   VI.   Duct system of the kidney   334
   VII.   Renal circulation   335
   VIII. Histophysiology of the kidney   337
   IX.   Renal nerve supply   338
   X.   Excretory passages of the urinary system   338

30   Pituitary Gland and Hypothalamus   **341**
   I.   Introduction to endocrine system   341
   II.   Pituitary gland   341
   III. Adenohypophysis   344
   IV.   Neurohypophysis   346
   V.   Hypothalamic regulation of hypophysis   348

31   Thyroid and Parathyroid Glands   **351**
   I.   Introduction   351
   II.   Thyroid gland   351
   III. Parathyroid glands   354

32   Adrenal Gland   **359**
   I.   Introduction   359
   II.   Development and structure   359
   III. Adrenal cortex   359
   IV.   Adrenal medulla   362
   V.   Fetal adrenal gland   364

33   Islets of Langerhans   **367**
    I.   Introduction   367
    II. Structure and development   367
    III. Control of release of insulin and glucagon   369

34   Pineal Gland   **371**
    I.   Introduction   371
    II. Pineal parenchymal cells   371
    III. Pineal functions   371

35   Female Reproductive System   **373**
    I.   Introduction   373
    II. Ovaries, oocytes, and ovarian follicles   373
    III. Ovulation and corpus luteum formation   377
    IV. Mitosis and meiosis of the female germ cell   379
    V. Oviducts   380
    VI. Fertilization   381
    VII. The uterus   381
    VIII. The menstrual cycle   384
    IX. The vagina   385
    X. The mammary gland   386
    XI. The placenta   388

36   Male Reproduction System   **391**
    I.   Introduction   391
    II. Testes   391
    III. Spermatogenesis   395
    IV. Sertoli cells   400
    V. Intratesticular genital ducts   402
    VI. Extratesticular genital ducts   403
    VII. Accessory sex glands   404
    VIII. Penis   406

37   Eye   **409**
    I.   Introduction   409
    ii. Specific functions of ocular tissues   409
    III. Embryonic development   411
    IV. Cornea   413
    V. Sclera   415
    VI. Anterior chamber and associated structures   415
    VII. Posterior chamber and associated structures   416
    VIII. Vitreous body   418
    IX. Retina   419
    X. Blood–ocular barrier   421
    XI. Choroid   422
    XII. Eyelids   422
    XIII. Lacrimal apparatus   423
    XIV. Extraocular muscles   423

38   Ear   **425**

    I.   Introduction   425
   II. External ear   425
  III. Middle ear   425
  IV. Inner ear   426
   V. Functions of the inner ear   429

Comprehensive Exam   **433**

Index   **499**

Preface

Histology occupies an important place in the biomedical curriculum. The study of macromolecular components and organelles of the cell, the myriad of cells and cell products that are assembled to form tissues, and certain aspects of the macroscopic structure of organs are all in the realm of histology. Histology now encompasses much of cellular and molecular biology, and many aspects of physiology and biochemistry, as well as traditional microscopic anatomy. The techniques of electron microscopy, cytochemistry, and immunochemistry are now routinely used to study the histology of cells, tissues, and organs.

The purpose of this book is twofold:

- The **concise presentation** in **outline format** enables the student initially to gain an overview of histology and later to review the discipline. This is particularly important in today's biomedical curriculum because of the reduction in time devoted to basic sciences and the dispersal of specific disciplinary materials into evolving, nontraditional curricula.

- The inclusion of approximately **300 study questions, and integration of their answers with the text,** enables the student to review histology, in a timely and efficient manner, in the context of licensing and other comprehensive examinations.

Acknowledgment

The authors are indebted to Marilyn Dockum for her expert assistance in all aspects of the preparation of this book.

Chapter 1

Membrane Structure and Cell Surface

I. **INTRODUCTION.** The cell is the basic unit of structure and function of all tissues and organs. It is a small, membrane-bounded aqueous compartment that contains the molecules, macromolecules, and inclusions that permit the cell to carry out its myriad functions.

A. **Classification of cells.** Cells can be separated into two categories: **prokaryotic cells** (bacteria) and **eukaryotic cells** (protists, fungi, plants, and animals). Eukaryotic cells, by definition, contain a **nucleus** (Greek *karyon* = nucleus); prokaryotic cells do not. This chapter is concerned chiefly with eukaryotic cells, in particular mammalian cells.

B. **Membranous compartments of eukaryotic cells**

1. When a routinely prepared histologic section of a tissue or an organ is examined in the light microscope, the stain in the section is seen to be distributed in a regular pattern. The stain appears to be limited by a barrier, permitting single cells to be delineated, and within that barrier the stain is further distributed differentially.

   a. The **plasma membrane,** which surrounds a cell, is indicated by the barrier limiting the stain.

   b. Within the area defined by the plasma membrane, the differential distribution of the stain reflects the compartmentation of the cell's cytoplasm into many smaller, subcellular **organelles** (e.g., nucleus, endoplasmic reticulum, Golgi apparatus, mitochondria, lysosomes, endosomes, peroxisomes; see Chapter 2).

2. The plasma membrane and the membranes of the organelles have a similar basic structure and composition. Specific differences in composition reflect the functions of individual membranes.

II. **ORGANIZATION OF BIOLOGICAL MEMBRANES**

A. **Overview**

1. Biological membranes are composed of lipids and proteins, held together primarily by noncovalent interactions. A small amount of carbohydrate is covalently bound to membrane proteins and lipids.

2. The membrane lipids form the structural foundation of a membrane, whereas the proteins are primarily responsible for the active functions of membranes.

3. The current interpretation of how a biological membrane is organized at the molecular level is referred to as the **modified fluid-mosaic model** (Figure 1-1).

B. **Lipid bilayer.** The basic structure of a biological membrane is the lipid bilayer.

1. The lipids in biological membranes are **amphipathic:** they have a **hydrophilic** ("water-loving"), or **polar,** head end and a **hydrophobic** ("water-hating"), or **nonpolar,** tail end.

   a. The **hydrophilic polar head groups** orient toward the outside of the bilayer and interact with the aqueous environment.

   b. The **hydrophobic hydrocarbon tails** interact with each other to form the inner core of the bilayer.

2. This gives a constant orientation to the lipid layers in all membranes that surround a compartment: the plasma membrane and the membranes of all organelles within a cell have this arrangement.

A

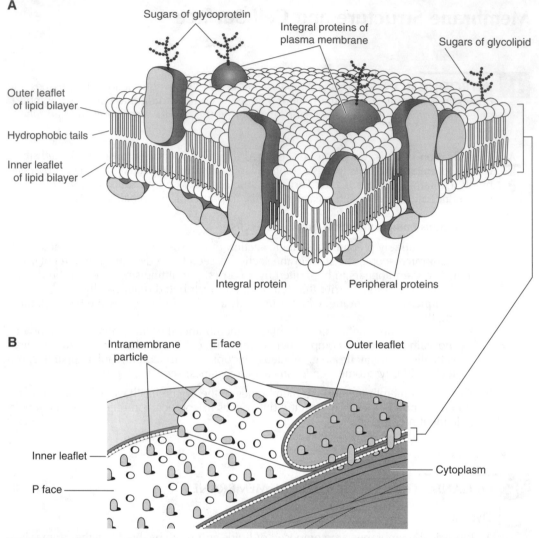

B

FIGURE 1-1. Structure of a biologic membrane. (*A*) The modified fluid-mosaic model. The biologic membrane is modeled as a continuum of phospholipids forming a bilayer, with proteins asymmetrically distributed in the bilayer. The proteins can be embedded within the membrane and completely traverse the bilayer, or they can be associated with only one side or the other of the bilayer. Carbohydrate moieties of glycoproteins and glycolipids are present on the external surface, facing the extracellular space. (*B*) The cleavage pathway in a freeze-fractured plasma membrane, showing the plasma membrane leaflets separated along the cleavage plane, which preferentially follows the hydrophobic interior of the bilayer. Proteins appear as particles on the internal faces of both separated layers of the membrane. The bracketed portions of the two diagrams indicate what would appear as the trilaminar image of the unit membrane in electron micrographs. *E face* = extracellular face; *P face* = protoplasmic (cytoplasmic) face.

3. The layer on the outside is called the **outer leaflet** and the layer on the inside is called the **inner leaflet.**
   a. The outer leaflet of the plasma membrane faces the extracellular environment and the outer leaflets of the organelles face the cytoplasm.
   b. The inner leaflet of the plasma membrane faces the cytoplasm and the inner leaflets of the organelles face an internal **cisternal** compartment.

C. **Membrane lipids.** There are three major types of lipids in biological membranes: phospholipids, cholesterol, and glycolipids.

1. **Phospholipids.** The most abundant lipid component in a biological membrane, phospholipids form the backbone of the membrane.
   a. Phospholipids at the appropriate concentration will spontaneously form a lipid bilayer when mixed with water. This bilayer will form a vesicle with no hydrophobic edges facing the aqueous environment.
   b. Phospholipids are diglycerides built on a glycerol backbone.
      (1) **Hydrophilic portion.** The polar head groups, either choline, serine, ethanolamine, or inositol, are linked to carbon 3 of glycerol to form the four major phospholipids: **phosphatidylcholine, phosphatidylserine, phosphatidylethanolamine,** and **phosphatidylinositol.**
      (2) **Hydrophobic portion.** Two hydrocarbon fatty acyl chains are linked to carbons 1 and 2 of glycerol; the fatty acyl tails interact with each other by weak van der Waals interactions.

2. **Cholesterol.** Like the phospholipids, cholesterol is amphipathic. Cholesterol contains a polar hydroxyl group, a hydrophobic planar steroid ring, and an attached hydrocarbon chain.
   a. Cholesterol inserts between the phospholipids in the lipid bilayer, with its hydroxyl group near the polar head groups and its steroid ring parallel to the acyl chains in the hydrophobic interior of the bilayer.
   b. Cholesterol plays a significant role in modulating the structure and fluidity of biological membranes.

3. **Glycolipids.** Glycolipids are lipids with sugar residues attached to them.
   a. Glycolipids are always present on the outer leaflet of the plasma membrane, with the sugar groups facing the outside of the cell. Their asymmetric distribution and orientation result from the way in which sugars are added during biosynthesis (see Chapter 2 II A 2 b; III B 2).
   b. Human and animal cell glycolipids are made from ceramide and are called **glycosphingolipids.** The glycosphingolipids are important for cell–cell and cell–matrix interactions, and contribute to the net negative charge of the cell surface.

D. Membrane proteins

1. Membrane proteins are of two classes: integral and peripheral.
   a. **Integral membrane proteins** are embedded within the phospholipid bilayer, and cannot be removed without disruption of the membrane (e.g., by extraction with organic solvents or treatment with detergent).
      (1) Some integral membrane proteins span the membrane, crossing it once (single-pass) or more than once (multiple-pass). Others are partially embedded in the membrane, on one side or the other. Integral membrane proteins can also be tethered to the phospholipid backbone via covalent interaction with fatty acid side chains that anchor them to the membrane.
      (2) Integral membrane proteins are amphipathic; portions directly interact with the hydrophobic interior of the bilayer, and hydrophilic regions interact with the aqueous environment, on one side or both sides of the membrane.
   b. **Peripheral membrane proteins** are defined as those proteins that can be removed without membrane disruption (e.g., by treatment of the membrane with solutions of high ionic strength or by shifting the pH of the solution that bathes the membrane).
      (1) These proteins are distributed asymmetrically on a membrane: they can be associated with one side or the other of the lipid bilayer.
      (2) Peripheral membrane proteins form this association by ionic interactions with integral membrane proteins, with other peripheral membrane proteins, or with the polar head groups of phospholipids.

2. **Membrane glycoproteins.** Most plasma membrane proteins are glycoproteins. Their sugar moieties are located on the outside surface of the cell, as are the sugar moieties of glycolipids.

E. **Mobility of membrane components.** Membranes are fluid structures. Membrane proteins and phospholipids can diffuse relatively freely within the plane of the membrane. However, their movements can be restricted in several ways.

1. Membrane proteins, both integral and peripheral, can have their movement restricted by attachment to other membrane proteins or to cytoskeletal elements.

2. Phospholipid movement within the bilayer can also be restricted by association with membrane proteins that are restricted in their movement.

3. A high cholesterol concentration (as is found in the eukaryotic plasma membrane) stiffens the membrane, thereby reducing membrane fluidity and restricting the diffusion of both phospholipids and proteins.

4. Membrane proteins and phospholipids do not spontaneously "flip-flop" from one leaflet to the other. They usually remain in the leaflet to which they were sorted during their biosynthesis and the assembly of the membrane.

F. **Microscopy of cellular membranes**

1. A biologic membrane cannot be **resolved** with the light microscope. It can be **detected,** however, and its presence inferred from the distribution of stain in a histologic section. A biologic membrane can be resolved by electron microscopy.

2. **Transmission electron microscopy** using thin sections of osmium tetroxide–fixed material shows a biologic membrane, when viewed in cross section, to be a **trilaminar structure:** two electron-dense layers with an electron-lucent layer between them (see Figure 1-1).
   a. This trilaminar structure has been designated the **unit membrane.**
   b. The total thickness of a biologic membrane is about 8 to 10 nm.

3. **Freeze-fracture electron microscopy** permits the examination of biologic membranes in the plane of the membrane. This procedure typically splits, or cleaves, the membrane along the hydrophobic plane between its two lipid layers (see Figure 1-1B).
   a. The cleavage exposes the interior of the membrane, revealing two faces of the membrane, the **E-face** (backed by the extracellular space) and the **P-face** (backed by the protoplasm, or cytoplasm).
   b. Numerous **intramembrane particles** seen on the two faces are considered to represent **integral membrane proteins.** The patterns of these particles can provide clues to the distribution of membrane proteins within the bilayer and can be related to functions of the particular membrane being examined.

III. **PLASMA MEMBRANE FUNCTIONS IN CELL REGULATION AND SIGNALING.** The plasma membrane is the interface between a cell and its external environment. The plasma membrane encloses a cell, governs what passes into and out of a cell, and responds to signals received from the external milieu.

A. **Classes of plasma membrane proteins.** Plasma membrane proteins have been categorized into several broad classes based on their function: pumps and carrier proteins, channels, receptors and transducers, enzymes, and structural proteins. Some proteins may serve more than one of these functions.

1. **Pumps** actively transport molecules across the plasma membrane. For example, **Na$^+$,K$^+$-ATPase,** the **sodium pump,** moves sodium and potassium ions across the plasma membrane. **Carrier proteins** also move ions across the membrane, as well as metabolites such as amino acids and sugars, usually by coupling their movement to the activity of the sodium pump.

2. **Channels** allow the passage of small ions and molecules across the plasma membrane in either direction. **Gap junctions** are intercellular junctions that contain channels [see Chapter 5 V C 2 b (2) (b)].

3. **Receptor proteins** bind specific extracellular signaling molecules (ligands) that initiate a response by a cell. A receptor is often a transmembrane protein with its ligand-binding site exposed to the external medium. Intracellular domains of receptor proteins are usually associated with some other molecule or complex that produces a signal. These receptors transfer information rather than ions or molecules across the membrane; thus, they act as **transducers.**

   a. **A ligand-gated receptor** is associated with a specific ion-selective aqueous channel. Binding of the ligand to the receptor induces a conformational change in the protein components of the channel. The channel then opens, permitting specific ions to move through it and thereby cross the membrane.

   b. **Enzymatic,** or **catalytic, receptors** contain a tyrosine kinase domain on the cytoplasmic surface of the membrane. This type of receptor activates a cell by phosphorylating tyrosine residues on intracellular proteins following binding by a ligand.

   c. **G protein–linked receptors** are associated with a guanosine triphosphate (GTP)-binding protein, or G protein, on the cytoplasmic surface of the plasma membrane. The binding of a ligand to this type of receptor activates the G protein.

      (1) Typically, G protein–linked receptors cause a change in the cytoplasmic concentration of one or more small intracellular signaling molecules, called **second messengers** (e.g., Ca^{2+}, cyclic AMP).

      (2) Some G protein–linked receptors activate the **inositol trisphosphate (IP_3) signaling pathway.** IP_3, a second messenger, induces the release of calcium, another second messenger, from stores in the smooth endoplasmic reticulum.

B. **Topographic distribution of membrane proteins.** The specific sites of proteins in a membrane can determine the function of the entire plasma membrane or of regions in the membrane. For example:

1. **Na^+,K^+-ATPase** is present on the surface of all cells and in this distribution plays a role in the regulation of intracellular volume.

2. In epithelia, tight junctions restrict Na^+,K^+-ATPase to the basolateral surface. Here it functions in the transport of Na^+ and K^+ across the basolateral membrane and the transport of salt and water across the entire epithelium (see Chapter 25 I C 1 c).

IV. ENDOCYTOSIS: TRANSPORT OF MACROMOLECULES AND PARTICLES

A. **Overview**

1. Proteins, macromolecules, and larger particles cannot be transported across the plasma membrane by the proteins that mediate the passage of small polar molecules and ions. Instead, the cell utilizes a process called **endocytosis,** in which a portion of the plasma membrane associates with the material to be taken up, invaginates, and is pinched off, producing an intracellular vesicle containing the ingested material.

2. Two types of endocytosis are recognized: **pinocytosis** and **phagocytosis.** Pinocytosis is a property of all cells. Phagocytosis is carried out by only a few cell types, the most notable being macrophages and neutrophils.

B. **Pinocytosis.** This process involves the ingestion of fluid and solutes via small vesicles (< 200 nm diameter).

1. There are two forms of pinocytosis: fluid-phase pinocytosis and receptor-mediated endocytosis.

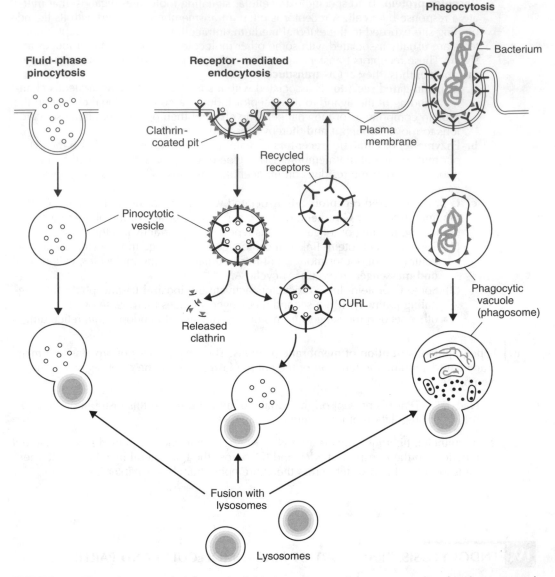

FIGURE 1-2. The major types of endocytosis: fluid-phase pinocytosis, receptor-mediated endocytosis, and phagocytosis. (See text for explanation.)

    a. Fluid-phase pinocytosis (Figure 1-2). In this form, small volumes of extracellular fluid and any solutes or small particles suspended in it are taken up nonspecifically in **noncoated pinocytotic vesicles.** The mechanisms involved in the formation of the vesicle are not well understood.

        (1) The concentration of the solute that is taken up in the vesicle is directly proportional to its concentration in the immediate extracellular fluid.

        (2) Although receptors are not involved in this process, in some instances, solute can interact with the charge on the plasma membrane by electrostatic interaction (e.g., positively charged, basic molecules are taken up more rapidly than negatively charged, acidic ones), making the uptake more selective.

    b. Receptor-mediated endocytosis (see Figure 1-2). In this form of pinocytosis plasma membrane receptors, occupied or not, are taken up in **coated vesicles.** The process requires that receptors be clustered in regions of the plasma membrane that are coated internally with a protein called **clathrin.**

(1) Formation of the vesicle. The material (ligand) to be endocytosed first binds to a receptor. The receptor may either be located in a coated region or moves to a coated region by lateral diffusion in the membrane after the ligand binds. A **coated pit** forms by invagination of the coated region, and the pit then becomes a **coated vesicle** as it is pinched off into the cytoplasm.

     (a) Clathrin molecules spontaneously assemble into a cage-like structure; this traps the overlying membrane and drives the formation of the vesicle.

     (b) The vesicle loses its clathrin coat soon after it is formed.

(2) Receptor–ligand interactions. Receptor-mediated endocytosis exhibits features that characterize basic receptor–ligand interactions.

     (a) The number of receptors for a specific ligand in the plasma membrane is limited ($\sim 10^5$ or fewer per cell). Thus, the uptake of ligand is saturable at low extracellular concentrations.

     (b) The high affinity of the ligand for the receptor, however, means that the ligand will be efficiently removed from the extracellular environment and concentrated in the cell.

     (c) Also, the number of ligand molecules taken up over a period of time can far exceed the number of receptors, because receptors are recycled via exocytosis and reutilized (see Figure 1-2).

2. Fate of endocytotic vesicles

  a. Some fluid-phase pinocytic vesicles carry their contents from one surface to another and release their content at that surface (e.g., pinocytic vesicles of vascular endothelium). Others sequester ions taken up from the extracellular medium (e.g., pinocytic vesicles in smooth muscle cells). Some may fuse with lysosomes.

  b. In receptor-mediated endocytosis, the vesicles are almost always targeted to **lysosomes,** where their contents are broken down.

     (1) In some instances of receptor-mediated endocytosis, the receptors are first dissociated from their bound ligand in a prelysosomal compartment known as **CURL** [compartment to uncouple receptor and ligand; see Chapter 2 III B 3 b (2)].

        (a) From the CURL, the receptor is recycled to the plasma membrane. The ligand is delivered to lysosomes and broken down.

        (b) The products of ligand digestion can serve in metabolic processes. For example, after the uptake and digestion of low-density lipoprotein (LDL), the released cholesterol is used by the cell for membrane synthesis.

     (2) In other instances the receptor–ligand complex is delivered to lysosomes intact and then broken down. This is one mechanism for **receptor down-regulation** used in some signaling processes (e.g., epidermal growth factor and its receptors).

  c. Some endocytic vesicles are not delivered to lysosomes but instead move to another domain of the plasma membrane, fuse with it, and release their contents. This process, called **transcytosis,** is involved in the mechanism for secretion of immunoglobulins A and M (see Chapter 25 I E 2).

C. **Phagocytosis** (see Figure 1-2). In phagocytosis, large regions of the plasma membrane extend around and engulf large particles such as microorganisms or cell debris. Vacuoles ($> 1 \ \mu m$ diameter) called **phagosomes** are formed.

1. Phagosome formation. The current interpretation of how phagosomes form is known as the **zipper hypothesis.**

  a. Phagocytosis is a receptor-mediated event: the phagocyte must have receptors on its plasma membrane that can recognize target molecules and bind to them. In addition, a particle or cell to be ingested must have binding sites distributed over its entire surface.

  b. Once the phagocyte has attached to its target, the plasma membrane of the phagocyte gradually surrounds the target, each receptor sequentially interacting with a binding site, much like the operation of a zipper.

  c. The cortical actin cytoskeleton in the phagocyte is reorganized, helping to facilitate the extension of the membrane around the target.

d. When the target is completely engulfed, the apposing portions of the membrane fuse to form the vacuole (phagosome).

2. Fate of phagocytic vacuoles. The completed phagosome fuses with lysosomes and its content is usually degraded (see Chapter 8 IV A 2).

3. Opsonization. When the immune system mounts a humoral antibody response against a pathogenic microorganism, the IgG molecules that are formed act as **opsonins,** which coat the microorganism to enhance its phagocytosis by macrophages.
   a. The IgG molecules coat the pathogen by interaction of their antigen binding sites with the microorganism's surface; the tails of the IgG molecules extend away from the surface.
   b. Phagocytes contain receptors for the IgG tail in their plasma membranes. These are called Fc receptors, and the binding of these receptors with the IgG tail facilitates the phagocytic uptake of the pathogen.

V. PLASMA MEMBRANE SURFACE STRUCTURES

A. **Glycocalyx.** This plasma membrane coating is found on the outer surface of cells (see Figure 1-3).

1. Composition. The glycocalyx consists of:
   a. Oligosaccharides covalently bound to plasma membrane glycoproteins and glycolipids
   b. Long polysaccharide chains of integral membrane proteoglycans
   c. Glycoproteins and proteoglycans that were secreted and readsorbed to the cell surface

2. Functions. The glycocalyx helps to protect the cell surface from mechanical damage. The oligosaccharides also mediate specific, transient cell–cell recognition and adhesion reactions (e.g., neutrophil binding to endothelial cells during inflammation; sperm–egg interactions; blood clotting).

B. **Plasma membrane specializations.** Certain cells, such as epithelial cells, exhibit surface modifications that facilitate their function. These modifications can take the form of stable extensions (microvilli, stereocilia, cilia, and flagella), folds and interdigitations, and specialized intercellular junctions. Intercellular junctions are discussed in Chapter 5 V; other surface specializations are discussed here.

1. Microvilli (Figure 1-3). These are finger-like extensions on the surface of epithelial cells that increase the area available for absorption.
   a. Light microscopic morphology. A single microvillus is not visible by light microscopy, but clumps of microvilli can be seen on the surface of a cell as fine striations that run parallel to the long axis of the cell. The striations have been named a **brush border,** or **striate border,** because of their brush-like appearance.
   b. Electron microscopic morphology. Single microvilli are seen as tubular extensions of the apical plasma membrane of epithelial cells.
      (1) Microvilli have a relatively constant diameter of approximately 0.1 μm. Their length can vary (1–3 μm) but is nearly constant for a given cell type.
      (2) Microvilli have a core of actin filaments that provide support and give rigidity to the microvilli, helping to maintain their parallel arrangement.
         (a) The actin core is anchored to the plasma membrane at the tip and sides of the microvillus. The core extends into the apical cytoplasm, where it interacts with the terminal web, a horizontal network of actin filaments.
         (b) Contractions of the terminal web are thought to increase the space between the microvilli by causing them to spread apart at their tips.
   c. Microvillar surface enzymes. Many digestive enzymes are inserted into the plasma membrane of the microvilli and have specific roles in digestion and absorption [see Chapter 25 I C 1 d (2) (a)].

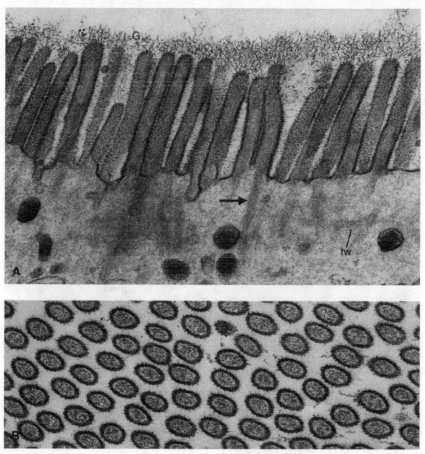

FIGURE 1-3. Electron micrographs of microvilli in longitudinal section (*A*) and cross-section (*B*). Note the uniformity of size and shape of the microvilli. The core of a microvillus is filled with bundles of actin filaments that extend out of the microvillus (*arrow*) into the apical cytoplasm, where they interact with the terminal web (*tw*). The fuzzy coating on the surface of the microvilli represents the glycocalyx (*G*).

2. **Stereocilia.** Stereocilia are elongated microvilli. They have no motile function and are not related to cilia, despite their name. Like microvilli, they contain actin filaments in their core. However, stereocilia are more restricted than microvilli in distribution.

   a. In the male reproductive system, stereocilia can be seen, in routine histologic sections, projecting into the lumen of the epididymis and the vas deferens, often in pyramid-shaped clumps. They may function in the absorption of substances from the tubular lumen.

   b. In the inner ear, stereocilia are found on the hair cells of the organ of Corti, semicircular canals, and maculae. Here, the stereocilia act as transducers, generating electrical potentials from the mechanical shearing forces that impinge on them during sound perception or body movements.

3. **Cilia and flagella.** Cilia and flagella are motile structures that project from the surface of a cell. They originate from basal bodies (see Chapter 3 III E). Cilia and flagella have similar structural elements and similar motile mechanisms, as well as origins. Cilia and flagella can move fluid and particles across the cell surface or propel the cell itself.

   a. **Light microscopic morphology**

      (1) With the light microscope, cilia appear as multiple short, hair-like structures projecting from the surface of a cell. Flagella are longer than cilia, and cells typically have only a single flagellum.

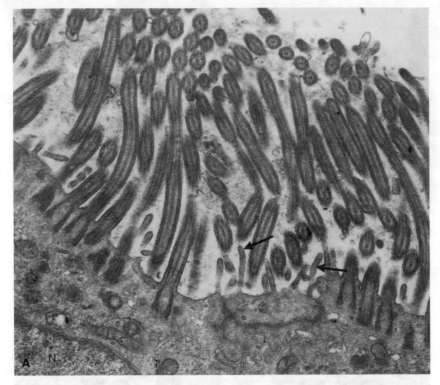

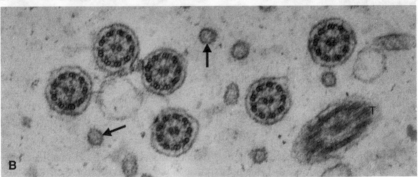

FIGURE 1-4. Electron micrographs of cilia in longitudinal section (*A*) and cross-section (*B*). The central core of each cilium is formed by bundles of microtubules. In each cilium, note the two central microtubules and the circular arrangement of nine peripheral doublets of microtubules. Microvilli (*arrows*) are visible in the interciliary space. *T* = tangentially sectioned cilium; *N* = nucleus.

       (2) When cilia are present in large numbers (e.g., on tracheal epithelium), their basal bodies are visible as a darkly staining band in the cytoplasm just beneath the cilia.

   b. Electron microscopic morphology. Cilia and flagella are composed of bundles of microtubules (Figure 1-4).

       (1) The **axoneme,** or core, of a cilium or flagellum consists of nine doublet microtubules in a ring around a pair of singlet microtubules (Figure 1-5).

       (2) Extending from each doublet in the outer ring are dynein side arms that give cilia and flagella their motility.

   c. Ciliary and flagellar motility

       (1) The dynein side arms of the doublet microtubules hydrolyze ATP to produce a sliding force between adjacent doublets. This sliding underlies the movements of cilia and flagella.

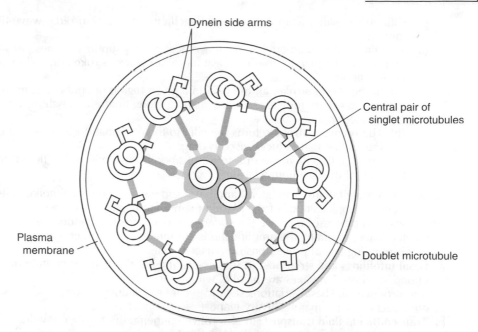

FIGURE 1-5. Diagram of the internal structure of a cilium.

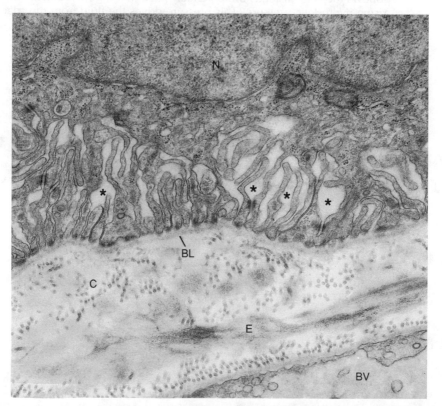

FIGURE 1-6. Electron micrograph of the basal surface of epithelial cells, showing extensive basal plications. The extracellular space (*) between the folds of the plasma membrane can increase in volume to accommodate transient increases in fluid volume as water moves across the epithelium. *Bl* = basal lamina; *N* = portion of nucleus; *C* = collagen fibrils; *E* = elastic fibrils; *BV* = capillary.

(2) Cilia move with a whip-like motion; flagella move in a sinusoidal wave-like motion.

(3) The many cilia on an epithelial surface beat rapidly (up to 15 times per second) in synchronized fashion. A beat has a fast power stroke and a slow recovery stroke.

    (a) In the **power stroke,** all the cilia in a given region of epithelium move in one direction, fully extended, sweeping along fluid and anything suspended in it.

    (b) The **recovery stroke** returns the cilia to their original position with a curling motion that reduces viscous drag.

(4) Unlike cilia, flagella move in a series of smooth undulations that flow from the base of the flagellum to its tip.

4. Folds and interdigitations. The lateral and basal surfaces of certain epithelial cells show extensive amplifications of the plasma membrane (Figure 1-6). These folds (plications) and processes increase the surface area and create a tortuous potential intercellular space. Laterally, the amplifications are interleaved or interdigitated with the corresponding lateral projections on adjacent cells.

  a. Basal infoldings and striations. In some cells, the basal processes contain mitochondria whose long axes are parallel with the long axis of the cell. This orientation produces the basal striations seen in sections of kidney tubules and the striated ducts of some major salivary glands.

  b. Transepithelial fluid transport. In absorptive epithelia, the highly convoluted lateral surface membranes are rich in Na^+,K^+-ATPase.

    (1) Na^+ is pumped from the cytoplasm across the lateral membrane, so that the space between the lateral interdigitations becomes hypertonic. The water that follows the Na^+ distends the potential space into an intercellular space with rising hydrostatic pressure. This pressure drives the fluid from the space into the adjacent connective tissue.

    (2) Mitochondria associated with the lateral plasma membrane provide the energy source for this process.

Chapter 2

Cytoplasmic Organelles and Inclusions

I. **INTRODUCTION.** The cytoplasmic compartment of a eukaryotic cell is the intracellular space situated between the plasma membrane and the nucleus.

A. **Cytoplasmic components.** The cytoplasm contains a variety of **membranous organelles, filamentous structures, particles,** and **inclusions.** These formed structures are surrounded by the **cytosol,** which is composed of water; ions; various metabolites, including amino acids and nucleotides; numerous proteins; and molecules such as glucose and adenosine triphosphate (ATP).

B. **Major biosynthetic pathways.** The cytoplasm of eukaryotic cells is elaborately subdivided into a series of functionally distinct, membrane-bounded organelles. A division of labor exists within the cell, whereby specific metabolic processes are localized to each organelle. The organelles in a major biosynthetic pathway are interconnected via vesicular transport.

1. **Vesicular transport.** A general mechanism of vesicular transport explains the movement of proteins and phospholipids between and within membrane-bounded organelles in a biosynthetic pathway.
   a. Vesicles form and pinch off from one membranous compartment, move to the next membranous compartment in the pathway (i.e., the target), fuse with it, and deliver their content.
   b. Vesicles then pinch off from the target membrane and return to and fuse with the original membrane to pick up more cargo. In this way, membranous organelles retain their unique identity as biosynthetic products pass through them.

2. **Protein biosynthetic pathway.** The intracellular pathway for protein synthesis and secretion links the **rough endoplasmic reticulum (rER), Golgi apparatus,** and **trans-Golgi network (TGN).** Certain proteins begin their synthesis in the rER; they are then transported to the Golgi apparatus, where they are further modified; and they are then sorted to their final location in the TGN.

3. **Membrane phospholipid biosynthetic pathway.** The intracellular pathway for membrane phospholipid synthesis and distribution links the **smooth endoplasmic reticulum (sER)** to the rER, from whence the phospholipids are distributed to other organelles in the protein biosynthetic pathway via vesicles. Cytoplasmic **phospholipid exchange proteins** carry phospholipids from the sER to other organelles that are not in the protein biosynthetic pathway.

II. **ENDOPLASMIC RETICULUM.** The ER plays major roles in cellular biosynthetic processes. It is a single membrane-bounded organelle in the cytoplasm that forms a large, continuous, interconnected network of compartments called the **ER cisternae.** The ER membrane accounts for more than 50% of the total membrane in a cell. The sER and the rER comprise two distinct regions of the ER. Although the membranes of these two regions are continuous, they are morphologically, compositionally, and functionally distinct.

A. **Smooth endoplasmic reticulum**

1. **Morphology.** The sER consists of a series of anastomosing, smooth-surfaced tubules (Figure 2-1).

2. **Function.** The sER is responsible for the biosynthesis of membrane lipids. This includes membrane phospholipids as well as cholesterol and ceramide. Ceramide

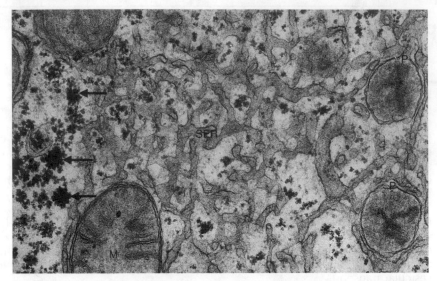

FIGURE 2-1. Electron micrograph of smooth endoplasmic reticulum (*sER*) in the cytoplasm of a hepatocyte. The sER is visible as a network of anastomosing tubules. Also in the field are peroxisomes (*P*), a portion of a mitochondrion (*M*), and glycogen (*arrows*).

can have a simple or complex carbohydrate side chain attached to it, to form a glycolipid.

   a. Location of biosynthesis. The enzymes involved in membrane lipid biosynthesis are localized in the cytoplasmic leaflet of the membrane, close to the cytoplasmic source of the substrates.

   b. Phospholipid translocation. Although membrane phospholipids are synthesized on the cytoplasmic side of the membrane, some are then moved to the cisternal leaflet. This accounts for the asymmetry of phospholipids observed in membrane compartments.

     (1) Flippases, enzymes which are present in the sER membrane, are responsible for this phospholipid translocation.

     (2) A particular flippase is responsible for the translocation of choline-containing phospholipid, but not for serine- or ethanolamine-containing phospholipids. Thus the **membrane lipid asymmetry** characteristic of biologic membranes is established within the sER.

   c. Transfer of sER-synthesized phospholipids to other membranous organelles

     (1) Transfer to the Golgi apparatus, lysosomes, and plasma membrane is accomplished by budding off of phospholipid-containing vesicles from sER and fusion of these vesicles with the target organelles.

     (2) Transfer to mitochondria and peroxisomes is accomplished by cytoplasmic phospholipid-exchange proteins.

3. Distribution. Because its role in phospholipid synthesis is essential for membrane maintenance, all cells contain some sER. However, it is particularly prominent in certain cell types.

   a. Hepatocytes. sER plays an important role in glycogen metabolism. In addition, the hepatocyte sER is the site for detoxification of lipid-soluble drugs, metabolic wastes, and ingested toxins.

   b. Striated muscle cells. sER sequesters cytoplasmic Ca^{2+} in most cells, and this function is highly developed in striated muscle cells. In these cells sER takes the form of the **sarcoplasmic reticulum,** an organelle that plays a major role in maintaining low concentrations of calcium in the sarcoplasm, and thus in the regulation of muscle contraction.

   c. Steroid hormone–producing cells. sER is well developed in cells that synthesize and secrete steroids, such as adrenal cortical cells, interstitial cells of the testes, and granulosa cells of the ovary.

B. **Rough endoplasmic reticulum**

    1. Morphology. The cytoplasmic leaflet of rER is studded with ribosomes and polyribosomes, giving it its rough appearance. It extends throughout the cytoplasm as a series of flattened membrane stacks or cisternae (Figure 2-2).

        a. The rER membrane is continuous with the membrane of the nuclear envelope.

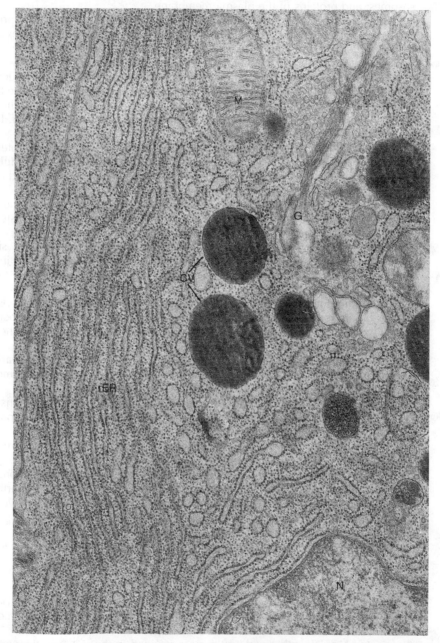

FIGURE 2-2. Electron micrograph of cisternae of rough endoplasmic reticulum (*rER*), part of a Golgi apparatus (*G*), and condensing vacuoles (*CV*) of a pancreatic acinar cell. This cell is specialized for protein synthesis and secretion. Also visible are a portion of a mitochondrion (*M*) and part of a nucleus (*N*).

    b. rER can be viewed by light microscopy by staining with basic dyes and with metachromatic dyes. This is because of the net anionic charge of the phosphate groups in the ribonucleic acids.

2. **Distribution.** rER is present in all cells, but it is abundant in cells specialized for protein secretion. It is prominent in the basal cytoplasm of some polarized secretory cells (e.g., exocrine pancreas) and in the perikarya of large neurons, where it is called **Nissl substance.**

3. **Function.** The rER is responsible for **protein biosynthesis,** including secretory proteins; lysosomal hydrolases; membrane proteins of the ER, Golgi apparatus and lysosomes; and proteins of the plasma membrane.

    a. Location of protein synthesis. Synthesis of all proteins begins on free polysomes in the cytoplasm (see VIII A). Polysomes that synthesize proteins on the rER are targeted to that organelle because the nascent protein contains a **signal sequence** near its amino terminus.

        (1) As the nascent protein emerges from the ribosome, the signal sequence is recognized by a cytoplasmic **signal recognition particle** (SRP). The SRP binds to the signal sequence, forming a complex that consists of the nascent protein, the ribosome, and the mRNA that is being translated. Protein synthesis is temporarily suspended.

        (2) The SRP complex binds to an **SRP receptor,** a transmembrane protein in the rER. Following docking, the ribosome binds to a **ribosome-binding protein** in the rER membrane, and the SRP dissociates and is recycled to the cytoplasm, and protein synthesis resumes.

    b. Translocation of proteins. As translation of the mRNA continues on the rER membrane-bound polysomes, the newly synthesized proteins are transferred across the rER membrane into the rER cisternae.

        (1) Secretory proteins. Following cleavage of the signal sequence by **signal peptidase,** an rER resident protein, secretory proteins are released into the cisternae. They are transported within vesicles from the rER to the Golgi apparatus.

        (2) Membrane proteins. Membrane proteins are also inserted into the rER membrane during synthesis. Membrane proteins, however, remain associated with the membrane of the vesicles as they move from the rER to the Golgi apparatus.

    c. Modification of proteins. Proteins synthesized on the rER undergo a variety of modifications. These can occur either during translocation across the membrane, or after the protein is released into the cisternae.

        (1) Cotranslational modifications involve modifications of, or additions to, specific amino acid residues in the primary sequence of the nascent proteins.

            (a) N-linked glycosylation

                (i) The addition of sugars to asparagine (Asn) residues is the most common modification.

                (ii) Most secretory and plasma membrane proteins are glycoproteins. Glycosylation of these glycoproteins begins in the rER. Further steps in the processing of N-linked oligosaccharides of glycoproteins occur in the Golgi apparatus (see III B 1).

            (b) Hydroxylation of proline and lysine residues in pro-α chains of collagen occurs while the nascent peptide is in transit across the rER membrane.

            (c) Cleavage of the signal sequence is itself a cotranslational modification of secretory proteins.

        (2) Post-translational modifications in the rER involve proper folding of proteins and association of protein subunits to form larger molecular complexes.

            (a) Newly synthesized proteins are retained in the rER until they either achieve proper conformation or they associate with the proper partner of an oligomeric complex.

(b) Several rER resident proteins serve this quality control function [e.g., binding protein (BiP), calnexin, protein disulfide isomerase].

4. **Vesicular transport from the rER to the Golgi apparatus.**
   a. **Transport vesicles** containing newly synthesized proteins pinch off the smooth-surfaced regions of the rER. These regions are called **transitional elements** of the rER.
   b. The vesicles move to and fuse with membranes of the **cis Golgi.**

5. **Vesicular transport to other membranous organelles.** Proteins that begin their synthesis in the rER move from the rER to the Golgi apparatus, move between and among Golgi stacks, and move from the *trans*-Golgi network to their final destinations by way of vesicles. The vesicles pinch off from one membrane, move to the next membranous compartment (target) in the pathway, fuse with it and deliver their content. They then pinch off from the target membrane and return to and fuse with the original membrane to pick up more cargo.

III. GOLGI APPARATUS

A. **Morphology.** The Golgi apparatus is an organelle that appears as a stack of 6–8 plate-like membranous compartments and associated vesicles and vacuoles, often located near the centrosome (Figure 2-3).

1. **Vesicles.** Large numbers of small vesicles are associated with the Golgi stacks. They are clustered on the *cis* **face** of the Golgi apparatus, which is the side nearest the rER. Vesicles are responsible for the directed movement of molecules from the rER to the Golgi apparatus.
   a. Vesicles are also arrayed along the outer rims of the Golgi cisternae.
   b. These small vesicles are responsible for the directed movement of molecules between the subcompartments of the Golgi apparatus.

2. **Vacuoles.** Vacuoles are located on the *trans* **face** of the Golgi apparatus, which is the side furthest away from the rER. Vacuoles are responsible for concentration and transport of finished products to their final destinations.

3. **Functional compartments of the Golgi apparatus.** The Golgi apparatus can be separated into four functionally distinct compartments: *cis* **Golgi stacks, medial Golgi stacks,** *trans* **Golgi stacks,** and the *trans* **Golgi network** (**TGN**). The first three are involved in post-translational modification of molecules transiting the stacks. The TGN is involved in sorting the molecules to their final destination (i.e., to lysosomes, to secretory vesicles, or to the plasma membrane).

B. **Function.** The Golgi apparatus functions in the further modification of proteins and lipids synthesized in the ER.

1. **Processing of N-linked oligosaccharide chains.** N-linked oligosaccharides synthesized in the rER are further processed in the Golgi apparatus in the *cis* and medial Golgi stacks.

2. **Synthesis of O-linked glycoproteins.** The addition of sugars to proteins at serine residues (O-linked glycoproteins) is accomplished in the medial and *trans* Golgi stacks by integral membrane proteins called **glycosyltransferases.** These enzymes also add sugars to the serine residues of glycolipids in the Golgi stacks.

3. **Processing of acid hydrolases.** Acid hydrolases destined for lysosomes are synthesized by polysomes of the rER. Further processing in the *cis* Golgi stacks targets them to the lysosomes.
   a. Targeting is accomplished by phosphorylating mannose residues on the enzymes, yielding **mannose-6-phosphate** (M-6-P).
   b. The hydrolases with M-6-P move through the Golgi stacks to the TGN, where

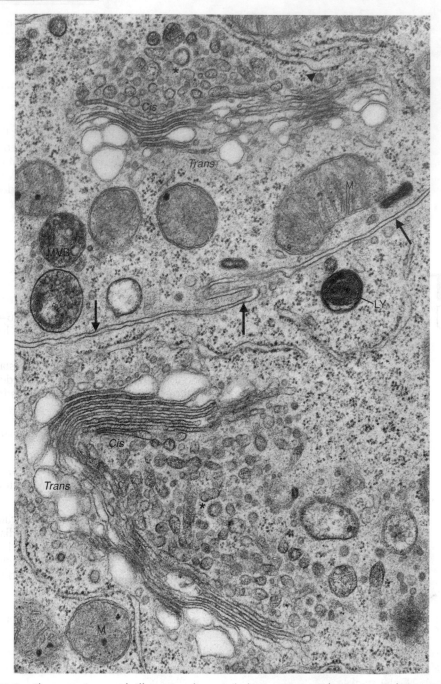

FIGURE 2-3. Electron micrograph illustrating the morphologic variations that may exist between examples of the Golgi apparatus. The profiles of two colonic epithelial cells show different views of the Golgi apparatus. The plasma membranes separating the two cells are indicated by *arrows*. In the upper cell, a portion of the rER containing transitional elements (*arrowhead*) is closest to the *cis* side of the Golgi apparatus. ER-to-Golgi transport vesicles are visible clustered between the rER and the cis Golgi (*). Smooth protrusions bud from the cisternae on the *trans* side of the Golgi apparatus. The profile of the Golgi apparatus in the lower cell is convex, in contrast with the flatter orientation of the Golgi cisternae in the upper cell. M = mitochondria, MVB = multivesicular bodies, LY = lysosome.

they bind to a mannose-6-phosphate receptor, a transmembrane protein in the TGN. This receptor aids in the sorting of the enzymes to lysosomes.

   (1) Receptor and hydrolase become localized to specialized regions of the TGN that are coated with the cytoplasmic protein **clathrin** (see Chapter 1 IV B 1 b).

   (2) Clathrin-coated vesicles, containing the receptor-bound hydrolases, pinch off the TGN and move to another membranous compartment in the cytoplasm called the **late endosome,** or **CURL** (compartment to uncouple receptor and ligand) [see Chapter 1 IV B 2 b (1)]. Here, the mannose-6-phosphate receptor and the hydrolase are uncoupled.

      (a) Hydrolases may remain in the late endosomal compartment to function there, or they may be packaged into lysosomes.

      (b) The mannose-6-phosphate receptor is cycled back to the TGN to be reused.

  4. Sulfation of proteins occurs in the *trans* Golgi stacks. The core proteins of proteoglycan of the extracellular matrix are extensively glycosylated and these sugars are heavily sulfated. Some tyrosine residues are also sulfated.

C. **Role of the Golgi apparatus in secretion.** Proteins and lipids that will become constituents of the plasma membrane, and proteins that will be secreted from the cell, move from the Golgi apparatus to the cell surface via transport vesicles. Some molecules are continuously transported to the cell surface and released, in a process called **constitutive secretion.** Other molecules are stored in secretory granules and released at a later time, following a stimulus. This process is called **regulated secretion. Sorting of these molecules occurs in the TGN.**

  1. Constitutive secretion is a function of all cells. Vesicles continuously move from the TGN to fuse with the plasma membrane, where they release their contents by **exocytosis.** The membrane of the vesicles is then taken back up by **endocytosis** and recycled to the Golgi apparatus. Examples of constitutive secretion include secretion of plasma proteins by hepatocytes, secretion of immunoglobulins by plasma cells, and delivery of proteins and lipids to the plasma membrane.

  2. Regulated secretion. Secretory proteins that follow this pathway are actively sorted to storage granules in the TGN by a process called **selective aggregation.** A signal sequence for sorting has not been identified for these proteins.

    a. Selective aggregation. These secretory proteins appear to aggregate in the presence of high Ca^{2+} concentration and a slightly acidic environment. Both of these conditions are met in regions of the TGN.

    b. Active sorting. The aggregated proteins become localized to regions of the TGN membrane that are coated with clathrin, which aids in the formation of coated vesicles.

    c. Post-translational modification of proteins in secretory granules. Secretory granules are not merely storage vesicles; active processing and maturation of content occur in them, as well. Newly formed vacuoles that pinch off of the TGN are large, with a dilute content. Such vacuoles are called **condensing vacuoles.** Subsequent modifications include **condensation** (i.e., concentration) of secretion, and **enzymatic modification** (i.e., cleavage) of secretory proteins.

    d. Stimulus of secretion. Increased cytoplasmic Ca^{2+} concentration is required to signal the secretory granules to move to the plasma membrane and release their contents via exocytosis.

IV. **MITOCHONDRIA.** Mitochondria are double-membrane organelles present in all cells (Figure 2-4). They are responsible for the production of ATP, and usually number about 1000 per cell. Mitochondria tend to accumulate in regions of the cell where metabolic activity is elevated and large amounts of ATP are required (e.g., apical mem-

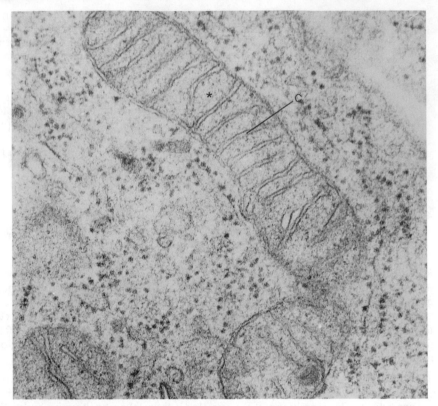

FIGURE 2-4. Electron micrograph of a mitochondrion. * = Matrix, C = crista.

brane of ciliated cells; basolateral membranes of cells involved in ion and water transport).

A. **Morphology.** Mitochondria are formed by two membranes that delineate two distinct compartments. They display a variety of shapes, including spheres, rods, and long filamentous structures.

1. **Outer membrane.** The outer membrane is smooth surfaced and contains a number of metabolic enzymes. The outer membrane also contains many molecules of **porin,** a transport protein. Porin is responsible for the outer membrane being **freely permeable** to solutes smaller than 5 kD.

2. **Inner membrane.** The inner mitochondrial membrane forms a variety of shelf-like and tubular folds called **cristae.** The numerous convolutions of the inner membrane greatly increase its surface area, enhancing its ability to generate ATP. The inner membrane is largely **impermeable** to ions. Thus, some form of **active transport** is required to move molecules across it.

3. **Mitochondrial compartments.** Two compartments are created by the two membranes.
   a. The **intermembrane space** is located between the inner and outer membranes.
   b. The **matrix** is located within the inner membrane. The matrix contains electron-dense matrix granules that contain accumulated Ca^{2+}, phosphate, and other divalent ions. The mitochondria are able to accumulate these ions against a concentration gradient.

B. **Function.** The mitochondrion is the organelle responsible for **ATP production.** A variety of metabolic pathways take place in the mitochondria, including β-oxidation of fatty acids, oxidative phosphorylation, and the Krebs cycle. Both the Krebs cycle and fatty acid oxidation produce substrates used by ATP synthase to form ATP.

1. **Mitochondrial enzymes**
   a. **Membrane enzymes.** The cristae contain ATP synthase and the enzymes of oxidative phosphorylation and the electron transport chain. ATP synthase is present in the form of **elementary particles,** lollipop-like structures whose "sticks"are embedded in the inner membrane, with the heads extending into the matrix.
   b. **Matrix enzymes.** The matrix contains the enzymes of the Krebs cycle and enzymes involved in the oxidation of fatty acids.

2. **Proton gradients.** The activity of the enzymes of the electron transport chain located in the inner mitochondrial membrane establishes an electrochemical proton (H^+) gradient across the inner membrane. This creates a large **proton motive force** (PMF), which causes the movement of H^+ down its electrochemical gradient through the ATP synthase. This movement of protons, called **chemiosmotic coupling,** drives ATP synthesis.
   a. The ATP that is produced is transported out of the matrix by an ADP–ATP antiport system in the inner membrane.
   b. The newly synthesized ATP then diffuses into the cytoplasm through the porous outer membrane.

C. **Mitochondrial genome.** Mitochondria contain their own DNA and protein synthesizing machinery. The genome is small, however, compared with the nuclear genome (see Chapter 4 II A).

1. Mitochondrial DNA is a closed, circular molecule that codes for 13 polypeptides, 2 rRNAs, and 22 tRNAs. All of the polypeptides encoded by mitochondrial DNA are subunits of the oxidative phosphorylation pathway. The tRNAs and rRNAs are used in the translation of the mitochondrial mRNAs that code for the polypeptides.

2. All of the rest of the mitochondrial proteins are coded for in the nuclear genome and are translated on polysomes free in the cytoplasm. They are post-translationally translocated across the mitochondrial membranes to reside in the appropriate mitochondrial membranes and compartments.

D. **Mitochondrial growth and division.** Mitochondria are never synthesized de novo. Rather, they arise from the growth and division of other mitochondria.

1. Mitochondria divide, increasing in number throughout interphase. The division of mitochondria is not in synchrony with the cell cycle. Replication of mitochondrial DNA is not restricted to the S phase but continues throughout the cell cycle.

2. The number of mitochondria appears to be regulated according to need. For example, when resting muscle is repeatedly stimulated to contract over a prolonged period of time, a 5- to 10-fold increase in mitochondrial number has been observed.

E. **Origins of mitochondria.** Mitochondria are believed to have originated during evolution from a relationship in which a prokaryote lived symbiotically in primitive eukaryotes. The following observations support this notion.

1. Mitochondria divide and contain their own genome. They synthesize rRNAs, tRNAs, and mRNAs, and they translate their messenger RNAs into mitochondrial proteins.

2. Mitochondrial ribosomal subunits more closely resemble those of bacteria than of eukaryotes.

3. Mitochondrial protein synthesis is sensitive to inhibitors of bacterial protein synthesis and not to inhibitors of eukaryotic protein synthesis.

V. **PEROXISOMES.** Peroxisomes are present in almost all eukaryotic cells as single membrane-bounded vesicles (see Figure 2-1).

A. **Morphology.** Peroxisomes are spherical or slightly ovoid structures that measure from 0.3 to 1.0 μm in diameter. Electron microscopy reveals a characteristically dense amorphous matrix. In some species (but not humans) they contain a crystalloid inclusion containing urate oxidase.

B. **Functions**

1. **β-oxidation of fatty acids.** The major function of peroxisomes is the breakdown of long-chain fatty acids via β-oxidation. Peroxisomes contain a variety of oxidative enzymes, and may be responsible for as much as 50% of this activity, with mitochondria accounting for the remainder.

2. **Hydrogen peroxide degradation.** β-oxidation produces hydrogen peroxide (H_2O_2), a potentially toxic substance to cells that must be eliminated.
   a. Peroxisomes contain the enzyme **catalase,** which destroys the H_2O_2 produced.
   b. Excess H_2O_2 that accumulates in a cell from other sources can also be eliminated by peroxisomes.

C. **Biogenesis.** Like the mitochondrion, the peroxisome is not in the protein biosynthetic pathway involving the rER and Golgi apparatus. Thus, all of the proteins and lipids of the peroxisome must be imported.

1. Proteins (both enzymes and membrane proteins) are synthesized on free polysomes in the cytoplasm and post-translationally imported into the peroxisome.

2. Phospholipids are made in the sER and transferred to peroxisomal membranes by phospholipid exchange proteins.

3. New peroxisomes arise from preexisting ones by growth and fission.

VI. **LYSOSOMES.** Lysosomes are membrane-limited organelles that are present in all cells. They contain a large number of acid hydrolases that are used in the **intracellular degradation of macromolecules.**

A. **Morphology.** Lysosomes are morphologically heterogeneous. This has resulted in a classification system based on ultrastructural characteristics in combination with enzyme histochemistry. Lysosomes are classified as **primary, secondary,** and **tertiary** (Figure 2-5).

1. **Primary lysosomes** are newly produced organelles that have not yet participated in any degradative process. These small vesicles, which measure 0.1 to 0.3 μm in diameter, stain homogeneously. They can be identified as lysosomes by staining for the enzymes they contain using appropriate histochemical reactions (e.g., for acid phosphatase).

2. **Secondary lysosomes** are usually much larger than primary lysosomes and have heterogeneous interiors indicative of the degradative processes taking place within the lysosomes.
   a. Material to be digested by lysosomal hydrolases can be delivered to the lysosomal compartment by several pathways.
      (1) **Endocytosis** and **phagocytosis** bring materials into the cell from the outside in vesicles that fuse with lysosomes (see Chapter 1 IV).
      (2) **Autophagocytosis** is a process by which the cell forms a membranous vacuole around cytoplasmic components. The vacuole subsequently fuses with lysosomes to expose its contents to hydrolytic enzymes.
   b. Secondary lysosomes contain partially digested material, the source of which sometimes can be identified by its residual structure. For example, an autophagic vacuole may contain recognizable fragments of mitochondria or rER; a phagocytic vacuole may contain a partially digested bacterium.

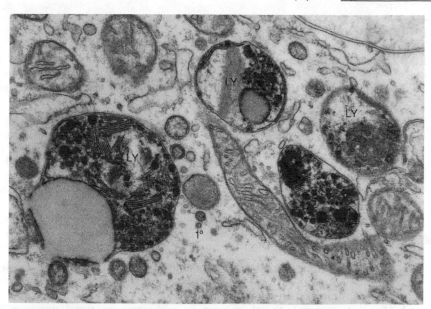

FIGURE 2-5. Electron micrograph of lysosomes (LY). These are either secondary or tertiary lysosomes. They contain material that is heterogeneous both in morphologic features and staining density. The material represents partially digested substances that could have originated from either endocytic or autophagocytic activity. A single primary (1°) lysosome is visible. It can be recognized by its small size and homogeneous contents.

3. **Tertiary lysosomes.** Morphologically, tertiary lysosomes resemble secondary lysosomes. Tertiary lysosomes, however, lack enzyme histochemical activity for acid hydrolases.
   a. Tertiary lysosomes accumulate in the cytoplasm with age. They may also be called **residual bodies.**
   b. In long-lived cells such as neurons, residual bodies are also known as **lipofuscin** (old-age pigment).

B. **Function.** More than 40 hydrolytic enzymes have been identified in lysosomes. These include proteases, lipases, nucleases, glycosidases, phophatases, phospholipases, and sulfatases. Almost any biologic substance, therefore, may be degraded by lysosomes. No single lysosome, however, contains all of the identified hydrolases.

1. **Acidic nature of the lysosome.** All of the lysosomal enzymes function at an acid pH (around 5.0). A proton pump (an H^+-ATPase) present in the lysosomal membrane lowers the pH by actively pumping H^+ into the lysosomal interior.

2. **Sites of lysosomal activity.** Most lysosomal function occurs intracellulary. However, some cells release lysosomal enzymes that function in the extracellular matrix.
   a. **Osteoclasts** actively secrete lysosomal enzymes into the extracellular milieu during bone resorption. These enzymes break down hydroxyapatite and release Ca^{2+} and phosphate into the blood.
   b. At sites of infection and inflammation, **neutrophils** often release their lysosomes into the extracellular matrix.

3. **Lysosomal storage diseases.** Several hereditary diseases have been identified that result from the absence of one or more specific acid hydrolases. The enzyme deficiency results in the intracellular accumulation of the normal substrates of those missing enzymes. For example, in Tay Sach, Fabray, and Gaucher diseases, glycolipids accumulate in lysosomes, eventually filling the cytoplasm and disrupting normal cell function.

VII. PARTICLES AND INCLUSIONS

A. **Ribosomes and polysomes.** All protein synthesis begins on ribosomes free in the cytoplasm. Messenger RNA, transfer RNA, and ribosomal subunits that were transported out of the nucleus into the cytoplasm assemble into functional protein-translating complexes.

1. **Morphology and distribution.** Ribosomes appear as angular particles with diameters ranging from 15 nm to 25 nm. They may occur singly (monoribosomes) or as polysomes, in clusters, spirals, rosettes, or helices. They may exist free in the cytoplasm or attached to rER membranes. Metabolically active cells have both free and bound polysomes.
   a. Cells specialized for protein secretion have a greater proportion of ribosomes as bound polysomes (i.e., fibroblasts).
   b. Undifferentiated cells and cells that synthesize large amounts of cytoplasmic proteins usually have more free polysomes (e.g., smooth muscle cells).

2. **Protein synthesis**
   a. **Bound ribosomes.** If a signal sequence is encoded by mRNA, this complex will be bound by a signal recognition particle and directed to the rER for continuation of translation.
   b. **Free ribosomes.** In the absence of a signal sequence, translation continues in the cytoplasm.

B. **Glycogen and lipid.** Cells store carbohydrates and lipids in forms that are readily available for use as intermediates in synthetic processes or as metabolic substrates.

1. **Glycogen** is a large branched polymer of glucose present in the cytoplasm as particles that are not enclosed by membranes. Particles measure about 30 nm in diameter, and may occur singly or in clusters (see Figure 2-1).
   a. Glycogen is abundant in hepatocytes and striated muscle cells but occurs sparingly in most other cell types. It is often associated with the sER.
   b. Glycogen synthesis and catabolism are highly regulated. When cells break down glycogen, glucose-1-phosphate is released and used in several metabolic pathways.

2. **Lipid droplets** are composed of triglycerides that have coalesced into droplets in the cytoplasm of cells. Triglycerides provide fatty acids to be used as an energy source in cells.
   a. During dehydration of tissue in preparation for light microscopy, lipid droplets are extracted, producing empty holes in routine histologic sections (see Figure 9-1). Fixation with osmium tetroxide, or preparation of frozen sections stained with lipid-soluble dyes, will readily demonstrate the droplets (see Figure 9-2).
   b. Steroid hormone–producing cells contain large numbers of lipid droplets, the contents of which serve as intermediates in the synthesis of steroid hormones.
   c. Accumulation of lipid droplets is a sign of a pathologic process in some cells (e.g., fatty degeneration of the liver).

Chapter 3

Cytoskeleton

I. **INTRODUCTION.** The cytoskeleton, in analogy to the bony skeleton of the body, provides a supporting framework for the cell, allowing it to adopt a variety of shapes. It also plays a role in organizing the content of a cell by maintaining the spatial distribution of organelles that is characteristic of a particular type of cell. In addition, the cytoskeleton provides the machinery for the movement of cells, and organelles within cells.

A. **Filamentous elements.** The cytoskeleton depends on three principal types of protein filaments: **actin, microtubules,** and **intermediate filaments,** plus a variety of **associated proteins.** Each type of filament is composed of a different protein subunit.

1. **Conservation of structure.** Actin and microtubule subunit proteins are highly evolutionarily conserved. Intermediate filaments, on the other hand, are diverse in size and molecular weight.

2. **Intracellular coexistence.** All three types of cytoskeletal filaments are found in most cells, sometimes independent of each other, but more often associated with one another through **accessory proteins.**

3. **The cytoskeleton is not a rigid super-structure.** In non-muscle cells, cytoskeletal elements are in a state of dynamic equilibrium between a pool of unassembled subunits and polymerized filaments. In muscle cells, the filamentous elements are found primarily in the assembled state (see Chapter 7).

B. **Organization of cytoplasm.** While membranous organelles (e.g., endoplasmic reticulum, Golgi complex, mitochondria, nuclei) provide for a division of function for many metabolic processes, the cytoskeleton provides for a higher order of organization by maintaining the placement of these organelles within the cytoplasm. Several examples follow.

1. **Cortical actin network.** A filamentous network of actin and **actin-binding proteins** is found just beneath the plasma membrane, forming a complex called the **cell cortex.** It controls cell shape and surface movement (see II C 1).

2. **Cytoplasmic scaffold.** The endoplasmic reticulum and Golgi membranes are positioned along an array of microtubules emanating from the **centrosome.**
   a. Golgi stacks are usually located closer to the centrosome than is the endoplasmic reticulum. The endoplasmic reticulum, which forms an extensive membranous network throughout the cytoplasm, is strung out along a scaffolding of microtubules.
   b. **Motor proteins,** which have attachment sites for cellular organelles and for microtubules, are responsible for moving organelles to their appropriate positions.

3. **Integrators of cytoplasmic space.** In most animal cells an extensive network of intermediate filaments surrounds the nucleus, extends out to the cell periphery, and contacts the plasma membrane. In epithelial cells this intermediate filament cytoskeleton attaches to **desmosomal plaques** to rigidify cell–cell contact (see Chapter 5).

II. **ACTIN.** Actin is the most abundant protein in most eukaryotic cells, comprising up to 5% or more of the total protein in non-muscle cells, and up to 20% of the weight of muscle cells.

A. Types of actin
1. **Filamentous actin (F-actin)** is a tight linear helix of polymerized globular subunits (monomers) called G-actin.

    2. Monomeric actin (G-actin), molecular weight of 42 kD, has binding sites for the nucleotides adenosine triphosphate (ATP) or adenosine diphosphate (ADP), and for both monovalent (K^+) and divalent (Mg^{2+}) cations.

B. **Actin polymerization.** When G-actin monomers are mixed in vitro with K^+, Mg^{2+}, and ATP, they polymerize into long filaments of F-actin.

    1. Polymerization begins with a lag phase (nucleation period), after which F-actin forms rapidly (elongation phase) until a plateau level of polymerization (steady-state phase) is reached.

        a. Nucleation period. The lag phase represents a kinetic barrier, as monomers associate first to form dimers and then trimers. The trimer is the **nucleating structure** for the spontaneous addition of monomer into the growing filaments.

        b. Elongation. Monomers are added to each end of the trimer, producing an elongated filament of 7 to 9 nm diameter and of indeterminate length.

        c. Steady state. At the steady-state phase, the rate of addition of monomer is equal to the rate at which monomer leaves the filament.

    2. ATP hydrolysis. Shortly after addition of monomers to the growing actin filament, the terminal phosphate of the ATP bound to the actin molecules is hydrolyzed.

        a. Hydrolysis of ATP results in a change in conformation of each actin subunit in the filament.

        b. While hydrolysis of ATP is not necessary for polymerization, the change in conformation modifies the rate of addition of G-actin at the two ends of the growing filament.

    3. Polymerization rate. The difference in the polymerization rate at the two ends of the forming filaments confers a **polarity** on the growing filament.

        a. The faster-growing end is the **plus end.** Growth at this end is up to 10 times faster than at the slower-growing **minus end.**

        b. At each end there is a **critical concentration** (C_c) of free actin monomer at which the rate of association is equal to the rate of dissociation.

            (1) The C_c at the plus end is approximately 1 μmol/l, while at the minus end it is approximately 8 μmol/l.

            (2) At G-actin concentrations between these values, monomer will add to the plus end and be subtracted from the minus end at the same rate, resulting in a condition called **treadmilling.** This is the steady-state condition.

                (a) At concentrations below 1 μmol/l, depolymerization is favored at both ends of the actin filaments. Disassembly will continue until the free monomer concentration reaches the C_c, whereupon steady-state conditions will be re-established.

                (b) At concentrations above 8 μmol/l, polymerization will be favored at both ends of the filaments. Growth will continue until the free monomer concentration drops to the C_c, whereupon steady-state conditions will be re-established.

                (c) During treadmilling, the filament will remain at a constant length, even though there is net flux of subunits through the filament.

    4. Regulation of polymerization. In non-muscle cells, the concentration of G-actin in the cytoplasm is in the range of 50 to 200 μmol/l. At these concentrations, one would expect all of the G-actin to be in the form of filaments, given the low C_c of actin. This is not the case, however, because most of the actin monomers are sequestered by a group of small actin-binding proteins (see II C), examples of which are **profilin** and **thymosin β_4.**

        a. Interaction of profilin and G-actin blocks participation of the monomer in the nucleation step that initiates polymerization.

        b. This interaction is a regulated process, so that monomers can be made available when needed. In platelet activation, for instance, this results in the extreme shape change essential for thrombus formation (see Chapter 12 VIII C 1).

C. **Actin-binding proteins.** Actin is found in a variety of structures within a cell, from stiff protrusions of the cell surface, such as microvilli, to the dynamic, three-dimensional

TABLE 3-1. Functions of Major Actin-Binding Proteins

Functions of Actin-Binding Proteins (ABPs)	Examples of ABPs
Bundle actin filaments: side to side or end to end	Fimbrin, villin, α-actinin
Strengthen actin filaments	Tropomyosin
Cross-link actin filaments into a gel	Filamin
Fragment actin filaments	Gelsolin
Attach sides of actin filaments to plasma membrane	Spectrin, ankyrin
Slide actin filaments in muscle	Myosin II
Move vesicles on actin filaments	Myosin I
Sequester actin monomers	Profilin, thymosin β_4

actin matrix in the **cell cortex.** Although the structure of the actin filaments is constant, the organization and motile function associated with them result from a large variety of actin-binding proteins that bind to F-actin, helping to organize and modulate its functions. Other actin-binding proteins bind to G-actin, regulating polymerization. Table 3-1 presents a summary of the major classes of actin-binding proteins. Examples of interactions between actin and actin-binding proteins include the following:

1. **Cell cortex.** Just beneath the plasma membrane in the cortical cytoplasm is a three-dimensional network of actin filaments that excludes organelles.
   a. The long filaments of actin are cross-linked into the network by two filamentous actin-binding proteins, fimbrin and spectrin II, forming a viscous gel.
   b. This gel can be made more liquid (i.e., sol-like). **Gelsolin,** another actin-binding protein present in this network, becomes a severing protein when cytoplasmic Ca^{2+} exceeds 10^{-6} mol.
      (1) When a **macrophage** comes in contact with a particle that it will engulf, intracellular Ca^{2+} levels increase and gelsolin cuts the actin filaments into short fragments. Gelsolin remains tightly bound to the newly created plus ends, blocking monomer growth. The resulting disassembly of the actin net permits the cell surface to restructure so that it can take up the particle.
      (2) During **regulated secretion,** cortical actin is made less viscous by gelsolin, following a stimulus that produces a transient increase in cytoplasmic Ca^{2+} levels. Secretory granules stored in the cytoplasm are then able to move to the plasma membrane, fuse with it, and release their contents by exocytosis.
   c. In motile cells, cortical actin can readily be reorganized to permit the extension of **lamellipodia.** A lamellipodium is a sheet-like extension of the cell's leading edge that makes contact with the underlying substratum and pulls the cell along.

2. **Microvilli.** The surface membrane of some epithelial cells has finger-like projections, called microvilli, that increase the surface area for absorption.
   a. Each microvillus has a central core of 20 to 30 tightly bundled actin filaments that run parallel to its long axis and that attach to the surface membrane at the tip (see Figures 1-3, 5-4).
   b. The filaments are crosslinked by two actin-binding proteins, **fimbrin** and **villin.** They are attached to the plasma membrane by **myosin I** and a **calmodulin,** and they are attached to the tip by another actin-binding protein of unknown composition.

D. **Actin-disruptive toxins.** Two toxins, **cytochalasin** and **phalloidin,** have been used to study actin monomer–polymer equilibrium.

   1. **Cytochalasin.** The fungal alkaloids cytochalasin A and B, and the more potent derivative cytochalasin D, bind to the plus ends of actin filaments in a cell, causing them to depolymerize.
      (a) Cytochalasin blocks the addition of subunits to the plus end, causing the C_c for actin monomers to shift to that of the minus end, causing subunits to dissociate from the filament.

(b) When cytochalasin is added to live cells, the actin cytoskeleton disappears. Cell locomotion and cytokinesis are thus inhibited and cells change shape.

2. **Phalloidin.** The phalloidins, derived from the *Amanita* mushroom, have the opposite effect; they stabilize actin filaments in the cell.
   (a) Phalloidin binds at the interface between subunits in F-actin, locking them together.
   (b) Because phalloidin binds only to F-actin, fluorescent-tagged phalloidin is used as an F-actin–specific stain in light microscopy.

III. MICROTUBULES.

III. **MICROTUBULES.** Microtubules are stiff, hollow cylinders with a diameter of 25 nm. Because they extend throughout the cytoplasm, they govern the location of membranous organelles and are involved in a variety of cellular motile functions, including movement of cilia and flagella, intracellular vesicle transport, and movement of chromosomes during meiosis and mitosis (Figure 3-1).

A. **Composition of microtubules.** Microtubules are long, filamentous polymers of **tubulin subunits.**

1. The tubulin subunit is a heterodimer of two non-identical globular monomeric proteins: α-**tubulin,** at the head of the subunit, and β-**tubulin,** at its tail. Each monomer has a molecular weight of approximately 50 kD.

2. Each heterodimer has two nucleotide binding sites, one on each monomer. The binding site on α-tubulin binds guanosine triphosphate (GTP) irreversibly but does not hydrolyze it. In contrast, the binding site on β-tubulin binds GTP reversibly and can hydrolyze it to guanosine diphosphate (GDP).

B. **Polymerization of tubulin.** Tubulin heterodimers add to one another head to tail, in a linear column to form **protofilaments.** Thirteen protofilaments, through lateral interactions, associate side to side to form long, hollow cylinders.

1. The assembly of microtubules follows a kinetic course similar to the polymerization of G-actin to form filamentous actin: nucleation, elongation, and steady state.

2. Because tubulin subunits are polarized, the protofilaments and microtubules that are formed from them are also polarized structures. The **plus end** grows faster than the **minus end.**
   a. As with F-actin, a different C_c of free tubulin subunits exists for each end of the microtubule.
   b. The minus end of a microtubule is usually capped. It is associated with the **cen-**

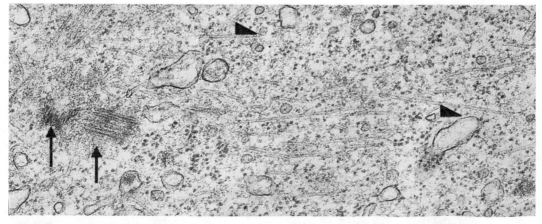

FIGURE 3-1. Microtubules (*arrowheads*) forming part of a mitotic spindle. The associated centrioles, which are microtubule organizing centers (MTOCs), are also visible (*arrows*). The microtubule triplets forming the walls of the centrioles are indistinct because of the plane of section.

trosome (see III E 1). Thus, only the plus end is available for the addition of tubulin dimers, thereby determining the polar orientation of microtubules in a cell.

C. **Dynamic instability of microtubules.** Microtubules undergo rapid assembly and disassembly. When monitored with morphologic cell culture techniques, individual microtubules can be observed growing steadily at a constant rate and then, suddenly, shrinking rapidly back toward the centromere. This behavior of microtubules has been termed dynamic instability. The current model to explain this phenomenon involves a relationship between the addition of GTP–tubulin dimers and the timing of the subsequent hydrolysis of the GTP to GDP.

1. The GTP–tubulin dimers add to the plus end of a rapidly growing microtubule faster than the rate of GTP hydrolysis.

2. This results in the formation of a GTP cap. Because GTP-bound tubulin dimers bind to one another more efficiently than to GDP dimers, the microtubule continues to grow.

3. If the rate of polymerization slows, allowing GTP hydrolysis to catch up, the GTP cap is lost and the microtubule, now containing only GDP–tubulin dimers, rapidly shrinks.

4. This catastrophic shrinkage occurs because GDP-capped microtubules are very unstable and the addition of GTP-tubulin to GDP-tubulin is very inefficient.

D. **Microtubule-associated proteins (MAPs).** If the process of dynamic instability were the sole determinant of polymerization of microtubules within a cell, at any one time some microtubules would be growing rapidly while others would be collapsing catastrophically. To assure some constancy in the microtubule cytoskeleton, however, MAPs stabilize microtubules and promote their interaction with other cellular components.

1. **Classification of MAPs.** MAPs are classified into two major groups: **HMW-MAPs** (high molecular weight proteins, > 200 kD) and **LMW-MAPs** (low molecular weight proteins, 55–62 kD). LMW-MAPs are also called **tau proteins.**

2. **Functions of MAPs**
   a. **Cellular structure.** Some MAPs act as structural components, providing connections to other cellular components. MAPs link microtubules to cellular components and inhibit microtubule depolymerization. MAPs also bind along the entire length of cytoplasmic microtubules, thus stabilizing them.
   b. **Molecular motors.** Other MAPs move membranous structures along microtubules.
      (1) The molecular motors **kinesin** and **cytoplasmic dynein** are a diverse group of microtubule-dependent motor proteins that are involved in organelle transport and in vesicular transport in axons [see Chapter 6 II C 3 e (4) (b) (i), (ii)]. Cytoplasmic dynein was so named because of its resemblance to ciliary dynein (see III F 2).
      (2) Both molecular motors are composed of two heavy chains and several light chains.
         (a) The heavy chains are similar to myosin in that they have a rod-like alpha-helical tail domain and a globular head that binds ATP.
         (b) Two tails intertwine to form a coiled coil, with which the light chains associate.
      (3) The globular heads bind to the microtubule and convert the hydrolysis of the bound ATP into movement of the molecular motor along the microtubule. Vesicular components of the cytoplasm interact with the tails and are thus carried along.
      (4) In general, cytoplasmic dyneins move their cargo toward the minus end of the microtubule, while kinesins move their cargo toward the plus end.

E. **Microtubule organizing centers.** These are regions in the cytoplasm that are preferred nucleation sites for the assembly of microtubules. They protect the minus end of microtubules and foster growth by the addition of tubulin dimers at the plus end.

1. **Centrosome.** The centrosome is the major site of microtubule nucleation in a cell. When the microtubules in an interphase cell are stained, they can be observed radiating outward from the centrosome, a region of the cytoplasm located near the nucleus.

   a. At the center of the centrosome are two hollow cylindrical structures called **centrioles.** These are oriented perpendicular to each other and are surrounded by a darkly staining, amorphous material (see Figure 3-1).

   b. The wall of each centriole is composed of nine triplet **microtubules.** Each triplet is formed by the lateral fusion of three adjacent microtubules.

      (1) The ends of the cytoplasmic microtubules do not interact directly with the triplet-microtubules of the centrioles, but with the associated amorphous material.

      (2) One component of this material, γ-**tubulin,** interacts with α and β-tubulins to foster nucleation of microtubules.

   c. Centrioles duplicate during interphase, producing two pairs of centrioles that migrate to opposite sides of the nucleus at the start of mitosis. They form the two poles of the mitotic spindle (see Chapter 4 VIII B 1 a).

2. **Basal bodies.** MTOCs also occur within basal bodies. The microtubules in cilia and flagella assemble from basal bodies, structures that resemble centrioles (see III F 3).

F. **Cilia and flagella.** Cilia and flagella of eukaryotic cells are specialized structures that are composed of bundles of **doublet microtubules.** They provide motility to the cells that possess them (e.g., swimming movement of sperm, directional beating of cilia of respiratory epithelial cells).

1. **Ultrastructure.** The ultrastructure of cilia and flagella are similar (see Chapter 1 V B 3 c).

2. **Ciliary and flagellar motility.** The dynein side arms hydrolyze ATP to produce a sliding force between the doublets.

3. **Cilia and flagella grow from basal bodies.** Basal bodies are cylindrical structures in the cytoplasm near the plasma membrane. They are composed of nine triplet microtubules. Adjacent triplets are joined by linker proteins along their length.

   a. During development of a cilium or flagellum, each doublet microtubule of the axoneme grows out from two of the microtubules in the triplet, maintaining the nine-fold symmetry of the basal body. It is not known how the two central microtubules of the axoneme grow.

   b. The cilia in a cell are usually the same length, but the mechanism for the establishment of this set length is also not known.

   c. In some instances, basal bodies and centrioles have been reported to interconvert from one to the other.

G. **Microtubule-disruptive toxins.** The drugs **colchicine** and **taxol** are used as anti-mitotic agents. They bind to tubulin or to microtubules, interfering with the exchange of tubulin subunits between microtubules and the cytoplasmic pool of tubulin dimers.

1. **Colchicine** inhibits microtubule assembly and promotes disassembly of existing microtubules. It binds directly with unpolymerized tubulin dimers, preventing their assembly.

2. **Taxol** has the opposite effect. It stabilizes microtubules when bound to them. It also promotes polymerization, thus depleting the tubulin pool.

3. In medicine, colchicine and taxol have been used to reduce growth of both benign and malignant tumors. By interfering with the mitotic spindle, they slow or stop uncontrolled cell division.

IV. **INTERMEDIATE FILAMENTS.** Intermediate filaments are the third set of cytoskeletal filaments. They are so named because in electron micrographs their apparent diameter (10 nm) lies between that of actin (7 nm) and microtubules (25 nm). In most cells, inter-

TABLE 3-2. Major Types of Intermediate Filament Proteins: Distribution and Properties

Intermediate Filament Protein	Intermediate Filament Type	Average Molecular Weight ($\times 10^3$)	Number of Polypeptides	Primary Tissue Distribution
Keratin	I	40–56.5	20	Epithelia
Keratin	II	53–70	20	Epithelia
Vimentin	III	57	1	Mesenchymal cells
Desmin	III	53–54	1	Muscle cells
Glial Fibrillary Acidic Protein (GFAP)	III	57	1	Astrocytes in CNS; some Schwann cells in PNS
Neurofilament proteins				
NF-L	IV	60	1	Axons,
NF-M	IV	140	1	dendrites, and
NF-H	IV	210	1	cell bodies of all CNS and PNS neurons
Nuclear lamins				
Lamin A and C	V	60–70	1	Nucleus of all
Lamin B	V	67	1	nucleated cells

CNS = central nervous system; PNS = peripheral nervous system.

mediate filaments form a meshwork surrounding the nucleus and extend out to the cell periphery, forming a network of filaments within the cytoplasm.

A. **Types of intermediate filaments.** In vertebrate cells, intermediate filaments are composed of a heterogeneous group of proteins that vary greatly in molecular weight and diverge widely in sequence. They are classified into five major classes or types (Table 3-2) Each type is characteristic of certain tissues and cells.

1. **Type I and type II intermediate filaments: keratin filaments.** Keratin intermediate filaments (also called cytokeratins) are found in epithelial cells (Figure 3-2).
   a. These are obligate heterodimers comprising a 1:1 mixture of type I (acidic) cytokeratins and type II (neutral/basic) cytokeratins. Neither subunit alone can form a filament.
   b. In human epithelia there are more than 20 different keratins that vary in molecular weight from 40 to 70 kD.

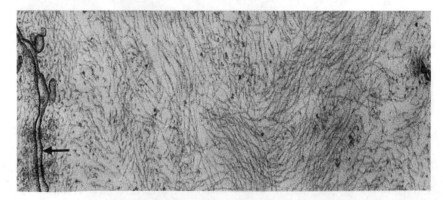

FIGURE 3-2. Keratin intermediate filaments in epidermal cells. *Arrow* indicates plasma membranes.

    c. A single epithelial cell can make a variety of keratins.
        (1) The simplest epithelia contain only two types of keratin: a type I and a type II (e.g., embryonic ectoderm and adult hepatocytes).
        (2) Other epithelia contain six or more different types of keratin (e.g., epithelia of tongue, urinary bladder, sweat glands).
        (3) Epidermis is the most heterogeneous, where distinct sets of keratins are contained by cells in the different layers of that stratified squamous epithelium (see Chapter 20).

2. Type III intermediate filaments. The proteins **vimentin, desmin,** and **glial fibrillary acidic protein** (GFAP) constitute the type III intermediate filaments. These proteins, which vary in molecular weight from 50 to 57 kD, are homopolymers (i.e., formed by polymerization of one type of intermediate filament protein).
    a. Vimentin intermediate filaments are the most widely distributed. They are found in most mesodermally derived cells (e.g., fibroblasts, endothelial cells, white blood cells) and are also transiently expressed during embryonic development in all cells.
    b. Desmin intermediate filaments are found in muscle cells. They are found throughout the cytoplasm of smooth muscle cells. In striated muscle cells, they link myofibrils to one another at the Z disks.
    c. GFAP forms **glial filaments** in astrocytes in the central nervous system and in some Schwann cells in the peripheral nervous system.

3. Type IV intermediate filaments: neurofilaments. Type IV intermediate filaments are found in the axons, dendrites, and perikarya of neurons (Figure 3-3).
    a. Neurofilaments are heteropolymers composed of three subunits: NF-L, NF-M, and NF-H. They are named for their low, medium, and heavy molecular weights: 60, 140, and 210 kD, respectively.
    b. All three subunits are usually found in a single neurofilament.
    c. The NF-M and NF-H subunits are found on the outside of the neurofilament, where their long carboxy-terminal tails extend outward from the central filament.

4. Type V intermediate filaments: nuclear lamins. Type V intermediate filaments are found in all nucleated cells.
    a. The lamins are composed of three polypeptides: lamins A and C, which are alternatively spliced products from the same gene, and lamin B.
    b. The lamins form the **nuclear lamina,** a fibrous protein meshwork that lines the inner surface of the nuclear envelope.

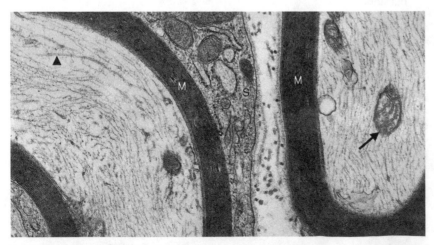

FIGURE 3-3. Type IV intermediate filaments (neurofilaments) in myelinated peripheral nerve. *M* = myelin; *S* = Schwann cell cytoplasm; *arrow* = mitochondrion; *arrowhead* = microtubule.

(1) The meshwork provides a framework for organizing nuclear envelope structure, and a site for attachment of chromatin during interphase.

(2) The nuclear lamina is attached to the nuclear envelope through lamin B.

B. **Ultrastructure of intermediate filaments.** In contrast to actin and tubulin subunits, which are globular proteins, intermediate filament subunits are **fibrous proteins.**

1. All intermediate filament subunits are elongated fibrous proteins with a central alpha-helical rod domain, and non-helical globular domains at the amino-terminal head and the carboxy-terminal tail.

2. The alpha-helical central domain, which is conserved among all intermediate filaments, plays a major role in their assembly.

3. The non-helical head and tail domains vary in length and amino acid sequence. These domains, because they protrude along intermediate filament surfaces, may participate in interactions between intermediate filaments and other cell components. The head and tail domains are also sites for post-translational modifications, such as phosphorylation.

C. **Assembly of intermediate filaments**

1. **Dimer formation.** The first step in the assembly of intermediate filaments involves the in-register, side-to-side association of intermediate filament proteins at the alpha-helical domains, forming a coiled-coil dimer.
   a. The information to guide assembly of intermediate filaments is inherent in the primary amino acid sequences of intermediate filament proteins.
   b. The assembly of intermediate filaments does not require the presence of bound nucleotides, as is the case for assembly of F-actin and of microtubules.

2. **Tetramer Formation.** Two coiled-coil dimers then associate side to side in an antiparallel fashion, forming a tetramer. The dimers are staggered with respect to one another.
   a. The tetramer is found in small amounts, soluble in the cytoplasm, suggesting that it is the basic stable structure from which intermediate filaments assemble.
   b. The tetramer is a nonpolarized structure—it is the same at both ends, a result of the antiparallel arrangement and the axial symmetry of the dimers. This is in contrast with actin filaments and microtubules, which are polarized molecules.

3. **Formation of protofilaments and final assembly.** Tetramers aggregate end to end, forming a protofilament. Protofilaments associate laterally to form a rope-like cylinder composed of eight tetramers. This process, which involves several steps, is not well understood.

4. **The intracellular pool of intermediate filament proteins is small.** In most cells, the intermediate filament proteins are found almost entirely in the polymerized state. This is, again, in contrast to the actin and microtubule cytoskeleton, in which the respective elements are in a state of dynamic equilibrium between a pool of unassembled subunits and polymerized filaments.

D. **Functions of intermediate filaments.** Intermediate filaments exhibit a highly organized structure and participate in a variety of cellular interactions. It has been proposed that the major functions of intermediate filaments are to organize and integrate cytoplasmic space, and to provide mechanical stability to cells and their components. Following are examples of intermediate filament functions in these contexts.

1. **Integration of cytoplasmic space.** Perhaps the best example of this function is that of neurofilaments, in which the long side-arms of NF-M and NF-H maintain the regular side-to-side spacing of neurofilaments in the axon, contributing to the structural stability of the axon and the regulation of axonal caliber.

2. **Mechanical stability.** Keratin intermediate filaments are associated with desmosomes and hemidesmosomes, where they form a flexible and resilient intracellular framework that provides support to the epithelium.

3. **Dynamic function of nuclear lamins.** In the interphase nucleus, lamins impart integrity to the nuclear envelope, providing structure and stability. During mitosis, the nuclear lamins play a role in the cyclic disassembly and reassembly of the nuclear envelope (see Chapter 4 VI B).

   a. During mitosis the nuclear envelope is disassembled, permitting the duplicated chromosomes to separate into daughter cells. Hyperphosphorylation of the nuclear lamins leads to the disintegration of the nuclear envelope.

      (1) Lamins A and C are dispersed into the cytoplasm.

      (2) Lamin B remains associated with vesicular fragments of the nuclear envelope.

   b. At the end of mitosis, nuclear envelope reassembly follows dephosphorylation of the lamins. Specific interactions between lamins and chromosomes are followed by lamin polymerization and restoration of nuclear integrity.

Chapter 4

Nucleus

I. **INTRODUCTION.** The nucleus is the most prominent structure in a histologic section of any interphase (nondividing) cell. It is the **center of cellular activity,** the repository of the **chromosomal deoxyribonucleic acid** (DNA), and the site of synthesis and processing of **ribonucleic acid** (RNA).

II. **CHROMOSOMES.** The double-stranded DNA in the nucleus of eukaryotic cells is packaged into linearly arranged units called chromosomes. The total amount of genetic information within an organism is called the **genome.** In human cells, the great bulk of genetic information is contained within the nucleus; however, there is a second, simpler, very small genome in mitochondria (see Chapter 2 IV C).

A. **General appearance**

1. **Mitotic cells.** Chromosomes are most obvious in a dividing cell in which the DNA is condensed into morphologically discrete structures.

2. **Interphase cells.** During interphase, the appearance of chromosomal DNA is amorphous, and varies depending on its degree of condensation (see II C 4).
   a. Female interphase cells contain a **Barr body,** a permanently condensed X chromosome that is usually visible adjacent to the nuclear envelope. This chromosome is a discrete, recognizable structure in the interphase nucleus.
   b. No other chromosomes are recognizable as discrete structures in the interphase nucleus.

B. **Chromosome number**

1. **Haploid cells.** In normal egg and sperm cells there is a single copy of the genome (1N). These cells are considered to be haploid cells. The genome in a haploid cell contains about 3×10^9 base pairs, packaged into **23 single chromosomes:** 22 autosomes and a single sex chromosome, X or Y.

2. **Diploid cells.** Somatic cells contain the diploid number of chromosomes (2N) comprised of **46 chromosomes:** 22 pairs of autosomes and two sex chromosomes: females normally have two X chromosomes, and males normally have one X and one Y chromosome.

C. **Chromatin.** Chromosomes are made of chromatin, which is a complex of **DNA, histones,** and **nonhistone proteins** found in the nucleus of eukaryotic cells.

1. **Histones.** Histones are the most abundant proteins associated with nuclear DNA.
   a. Histones are a family of basic proteins comprising five major types: H1, H2A, H2B, H3, and H4. The latter four histones are also called **nucleosomal histones.**
   b. Histones are rich in lysine and arginine and are thus positively charged. This allows them to bind tightly to the negatively charged phosphate groups in DNA.

2. **Nonhistone proteins.** Nonhistone proteins are a heterogeneous group of proteins that includes structural proteins (e.g., scaffolding involved in condensation of mitotic chromosomes), regulatory proteins involved in gene regulation (e.g., regulation of oncogenes such as *Fos* and *Myc*), and enzymes involved in nuclear function (e.g., DNA polymerases and RNA polymerases).

3. **Chromatin organization.** If the DNA in a nucleus were stretched out fully, it would extend to about 1.5 meters in length. **Efficient packing** must therefore be accom-

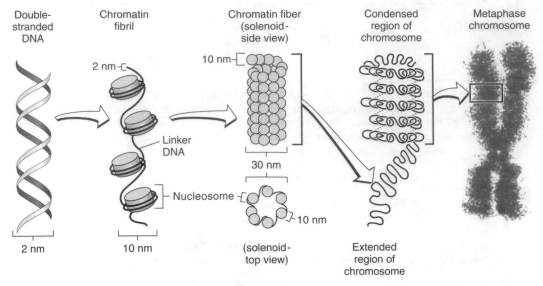

FIGURE 4-1. Representation of successive levels of chromatin packing, from the DNA double helix to the highly condensed metaphase chromosome.

plished to fit all of this material into the small volume of the nucleus. Histones play a major role in this packing of DNA (Figure 4-1).

  a. Nucleosomes. Extended DNA has the appearance in electron micrographs of "beads on a string." The "beads" are nucleosomes, and the "string" is **linker DNA.**

    (1) Nucleosome structure. Each nucleosome bead has two copies of each of the nucleosomal histones. Double-stranded DNA is wound 1.75 turns around this core of eight histone proteins.

    (2) Linker DNA. Nucleosomes are separated from each other by a short stretch of DNA called linker DNA.

    (3) Unit chromatin fibril. The string of nucleosome–linker DNA complexes forms a fibril about 10 nm in diameter.

  b. Unit chromatin fiber. A unit chromatin fibril twists into a solenoidal, helical fiber with a diameter of about 30 nm.

    (1) The solenoid helix has six nucleosomes per turn.

    (2) The non-nucleosomal histone H1 is bound to the DNA on the inside of the solenoid, stabilizing the fiber.

  c. Structure of condensed chromosomes. The mechanisms for the higher-order packing that are required to produce the highly condensed state of the mitotic chromosome are not well understood. They are speculated to involve further levels of looping of the 30-nm fiber.

    (1) Long loops of the 30-nm solenoid chromatin fiber are anchored to a scaffold of nonhistone proteins.

    (2) These looped structures in turn are arranged in a spiral that results in the tight packing characteristic of the mitotic chromosome.

4. Types of chromatin. Chromatin of the interphase nucleus is classified into **heterochromatin** and **euchromatin** based on the degree of condensation (Figure 4-2).

  a. Heterochromatin. Heterochromatin is highly condensed and is **transcriptionally inactive.** In a typical cell, 90% of the chromatin may be in this form.

    (1) Heterochromatin stains intensely with basic dyes and with hematoxylin.

    (2) Heterochromatin can also be readily demonstrated using propidium iodide, a fluorescent dye, or the Feulgen reaction, a specific histochemical staining process for the deoxyribose of DNA.

  b. Euchromatin. Euchromatin is more extended and dispersed than heterochroma-

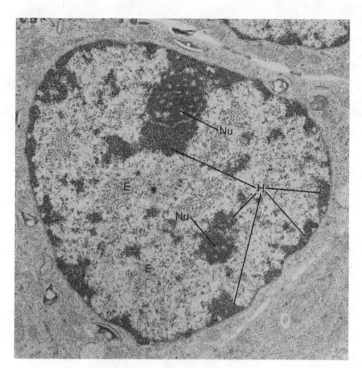

FIGURE 4-2. Electron micrograph of a nucleus from a transcriptionally active mammalian cell. Two nucleoli (*Nu*) are included in the section. The heterochromatin (*H*) is distributed primarily in clumps near the nuclear envelope. The nucleoplasm is filled with euchromatin (*E*).

tin and is **transcriptionally active.** Euchromatin is the template for the messenger RNA (mRNA) molecules that encode the proteins of a cell.

(1) Euchromatin is extensive in cells that are metabolically active in protein synthesis (e.g., neurons).

(2) Euchromatin is visible in routine hematoxylin–eosin (H&E)-stained nuclei as lightly stained regions interspersed with the intensely stained heterochromatin.

III. **NUCLEOLUS** (see Figure 4-2). The nucleolus is the site of transcription of **ribosomal RNA** (rRNA) and assembly of ribosomal subunits.

A. **Morphology.** The nucleolus is a nonmembranous intranuclear structure that stains intensely with hematoxylin and with basic dyes.

1. The nucleolus is present only in the interphase nucleus.

  a. Each cell usually has only one or two nucleoli. Because the genes that code for rRNA are located on five different chromosomes, the potential exists for many more nucleoli. They usually fuse to form fewer than five, however.

  b. The nucleolus varies in size. It is particularly well developed in cells active in protein synthesis.

2. By electron microscopy, the nucleolus appears as a heterogeneous structure with fibrillar, granular, and pale-staining regions.

B. **Functional regions.** Synthesis of rRNA and assembly of ribosomal subunits takes place in distinct regions of the nucleolus. Following assembly, the immature large and small ribosomal subunits undergo maturation as they are transferred out of the nucleus and into the cytoplasm through nuclear pore complexes.

1. Fibrillar regions are sites of active transcription of rRNA from the rRNA genes (ribosomal DNA).

2. **Granular regions** are sites of assembly of rRNA, 5S RNA, and ribosomal proteins into ribosomal subunits.
   a. 5S RNA is transcribed on DNA outside the nucleolus.
   b. Ribosomal proteins are synthesized in the cytoplasm on free polysomes (see Chapter 2 VIII A), and translocated into the nucleus via the nuclear pore complex.

3. **Pale-staining** regions contain DNA that is not being actively transcribed.

IV.   NUCLEAR ENVELOPE. The nuclear envelope is formed by two unit membranes that serve as the physical boundary between the cytoplasm and the nucleus (Figure 4-3).

A. The **outer nuclear membrane** faces the cytoplasm, is continuous with the rough endoplasmic reticulum, and is studded with ribosomes and polyribosomes.

B. The **inner nuclear membrane** faces the nucleoplasm and is covered by the meshwork of the **nuclear lamina.**

C. The **perinuclear space** is the compartment between the inner and outer nuclear membranes. It is continuous with the cisternal space of the endoplasmic reticulum.

1. Proteins that are synthesized on polysomes bound to the outer nuclear membrane are inserted into the membrane or are translocated across the membrane into the perinuclear space.

2. Those proteins that do not remain associated with the nuclear envelope follow the

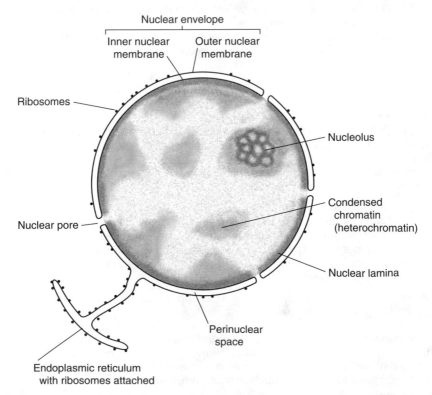

FIGURE 4-3. Cross-section of a typical cell nucleus. Note continuity between perinuclear space and the cisternae of the endoplasmic reticulum.

same fate as proteins synthesized on the rough endoplasmic reticulum (see Chapter 2 I B 2).

V. NUCLEAR PORES. Pores provide channels for direct communication between the nucleoplasm and the cytoplasm. The inner and outer membranes are continuous around the rim of the nuclear pore.

A. Structure. A nuclear pore is cylindrical in outline, with an outer diameter of 120 to 140 nm and an inner channel with a diameter of 9 nm. The cylindrical pore spans the distance between the inner and outer nuclear membranes.

1. The **nuclear pore complex** is a macromolecular assembly with octagonal symmetry. Each pore is composed of more than 100 globular proteins with an estimated total molecular mass of 125×10^6 D.

2. The nuclear envelope of a typical mammalian cell contains 3,000 to 4,000 nuclear pore complexes. This number is greater in more transcriptionally active cells.

B. Function. The nuclear pore complex functions in the selective transport of substances across the nuclear envelope. Transport through the pore is **bidirectional.** Molecules exported from the nucleus to the cytoplasm include transfer RNA, ribosomal subunits, and mRNA. Molecules imported from the cytoplasm into the nucleoplasm include DNA and RNA polymerases, gene regulatory proteins, ribosomal proteins, and histones.

1. **Passive diffusion.** Nuclear pores are freely permeable to ions and to small molecules with molecular radii approaching 4.5 nm (equivalent to approximately 60 kD). Proteins larger than 9 nm in diameter do not freely transit the nuclear pore.

2. **Active transport.** The transport of large molecules (> 9 nm diameter) and macromolecular complexes through the nuclear pore complex is a **receptor-mediated process** that **requires ATP.** To transit the nuclear pore complex, proteins must possess one or more **nuclear location sequences** (NLSs) in their primary amino acid sequence.
   a. The NLS is a short peptide sequence of 4 to 8 positively charged, basic amino acids (e.g., lysine, arginine, proline). The NLS can be located anywhere in the protein, and a protein may contain more than one NLS.
   b. **Mechanism of transport**
      (1) **Cytoplasm to nucleus.** Transport of proteins through the nuclear pore complex is a two-step process.
         (a) **Docking.** Proteins that possess a NLS bind to specific cytosolic proteins to form a complex. The complex then docks with a receptor on the periphery of the nuclear pore complex.
         (b) **Translocation**
            (i) The NLS-containing protein is transported through the nuclear pore and the cytosolic proteins are released back into the cytoplasm.
            (ii) Translocation is an **ATP-dependent process.** Some of the energy from ATP hydrolysis may be used in the transient dilation of the nuclear pore to accommodate the size and shape of proteins that are transported.
      (2) **Nucleus to cytoplasm.** The transport of RNA and ribosomal subunits out of the nucleus into the cytoplasm is also selective. Transport in this direction appears also to require a receptor. Details of the mechanism are lacking.

VI. NUCLEAR LAMINA. The nuclear lamina is a fibrous meshwork that lines the inner surface of the nuclear envelope. The lamina, which is 10 to 20 nm thick, provides structure and stability to the interphase nucleus and mediates the binding of chromatin to the nuclear envelope. It is interrupted by nuclear pores.

A. **Composition.** The nuclear matrix is composed of type IV intermediate filaments called **nuclear lamins A, B, and C** (see Chapter 3 IV A 3).

B. **Role in mitosis.** Lamins play a major role in the rapid breakdown of the nuclear envelope at the start of mitosis and its reassembly at the end of mitosis (see Chapter 3 IV D 3).

VII. **NUCLEAR MATRIX.** The ordered appearance of the nucleus results from an underlying substructure called the nuclear matrix. This is a fibrous network that contains approximately 10% of total nuclear proteins, 30% of nuclear RNA, 1% to 3% of total DNA, and 3% of nuclear phospholipid.

A. **Morphology.** Nuclear matrix preparations are made from isolated nuclei by dissolving the nuclear envelope, extracting most of the RNA and loosely associated proteins, and digesting most of the DNA.

1. Viewed by electron microscopy, such preparations reveal a fibrous network with the original shape of the nucleus.

2. Within the network are residual elements of the nucleolus, fibrils associated with nuclear pore complexes, and fibrils associated with the nuclear lamina.

B. **Function.** The nuclear matrix is believed to provide structure and organization to the internal nuclear compartment. It is proposed to serve as a solid phase to which are attached the enzyme complexes responsible for RNA transcription and DNA replication.

VIII. **CELL CYCLE.** The cell cycle is an ordered sequence of events during which the cell grows, duplicates its chromosomes, and divides into two cells. The normal somatic cell cycle can be divided into two histologically identifiable parts: interphase and mitosis.

A. **Interphase.** A cell in interphase continues to grow, during which time it doubles its size and replicates its DNA. Interphase has been divided into three phases: G_1 phase, S phase, and G_2 phase (Figure 4-4).

1. **G_1 phase.** Immediately following mitosis, the cell enters the G_1 phase (G = gap). This is a period of cell growth.
   a. **Activity.** During G_1, the cell synthesizes and accumulates RNA for protein synthesis, and regulatory proteins and enzymes for DNA synthesis.
   b. **Duration.** G_1 is the most variable phase of the cell cycle.
      (1) In some rapidly growing cells (e.g., embryonic cells), G_1 is so short that it is almost nonexistent.
      (2) In other cells (e.g., quiescent fibroblasts, prepubertal spermatogonia) G_1 is very long and the cells appear to have ceased cycling altogether. Cells in such a long G_1 are considered to be in a **G_0 phase,** during which the cells are neither growing nor dividing. G_0 can last for days, weeks, or years before cells resume proliferation (i.e., re-enter the cell cycle).

2. **S phase.** DNA synthesis occurs in the S phase, which normally lasts from 6 to 12 hours. During this time, the genome is replicated and protein and RNA synthesis continue as well.
   a. Doubling of DNA content (2N to 4N) is not apparent in routine histologic sections, but can be easily detected by microspectrophotometry of Feulgen-stained

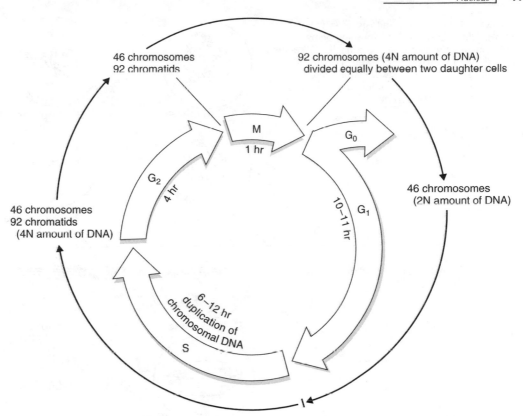

46 chromosomes
92 chromatids

92 chromosomes (4N amount of DNA)
divided equally between two daughter cells

M
1 hr

G₀

46 chromosomes
(2N amount of DNA)

G₂
4 hr

46 chromosomes
92 chromatids
(4N amount of DNA)

10–11 hr

G₁

6–12 hr
duplication of
chromosomal DNA
S

FIGURE 4-4. Human chromosomal DNA amount and number during the cell cycle.

sections, or by the use of DNA-specific fluorescent dyes and a fluorescence-activated cell sorter.

  b. After chromosomes have replicated in the S phase, they remain attached to each other and are referred to as **sister chromatids.**

3. G₂ phase. In this period between synthesis of DNA and mitosis, the cell continues to synthesize RNA and proteins in preparation for cell division.

  a. In the G_2 phase, the DNA content is exactly twice that of G_1 cells. (Cells in the S phase have an intermediate amount of DNA while replication proceeds.)

  b. G_2 phase lasts from 2 to 4 hours in most human cells.

B. **Mitosis.** In mitosis the nuclear and the cytoplasmic content are equally divided between the two daughter cells. Mitosis is divided into six stages: prophase, prometaphase, metaphase, anaphase, telophase, and cytokinesis (Figure 4-5). Mitosis averages 1 hour in duration.

1. Prophase. During prophase, the chromatin that was dispersed during interphase slowly condenses into discrete chromosomes. At the same time, the cytoskeleton rearranges: cytoplasmic microtubules begin to disassemble, and the **mitotic spindle** begins to form.

  a. The **mitotic spindle** is a bipolar structure composed of centrioles, microtubules, and associated proteins.

  b. Contained within each of the sister chromatids is a specific DNA sequence called a **centromere,** and associated with it is a structure called a **kinetochore.**

  (1) The kinetochore is the site of attachment for microtubules of the mitotic spindle.

  (2) The **centromere** is the primary constriction along the chromosome at which sister chromatids are held together.

FIGURE 4-5. Diagram of mitosis. E' = enlargement of one metaphase chromosome being pulled apart. c = centriole; n = nucleus. (Reprinted with permission from Kelly DE, Wood RL, Enders AC: *Bailey's Textbook of Microscopic Anatomy*, 18th ed. Baltimore, Williams & Wilkins, 1984, p. 89.)

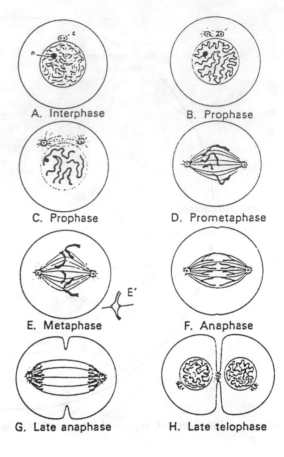

A. Interphase

B. Prophase

C. Prophase

D. Prometaphase

E. Metaphase

F. Anaphase

G. Late anaphase

H. Late telophase

2. **Prometaphase.** Prometaphase begins with disassembly of the nuclear envelope.
   a. Some of the spindle microtubules attach to the kinetochores and are called **kinetochore microtubules.** The remaining microtubules in the spindle are called polar microtubules. Those outside of the spindle are called astral microtubules.
   b. The kinetochore microtubules exert tension on the chromosomes and begin to organize the haphazardly arranged chromosomes.

3. **Metaphase.** In metaphase, the chromosomes are aligned in one plane, the equatorial plane, between the spindle poles in a structure called the **metaphase plate.** They are held there by the kinetochore microtubules.

4. **Anaphase.** Anaphase begins when the paired centromeres are split, allowing each chromatid (now considered a chromosome) to move toward the spindle pole it faces.
   a. The chromatids are slowly pulled toward the spindle poles by the shortening of the kinetochore microtubules and the elongation of the polar microtubules.
   b. Anaphase is very short, lasting only a few minutes.

5. **Telophase.** Telophase begins when the separated daughter chromosomes arrive at their respective poles.
   a. The **kinetochore microtubules disassemble** and a new array of interphase microtubules is formed.
   b. A **new nuclear envelope assembles** around each set of chromosomes which then begins to disperse. The nucleoli, which disappeared during prophase, reappear.
   c. This is the **end of mitosis.** Daughter nuclei are now recognized, but the formation of two separate cells occurs only upon completion of cytokinesis.

C. **Cell division.** The division of the cell is complete after karyokinesis and cytokinesis take place.

   1. Karyokinesis is nuclear division.
      a. Karyokinesis begins in anaphase and is completed in telophase, when new nuclear envelopes assemble around each set of daughter chromosomes to form the daughter nuclei.
      b. Replication of DNA without subsequent karyokinesis results in the formation of **polyploid** nuclei.
         (1) Polyploid nuclei contain any multiple of the haploid number of chromosomes other than the diploid number (i.e., 3N, 4N, etc.).
         (2) A megakaryocyte is an example of a polyploid cell.

   2. Cytokinesis. During cytokinesis, the cytoplasm divides by a process called **cleavage,** resulting in the production of two identical daughter cells.
      a. Cytokinesis begins in late anaphase, spans telophase, and is completed in early interphase when the daughter cells separate.
         (1) A thin ring composed of actin filaments and associated myosin II filaments forms at the midpoint of the cell, perpendicular to the spindle axis between the two daughter nuclei.
         (2) As the ring contracts, a **cleavage furrow** is formed. The cleavage furrow deepens until the two cells are separated from each other when the plasma membrane within the ring fuses with itself.
      b. Karyokinesis without subsequent cytokinesis results in a binucleate or multinucleate cell. An osteoclast is an example of a multinucleate cell.

IX. **MEIOSIS.** Meiosis is a special type of cell division that results in the production of **haploid** gametes (sperm and egg cells) from **diploid** cells. These haploid cells contain only a single copy of the genome.

A. Overview

   1. Nuclear events. Meiosis is divided into two stages: **meiosis I** and **meiosis II.** Each stage has a prophase, metaphase, anaphase, and telophase. Prior to meiosis I, just as in somatic cell division, a cycle of DNA replication produces the 4N amount of DNA. In contrast with mitosis, however, in meiosis this duplication of chromosomal DNA is followed by **two separate cell divisions** that produce four progeny, each with 1N amount of DNA. There is no S phase between meiosis I and meiosis II (Figure 4-6).
      a. Homologous chromosomes (homologs). Except for the sex chromosomes, a diploid nucleus contains two similar sets of autosomes, one from the father (paternal) and the other from the mother (maternal).
      b. Meiosis versus mitosis. The duplicated homologous chromosomes behave differently in mitosis and meiosis.
         (1) In mitosis, the duplicated homologous chromosomes align on the metaphase plate **independently** of one another.
            (a) The sister chromatids separate during anaphase to become individual chromosomes.
            (b) Each daughter cell inherits one copy of each paternal chromosome and one copy of each maternal chromosome.
         (2) In meiosis I, prior to alignment on the metaphase plate, each duplicated homologous pair of chromosomes becomes **physically paired.** This process, called **synapsis,** is unique to meiosis. Each daughter cell receives two copies of one of the homologs, either a paternal copy or a maternal copy.

   2. Cytoplasmic events. Cytoplasmic events in meiosis differ for sperm and egg production.

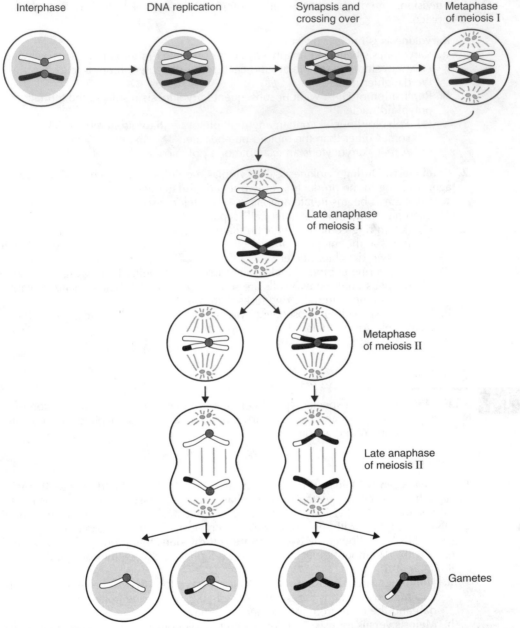

FIGURE 4-6. Diagram of meiosis in the male. One pair of homologous chromosomes (2N) and one cross-ing-over event are depicted. Four haploid (1N) gametes are produced from one diploid (2N) parent cell. In the female, only one haploid gamete is produced.

a. In the male, meiosis results in the production of four equally sized haploid **spermatozoa,** each capable of fertilizing an egg (see Chapter 36 III B 4).

b. In the female, a single large, functional haploid **oocyte** is produced that contains most of the cytoplasm. The other cells resulting from meiotic division are small haploid **polar bodies** that receive minimal amounts of cytoplasm. The polar bodies undergo degeneration (see Chapter 35 IV).

B. Meiosis I: first meiotic division

1. **Prophase I.** Prophase I is a prolonged stage during which the homologous chromosomes pair and genetic recombination can occur.

    a. Synapsis. The duplicated homologous chromosomes, each containing a pair of chromatids, undergo synapsis producing a **tetrad.** A tetrad contains four chromatids.

    b. Crossing over. During synapsis, small regions of the DNA of homologous chromosomes are reciprocally exchanged between the nonsister chromatids. This process, called crossing over, mixes the genetic make-up of the chromosomes in gametes, introducing genetic diversity.

2. **Metaphase I.** Tetrads align on the metaphase plate, having associated with the mitotic spindles during prometaphase.

3. **Anaphase I.** Homologous pairs of chromosomes separate and move toward the spindle poles that they face. Because the centromere did not divide, the chromatids in each homologous pair act as a unit.

    a. The maternal and paternal homologs segregate randomly and independently. They are not predisposed to move to one pole or another. This is called **random assortment.**

    b. The daughter cells thus acquire a different assortment of chromosomes. Both random assortment and crossing over contribute to **genetic diversity.**

4. **Telophase I.** As in mitosis, the chromosomes arrive at the spindle pole and daughter nuclei form.

    a. Reduction division. Each daughter nucleus contains the haploid number (1N) of chromosomes, each containing two chromatids.

    b. Each nucleus contains the 2N amount of DNA.

C. **Meiosis II: second meiotic division.** At the end of meiosis I a brief interphase begins. The chromosomes may decondense slightly during telophase I and in the brief interphase, but they recondense and prophase II begins. During the brief interphase, **DNA is not duplicated.**

1. **Prophase II** is brief. The nuclear envelope disassembles and a new mitotic spindle forms.

2. In **metaphase II,** the sister chromatids associate with kinetochore microtubules and are separated, as in mitosis.

3. **Anaphase II** and **telophase II** follow quickly in succession. The daughter cells produced in the second meiotic division contain the haploid number (1N) of chromosomes and the haploid amount (1N) of DNA.

Chapter 5

Epithelium

I. **INTRODUCTION.** Epithelium is **one of the four basic tissues** of the body. The other three basic tissues are **connective tissue, muscle, and nerve.**

A. Epithelia **cover body surfaces** (e.g., cutaneous and gastrointestinal) and **line most body cavities** (e.g., peritoneal and pleural cavities, but not synovial joint spaces).

B. Epithelia also form **exocrine** and **endocrine glands.**

1. The major exocrine glands are associated with the digestive system. Their general and specific characteristics are presented in the chapters describing the alimentary canal (see Chapters 21–27).

2. The endocrine glands are discussed primarily in relation to their regulatory and secretory functions in Chapters 26 and 30–34.

II. **GENERAL CHARACTERISTICS OF EPITHELIA**

A. **Embryonic origin.** All three embryonic **germ layers** give rise to epithelia. For example, epidermis forms from **ectoderm,** vascular endothelium forms from **mesoderm,** and the lining of the gastrointestinal tract forms from **endoderm.**

B. **Minimal extracellular space.** An epithelium is a **cell-rich tissue.**

1. Extracellular space and cellular secretions retained in the space account for only a very small fraction of the total mass of an epithelium.

2. Cell–cell junctions are highly developed in epithelia and help maintain the close proximity of epithelial cells to one another.

C. **Absence of blood vessels.** Epithelia are avascular. Blood vessels are found close to epithelia but are always separated from epithelial cells by a perivascular connective tissue space.

D. **Polarization.** Both epithelial cells and epithelial tissues are polarized.

1. **Cell surfaces.** An epithelial cell in a **simple epithelium** has three distinct surfaces.
   a. **Apical surface.** The apical surface of the cell forms the free surface of the epithelium. The apical surface faces a space.
   b. **Lateral surface.** The lateral surface faces adjacent epithelial cells.
   c. **Basal surface.** The basal surface is adjacent to the connective tissue substratum of the epithelium. The basal surface is attached to a basal lamina.

2. **Cell domains.** The surface of a cell in a simple epithelium has two domains relative to the membrane biochemistry of the epithelial cell.
   a. **Apical domain.** The apical surface is usually described as one membrane domain.
   b. **Basolateral domain.** The basal and lateral surfaces are considered a second functional domain.
   c. Maintenance of cellular domains is largely a function of tight junctions (see IV D 7).

3. **Tissue surfaces.** Both simple and stratified epithelia have two surfaces.
   a. **Free surface.** An epithelium has a free surface that faces either the external environment or an internal space.

       (1) **External environments** include that faced by the epidermis and that faced by the epithelial linings of tubular structures, such as the alimentary canal, whose lumens are continuous with the outside of the body.

       (2) **Internal spaces** are totally isolated from the outside of the body. These include the peritoneal and pleural cavities, and the lumen of the cardiovascular system.

    b. **Basal surface.** An epithelium also has a basal surface that is adjacent to the connective tissue substratum.

III. FUNCTIONS OF EPITHELIA

A. Absorption

1. Many epithelia are located at the interfaces between the body and the external and internal environments. Solvents, solutes, metabolic substances, and gases are passively absorbed or actively transported across these epithelia.

2. Examples of absorbing or transporting epithelia include the intestinal epithelium, pulmonary alveolar epithelium, vascular endothelium, and kidney tubule epithelium.

B. Protection

1. Epithelia are specialized to protect and maintain the consistency of the internal environment.
    a. Such epithelia present to the generally hostile environment a continuous, coherent cellular barrier.
    b. An epithelium may also present to the environment a layer of expendable squamous cells.

2. Examples of protective epithelia include the epidermis and the lining of the colon.

C. Secretion

1. **Unicellular glands.** An individual epithelial cell may be a secretory structure (e.g., intestinal goblet cells). Such cells are surrounded by nonsecreting epithelial cells.

2. **Secretory surfaces.** Multiple secreting epithelial cells may form a **homogeneous epithelial secretory layer** (e.g., lining of gastric pits).

3. **Multicellular glands.** Both exocrine and endocrine glands develop from invaginations of epithelial surfaces.
    a. In **exocrine glands,** the epithelial characteristics of the structure are seen in both the secretory regions and in the ducts that connect the gland to an epithelial surface (e.g., the parotid gland and its duct).
    b. In **endocrine glands,** the duct-like portion of the embryonic invagination is lost and the epithelial nature of the adult gland may be less obvious (e.g., adenohypophysis).

IV. CLASSIFICATION OF EPITHELIA. Epithelia are classified by **cell shape** and by the **number of cell layers** (Figure 5-1, Table 5-1).

A. Cell shape

1. A **squamous** epithelial cell is a flattened cell—height is much less than diameter.

2. A **cuboidal** epithelial cell is cube-shaped—height and diameter are similar.

3. A **columnar** epithelial cell is a tall cell—height is greater than diameter.

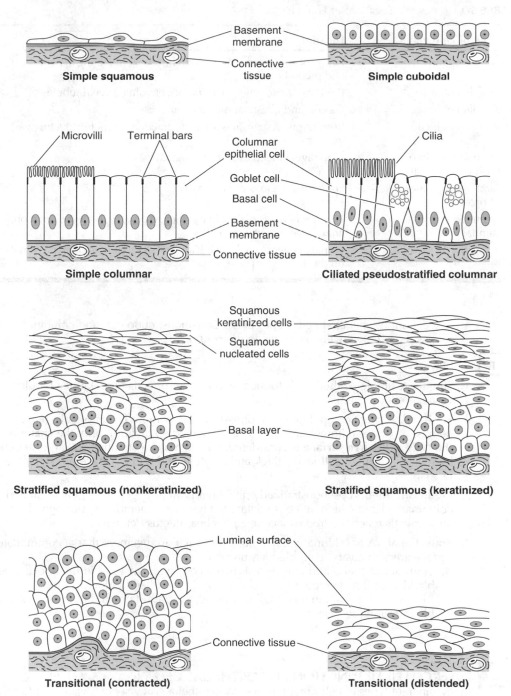

FIGURE 5-1. Schematic representation of various types of epithelia. In each example, the epithelium is shown with its substratum of connective tissue. (Adapted with permission from Kelly DE, Wood RL, Enders AC: *Bailey's Textbook of Microscopic Anatomy,* 18th ed. Baltimore, Williams & Wilkins, 1984, p. 116; and Junqueira LC, Carneiro J, Kelley RO: *Basic Histology,* 7th ed. Englewood Cliffs, NJ, Appleton & Lange, 1992, pp 76–77.)

TABLE 5-1. Types and Locations of Epithelia

Type of Epithelium	Locations
Simple squamous	Lining of cardiovascular system (endothelium); lining of peritoneal and pleural cavities
Simple cuboidal	Portions of exocrine gland ducts; convoluted renal tubules
Simple columnar	Gastric and intestinal mucosal surfaces
Pseudostratified	Respiratory system (nasal cavity, trachea, bronchi); ductus (vas) deferens
Stratified squamous (non-keratinized)	Esophageal mucosal surface; vagina
Stratified squamous (keratinized)	Epidermis; regions of oral cavity
Stratified cuboidal/columnar	Portions of ducts of exocrine glands; esophageal–gastric junction; anal canal; regions of urethra
Transitional	Urinary system (renal calyces and pelvis, ureter, bladder, proximal urethra)

4. A spectrum of epithelial cell shapes exists. Squamous, cuboidal, and columnar shapes represent convenient points in the continuum.

B. **Cell layers**

1. **Simple.** A simple epithelium is formed by one layer of cells (e.g., kidney tubules, vascular endothelium).

2. **Stratified.** A stratified epithelium is formed by two or more layers of cells (e.g., epidermis, esophageal lining). In describing a stratified epithelium, **only the shape of the cells at the free surface** is considered. For example, a stratified squamous epithelium is two or more cell layers thick and the cells at the free surface are squamous in shape.

3. **Pseudostratified.** A pseudostratified epithelium is an arrangement of cuboidal and columnar cells in which all cells contact the basement membrane, but only the columnar cells reach the free surface (e.g., trachea, ductus deferens).

4. **Transitional.** A transitional epithelium is a cellular arrangement that accommodates surface areas that vary (e.g., bladder, ureters).
   a. Transitional epithelium may appear many cell layers thick, as in the unexpanded bladder, or it may appear much thinner, as in the filled bladder.
   b. All cells in a transitional epithelium contact the basal lamina, but this is not visible in routine sections.

V. **INTERCELLULAR JUNCTIONS OF EPITHELIAL CELLS** (Figure 5-2, Table 5-2.) Many different types of cell junctions occur in epithelia. They serve a variety of functions that include cell adhesion; cell–cell communication; and, in transporting epithelia, the establishment of intraepithelial compartments.

A. **Desmosomes.** Cells are physically attached to one another by desmosomes—small, localized areas of contact between cells (Figure 5-3). Desmosomes are also called **maculae adherentes,** a term that emphasizes their punctate shape and adhesive characteristics.

1. **Location and distribution.** Desmosomes are found on all surfaces of epithelial cells except those surfaces facing a space or the connective tissue substratum.

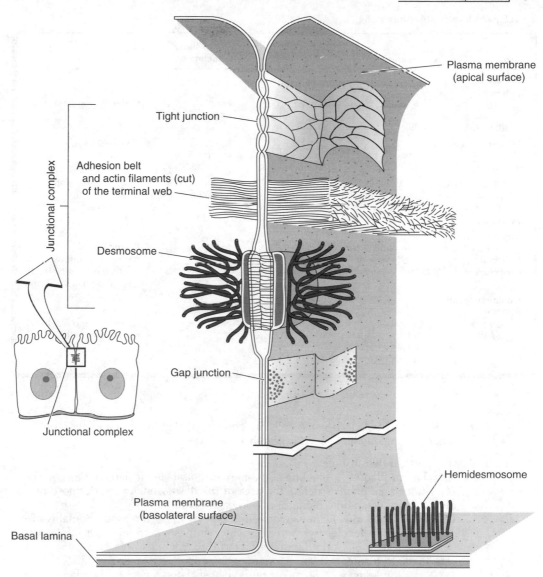

FIGURE 5-2. Schematic representation of the fine structure of several types of cellular junctions as depicted on the surface of cells forming a simple columnar epithelium. A junctional complex is formed by a tight junction, an adhesion belt, and a desmosome. (The junctional complex is enlarged relative to the height of the cell, to show details of junctions.) Visible on the lateral cell surface, deep to the junctional complex, is a gap junction. A hemidesmosome connects the basal plasma membrane to the basal lamina. Also depicted is the freeze-fracture view of a tight junction, showing its network of strands of intramembranous particles, and of a gap junction, showing its clustering of connexons. *Inset:* Schematic representation of a simple columnar epithelium. Enclosed in the rectangle are the lateral surfaces of two epithelial cells, showing the location of the junctional complex.

    a. Hundreds of desmosomes may be found over the surface of an epithelial cell in a stratified epithelium.

    b. Some regions of an epithelial cell surface in a stratified epithelium may appear nearly free of desmosomes, however.

2. Light microscopic appearance of desmosomes

    a. Desmosomes appear as tiny, button-like points of contact between adjacent cells. The size of a large desmosome places it close to the limit of resolution of the light microscope.

TABLE 5-2. Intercellular Junctions

Type	Shape	Extracellular Attachment	Intracellular Attachment	Function
Adherens junctions				
Desmosome (macula adherens)	Punctate (macular, spot-like)	Cadherin transmembrane linker proteins	Keratin intermediate filaments	Cell–cell adhesion
Hemidesmosomes	Punctate (macular, spot-like)	Integrin transmembrane linker proteins	Keratin intermediate filaments	Cell–basal lamina adhesion
Adhesion belt (zonula adherens)	Circumferential (zonular, belt-like)	Cadherin transmembrane linker proteins	Actin microfilaments	Cell–cell adhesion, morphogenetic movements
Occluding junction				
Tight junction (zonula occludens)	Circumferential (zonular, belt-like)	Focal connections of membrane proteins	None	Restriction of paracellular diffusion, maintenance of cell surface domains
Communicating junction				
Gap junction (nexus)	Punctate (macular, spot-like; extremely variable in size)	Connexon–connexon pairs	None	Metabolic and electric coupling of cells

    b. They are most obvious when cells are contracted slightly during fixation or when the intercellular space is slightly enlarged.

  3. Components of desmosomes
    a. Attachment plaques. Attachment plaques are intracellular parts of desmosomes.
      (1) Attachment plaques **define the area of the desmosome.** One desmosome has two attachment plaques, one in each cell.
      (2) Each filamentous plaque is formed in part by the **cytoplasmic domains of cadherin molecules** (see V A 3 c). The cytoplasmic proteins desmoplakins and plakoglobin form the major part of the attachment plaque.
    b. Intermediate filaments
      (1) Keratin intermediate filaments of the cytoskeleton attach to the plaque.
      (2) Keratin filaments appear to loop in and out of the attachment plaque. The attachment plaque thereby serves a role in the support of the cytoskeleton.
    c. Transmembrane linker proteins. The glycoproteins desmoglein and desmocollin are the adhesive components of desmosomes.
      (1) Desmogleins and desmocollins are members of the **cadherin family of calcium-dependent, cell–cell adhesion molecules.**
      (2) The transmembrane linker protein molecules have intracellular and extracellular domains.
        (a) The **intracellular domain** of the glycoprotein **extends into the attachment plaque** and contributes to the structure of the plaque.
        (b) The **extracellular domain** of the molecule **extends into the intercellular space** and binds with similar molecules from the neighboring, connected cell.
    d. Central dense layer. Evidence of the interaction of transmembrane linker proteins may be visible as a central dense layer in the intercellular space, between the apposed cells.
      (1) This is the **site of the adhesive reaction** that forms the basis of the mechanical joining of cells by desmosomes.

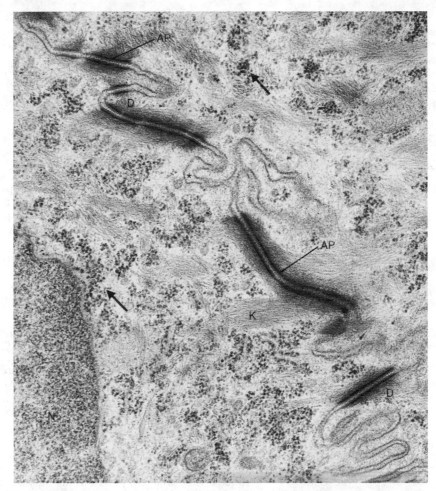

FIGURE 5-3. Electron micrograph showing several desmosomes (*D*) between epithelial cells in the basal layer of the epidermis. Note the keratin intermediate filaments (*K*) and the attachment plaques (*AP*) of the desmosomes. The fine structure of some of the desmosomes is indistinct because of the oblique plane of section through the structure. Also visible are a portion of the nucleus (*N*), ribosomes (*arrows*), and the intercellular space.

    (2) The **transmembrane linker proteins bind calcium,** and this ion is required for the functioning of desmosomes as cell–cell adhesion sites.

    (3) The central dense layer is not as regularly noted in routine electron microscopic preparations as are attachment plaques and their associated intermediate filaments.

B. **Hemidesmosomes.** These desmosomal junctions occur at the interface between epithelia and connective tissue—on the basal plasma membrane of epithelial cells, adjacent to the basal lamina.

    1. Components of hemidesmosomes
        a. Hemidesmosomes are formed by **attachment plaques, cytoskeletal intermediate filaments,** and **transmembrane linker proteins.**
        b. The transmembrane linker proteins of hemidesmosomes are in the **integrin** family of adhesion molecules, but have a role similar to the cadherins of desmosomes.

    2. Hemidesmosomes and basal laminae. Hemidesmosomes serve as points of attach-

ment of epithelial cells to a basal lamina (see VII B) and, thus, to the extracellular matrix.
    a. The **laminin** of a basal lamina is concentrated in the areas of the lamina opposite hemidesmosomes.
    b. **Laminin molecules interact with integrin molecules** to connect the basal lamina to the plasma membrane.

3. **Hemidesmosomes and desmosomes.** These two intermediate filament-associated junctions share some structural and functional similarities but have chemical dissimilarities.

C. **Gap junctions.** Cells are electrically and chemically coupled by gap junctions.

1. **Structure of gap junctions.** Gap junctions are not visible by light microscopy.
    a. This type of cell–cell junction appears with the electron microscope as the close apposition of plasma membranes of adjacent cells. The ''gap'' of a gap junction refers to a remarkably uniform 2–3 nm intercellular space in the junctional region.
    b. **Sample preparation techniques** that facilitate observation of gap junctions include lanthanum staining and freeze-fracture.
        (1) **Lanthanum staining.** The intercellular space of an epithelium can be demarcated by exposure of the intact tissue to colloidal suspensions of lanthanum salts during EM fixation.
            (a) After filling the intercellular region of the gap junction with lanthanum, the narrow gap is more sharply defined and is seen to be **interrupted by subunits** that appear to join the two cells.
            (b) The gap junction subunits are made visible by the **negative staining effect of the lanthanum.**
        (2) **Freeze-fracture.** The technique of freeze-fracture exposes the subunit structure of gap junctions (see Figure 5-2).
            (a) When the plasma membrane of a cell that is known to have gap junctions is cleaved by freeze-fracture, a characteristic **clustering of intramembrane protein particles** is seen. These clusters are **evidence of a gap junction.**
            (b) Freeze-fracture technique reveals that gap junctions are very **variable in size,** ranging from only a few particles to thousands of particles per junction.

2. **Components of gap junctions**
    a. **Connexons.** The subunits made visible by the lanthanum technique and the particles observed by freeze-fracture are different views of the connexon.
        (1) The connexon is a protein complex embedded in the plasma membrane of a cell. It projects out of the membrane into the extracellular space.
        (2) The connexon fuses end-to-end with a connexon from an adjacent cell, producing a **connexon pair.** The connexon pair is the **structural and functional unit of a gap junction.**
        (3) A gap junction may be formed by only a few connexon pairs or by thousands of connexon pairs.
    b. **Connexin molecules.** Connexons are formed by transmembrane connexin molecules.
        (1) High-resolution electron microscopy has shown that the connexon is a hexamer of connexin molecules. Each connexin molecule has four transmembrane segments.
        (2) The six connexin molecules enclose a narrow aqueous channel, approximately 2 nm in diameter.
            (a) This channel is in precise register with a similar channel in the other connexon of the connexon pair.
            (b) Therefore, a channel formed by 12 connexin molecules exists in each connexon pair, providing an aqueous bridge from the cytoplasm of one cell to the cytoplasm of the adjacent cell.

3. **Gap junction function.** Gap junctions are sites of metabolic and electric coupling of cells.
   a. **Basis of function.** The aqueous channels of connexon pairs provide continuity of the cytoplasm of one cell with the cytoplasm of an adjacent cell.
      (1) A large number of such channels may exist in one gap junction, and a cell may have many gap junctions over its surface.
      (2) Therefore, there is extensive cytoplasm–cytoplasm and membrane membrane coupling in a group of cells joined by gap junctions.
   b. **Metabolic coupling.** The junctions provide **avenues of diffusion** for ions and relatively small molecules from one cell to another through the channels in each connexon pair.
      (1) Diffusion can be demonstrated at the light microscopic level by **microinjecting fluorescently labeled molecules** of varying molecular weights into a cell and observing diffusion of the probe or a lack thereof—to adjacent cells. Such investigations have shown that the **maximum molecular weight** of a particle capable of diffusing from one cell to another is about 1200 daltons.
      (2) Intracellular messengers such as cyclic AMP may diffuse from cell to cell through gap junctions and, thus, propagate the stimulatory event through the tissue.
   c. **Electric coupling**
      (1) Gap junctions are also implicated in the electric coupling of cells in epithelia because ions move freely through the aqueous channel of the junction.
      (2) Potentials are able to spread through other tissues as well, such as smooth muscle and myocardium, and this electric coupling correlates closely with the presence or absence of gap junctions in the tissue.

4. **Gap junction regulation. Intracellular calcium concentration** and **cytosolic pH** control gap junction function. Epithelial cells that are coupled by gap junctions become uncoupled if the intracellular concentration of calcium is raised or if the pH is lowered. This is significant in the **response of the tissue to injury.**
   a. **Cell injury and solute loss.** Disruption of the plasma membrane of a cell that is part of a coupled cellular complex can result in the leaking of important low–molecular-weight solutes from the non-injured but coupled cells.
   b. **Uncoupling of cells reduces solute loss.** The influx of extracellular calcium into the ruptured cell causes the closing down of the aqueous channels of its connexon pairs. This prevents excessive loss of low molecular-weight cytosolic components from adjacent, coupled, uninjured cells.

D. **Tight junctions.** The tight junction encircles the cell, joining it to all immediately neighboring cells. The tight junction is also called a **zonula occludens** because of its belt-like, encircling nature, and because of its occlusion of the extracellular space.

1. **Location and distribution of tight junctions.** The presence of tight junctions may be inferred from light microscopy because they are one of the components of the **terminal bar** (see V E 2 c).
   a. Tight junctions are commonly present in **absorptive** and **secreting epithelia.**
   b. These junctions usually are found in simple cuboidal or simple columnar epithelia on the **lateral cell surface, close to the apical surface.**
   c. Generally, **only one tight junction is present on an epithelial cell,** in contrast to the numerous desmosomes and gap junctions that may be present on the same cell.

2. **Structure of tight junctions**
   a. **Transmission electron microscopy** of thin sections characterizes tight junctions as regions of **membrane contact** in the form of focal connections.
      (1) **Focal connections.** Tight junctions are visible as a series of focal connections of the unit membranes of the adjacent cells. Each focus of contact has been called a membrane kiss.
      (2) **Junction depth.** The depth of the junction is variable. There may be just a few or there may be many focal connections forming the tight junction.

    b. Freeze-fracture characterizes tight junctions as networks of strands of intramembrane particles.

      (1) Networks of strands and grooves. The junction appears as a continuous net-like arrangement of rows of particles that form **intramembranous strands,** or ridges, and **complementary grooves.**

      (2) Strands, grooves, and kisses. The strands and grooves are intramembranous indications of the points of membrane contact visible in thin sections of tight junctions.

      (3) Structural variation. The net-like tight junctions visible by freeze-fracture vary from narrow and relatively simple arrangements of a few strands and grooves, to wide and geometrically complex configurations consisting of many strands and grooves.

    c. Tight junction proteins. Some tight junction proteins have been characterized. None of these proteins, however, corresponds to the intramembranous strands demonstrated by electron microscopy after freeze-fracture.

  3. Functions of tight junctions

    a. Occlusion of the intercellular space. Tight junctions function as **intraepithelial gaskets** by blocking the intercellular space of an epithelium.

      (1) This prevents or retards the flow of materials from one side of an epithelium to the other via the paracellular pathway.

      (2) The effectiveness of a tight junction as a barrier to diffusion across the epithelium is a function of the **depth and complexity** of the junction.

        (a) Narrow junctions—those with few anastomosing strands—are classified as leaky.

        (b) Wide junctions—those with many anastomosing strands—are more effective barriers.

    b. Transport. Directional transport of water and solutes across an epithelium depends upon occlusion of the apical end of the intercellular space by tight junctions.

      (1) Tight junctions are an essential component of the mechanism that is responsible for movement of solutes and water across an epithelium.

      (2) In the absence of tight junctions, free diffusion would occur through the paracellular pathway (i.e., intercellular space), and no net flux of solutes or water could occur across the epithelium.

    c. Cell polarity. The tight junction has an important role in the maintenance of the **apical** and **basolateral chemical domains** of the epithelial cell membrane.

      (1) The phospholipids and proteins present in the two membrane domains are different. Segregation of these components is essential for cell and tissue function.

      (2) A tight junction functions as a **molecular fence,** preventing the intermixing of the two membrane domains.

E. **Adhesion belt.** This type of junction is found in the junctional complex **deep to the tight junction.** The adhesion belt is also called a **zonula adherens** because it is a circumferential adhering junction (see Figure 5-2).

  1. Cadherin transmembrane linker proteins are components of the adhesion belt and function in cell–cell attachment.

  2. The adhesion belt is associated with **actin filaments.**

    a. The adhesion belt is attached to a **cytoplasmic band** of actin filaments, which also follow a **circumferential pathway** on the cytoplasmic side of the junctional complex.

    b. The adhesion belt also functions as an attachment site for the actin filaments of the **terminal web.**

F. **Junctional complex.** A junctional complex is a grouping of certain cell–cell junctions. Junctional complexes are present in many epithelia.

  1. Location and distribution of the junctional complex

    a. The complex is located on the lateral surface of epithelial cells close to the apical surface.

    b. Junctional complexes are usually present in simple epithelia, and are most obvious in simple cuboidal and simple columnar epithelia. The complex is most often observed in:

        (1) Absorbing epithelia (e.g., the simple columnar epithelium of the intestines)

        (2) Secreting epithelia (e.g., acinar cells of the exocrine pancreas)

2. Components of a junctional complex. The complex usually is formed by a **tight junction,** an **adhesion belt,** and a **desmosome.** Some histologists include a **gap junction** in a junctional complex.

3. Terminal bar. The two zonular junctions of the junctional complex (i.e., the tight junction and the adhesion belt) encircle the cell in a belt-like fashion. At the resolution afforded by light microscopy, these zonular junctions are detected as a single structure, called the terminal bar.

    a. In transverse section, the terminal bar appears as a dot on the lateral surface of the epithelial cell, close to the free surface.

    b. In sections parallel to the plane of the terminal bar, the terminal bar appears as a polygonal structure, sharply outlining the cell. This view clearly demonstrates that zonular junctions encircle the cell.

4. Terminal web. The terminal web is anchored to the adhesion belt of the junctional complex.

    a. The terminal web is a **mat of filaments** in the apical cytoplasm of the epithelial cell. It is formed by actin and spectrin, and rests on a layer of intermediate filaments (Figure 5-4).

    b. The terminal web functions as an **attachment point** for the **bundles of actin filaments** that support microvilli. The actin filaments extend out of the microvilli into the apical cytoplasm to insert into the terminal web.

    c. The terminal web, together with its associated circumferential band of actin filaments, may be a **contractile structure.**

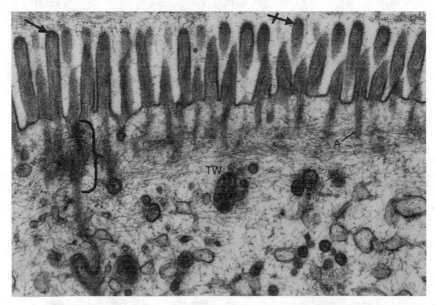

FIGURE 5-4. Electron micrograph of the apical surface of colonic epithelial cells. The epithelial surface is covered by microvilli (*arrow*), some of which have been sectioned obliquely (*crossed arrow*). Actin bundles (*A*) extend from the microvilli into the apical cytoplasm to insert into the filamentous terminal web (*TW*). A junctional complex (*bracket*) is visible in the field but it is indistinct because of the plane of section.

(1) It functions during embryonic development in the morphogenetic movements of epithelial layers.

(2) It may also function in adult epithelia to seal the epithelial surface after loss of senescent cells.

VI. EPITHELIAL CELL MITOSIS AND TISSUE RENEWAL

A. Turnover of the tissue. A general characteristic of epithelia is the **gradual replacement of the tissue** over a period of time.

1. Turnover times vary from a **few days** in the epithelial lining of the small intestine to approximately **one month** in the epidermis.

2. Some epithelia, however, have an **extremely slow rate of replacement** (e.g., ependymal cells of the central nervous system, kidney tubule epithelial cells).

B. Intraepithelial site of mitosis. Epithelia often have identifiable **mitotic** and **postmitotic compartments.**

1. Mitotic compartment. In renewing epithelia, dividing cells are often restricted to particular regions of the epithelium (e.g., basal layer of the epidermis, lower third of the intestinal crypt).
   a. Stem cells remain in the most restricted portion of the mitotic compartment.
   b. Cells may undergo more than one division as they migrate through the mitotic compartment to the site of postmitotic differentiation.

2. Postmitotic compartment. Recently divided cells migrate from the mitotic compartment to other regions of the epithelium where cell divisions normally are not seen.

C. Stages in renewal cycle of an epithelium. The stages and events that usually take place during the process of renewal include the following: **cell division, migration, differentiation, senescence,** and **cell loss.**

VII. EPITHELIA–CONNECTIVE TISSUE INTERFACE

A. Basement membrane. The basement membrane is a thin **connective tissue layer** underlying an epithelium. It consists of a superficial layer called the **basal lamina,** which is recognized only by electron microscopy, and a deeper layer called the **reticular lamina,** which is visible by light microscopy.

1. Components. The basement membrane is composed of small collagen fibers, reticular fibers, proteoglycans, and glycoproteins.

2. Histologic characteristics. The basement membrane is generally not visible after routine hematoxylin–eosin (H&E) staining. **Special staining of the polysaccharide components of the reticular lamina** (e.g., periodic acid–Schiff stain) is required to visualize the basement membrane.
   a. The deep boundary of the basement membrane is poorly defined and it merges with the extracellular matrix, which is not part of the basement membrane.
   b. The basement membrane may thicken in certain **pathologic states,** such as nephropathies, vasculopathies, and autoimmune diseases. A basement membrane affected by these conditions is identifiable following H&E staining.

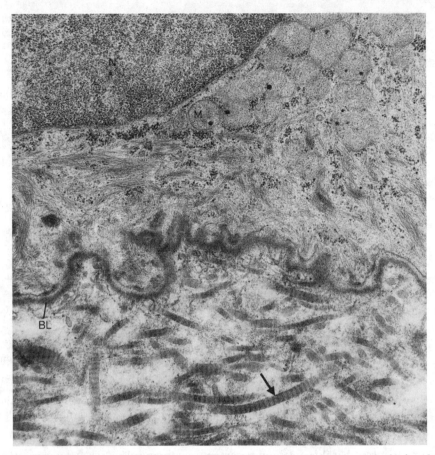

FIGURE 5-5. Electron micrograph depicting an epithelium–connective tissue junction: the basal surface of epidermis and the papillary layer of dermis. A distinct basal lamina (*BL*) follows the contours of the epidermal cell. In the epidermal cell are seen a portion of a nucleus (*N*), mitochondria (*M*) with matrix granules, and keratin intermediate filaments that are beginning to aggregate into tonofibrils. Visible in the dermis are banded fibrils of type I collagen (*arrow*) and, in the interfibrillar space, fine granular material that is evidence of the macromolecules of the ground substance.

B. **Basal lamina** (Figure 5-5). The basal lamina is a component of the basement membrane.

    1. Components. The basal lamina is a **30–100 nm thick, filamentous meshwork** that contains type IV collagen, laminin, other glycoproteins, and proteoglycans.

        a. The electron-dense layer of the basal lamina is called the **lamina densa.** The clear, electron-lucent zone between the lamina densa and the basal plasma membrane is called the **lamina rara,** or **lamina lucida.**

        b. The molecular composition of the basal lamina varies from region to region, but it appears that **type IV collagen, type VII collagen, and laminin are common constituents** of basal laminae in different sites in the body.

            (1) **Laminin** is concentrated in the lamina rara and functions to attach the lamina densa to the basal surface of the epithelial cell (see V B 2 a).

            (2) **Type VII collagen** connects the lamina densa to the underlying reticular lamina. These collagen filaments have been termed **anchoring filaments.**

    2. External laminae. Histologists sometimes reserve the term basal lamina for use exclusively with epithelia, and use the term external lamina to describe a basal lamina–like layer in muscle and nerve tissue. External laminae are found at the following locations:

      a. The junction of a peripheral nerve–Schwann cell complex and endoneurial connective tissue.

      b. The junction of muscle cells (fibers) and endomysial connective tissue.

3. Functions of the basal lamina

  a. Barrier

    (1) Throughout the body, basal laminae (and external laminae) form a barrier between connective tissue and the other basic tissues (i.e., epithelium, nerve, and muscle). The barrier defines tissue compartments and normally restricts free movement of most cells between compartments.

    (2) Connective tissue cells, however, may normally cross the barrier to enter an epithelial compartment (e.g., movement of lymphocytes into and out of epithelia during immune surveillance).

    (3) In pathologic situations, the barrier is necessarily breached.

      (a) In inflammation, all types of blood cells cross the basal lamina of postcapillary venules to enter loose connective tissue.

      (b) In cancer, neoplastic cells cause focal damage to basal and external laminae when they become invasive.

  b. Filtration

    (1) In addition to restricting passage of cells, basal laminae and external laminae filter noncellular materials based on size and charge.

    (2) The renal glomerular basement membrane, for example, is an unusually thick basal lamina that serves as the major filter in the formation of the glomerular filtrate.

  c. Regeneration

    (1) The basal lamina provides a surface along which epithelial cells migrate during cell renewal and wound healing.

    (2) The external lamina often persists after its associated nerve or muscle cell has been destroyed by a traumatic event. The resilient external lamina guides regenerating nerve or muscle cells back into normal cell–cell relationships.

C. **Comparison of basal lamina and basement membrane.** The two terms basal lamina and basement membrane often are incorrectly used synonymously. The basal lamina and the basement membrane are related, but they are not identical structures.

1. Relative dimensions. The **basal lamina** is a structure visible only with the electron microscope. The **basement membrane,** after appropriate staining, is visible with the light microscope.

2. Structural overlap. The most superficial part of the basement membrane is formed by the basal lamina. The deeper part of the basement membrane, the reticular lamina, can be visualized by light microscopy after the appropriate staining and is quite distinct from the much thinner basal lamina.

3. Synthesis. The basal lamina or external lamina is synthesized by its associated epithelial cell, Schwann cell, or muscle cell. The reticular lamina is synthesized by fibroblasts.

Chapter 6

Nerve

INTRODUCTION. Nerve is one of the four basic tissues of the body.

A. **Nervous system components**

1. The **central nervous system (CNS)** consists of the brain and spinal cord. The neural substance forming the brain and spinal cord may be divided into white and gray matter.

   a. **White matter.** This is characterized by the presence of large myelinated nerve fibers (axons) and the absence of nerve cell bodies. Its whitish appearance in fresh tissue is due to myelin.

   b. **Gray matter.** This is characterized by the presence of many nerve cell bodies and dendrites and the absence of heavily myelinated nerve processes. Sparsity of thick myelin sheaths produces a grayish color in fresh tissue.

2. The **peripheral nervous system (PNS)** consists of the spinal and cranial nerves (except the olfactory and optic nerves), and associated ganglia.

   a. **Spinal and cranial nerves.** These are the large named and small unnamed nerves of the PNS. They contain myelinated and unmyelinated axons, and sensory and motor axons.

   b. **Ganglia.** These are assemblies of nerve cell bodies outside the CNS.

3. The **autonomic nervous system** consists of the sympathetic, parasympathetic, and enteric systems.

B. **Nerve tissue components.** Nerve tissue is formed by **neurons** (nerve cells) and **supporting cells.**

1. **Glial cells** are the supporting cells of the CNS. These include oligodendrocytes, astrocytes, microglia, and ependymal cells (see IV A).

2. **Schwann cells** and **satellite cells** are the supporting cells of the PNS (see IV B)

C. **Function of the nervous system.** The ability to **perceive and respond** to events in our **internal and external environments** depends on the nervous system.

1. Neurons react to mechanical or chemical stimuli and the effect of stimulation is transmitted to other parts of the same cell.

2. Subsequently, the effects of stimulation are conveyed to other nerve cells, muscle cells, or gland cells.

II. **NEURONS.** The cellular units of structure and function in the nervous system are neurons (nerve cells). The number of neurons in the nervous system is estimated to be in the range of 9–15 billion. Nerve cells show the **greatest variation of size and shape** of any group of cells in the body (Figures 6-1, 6-2).

A. **Cell body** (perikaryon, soma). The dilated, nucleus-containing region of the neuron is the cell body. The cell body is the center of the metabolic and integrative functions of the neuron.

1. **Size.** The cell body often is recognized in histologic sections because it is **larger** than most nearby cells.

   a. Some nerve cell bodies may be as large as 125 μm in diameter and, therefore, can be seen with the naked eye.

   b. Most nerve cell bodies, however, are smaller.

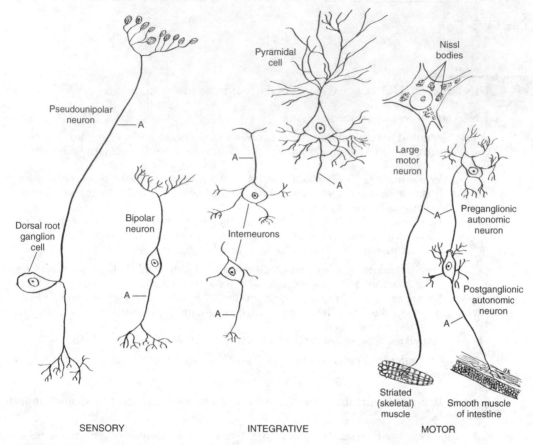

FIGURE 6-1. Diagram of various types of neurons found in the central and peripheral nervous systems. Pseudounipolar and bipolar neurons are examples of sensory neurons. Interneurons, Purkinje cells, and pyramidal cells are examples of integrative neurons (see also Figure 6-2). Spinal motor neurons and autonomic neurons are examples of motor neurons. *A* = axon. (Adapted from Ross MH, Romrell LJ, Kaye GI: *Histology: A Text and Atlas,* 3rd ed. Baltimore, Williams & Wilkins, 1995, p 259.)

    2. Shape. The nerve cell body in histologic section generally has a **round or ovoid shape.**
       a. Large spinal motor neurons have a characteristic **stellate shape.**
       b. This characteristic shape is due to the many processes (axons and dendrites) originating from the nerve cell body.

    3. Nucleus. The nucleus is large, spheroidal, and euchromatic, with a prominent nucleolus (Figure 6-3).

    4. Cytoplasmic components. The cytoplasm of the neuron contains a large Golgi apparatus, considerable rough endoplasmic reticulum (Nissl bodies), neurofilaments, mitochondria, and lysosomes.

  B. **Nissl bodies and Golgi apparatus.** These organelles, which are highly developed in nerve cells, are indicative of a metabolically and synthetically active cell.

    1. Nissl bodies (Nissl substance). These are **basophilic particles that vary in size and number** (see Figure 6-3). They stain intensely with basic dyes and metachromatically with thiazin dyes.
       a. Electron microscopy reveals that each Nissl body consists of a stack of **rough endoplasmic reticulum cisternae** and associated **polyribosomes.**

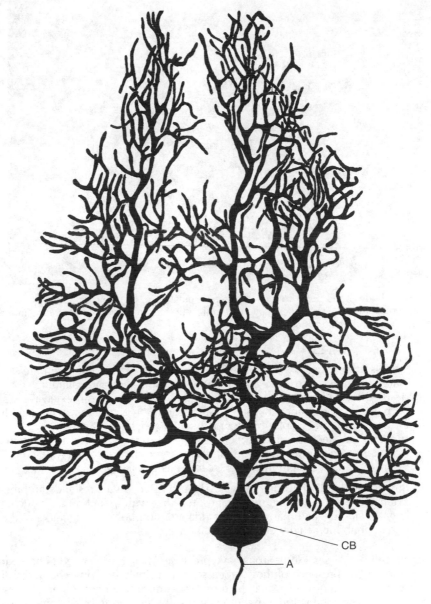

FIGURE 6-2. Diagram of a Purkinje cell of the cerebellum. Note the elaborate dendritic arborization. Thousands of synapses are formed over this large surface area. The dendritic, or receptor, region of the neuron contrasts with the solitary unbranched axon (*A*) that arises from the opposite side of the cell body (*CB*). (Modified with permission from Pentney RJ: *Neurobiol. Aging* 11:112, 1990.)

      (1) Most polyribosomes are attached to the cisternal membrane, but some polyribosomes appear to be unattached and are free in the intercisternal space.

      (2) Nissl bodies vary in size from fine, dust-like particles, formed by only a couple of cisternae, to large, angular chunks, formed by many cisternae.

   b. The presence of large numbers of Nissl bodies indicates that the nerve cell has considerable **protein synthetic capacity.**

   c. Nissl bodies, free polyribosomes, and, occasionally, parts of the Golgi apparatus **extend into the dendrites of the neuron but not into the axon** (see II C 3 c).

  2. Golgi apparatus (Golgi zone, Golgi membranes; see Chapter 2 III). The Golgi appa-

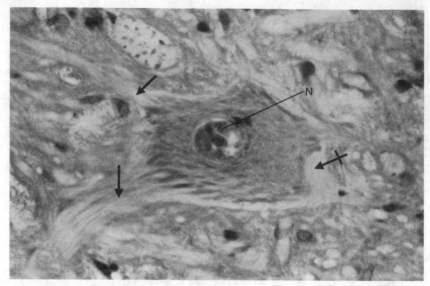

FIGURE 6-3. Cell body of motor neuron, gray matter of spinal cord, light micrograph. Nucleus (*N*) with a prominent nucleolus, many Nissl bodies scattered throughout the cytoplasm and extending into dendrites (*arrows*), and an axon hillock (*crossed arrow*).

ratus is a large organelle. Its size and distribution in the perikaryon are best appreciated by light microscopy after silver- or osmium-reduction staining.

   a. By these techniques, the Golgi apparatus is seen to be an extensive system of particles and strands that spread throughout the cytoplasm of the cell. It is as extensive in the cytoplasmic compartment as Nissl substance.

   b. With the electron microscope, the Golgi apparatus is seen as a system of agranular membranes similar to that encountered in most eukaryotic cells. This membranous system, however, reaches its greatest size in neurons.

3. **Biochemical activity of nerve cells.** The extensive Nissl substance and the equally extensive system of Golgi membranes, together with a euchromatic nucleus, a large nucleolus, and many mitochondria are morphologic indicators of the high rate of anabolic activity characteristic of nerve cells.

C. **Nerve cell processes.** All neurons have processes, which are called either **axons** or **dendrites.** The presence of these processes is the **single unifying characteristic** of nerve cells. Some processes may be a **meter or more in length;** other processes are quite short. The total volume of the processes of a neuron may be considerably greater than the volume of the cell body.

1. **Nerve cell classification.** Neurons are classified on the basis of their processes (see Figure 6-1).

   a. **Unipolar (pseudounipolar) neurons** (e.g., sensory neurons of the spinal cord). This type of neuron has a single, short process that divides close to the cell body into a peripherally running dendrite and a centrally running axon. The processes are continuous without an intervening cell body.

   b. **Bipolar neurons** (e.g., olfactory neurons). This type of neuron has an axon and a dendrite.

   c. **Multipolar neurons** (e.g., motor neurons of the spinal cord). This type of neuron has many processes; usually a large number of dendrites and only one axon are present.

2. **Dendrites are receptor processes.** Dendrites are processes whose main function is to receive information from other nerve cells and to carry that information to the cell body.

a. Cytologic characteristics of dendrites
   (1) Dendrites are usually of **larger diameter than axons** at their sites of origin from the cell body.
   (2) Dendrites are **unmyelinated** and generally are distinctly **tapered.**
b. Neurons often have **many dendrites** (see, for example, the Purkinje cell depicted in Figure 6-2).
   (1) Dendrites may form an **extensive and elaborate arborization** (dendritic tree) with successive branches of decreasing diameter. The pattern of the arborization may be used to classify the neuron.
   (2) Such dendritic arborization **increases the receptor surface area** of the neuron.

3. **Axons are effector processes.** Most axons convey the nerve impulse away from the cell body to another neuron or to an effector structure, such as a muscle cell. Neurosecretory axons, however, such as those that end in the neurohypophysis, convey peptide hormones from the cell body to an axon terminal near fenestrated capillaries (see Chapter 30 IV A 1).
   a. Cytologic characteristics of axons
      (1) Axons usually are of a finer diameter and are less conspicuous than dendrites (see Figure 6-2).
      (2) Neurons generally have only one axon.
      (3) Larger axons (>1 μm diameter) generally are myelinated. Smaller axons are unmyelinated.
   b. Axon length. The length of an axon is extremely variable depending on the neuron type.
      (1) Golgi type I neurons have long axons that may be a meter or more in length.
         (a) Pyramidal cells of the cerebral cortex and motor neurons of the spinal cord are typical Golgi type I cells.
         (b) Golgi type I neurons are called **projection neurons** because they carry information to distant points.
      (2) Golgi type II neurons have short axons.
         (a) Interneurons of the cortex or spinal cord are typical Golgi type II neurons.
         (b) Golgi type II neurons are called **local circuit neurons** because they convey information to other cells in their immediate vicinity.
   c. Axon hillock. This is the point of origin of the axon from the nerve cell body (see Figure 6-3).
      (1) The axon hillock is **free of Nissl substance.** The junction between the Nissl-containing cytoplasm of the nerve cell body and the Nissl-free cytoplasm of the hillock is often abrupt.
      (2) Microtubules and neurofilaments (see Chapter 3 III; IV A 3) pass through the hillock into the axon.
   d. Initial segment of the axon. This is a short region of the axon immediately distal to the axon hillock.
      (1) The initial segment is that part of the axonal process between the **apex of the hillock and the beginning of the myelin sheath.**
      (2) The initial segment is the **site of initiation** of an action potential in response to the summation of impulses received on the dendrites and cell body of that neuron.
   e. Axonal transport. Bidirectional intracellular movement of materials occurs between the cell body and its axon.
      (1) Axonal transport is a means of **intracellular communication.**
         (a) The Nissl substance and Golgi apparatus are restricted to the cell body and dendrites, often hundreds of centimeters distant from the point of use of the newly synthesized materials.
         (b) Thus, mechanisms must exist to transport them from the cell body distally to the end of the axon.
      (2) Anterograde and retrograde transport

    (a) **Anterograde (orthograde) transport** is the movement of materials from the cell body to distal parts of the axon.

    (b) **Retrograde transport** is the movement of materials from distal parts of the axon to the cell body.

      (i) This includes transport of growth factors and recycled membrane.

      (ii) Transport of viruses, toxins, and other noxious agents also occurs by the retrograde process.

  (3) **Slow and fast transport**

    (a) **Slow transport.** Some materials move at relatively slow rates, ranging from 0.1 to 10 mm per day. Slow transport is also called **axoplasmic flow.**

      (i) Structural elements needed for cell maintenance and cell growth (e.g., subunits of microtubules and neurofilaments) are carried by slow transport.

      (ii) Slow transport occurs only in an anterograde direction.

    (b) **Fast transport.** Other materials move at faster rates, ranging from 200 to 400 mm per day. Fast transport is also called **axoplasmic transport.**

      (i) Membrane components and neurotransmitters are carried by fast transport in vesicles that are associated with microtubules.

      (ii) Fast transport occurs in both anterograde and retrograde directions.

  (4) **Microtubule-associated proteins in axonal transport**

    (a) Transport mechanisms are closely related to **microtubules** and a class of microtubule-associated proteins (MAPs) called **microtubule motor proteins** that are found in neuronal processes.

    (b) These microtubule motor proteins are also called **molecular motors** in recognition of their role in fast transport.

      (i) **Kinesin** is a MAP that functions in anterograde transport.

      (ii) **Cytoplasmic dynein** is a MAP that functions in retrograde transport.

  (5) **Experimental application of axonal transport.** Retrograde and anterograde axonal transport of experimentally applied tracer materials (e.g., horseradish peroxidase or radioactive amino acids) may be used as a non-destructive means of delineating neural pathways. This has largely replaced neuron degeneration as a research method.

III. **SYNAPSES.** Synapses are points of functional contact between two neurons or between a neuron and a muscle cell or gland cell. Synapses may be subclassified into **chemical synapses** or **electrical synapses.**

A. **Chemical synapses** (Figures 6-4 and 6-5)

  1. **General characteristics**

    a. **Proximity of cells.** There is **close apposition** between cells at the site of synaptic interaction. A **synaptic cleft,** a space of 20–30 nm, separates two cells at a chemical synapse.

    b. **Cell–cell communication.** At a chemical synapse, a chemical **neurotransmitter** released from one cell affects the adjacent cell.

    c. **Cellular components of a synapse**

      (1) The **presynaptic component** is that part of the synapse from which the neurotransmitter is released.

      (2) The **postsynaptic component** of the synapse is that region of a cell surface that is affected by the released neurotransmitter.

  2. **Light microscopy of chemical synapses.** Synapses are not usually visible in routinely prepared sections for light microscopy. Synapses can be seen, however, in sections stained by the **Golgi method,** which is based on the precipitation of reduced silver in a small number of neurons in a particular sample of nerve tissue.

    a. Synapses may appear as button-like swellings, called **boutons,** either at the end

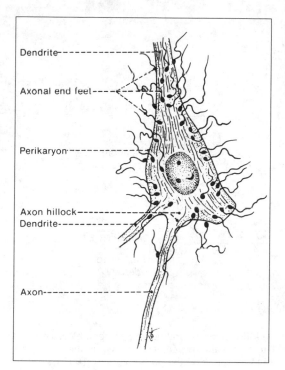

Dendrite

Axonal end feet

Perikaryon

Axon hillock
Dendrite

Axon

FIGURE 6-4. Cell body of a neuron showing synapses over its surface and also on its dendrites and axon. Terminal portions of incoming axons and boutons terminaux are illustrated. (Reproduced from DeMyer W: *NMS Neuroanatomy.* Baltimore, Williams & Wilkins, 1988, p 14.)

of an axon (boutons terminaux) or at points along the axon (boutons en passant). Other specialized synapses, such as the neuromuscular junction, have a more complex appearance.

   b. The Golgi method also demonstrates the overall shape of the neuron.

3. Number of synapses (see Figure 6-4)

   a. The number of synapses found over the surface of a neuron and its processes generally **varies from hundreds to tens of thousands.** In some organs of special sense, however (e.g., the eye), some neurons may have only a **single synapse.**

   b. The number of synapses on a cell body or its processes is directly related to the **amount of input** that neuron is receiving and integrating.

4. Distribution of synapses

   a. Any part of a neuron may form a synapse with any part of a second neuron.

   b. **Axodendritic** and **axosomatic** synapses are the most numerous. Axoaxonal and dendrodendritic synapses are also found. Other types of synapses (e.g., somatosomatic) occur but are only rarely observed.

5. Ultrastructure of chemical synapses. Electron microscopy reveals structural details of the presynaptic and postsynaptic components (Figure 6-5).

   a. Presynaptic component. This is the transmitter region of the synapse.

   (1) Synaptic vesicles. At the electron microscopic level, the presynaptic component of the synapse is characterized by the presence of **synaptic vesicles.** A synaptic vesicle is a membrane-bounded structure that contains neurotransmitter.

   (a) Synaptic vesicles are usually **spheroidal** and **appear empty.** They range in diameter from about 30 nm to 100 nm.

   (b) Some synaptic vesicles, especially those containing **catecholamines,** have an electron-opaque core (dense-core vesicles).

   (c) The flattened or ovoid appearance of some vesicles may result from the use of hyperosmotic fixatives.

   (2) Exocytotic release. Synaptic vesicles release their contents of neurotransmitter by **exocytosis into the synaptic cleft.**

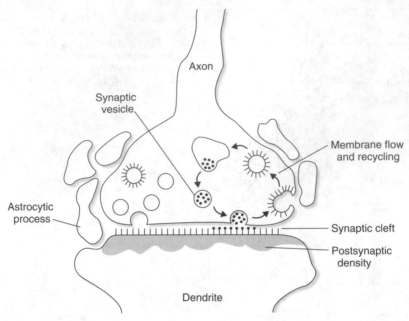

FIGURE 6-5. Diagram of a synapse (chemical, axo-dendritic) of the central nervous system. Neurotransmitter release by exocytosis of synaptic vesicles and vesicle membrane recycling are shown in the axonal presynaptic component. Neurotransmitter is shown bound to receptors on the postsynaptic surface. Astrocytic processes surround the synapse and form a cellular dam around the synaptic cleft.

  (3) Recycling of synaptic vesicle membrane. Exocytosis of synaptic vesicles results in the addition of **patches of membrane to the presynaptic surface.** Each patch is derived from one synaptic vesicle. The presynaptic surface area, however, normally does not increase.
   (a) Membrane flow occurs from the area of vesicle release, facing the synaptic cleft, to the periphery of the presynaptic ending.
   (b) Membrane is retrieved or internalized there by **endocytosis.**
   (c) Retrieved membrane fuses with the smooth endoplasmic reticulum in the presynaptic compartment and is **reused in the formation of new synaptic vesicles.**
 b. Postsynaptic component. This is the **receptor region** of the synapse.
  (1) Location. The region on the surface of a neuron on the opposite side of the synaptic cleft from the presynaptic component is the postsynaptic component. It is similar in shape and area to the presynaptic component.
  (2) Postsynaptic density. The postsynaptic density is a layer of dense material of variable thickness attached to the cytoplasmic side of the postsynaptic membrane.
  (3) Receptor site. Receptors in the postsynaptic membrane bind neurotransmitter, causing changes in the electrical potential across the membrane at the postsynaptic site. The cytoplasmic domains of the receptor molecules are anchored in the postsynaptic density.
6. Functions of chemical synapses
 a. One neuron is able to affect the functional state of another by synaptic contact. Neurotransmitter released from one neuron binds to receptors in the adjacent, postsynaptic neuron and alters the membrane potential of the postsynaptic cell.
  (1) Excitatory synapses. The neurotransmitter causes depolarization of the postsynaptic membrane. Acetylcholine is an example of an excitatory neurotransmitter.
  (2) Inhibitory synapses. The neurotransmitter produces a hyperpolarizing effect

on the postsynaptic membrane. γ-aminobutyric acid (GABA) is an example of an inhibitory neurotransmitter.

b. Summation of the effects of many excitatory and inhibitory synapses occurs in a postsynaptic cell and results in either the generation of a nerve impulse or inhibition of impulse generation.

B. Electrical synapses

1. Electrical synapses provide **low-resistance pathways** between neurons. Chemical neurotransmitters do not function at these synapses. Electrical synapses are equivalent to the **gap junctions** of non-nerve tissue (see Chapter 5 V C).

2. Electrical synapses are **not widely distributed in the mammalian nervous system.** Gap junctions, however, are commonly found in the impulse conducting system of the heart and in the intercalated disks of the myocardium, where they are essential for the transmission of electrical activity.

IV. SUPPORTING CELLS OF THE NERVOUS SYSTEM

A. Supporting cells of the CNS. The non-neural supporting cells of the CNS are **glial cells,** which are more numerous than neurons. In routine histologic sections, only the nuclei of glial cells are visible. Immunocytochemical methods or impregnation of the tissue with heavy metals reveal the entire glial cell.

1. **Oligodendrocytes**
   a. **Characteristics.** These cells have **few processes.** Oligodendrocytes are often **aligned in rows** between axons in the white matter.
   b. **Function.** These are the **myelin-forming cells** of the CNS.

2. **Astrocytes**
   a. **Characteristics.** Astrocytes are characterized by the presence of **many processes.**
      (1) The intermediate filaments of astrocytes are formed by **glial fibrillary acidic protein** (GFAP).
      (2) Astrocytic processes develop **end-feet** at the junction of nerve tissue and non-nerve tissue.
         (a) Astrocytic end-feet are found along blood vessels. It was once thought, incorrectly, that the perivascular end-feet formed the blood–brain barrier.
         (b) The end-feet also form a layer called the glia limitans at the outer surface of the brain and spinal cord. End-feet also underlie the ependymal lining of the ventricles.
      (3) Astrocytes are joined to one another by **gap junctions.**
   b. **Types.** Astrocytes are usually described as either **fibrous** or **protoplasmic astrocytes.**
      (1) These two types probably represent developmental variants of a single cell type.
      (2) Fibrous astrocytes predominate in white matter and protoplasmic astrocytes are more numerous in gray matter.
   c. **Function**
      (1) Bare areas of myelinated axons, at nodes of Ranvier and at synapses, acquire an **astrocyte sheath.** Perisynaptic astrocytes may function to confine neurotransmitters to the synaptic cleft and to metabolize excess neurotransmitters.
      (2) Astrocytes **regulate potassium concentration** in nerve tissue.

3. **Microglia**
   a. **Characteristics.** Microglia, as their name indicates, are the **smallest glial cells.**

        (1) Their processes are **shorter and less elaborate** than those of oligodendrocytes and astrocytes.

        (2) Microglia are members of the **mononuclear phagocyte system.**

   b. Function. Microglia are normally present only in small numbers in the CNS. Their numbers increase at sites of injury and disease, where their phagocytic nature becomes evident.

  4. Ependymal cells. Ependymal cells are epithelial glial cells that line the ventricles of the brain and the central canal of the spinal cord.

  5. Note on current terminology. Once, the term glial cell was reserved for non-neuronal supporting cells found exclusively in the CNS. In current usage, however, the term glial cell is also applied by some investigators to Schwann cells and satellite cells of the PNS.

B. **Supporting cells of the PNS.** Schwann cells and satellite cells form a continuous, uninterrupted layer over the surface of most neurons of the PNS.

  1. Schwann cells are the **myelin-forming cells** of the PNS. They form myelin around the large axons of peripheral nerve cells. They also ensheath the smaller, unmyelinated axons of peripheral nerves (see VIII A).

   a. Schwann cells derive from the cells of the neural crest and continue to increase in number during development and growth of the nervous system.

   b. Because Schwann cells cover most of the surface of peripheral nerves, they are in a position to regulate metabolic exchanges between the axon and the periaxonal space.

  2. Satellite cells form an epithelioid layer around nerve cell bodies (ganglion cells) in the PNS. As the Schwann cells do for the axon, the satellite cells probably establish and maintain a favorable environment around the nerve cell body.

   a. Satellite cells are also derived from the cells of the neural crest, as are most ganglion cells themselves.

   b. The layer of satellite cells covering the cell body is continuous with the Schwann cells covering the axon.

   c. Satellite cells generally **do not form myelin** around the nerve cell body. An exception to this, however, is the myelin formed by satellite cells around the ganglion cells of the eighth cranial nerve and at a few other sites.

V. **MYELIN SHEATH OF THE PERIPHERAL NERVOUS SYSTEM.** Layering of Schwann cell plasma membrane around an axon forms myelin. Myelin insulates the axon from the extracellular space. Myelin also increases the conduction velocity of the nerve impulse.

A. **General characteristics**

  1. Staining characteristics

   a. Routine tissue processing. Myelin is **not retained** by routine tissue processing. The myelin sheath is a lipid-rich layer that is extracted by the organic solvents used in routine microscopic techniques. Evidence of the myelin sheath, after routine tissue processing, is seen as a clear space around the axon.

   b. Non-routine techniques. Myelin can be demonstrated by non-routine techniques.

    (1) Fixatives that preserve the myelin sheath can be used.

     (a) Such fixatives are based on the stabilization of the fatty acid components of the myelin lipids by heavy metal oxides such as osmium tetroxide.

     (b) The reduced metal oxide also serves as a stain for the myelin sheath.

    (2) Lipid-soluble stains such as Sudan black B may also be used after appropriate fixation and avoidance of lipid solvents during processing.

2. **General structure**
   a. Myelin is **segmented.**
      (1) Each myelin segment is called an **internodal segment** and is the amount of myelin formed by one Schwann cell (see V C).
      (2) The gap between internodal segments is a **node of Ranvier** (see V D).
   b. An **external lamina** surrounds the Schwann cell–axon complex.

B. **Ultrastructure of the myelin sheath**

1. **Lamellae**
   a. Using electron microscopy, the myelin sheath appears as a complex of **concentrically arranged, electron-opaque (dark) lamellae** and **electron-lucent (light) spaces** around an axon.
   b. The **number of lamellae varies** from just a few lamellae around a small axon, to 50 or more lamellae around the largest diameter axons.
   c. The lamellae are referred to as **major dense lines** and **intermediate lines** (intraperiod lines) (see V C 3).

2. **Landmarks** of the myelin sheath–axon complex (see Figure 6-6)
   a. **Outer mesaxon.** This is a double layer of plasma membrane connecting the outermost surface of the Schwann cell, adjacent to the surrounding external lamina, to the myelin lamellae.
   b. **Inner mesaxon.** This is also a double layer of plasma membrane. It connects the innermost surface of the Schwann cell, adjacent to the axon, to the inner aspect of the myelin lamellae.
   c. **Schwann cell cytoplasmic compartments**
      (1) **Inner compartment.** A layer of Schwann cell cytoplasm lies between the axon and the inner aspect of the myelin lamellae.
      (2) **Outer compartment.** A layer of Schwann cell cytoplasm surrounds the myelin sheath. In older literature, the complex consisting of this cytoplasmic layer, the outermost plasma membrane of the Schwann cell, and the external lamina was called the **neurilemma,** or **Schwann sheath.**

C. **Development of the peripheral myelin sheath** (Figures 6-6, 6-7). The myelin sheath is synthesized by Schwann cells.

1. **Early in development,** Schwann cells become sequentially arranged along axons. Grooves develop on the surface of the Schwann cell and nerve bundles fit into the grooves.

2. **Later in development**
   a. Eventually, only one axon is found in a single groove on the surface of a Schwann cell. This is presumably the result of an increase in number of Schwann cells, together with a sorting process.
      (1) An intercellular space of uniform width separates the axon and the Schwann cell.
      (2) The axon–Schwann cell complex is surrounded by an external lamina that is synthesized by the Schwann cell.
   b. Close apposition of the edges of the groove to enclose the axon produces the **mesaxon.**
   c. A single axon may have thousands of Schwann cells aligned along it. **Each Schwann cell elaborates one internodal segment** of myelin on that axon.

3. **Formation of lamellae.** The first few myelin lamellae that form are loosely arranged (see Figure 6-6). Later, the lamellae become compact and the characteristic laminated structure of myelin can be recognized. Two types of electron-opaque lamellae are visible in electron micrographs of myelin.
   a. **Major dense line.** This is the darker, more prominent lamella. It is formed by the close apposition of the cytoplasmic sides of the Schwann cell plasma membranes. Schwann cell cytoplasm is squeezed out as compaction proceeds.
   b. **Intermediate line.** This is a less darkly stained lamella. It is formed by the ap-

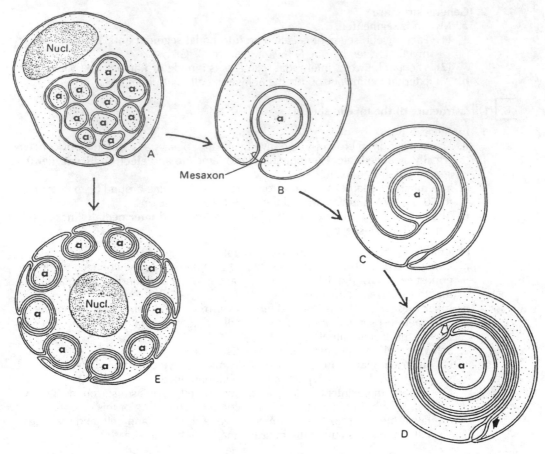

FIGURE 6-6. Forms of ensheathment in peripheral nerve. (*A*) During development, the small embryonic nerve fibers are surrounded in groups by Schwann cells. (*B*) The fibers that will ultimately become myelinated enlarge and become ensheathed by individual Schwann cells. (*C*) The encircling lips of the Schwann cell slide by one another, and the mesaxon is elongated. (*D*) As the mesaxon is compacted, myelin is formed. Note that the apposition of the cytoplasmic surfaces of the plasma membrane forms the major dense line of the myelin sheath; the apposition of the external surfaces of the plasma membrane forms the intraperiod line. (*E*) Axons that do not become myelinated remain small and become ensheathed within individual troughs in the Schwann cell. The *open arrow* in (*D*) indicates the inner mesaxon; the *black arrow* indicates the outer mesaxon. *a* = axon; *nucl* = nucleus. (Reproduced with permission from Kelly DE, Wood RL, Enders AC: *Bailey's Textbook of Microscopic Anatomy,* 18th ed. Baltimore, Williams & Wilkins, 1984, p 341.)

           proximation of the external surfaces of the apposed Schwann cell plasma membrane.

    4. Mechanisms of myelin formation. Two mechanisms have been proposed for the formation of the myelin sheath by the Schwann cell.
      a. Rotating cell model. The Schwann cell is fixed to the surface of the axon and the nucleus-containing region of the cell rotates around the axon.
        (1) During this process, the mesaxon elongates and forms myelin lamellae.
        (2) This model is based on observations of peripheral nerve myelination in organ culture.
      b. Extended tongue model. The nucleus-containing region of the Schwann cell remains fixed while a tongue of its surface insinuates itself between the Schwann cell and the axon.
        (1) Continued spiral growth of the Schwann cell tongue produces myelin lamellae.

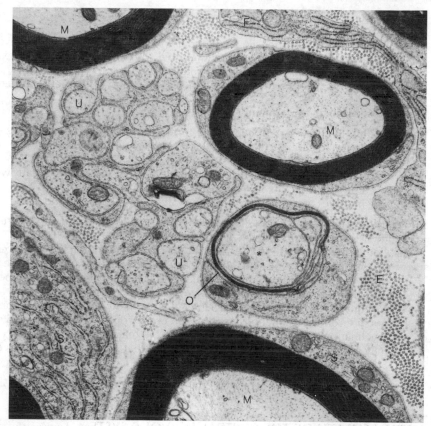

FIGURE 6-7. Electron micrograph of a peripheral nerve illustrating the heterogeneity that is typical of a peripheral nerve. Present in this field are axons with myelin sheaths (*M*), unmyelinated axons (*U*), an axon in process of myelination (*), outer mesaxons (*O*), Schwann cell cytoplasm (*S*), endoneurial collagen (*E*), and a portion of an endoneurial fibroblast (*F*), which is infrequently encountered.

        (2) While this has not been observed directly in peripheral nerve myelination, it is the model that describes myelination in the CNS.

D. **Nodes of Ranvier in the PNS**

  1. **Interruption in myelin sheath.** A node of Ranvier is located at the junction of two internodal segments of myelin.
    a. The bare area of the axon at the node is partially bridged by delicate processes from the two adjacent Schwann cells.
    b. The external lamina is continuous across the node.
    c. Myelin is less compactly arranged in the paranodal areas, that is, the parts of two internodal segments that abut to form the node of Ranvier. Lamellae appear to partially unravel adjacent to the node.

  2. **Rapid impulse conduction.** Myelinated axons conduct impulses more rapidly than unmyelinated axons.
    a. The internodal length of myelin is proportional to axon diameter. Larger diameter axons conduct more rapidly than smaller diameter axons and have longer internodal segments of myelin.
    b. The rapid impulse conduction by myelinated axons is explained partially by the presence of nodes of Ranvier and partially by the insulating properties of myelin.

  3. **Saltatory conduction.** As it passes down a myelinated nerve, a nerve impulse

jumps from node to node. This saltatory (discontinuous) conduction does not occur in unmyelinated axons.

    a. The nodes are the only site along the myelinated axon at which the **axon membrane is in contact with extracellular fluid.** At these sites, the ionic exchanges necessary to propagate the action potential can occur.

    b. Nodes of Ranvier are thus sites for the **regeneration of the action potential.**

E. **Incisures of Schmidt-Lantermann**

  1. Definition. In an internodal expanse of myelin, several adjacent major dense lines may open in a diagonal path across the layers of myelin. These are incisures (clefts) of Schmidt-Lantermann.

    a. Small amounts of Schwann cell cytoplasm may be found in the narrow incisures or openings.

    b. The incisures are more frequently found in the PNS than in the CNS.

  2. Function. There are two possible explanations for the existence of incisures of Schmidt-Lantermann.

    a. Communication pathway. An incisure of Schmidt-Lantermann produces a continuous helical cytoplasmic channel across the myelin. An incisure thereby connects the inner and outer compartments of Schwann cell cytoplasm, potentially providing a communication pathway between them.

    b. Myelination error. Incisures of Schmidt-Lantermann may also be a nonfunctional error in myelination. As Schwann cell cytoplasm is compressed during myelination, prior to the establishment of the major dense line, some cytoplasm may remain behind to produce irregularities that are seen as incisures of Schmidt-Lantermann.

VI. **MYELIN SHEATH OF THE CENTRAL NERVOUS SYSTEM.** Layering of oligodendrocyte plasma membrane forms myelin in the CNS.

A. **Light microscopic appearance of the myelin sheath**

  1. The sheath in the CNS has many similarities to the myelin sheath of the PNS. It, too, is largely extracted by the organic solvents used in the routine preparation of tissues for histologic examination.

  2. The white matter of the CNS is formed predominantly of myelinated nerves. The fatty myelin appears white in unfixed and unstained specimens, hence the name white matter.

B. **Ultrastructure of the myelin sheath.** Electron microscopy reveals that CNS myelin is similar to PNS myelin in many ways. It surrounds axons and has major dense lines, intermediate lines, and electron-lucent layers. However, there are two major differences in the fine structure of CNS myelin as compared with PNS myelin.

  1. External laminae do not surround myelinated axons in the CNS.

  2. Adjacent axons in the CNS are often so tightly packed that their myelin sheaths may form a common intermediate line over part of their circumferences (see V C 3 b).

C. **Development of the central myelin sheath**

  1. Location of myelin-forming cell. The central part of the oligodendrocyte (i.e., the nucleus-containing region of the cell) is distant from the axon that it is myelinating.

  2. Extension of a tongue-like process. A tongue-like process is produced by the oligodendrocyte. The process finds its way to an axon and, in a manner not well understood, wraps itself around the axon to produce lamellae of myelin. One oligodendrocyte usually sends out **several tongue-like processes,** probably simultaneously.

3. **Formation of internodal segment.** Each process forms an internodal myelin segment. Each internodal segment may be on a different axon.

D. **Nodes of Ranvier in the CNS.** As in the PNS, nodes in the CNS are interruptions between successive segments of myelin.

   1. The nodal region in the CNS is more exposed than the nodal region in the PNS.

   2. Nodes of Ranvier in the CNS function in the regeneration of the action potential, as do nodes in the PNS.

VII. COMPARISON OF PERIPHERAL MYELIN AND CENTRAL MYELIN

A. Myelin-forming cells

   1. **Schwann cells** form myelin in the PNS and **oligodendrocytes** form myelin in the CNS.

   2. Schwann cells are derived from **neural crest** after it separates from the neural tube and oligodendrocytes are derived directly from the **neural tube.**

B. Relationships of myelin-forming cells to internodal segments and to axons

   1. **One Schwann cell** elaborates only **one internodal segment** of myelin. **One oligodendrocyte** elaborates **several internodal segments.**

   2. **One Schwann cell** myelinates part of only **one axon.** **One oligodendrocyte** may myelinate parts of **several axons.**

C. Individuality of myelinated axons

   1. **Peripheral myelinated axons** are **sharply defined** structures, each delimited by a layer of Schwann cell cytoplasm, an external lamina, and connective tissue of the endoneurium (see IX A).

   2. **Central myelinated axons** may abut one another so closely that they **share an interperiod line.** There is no complete cytoplasmic layer, external lamina, or endoneurium around nerves in the CNS.

D. Mesaxons

   1. Inner and outer mesaxons regularly occur in the PNS but may be indistinct because of the plane of section.

   2. There may be **no outer mesaxon** in myelinated nerves of the CNS because of the frequent absence of a complete circumferential cytoplasmic layer on the outer side of the myelin sheath.

VIII. UNMYELINATED NERVES IN THE PERIPHERAL AND CENTRAL NERVOUS SYSTEMS

A. **Unmyelinated nerves in the PNS.** Large numbers of small axons of the PNS lack a myelin sheath but do associate with Schwann cells (see Figure 6-7).

   1. **Role of Schwann cells.** One Schwann cell usually ensheaths multiple unmyelinated axons (see Figure 6-6).
      a. Schwann cells are elongated parallel to the long axis of the axons. **Axons fit into grooves** in the surface of each Schwann cell.
         (1) Schwann cells may have 20 or more grooves, each containing one unmyelinated axon.

(2) Close to the termination of a nerve, a Schwann cell may ensheath only one
unmyelinated axon.

b. The **lips of the groove may be separated,** so that part of the circumference of
the axon is exposed to the extracellular space, or the **lips may be closely apposed,** forming a **mesaxon.**

c. An **external lamina** surrounds the Schwann cell and its unmyelinated axons.

2. Schwann cells in autonomic plexuses

a. Bundles of unmyelinated axons in the autonomic nervous system occupy one
groove in a Schwann cell.

b. This relationship is reminiscent of the axon–Schwann cell arrangement in the
developing somatic portion of the PNS (see V C 1).

B. **Unmyelinated nerves in the CNS.** The large numbers of unmyelinated axons in the
CNS are not sheathed by any glial elements.

IX. **CONNECTIVE TISSUE SHEATHS OF PERIPHERAL NERVE.** Peripheral nerve tissue is closely associated with connective tissue (Figure 6-8). No such association is
seen in the CNS.

A. **Endoneurium.** This is the finest level of the connective tissue sheathing and it surrounds individual Schwann cell–axon complexes.

1. Endoneurium is usually not visible in routine light microscopic preparations. However, connective tissue–specific stains do demonstrate endoneurium.

2. Endoneurium is readily identified in routine electron micrographs of peripheral
nerve (see Figure 6-7). It consists of the external lamina of the Schwann cells and
of fine collagen fibrils and ground substance, which are secreted by Schwann cells
and the occasional fibroblast.

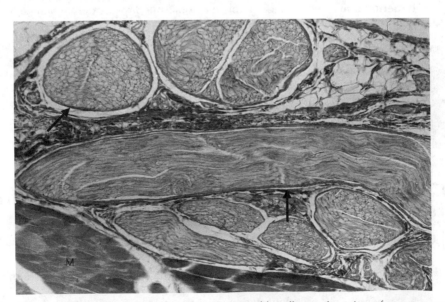

FIGURE 6-8. Light micrograph of a peripheral nerve. Several bundles, or fascicles, of axons are each defined by a perineurium (*arrows*). The nerve bundles are bound into a single, multifascicular nerve by epineurium. Within a nerve bundle, the larger myelinated axons can be identified but smaller myelinated
axons and unmyelinated axons cannot readily be discerned. *M* = skeletal muscle.

B. **Perineurium.** This is a sleeve-like layer of connective tissue that sharply defines nerve bundles (fascicles).

1. The perineurium is formed by an **epithelioid arrangement of flattened cells** that are joined by tight junctions. The perineurial layer is usually stratified (see Figure 9-2).

2. The perineurium appears to have a **barrier function** in establishing a protected intrafascicular environment for axons and Schwann cells.

C. **Epineurium.** The epineurium is visible by eye in the gross anatomy laboratory as the fascial covering of peripheral nerves.

1. The epineurium is **dense irregular connective tissue.**

2. Two or more nerve fascicles are **bound into a common bundle** by the epineurium, which also extends into the interfascicular spaces.

X. **BLOOD–BRAIN BARRIER.** The blood–brain barrier is a functional and morphologic barrier that restricts free passage of all but a few lipid-soluble materials from the circulation to the parenchyma of the CNS.

A. **The blood–brain barrier resides in vascular endothelium.** Electron microscopic studies using electron-opaque probes have shown that the barrier is formed by tight junctions between endothelial cells.

1. The tight junctions of capillary endothelial cells in the cerebral cortex are among the most complex junctions in the body, having many anastomosing strands of intramembrane junctional particles.

2. Also, the capillary endothelial cells are nonfenestrated and have very few pinocytotic vesicles.

B. **The blood–brain barrier is not absolute.** In some areas of the CNS (e.g., the neurohypophysis), the barrier is less effective and some tracer molecules cross vascular endothelium to penetrate brain tissue.

XI. **DEGENERATION AND REGENERATION IN THE NERVOUS SYSTEM.** Injured nerves degenerate. Regeneration may occur in the PNS but does not occur in the CNS.

A. **Anterograde (wallerian) degeneration.** This occurs in a PNS or CNS axon distal to the site of injury.

1. The axon distal to the injury undergoes degeneration because of interrupted axonal transport.

2. Phagocytic cells derived from Schwann cells and blood monocytes in the PNS, and microglia in the CNS, remove the fragments of myelin and degenerated axons.

B. **Retrograde degeneration.** This occurs proximal to the site of injury, i.e., between the site of injury and the nerve cell body. Evidence of retrograde degeneration extends proximally for only a few myelin segments.

C. **Chromatolysis** (axon reaction). This is a series of changes that occurs in the nerve cell body of an injured neuron. A nerve cell body undergoing chromatolysis exhibits the following characteristics:

1. **Reduction in Nissl substance,** producing unstained regions in the cytoplasm

  2. Increase in cell volume resulting from increased fluid uptake

  3. Relocation of the nucleus from a central to an eccentric position in the cell

D. Scar formation

  1. PNS. A connective tissue scar develops in the gap between the cut ends of a severed nerve.

   a. If the amount of scar tissue is not excessive, the cut nerve will probably regenerate.

   b. Surgical apposition of the cut ends of the nerve will increase the probability of successful regeneration.

  2. CNS. Scar tissue derived from proliferated astrocytes prevents regeneration in the CNS.

E. Regeneration

  1. Regeneration in PNS. Regeneration and restoration of nerve function can occur in the PNS.

   a. Proliferation of Schwann cells

    (1) Following wallerian degeneration, Schwann cells divide and produce cellular bridges that cross the injured region.

    (2) A wide gap or an unusually dense connective tissue scar impedes the formation of Schwann cell bridges.

   b. Development of nerve sprouts

    (1) New nerve processes, or neurites, arise from the proximal stump. The Schwann cell bridges serve as guides through the connective tissue scar for the regenerating nerve processes.

    (2) The large quantity of nerve sprouts that initially develop increases the probability of re-establishing sensory and motor connections. Many of the new nerve processes degenerate, however.

   c. Schwann tubes. External laminae and Schwann cells of nerve fibers distal to the injury remain as tubular structures after wallerian degeneration of the myelin sheath and axon.

    (1) Schwann cells survive wallerian degeneration and initially participate in regeneration by dividing and bridging the injured area.

    (2) The regenerating axons enter the Schwann tubes. The tubes help guide the growing axon to the correct sensory or motor ending.

  2. Regeneration in CNS. Regeneration usually does not occur in the CNS. The presence of glial scar formation, the absence of guiding cellular bridges, and the absence of anything comparable to Schwann tubes are important factors in the relative ineffectiveness of regeneration in the CNS.

XII. **AFFERENT RECEPTORS** (sensory receptors). Afferent receptors are specialized structures that are able to **initiate a nerve impulse** in response to a stimulus. The terminals are the **distal tips** of the peripheral axons of sensory neurons. **Exteroceptors** react to stimuli from the external environment, and **proprioceptors** and **enteroceptors** react to stimuli from within the body. Receptors are usually described as having a connective tissue capsule (encapsulated) or lacking a capsule (nonencapsulated).

A. Nonencapsulated receptors

  1. Free nerve endings. These are pain receptors found in epithelia and connective tissue.

  2. Merkel's corpuscles. These are light touch receptors found in epidermis.

B. Encapsulated receptors

1. **Meissner's corpuscles.** These are touch receptors found in the papillary layer of the dermis.
2. **Pacinian corpuscles.** These are pressure and vibration receptors found in the deep dermis, joint capsules, and internal organs.
3. **Ruffini's corpuscles.** These are mechanoreceptors found in skin and joint capsules.
4. **Muscle spindles.** These are proprioceptors found in skeletal muscle.
5. **Golgi tendon organs.** These are proprioceptors found at muscle–tendon junctions.

Chapter 7

Muscle Tissue

I. **INTRODUCTION.** Muscle tissue is one of the four basic tissue types. The primary function of muscle is **contraction** for the purpose of performing **mechanical work.**

A. The cells in muscle tissue are specialized for contraction because of the abundance and the regular arrangement of the major contractile proteins **actin** and **myosin.**

B. The arrangement of these contractile elements allows the histologic classification of muscle into two categories: **striated** muscle, which includes skeletal and cardiac muscle, and **smooth** muscle.

II. **CONTRACTILE PROTEINS.** Actin and myosin are the major contractile proteins of striated and smooth muscle. These filamentous proteins, often referred to as **myofilaments,** can constitute as much as 20% of the total mass of striated skeletal muscle cells.

A. Actin

1. **F-actin** is a helical polymer of uniformly oriented globular actin (G-actin) monomers that assemble into long, flexible, **thin filaments,** which vary in diameter from 7–9 nm.

2. **G-actin** monomers each have two binding sites:
   a. One binding site is a **nucleotide-binding site** that must be occupied by adenosine triphosphate (ATP) or adenosine diphosphate (ADP) in order for the assembly of G-actin into an F-actin filament to take place.
   b. The other binding site is a **myosin-binding site** that functions in the crossbridging of actin and myosin needed for contraction.

B. **Myosin.** Muscle myosin (myosin II) is a large asymmetric protein with a long filamentous tail domain and a domain with two globular heads. Two heavy chains and four light chains assemble into myosin II molecules, which measure 15–18 nm in diameter by 325 nm in length.

1. The carboxy terminal region of each heavy chain is a long alpha helix, and the amino terminal portion forms the globular head with which two light chains associate.

2. Two heavy chains then join by intertwining their alpha-helical tail domains, thus forming a stable dimeric protein with a single rod-like tail and with the two heads sticking out at one end of the molecule.
   a. The head domain is an actin-activated ATPase that is able to couple the hydrolysis of ATP with motility.
   b. The tail domain regulates the assembly of myosin molecules into the **thick filaments** of striated muscle cells.
      (1) Several hundred myosin molecules assemble tail to tail, in a staggered fashion, to produce this bipolar macromolecular complex.
      (2) The heads project outward from the sides of the thick filament. There is a central bare zone in which there are no heads (see Figure 7-2).

C. Additional proteins help to organize actin and myosin into functional units and play a role in regulating the interaction between these two proteins (see IV D 7, E 3 a, b).

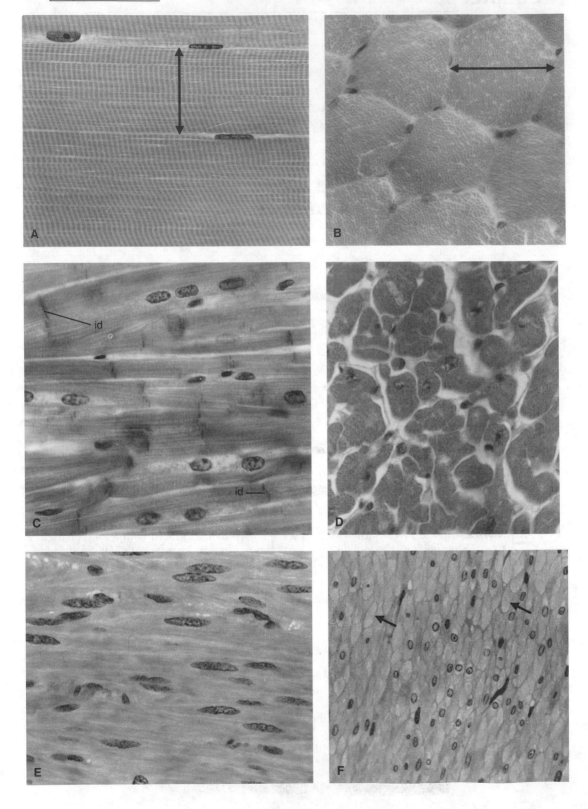

III. **CLASSIFICATION OF MUSCLE.** Muscle is classified on the basis of the appearance of the individual muscle cells in a histologic section. Two general categories are recognized: **striated muscle** and **smooth muscle** (Figure 7-1).

A. **Striated muscle.** Striated muscle cells exhibit cross-striations at the light microscopic level. On the basis of location, striated muscle tissue is further subdivided into **skeletal muscle** and **cardiac muscle.**

1. **Skeletal muscle** is attached to bone and is responsible for movements of the axial and appendicular skeleton. **Visceral striated muscle** is morphologically identical to skeletal muscle but is restricted to soft tissues (e.g., the tongue, pharynx, diaphragm, and upper part of the esophagus).

2. **Cardiac muscle** is the muscle of the heart, forming the myocardium.

B. **Smooth muscle.** Smooth muscle cells do not exhibit cross-striations (see Figure 7-1).

1. Smooth muscle is the intrinsic muscle of the alimentary canal, blood vessels, genito-urinary tract, respiratory tract, and other hollow and tubular organs.

2. Smooth muscle is also found as organized muscle bundles of the iris and ciliary body of the eye, as a thin sheet of muscle in the scrotum (the dartos muscle) and as isolated fibers in association with hair follicles in the skin (the arrector pili muscles).

IV. **SKELETAL MUSCLE.** Striated skeletal muscle tissue is the major muscle component of the body. It consists of bundles of striated muscle fibers, called **fascicles,** held together by connective tissue and attached by connective tissue to bone. It is responsible for gross and fine movements of limbs and digits, maintenance of body position, variations in facial expression, and the precise movement of the eye.

A. **General characteristics of skeletal muscle fibers.** The skeletal muscle cell—usually called a muscle fiber—is an elongated, cylindrical, multinucleate syncytium.

1. Fibers form during embryonic development by the fusion of small individual muscle cells called **myoblasts.**

2. Skeletal muscle fibers have a diameter of 10–100 μm and, in some instances, can extend the entire length of a muscle, from origin to insertion.

3. The **myofibril** is the major structural and functional subunit of the muscle fiber.
   a. Myofibrils are composed of bundles of actin and myosin filaments.
   b. Each myofibril is surrounded by a loose network of specialized smooth endoplasmic reticulum, called the **sarcoplasmic reticulum** (SR), along with mitochondria and glycogen, which provide energy for contraction.

4. The cytoplasm of muscle cells is traditionally called the **sarcoplasm** and the plasma membrane and its external lamina are called the **sarcolemma.**

FIGURE 7-1. Photomicrographs of the three muscle types. Skeletal muscle (A, B) is composed of long, cylindrical multinucleate cells (fibers) arranged in parallel arrays. *Double-headed arrow* in A and B indicates the diameter of a muscle cell. Cardiac muscle (C, D) is composed of single cells joined end to end by intercalated disks (*id*) and organized into long, branching fibers. Both skeletal and cardiac muscle cells are striated. Smooth muscle (E, F) occurs as bundles or sheets of elongate fusiform cells. The small cells in F, indicated by *arrows,* appear to be without a nucleus; these cells have been sectioned through their tapered ends. Because all micrographs are at the same magnification, it can be readily appreciated how much larger striated muscle cells are compared with cardiac and smooth muscle cells. Left panels are longitudinal sections, right panels are cross sections.

B. **Types of skeletal muscle fibers.** Based on an aggregate of morphologic, enzymatic, and functional characteristics, skeletal muscle fibers are classified into three types: red fibers, white fibers, and intermediate fibers. Most human muscles contain mixtures of these fiber types in various proportions.

1. **Red fibers.** Red fibers are small fibers with a high content of myoglobin and cytochromes and many mitochondria.
   a. **Myoglobin** is an oxygen-binding protein that closely resembles hemoglobin and occurs in varying amounts in muscle fibers. The higher content of myoglobin in red fibers accounts for the reddish appearance of this fiber type in freshly cut muscle tissue.
   b. Red muscle fibers, also called **slow twitch** fibers, are specialized for prolonged, sustained activity. They contract more slowly than white muscle fibers, and have a greater resistance to fatigue.
      (1) Myosin ATPase activity is greatest in red fibers.
      (2) Red fibers derive most of their energy from oxidative phosphorylation.
   c. In humans and other higher primates, red fibers are the major fibers of the long muscles of the back, where they are responsible for the long, slow contractions required to maintain an erect posture. They are also found in the long muscles of the limbs.

2. **White fibers.** White fibers are large fibers with less myoglobin and fewer mitochondria than red fibers.
   a. White fibers are adapted for rapid contraction and precise movements, and are thus called **fast twitch** fibers.
   b. They fatigue more easily than red fibers, and thus are not as suited for prolonged work. White muscle fibers derive their energy mostly from anaerobic glycolysis.
   c. White fibers constitute the primary fiber of the extraocular muscles and the muscles that control movement of the digits.

3. **Intermediate muscle fibers.** Intermediate muscle fibers are smaller than white fibers and have a pigment content and quantity of mitochondria between those of red and white fibers.

C. **Connective tissue associated with skeletal muscle.** The connective tissue of muscle has a distinct set of names that describes its relationship with the muscle fibers.

1. **Endomysium.** This is a delicate layer of reticular fibers and loose connective tissue that surrounds each muscle fiber. Small-caliber capillaries and fine branches of peripheral nerves run in this connective tissue.

2. **Perimysium.** This is a thicker layer of connective tissue that surrounds a group of muscle fibers to form a bundle or **fascicle.** Larger blood vessels and nerves run in the perimysium.

3. **Epimysium.** This is the outermost sheath of dense connective tissue that surrounds the entire collection of fascicles in the muscle.
   a. The major vascular and nerve supply of the muscle (i.e., the named vessels and nerves) passes through the epimysium.
   b. The epimysium is the fascia observed during dissection in the gross anatomy laboratory.

4. **Myotendon junction.** The connective tissue that surrounds the muscle fibers and fascicles is continuous with tendons and aponeuroses, thus providing a connection to the skeleton.

D. **Histologic characteristics of skeletal muscle**

1. **Cross-striations.** The cross-striations characteristic of histologic sections of striated muscle cells result from the regular arrangement of the contractile elements actin and myosin within the cytoplasm of these cells.
   a. Cross-striations are evident in hematoxylin–eosin (H&E)-stained longitudinal sections of muscle fibers as **alternating dark and light bands** (see Figure 7-1). They

are also visible in unstained sections when viewed with phase-contrast or polarization microscopy.

   (1) A bands. The **dark bands** are called A bands because they appear **aniso-tropic** in polarized light. They are birefringent (i.e., their refractive index changes with the plane of polarization).

   (2) I bands. The **light bands** are called I bands because they are **isotropic** in polarized light. In contrast to the A bands, they are monorefringent.

   b. Each of the major bands, the A band and I band, is bisected by a **narrow zone of contrasting density.**

   (1) The **Z disk** is a **dense zone** that appears as a line bisecting the I band.

   (2) The **H zone** is a **light zone** that bisects the A band; in ideal preparations, a dense **M line** can be seen to bisect the H zone.

   (3) The H zone and M line are demonstrated best in electron micrographs of striated muscle.

2. **Sarcomere.** The sarcomere is the segment of a myofibril between two adjacent Z disks. It is the basic contractile unit of striated muscle.

   a. It measures 2–3 μm in relaxed mammalian striated muscle.

   (1) It may be stretched to more than 4 μm.

   (2) In extreme contraction, it may be reduced to as little as 1 μm.

   b. Cross-striations are visible in striated muscle because sarcomeres in adjacent myofibrils and in adjacent myofibers are in register.

3. **Ultrastructure of cross-striations.** Electron microscopy reveals that cross-striations result from the highly ordered arrangement of the **thick (myosin)** and **thin (actin) filaments** within the sarcomere (Figure 7-2).

   a. Thick filaments average 1.5 μm in length and are restricted to the central region of the sarcomere (i.e., the A band).

   (1) Thick filaments are bound together at their centers by several structural proteins, one of which is **myomesin.**

   (2) This accumulation of structural proteins constitutes the M line.

   b. Thin filaments attach to the Z disk and extend into the A band where they interdigitate with the thick filaments.

   (1) The I band is composed almost entirely of thin actin filaments.

   (2) Thin filaments extend into the A band as far as the edge of the H zone.

   c. The three-dimensional organization of myofilaments is clearly illustrated when ideal cross-sections through different parts of the sarcomere are examined (see Figure 7-2).

   (1) A section through the I band reveals only cross-sections of thin actin filaments, arranged in an hexagonal array.

   (2) A cross-section through the H zone of the A band shows only thick filaments, also in an hexagonal pattern.

   (3) A cross-section through the M line shows thick filaments held in a precise array by myomesin.

   (4) A cross-section through the A band where the thick and thin filaments overlap shows a thick myosin filament surrounded by an hexagonal array of thin filaments.

4. **Sarcoplasmic reticulum.** The SR is arranged in networks around bundles of myofilaments, thereby defining the myofibrils (Figure 7-3).

   a. The SR resembles a sleeve of interconnecting flattened tubules surrounding a short portion of the myofibril, extending from A–I band junction to A–I band junction in mammalian skeletal muscle.

   (1) The lace-like network of tubular elements is particularly abundant over the A band.

   (2) Repeating units of the SR are stacked end to end along each myofibril.

   b. The ends of each sleeve balloon out, forming large compartments called **terminal cisternae.** Terminal cisternae store Ca^{2+} ions.

5. **T system.** Transverse tubules, or **T tubules,** which make up the T system, are

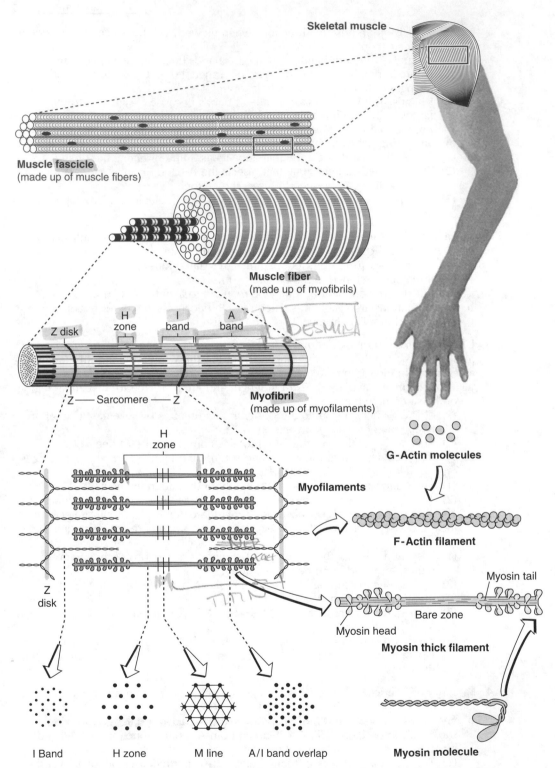

Skeletal muscle

Muscle fascicle
(made up of muscle fibers)

Muscle fiber
(made up of myofibrils)

H zone   I band   A band

Z disk

Z — Sarcomere — Z

Myofibril
(made up of myofilaments)

H zone

Z disk

Myofilaments

G-Actin molecules

F-Actin filament

Myosin tail

Bare zone

Myosin head

Myosin thick filament

Myosin molecule

I Band   H zone   M line   A/I band overlap

FIGURE 7-2. A diagram of the organization of skeletal muscle from the gross anatomic level to the molecular level. Illustrated are the four levels of structural organization in striated muscle: fascicles, fibers, myofibrils, and myofilaments. Thin (F-actin) filaments are composed of long polymers of G-actin molecules. Thick filaments are macromolecular assemblies of myosin molecules. (Adapted from Bloom W, Fawcett DW: *A Textbook of Histology,* 11th ed. Philadelphia, WB Saunders, 1986, p 282; and Ross MH, Romrell LJ, Kaye GI: *Histology: A Text and Atlas,* 3rd ed. Baltimore, Williams & Wilkins, 1995, p 218.)

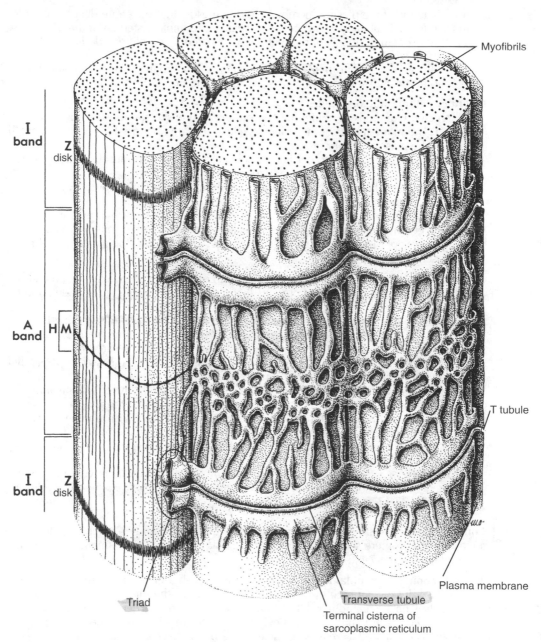

FIGURE 7-3. Diagram of part of a mammalian striated muscle fiber, illustrating the organization of the sarcoplasmic reticulum (SR) and its relationship to the myofibrils. In the myofibril at the left, the A, I, and H bands, and the Z disks, are indicated. The SR is shown surrounding the myofibrils at the middle and right of the illustration. Note that in mammalian striated muscle fibers, two T tubules supply a sarcomere. Each T tubule is located at an A–I band junction, where it is associated with two terminal cisternae of the SR, one cisterna on either side of the T tubule. The triple structure as seen in cross section, where the two terminal cisternae flank a T tubule at the A–I band junction, is referred to as a triad. (Courtesy of C. P. Leblond.)

invaginations of the plasma membrane of the muscle that penetrate deeply into the muscle fiber. T tubules extend between adjacent terminal cisternae of the SR.

    a. The association of a T tubule with the two cisternae on either side is called a **muscle triad.**

    b. Triads are located at the A–I band junction in mammalian skeletal muscle fibers, and at the Z disk in mammalian cardiac muscle fibers.

6. Other cytoplasmic organelles

    a. Nuclei. Hundreds of nuclei may be present in one skeletal muscle fiber.

        (1) The many nuclei of the striated skeletal muscle fiber are located just beneath the plasma membrane.

        (2) This is in contrast to cardiac muscle cells and smooth muscle cells, in which the single nucleus is centrally located.

    b. Cisternae of the **rough endoplasmic reticulum** and the **Golgi complex** are present near the nuclei.

    c. Mitochondria are abundant and are present beneath the plasma membrane and between the myofibrils. They are especially abundant in red muscle fibers.

    d. The sarcoplasm is rich in **glycogen granules,** a polymeric storage form of glucose.

7. Supporting proteins of the sarcomere. The sarcomere is held together by an elaborate scaffolding of filamentous proteins that regulate the spacing, attachment, and precise alignment of the myofilaments.

    a. Titin, a large elastic protein, connects the Z disk to the M line. Its spring-like character appears to help stabilize the thick filaments, keeping them centered in the sarcomere, and helps prevent excessive stretching of the sarcomere.

    b. Nebulin, an inelastic filamentous protein, attaches to the Z disk and runs parallel to the thin filaments, serving as an interfilament spacer.

    c. α-Actinin, a short, bipolar, rod-shaped molecule, bundles thin filaments into parallel arrays at the Z disk and helps anchor thin filaments at the Z disk.

    d. Desmin, one type of intermediate filament, forms a lattice surrounding the sarcomere at the level of the Z disks, attaching them to one another and to the plasma membrane. This serves to form crosslinks between myofibrils, stabilizing them within the muscle cell.

    e. Myomesin, a structural protein, forms a transversely oriented network of fine filaments at the middle of the H zone (i.e., the M line). This holds the thick myosin filaments in register and binds them together.

E. **Contractile mechanism of striated muscle: sliding filament model.** When muscle contracts, each sarcomere shortens and becomes thicker, but the myofilaments remain the same length (Figure 7-4).

1. Overlapping of myofilaments. To accomplish the shortening, there must be an increase in the overlapping of the myofilaments; that is, the thick and thin filaments must slide past one another. Ultrastructural examination of the sarcomere in various states of contraction has provided evidence for this mechanism. When contracted muscle is compared to relaxed muscle, it has been observed that:

    a. The I band shortens in length while the A band remains the same length.

    b. The H zone becomes narrower, with the thin filaments penetrating the H zone.

    c. These observations suggest that the **thin filaments slide past the thick filaments** during contraction.

2. Interaction between myosin and actin filaments during contraction. A myosin head binds to an adjacent actin filament and a conformational change in the head ratchets the myosin along the actin filament. An ATP-dependent cyclic interaction between myosin heads and the adjacent actin filaments generates a force that causes the filaments to move past one another (Figure 7-5).

    a. Steps in contraction. The cyclic interaction can be divided into sequential steps.

        (1) Step 1: myosin dissociates from actin

            (a) At the start of a cycle, the head of the myosin filament, lacking a bound nucleotide, is tightly attached to an adjacent actin filament.

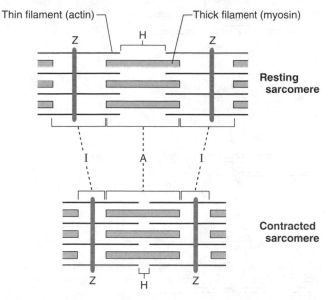

Thin filament (actin)⌐   ⌐Thick filament (myosin)

Resting sarcomere

Contracted sarcomere

FIGURE 7-4. Relaxed and contracted sarcomeres. During contraction, interdigitation of the actin and myosin filaments is increased and the length of the I band is decreased. Thus, the length of the sarcomere is decreased. The length of the actin (thin) and myosin (thick) filaments remains constant, as does the length of the A band.

- **(b)** When ATP binds to the myosin head, the affinity of the head for the actin is reduced and the head detaches.
  - **(i)** ATP binding is essential for the release of myosin from the actin filament.
  - **(ii)** In the absence of ATP, the actin–myosin interaction will not be terminated and the muscle will not relax. This is the basis for **rigor mortis,** the muscular rigidity that develops after death.
- **(2) Step 2: conformational change in myosin**
  - **(a)** Following release of the myosin head from the actin, the bound ATP is hydrolyzed by myosin ATPase, inducing a conformational change in the myosin that causes the head to be displaced along the actin filament a distance of about 5 nm.
  - **(b)** The products of ATP hydrolysis, ADP and inorganic phosphate (P_i), remain attached to the myosin head.
- **(3) Step 3: myosin binds to actin**
  - **(a)** The myosin head—with the still-attached ADP and P_i —binds to a new site on the actin filament.
  - **(b)** The initial contact of the myosin head causes the release of the P_i molecule and leads to a tight binding of the head to actin.
- **(4) Step 4: second conformational change in myosin**
  - **(a)** The tight binding induces a conformational change in the myosin head, such that it pulls against the actin filament, causing the actin filament to slide along the myosin filament. This is the **power stroke.**
  - **(b)** This change in shape in the myosin head is accompanied by the release of the ADP molecule, opening up a site for an ATP molecule. The subsequent binding of another ATP molecule to the myosin head induces its release from the actin filament, setting another cycle in motion.
- **b. Contraction symmetry**
  - **(1)** The myosin thick filaments are bipolar; thus the same cyclic interaction of myosin heads and actin filaments occurs at each end of the filament.
  - **(2)** The Z disks in a sarcomere are thus pulled toward one another, resulting in shortening of the sarcomere.

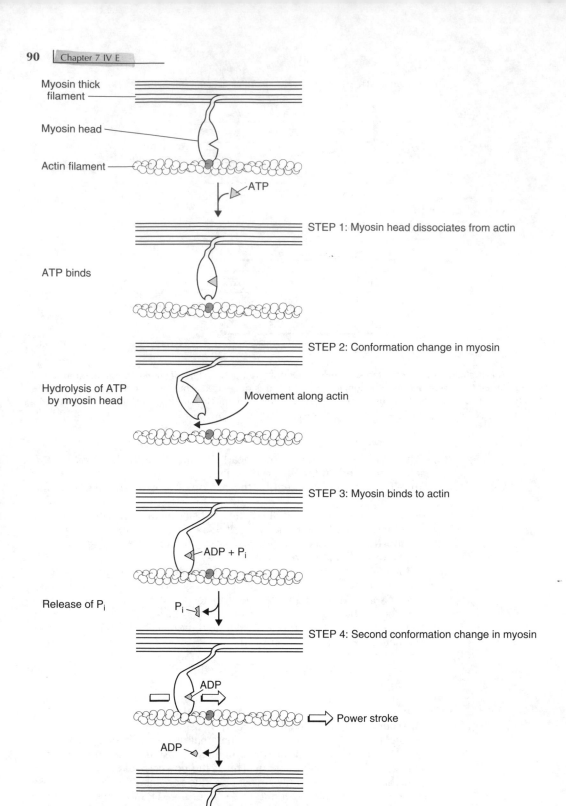

Myosin thick filament

Myosin head

Actin filament

ATP

STEP 1: Myosin head dissociates from actin

ATP binds

STEP 2: Conformation change in myosin

Hydrolysis of ATP by myosin head

Movement along actin

STEP 3: Myosin binds to actin

ADP + P$_i$

Release of P$_i$

P$_i$

STEP 4: Second conformation change in myosin

ADP

Power stroke

ADP

   c. Contraction dilemma. Although the sliding filament model can explain contraction in a single sarcomere, it cannot adequately explain the shortening of an entire myofibril.

     (1) If the aforementioned activity were to occur simultaneously in adjacent sarcomeres, no contraction would occur, because equal and opposite forces would be exerted on either side of the Z disk. The contraction of any given sarcomere would be prevented by the contraction of its two adjacent neighbors.

     (2) However, ultrahigh-speed photography has demonstrated that there is an **extremely small temporal delay** in the contraction of adjacent sarcomeres. This creates a wave-like contraction in each myofibril and, consequently, in each muscle fiber.

3. Regulation of contraction. The regulation of contraction in striated muscle is a function of the regulation of the interaction between myosin and actin. This interaction depends upon the presence of the regulatory proteins **tropomyosin** and **troponin,** which are associated with F-actin, and upon the availability of **calcium ions** in the sarcoplasm.

   a. Tropomyosin. Tropomyosin is a rod-shaped protein that sits in the groove of the alpha helix of F-actin.

     (1) It consists of a double helix of two polypeptides.

     (2) In resting muscle, it masks the myosin binding site on the actin molecule.

   b. Troponin. Troponin is a complex of three globular proteins (troponins T, C, and I). Troponin is present in a one-to-one stoichiometry with tropomyosin.

     (1) Troponin T, named for its **tropomyosin-binding activity,** is believed to be responsible for the positioning of the complex on the actin filament.

     (2) Troponin C binds **calcium** ions, the essential step in the initiation of contraction. Troponin C can bind up to four molecules of Ca^{2+}.

     (3) Troponin I inhibits the binding of myosin with actin.

   c. Role of calcium ions. When all three subunits of troponin are present as a complex, their combined function becomes sensitive to Ca^{2+}. When Ca^{2+} is bound to troponin C, the conformation of the troponin complex changes, permitting the tropomyosin molecules to shift their position slightly so that the myosin heads can bind to the actin filament.

   d. Regulation of calcium levels. Calcium levels in the sarcoplasm are regulated by the SR.

     (1) Calcium is sequestered in the terminal cisternae of the SR.

       (a) The SR membrane contains Ca^{2+}-ATPase, an integral membrane protein that actively pumps Ca^{2+} from the sarcoplasm into the SR, maintaining the sarcoplasmic concentration of Ca^{2+} to levels usually below 10^{-7} mol/L. At this low level, the actin–myosin interaction is blocked by the regulatory proteins.

       (b) The Ca^{2+} ions in the SR are bound to membrane-associated proteins that face the interior of the terminal cisternae.

     (2) Calcium is released from the SR cisternae.

       (a) Following stimulation of the muscle fiber by the innervating motor neuron, the stored Ca^{2+} floods into the surrounding sarcoplasm, raising the cytoplasmic concentration to as high as 10^{-5} mol/L.

       (b) At these elevated levels, Ca^{2+} binds to troponin C, releasing the inhibition of actin–myosin interaction and initiating contraction.

FIGURE 7-5. Schematic representation of the interaction between myosin and actin during contraction. This model emphasizes the role of ATP hydrolysis in conformational changes induced in the myosin head that bring about actin and myosin interaction during the contraction cycle. A single myosin head is depicted extending from the backbone of a thick filament. The actin subunit to which the myosin head is initially bound is darkly colored and is used as a frame of reference to show that the myosin head binds to a different actin subunit in step 3. (Adapted from Lodish H, Baltimore D, Berk A, et al: *Molecular Cell Biology,* 3rd ed. New York, Scientific American Books, 1995, p 1020; and Rayment I, Holden HM: The three-dimensional structure of a molecular motor. *Trends in Biochemical Sciences* 19: 129–134, 1994.)

(3) Calcium is re-sequestered in the SR cisternae.
  (a) When nervous stimulation ceases, Ca^{2+} is pumped back into the SR, thus lowering the cytoplasmic concentration to the normally low level of less than 10^{-7} mol/L.
  (b) Relaxation ensues.

F. **Neuromuscular junction.** The point of functional association between the nervous system and skeletal muscle tissue is the neuromuscular junction, also called the **motor end plate.**

1. **Structure of the neuromuscular junction**
   a. **Motor innervation.** Striated skeletal muscle is richly innervated by motor neurons that are located in the spinal cord or brain stem.
      (1) As motor axons near the muscle they branch, sending fine fibers that end on individual skeletal muscle fibers.
      (2) At the point of contact, the myelin sheath ends but the axon terminal remains covered by thin Schwann cell processes and their external laminae.
   b. **Axon terminal.** The axon terminal further splits into a number of fine branches that lie in a shallow depression on the surface of the muscle fiber.
      (1) The axon ending contains numerous mitochondria and synaptic vesicles that contain **acetylcholine (ACh),** a neurotransmitter.
      (2) The axon ending and the muscle cell plasma membrane (the sarcolemma) are separated by a synaptic cleft.
   c. **Junctional folds.** The sarcolemma that underlies the synaptic cleft has many deep junctional folds. The synaptic cleft is filled with an external lamina.
      (1) Acetylcholine receptors (AChR) are located in the sarcolemma on the top of these folds.
      (2) Acetylcholinesterase is present in the external lamina throughout the synaptic cleft and the junctional folds.
      (3) The sarcoplasm beneath the junctional folds contains nuclei, cisternae of rER, ribosomes, and glycogen granules. These organelles are responsible for synthesis of AChR proteins and acetylcholinesterase.

2. **Initiation of contraction.** Synaptic activity of the motor neuron is ultimately responsible for initiating contraction of skeletal muscle.
   a. **Neurotransmitter release.** The arrival of the action potential at the presynaptic ending induces the exocytosis of ACh by the neuron.
   b. **Neurotransmitter binding.** ACh diffuses across the synaptic cleft and binds to the AChR on the sarcolemma at the top of the folds.
   c. **Depolarization.** Depolarization of the sarcolemma follows the binding of ACh to its receptor.
      (1) The AChR is a ligand-gated ion channel. When ACh binds to the receptor the channel opens, allowing the cations Na^+, K^+, and Ca^{2+} to enter the muscle cell.
      (2) The influx of sodium is primarily responsible for the depolarization of the muscle membrane.
   d. **Propagation of depolarization.** A wave of depolarization is propagated across the entire muscle fiber surface and is conducted deep into the muscle fiber by the T tubules.
   e. **Calcium release.** The depolarization signal is relayed across the gap between the T tubule and the terminal cisternae of the SR (i.e., the muscle triad) by calcium channels formed by membrane proteins that connect the membranes (see IV E 3 d).
   f. **Neurotransmitter breakdown.** To prevent continued stimulation, ACh is rapidly removed from the cleft by diffusion and by inactivation by acetylcholinesterase present in the external lamina.

3. **Motor unit.** A single motor neuron may innervate only a few muscle fibers or a few hundred muscle fibers. The motor neuron and all the muscle fibers it innervates is called the motor unit.
   a. All of the muscle fibers in a single motor unit are either red, white, or intermedi-

ate fibers. Thus, three types of motor units can be distinguished according to fiber type.

b. The innervating neuron in a motor unit determines the type of muscle fiber in the unit.

c. The muscle fibers of any one motor unit are widely distributed within the muscle.

d. Loss of innervation produces fiber atrophy. Such loss in a large motor unit can produce significant weakness in a muscle because of the large number of fibers innervated by that neuron.

V. **CARDIAC MUSCLE.** Cardiac muscle (myocardium) is the striated muscle of the heart. It may also be present in the great veins close to the heart.

A. **Morphologic characteristics of cardiac muscle.** Cardiac muscle tissue consists of single, mononucleated cells organized as long fibers that branch and anastomose with neighboring fibers. Because cardiac muscle has the same types and arrangements of contractile elements as skeletal muscle, it also exhibits cross-striations (see Figure 7-1).

1. **Intercalated disks.** Cardiac muscle fibers are joined one to the other in linear arrays by specialized intercellular junctions called intercalated disks. Intercalated disks are characteristic of cardiac muscle.

    a. **Light microscopic appearance.** Intercalated disks are visible by light microscopy as darkly staining bands oriented perpendicular to the long axis of the fiber.

    b. **Electron microscopic appearance.** Electron microscopy reveals that intercalated disks take an irregular, step-like path. The **lateral portion** of the junction is oriented parallel to the fiber, and the **transverse portion** is oriented perpendicular to the fiber.

    c. **Components of the intercalated disk.** The various regions of the intercalated disk contain specific types of junctions.

        (1) **Fasciae adherentes** are the major component of the transverse portion.

            (a) The adhering plate in this junction serves to bind cardiac muscle cells to each other at their ends to form the fiber. The fascia adherens is analogous in structure to the zonula adherens, a component of the junctional complexes that link epithelial cells.

            (b) Actin filaments in the terminal sarcomeres anchor in the dense material on the cytoplasmic side of the plasma membrane.

        (2) **Gap junctions** are the major component of the lateral portion.

            (a) Gap junctions provide a path for ionic conductivity between adjacent muscle cells, allowing contractile signals to pass between them.

            (b) This arrangement, whereby all cardiac muscle cells are electrotonically coupled to one another, allows them to behave as a **functional syncytium** while retaining their cellular integrity.

        (3) **Desmosomes** are present in both the transverse and lateral portions of the intercalated disk.

2. **Cytoplasmic organelles.** The single nucleus of the cardiac muscle cell is located in the center of the cell. Myofibrils pass around the nucleus, producing a biconical juxtanuclear region in which the other organelles are concentrated.

    a. This perinuclear region is rich in mitochondria and contains a Golgi apparatus, glycogen granules, and lipofuscin granules.

    b. Atrial muscle cells also contain **atrial granules** [see Chapter 14 II B 1 b (3)], which contain the polypeptide hormone atrial natriuretic factor (ANF), which affects urinary excretion of sodium and the contraction of vascular smooth muscle.

3. **Sarcomeres.** The myofilaments of cardiac muscle cells are organized into sarcomeres like those in skeletal muscle cells.

4. **Mitochondria.** As in skeletal muscle cells, mitochondria are found between the sarcomeres, with their long axes parallel to the filaments in the sarcomere. Cardiac mitochondria are often much longer than their skeletal muscle counterparts.

5. **Sarcoplasmic reticulum.** The cardiac SR and T system are not as well organized as they are in skeletal muscle.
   a. The SR does not usually separate bundles of myofilaments into discrete cylindrical myofibrils.
   b. T tubules penetrate into muscle cells at the level of the Z disk.
   c. T tubules associate with only one terminal cisterna of the SR, forming a structure called a **diad.**

B. **Regulation of contraction in cardiac muscle**

1. **Cardiac conduction system.** All cardiac muscle cells exhibit an intrinsic rhythmic contraction or beat. This beat is coordinated by specialized, modified cardiac muscle cells that form the cardiac conduction system (see Chapter 14 II C). The cells are organized into nodes and bundles to transmit the contractile impulse to various parts of the myocardium in proper sequence.

2. **Neural regulation.** Many unmyelinated nerves, mostly derived from the vagus nerve (cranial nerve X), end near the nodes. The action of these nerves only modifies the rate of intrinsic cardiac muscle contraction.

VI. **SMOOTH MUSCLE.** Smooth muscle generally occurs as bundles or sheets of elongated fusiform cells. It is specialized for slow, prolonged contraction.

A. **Morphologic characteristics of smooth muscle cells.** Smooth muscle cells do not contain a highly ordered arrangement of thick and thin filaments, thus they **do not appear striated.** In routine H&E-stained sections, smooth muscle cells appear uniformly acidophilic (see Figure 7-1).

1. **Nucleus.** Smooth muscle cells have a single nucleus that is centrally located. It often has a corkscrew appearance in longitudinal section, probably resulting from contraction of the muscle cell at the time of fixation.

2. **Cytoplasmic organelles.** As in cardiac muscle cells, cytoplasmic organelles are concentrated at either end of the nucleus. The remainder of the cytoplasm is filled with actin filaments, intermediate filaments, and myosin filaments.

3. **Dense bodies.** Electron microscopy reveals numerous densely staining regions, called dense bodies, located throughout the cytoplasm and on the inner aspect of the plasma membrane.
   a. Dense bodies contain α-actinin. This suggests that they serve as the functional counterpart of the Z-disk; that is, as a site for insertion of thin filaments.
   b. Also associated with dense bodies are the intermediate filaments **desmin** and **vimentin.** These proteins interconnect the dense bodies, forming a cytoskeleton and helping to maintain the positioning of the dense bodies.

4. **Filamentous proteins**
   a. **Actin.** These thin filaments are similar to the actin filaments of striated muscle. Actin filaments align approximately along the long axis of the cell as they interact with the dense bodies.
   b. **Myosin**
      (1) Smooth muscle myosin is similar in molecular structure to striated muscle myosin.
      (2) In striated muscle, myosin is always arranged in thick filaments. In contrast, smooth muscle myosin is more like non-muscle myosin, and appears to form thick filaments only when necessary for contraction.
   c. **Filament ratio.** The ratio of actin filaments to myosin filaments is higher in

smooth muscle (12:1) than in striated muscle (6:1). The overall content of actin is also higher in smooth muscle.

5. **Smooth muscle has no T system.** Instead, a large number of pinocytic vesicles associated with the plasma membrane and the smooth ER are believed to be responsible for sequestration and release of Ca^{2+}.

B. **Contraction of smooth muscle**

1. **Contractile mechanisms.** Contraction of smooth muscle depends upon calcium and myosin-based mechanisms. A modified version of the sliding filament hypothesis as described for striated muscle can also explain contraction in smooth muscle. In the case of smooth muscle, however, the interaction between myosin heads and actin is dependent upon a cyclic pattern of phosphorylation and dephosphorylation of myosin light chains.

   a. **Phosphorylation**
      (1) Following a rise in intracellular Ca^{2+} concentration that is produced by any one of several possible stimuli, a **calmodulin-dependent myosin light chain kinase** is activated.
      (2) This activated enzyme catalyzes the phosphorylation of myosin . This allows myosin to form into thick filaments, which can interact with adjacent actin thin filaments and effect contraction.
      (3) Phosphorylation occurs slowly, so contraction often takes up to a second to reach its maximum level. Thus, contraction is slow in onset and can be prolonged.

   b. **Dephosphorylation** of the myosin light chain by a phosphatase leads to dissociation of actin and myosin and to muscle relaxation.

2. **Regulation of contraction in smooth muscle**
   a. **Neural control of contraction**
      (1) Smooth muscle is usually under the control of postganglionic neurons of the **autonomic nervous system.**
         (a) In most sites, smooth muscle is directly innervated by both sympathetic and parasympathetic nerves.
         (b) In the gastrointestinal tract, however, the enteric branch of the autonomic nervous system is the primary source of nerves to the muscular layers.
      (2) **There are no specialized neuromuscular junctions in smooth muscle.** Nerve terminals in smooth muscle tissue are located in connective tissue adjacent to the muscle cells.
         (a) The terminals contain synaptic vesicles with neurotransmitter. On stimulation of the nerve, neurotransmitter is released into the surrounding connective tissue, where it diffuses to receptors on the nearby smooth muscle cell plasma membranes.
         (b) Smooth muscle cells are connected to each other by **gap junctions.** Thus, stimulation of one or more smooth muscle cells near a nerve ending will be transmitted to distant smooth muscle cells via **electrotonic conduction.**
   b. **Hormonal control of contraction.** Smooth muscle contraction may be regulated by a number of hormones.
      (1) Oxytocin and, to a lesser degree, vasopressin, both of which are released from the posterior lobe of the pituitary gland, can stimulate contraction.
      (2) The adrenal medullary hormones epinephrine and norepinephrine can either stimulate or inhibit contraction, as can peptide secretions of the enteroendocrine cells.
   c. **Intrinsic contractile activity.** In some instances, smooth muscle displays intrinsic contractile activity in the absence of nerve or hormonal stimuli.

C. **Noncontractile functions of smooth muscle**

1. **Matrix secretion.** Smooth muscle cells are responsible for the synthesis and secre-

tion of several extracellular matrix components, including type IV (basal lamina) collagen, type III (reticular) collagen, laminin, elastin, and proteoglycans.

2. **Hormone secretion.** Modified smooth muscle cells in the walls of the afferent arteriole of the **juxtaglomerular apparatus** in the kidney secrete the hormone **renin,** which, as part of the renin–angiotensin system, plays a role in regulation of blood pressure (see Chapter 29 V G).

VII. **REPAIR AND RENEWAL IN MUSCLE TISSUE.** The three muscle types differ in their capacity for repair and renewal.

A. **Skeletal muscle cells** are postmitotic, but retain some regenerative capacity. Injured skeletal muscle tissue can regenerate by recruitment of a **satellite cell,** a specialized cell that lies interposed between the plasma membrane of the muscle cell and its basement membrane.

1. **Stem cells.** Satellite cells are stem cells that may proliferate after minor injury to give rise to new myoblasts.

2. **Myotube formation**
   a. If the basal lamina remains intact, the new myoblasts will fuse to form myotubes, which then mature to form new multinucleate muscle fibers.
   b. If the basal lamina is disrupted, fibroblasts proliferate and secrete collagen, thus forming scar tissue that prevents regeneration of muscle tissue.

B. **Cardiac muscle cells** have no regenerative capacity.

1. Cardiac muscle cells do not divide.

2. Damaged cardiac muscle is always replaced by scar tissue. **Myocardial infarctions** thus produce permanent loss of myocardium.

C. **Smooth muscle cells** are capable of dividing to maintain or increase their number.

1. **Repair.** In response to injury, smooth muscle cells may undergo mitosis.
   a. New smooth muscle cells have been shown to develop from undifferentiated cells in the adventitia of blood vessels.
   b. Smooth muscle cells have also been shown to develop from the division and differentiation of endothelial cells and **pericytes** in blood vessels.

2. **Regular renewal.** In addition, there are regularly replicating populations of smooth muscle cells.
   a. Smooth muscle cells in the **uterus** proliferate during the normal menstrual cycle and during pregnancy. Both activities are under hormonal control.
   b. The smooth muscle of **blood vessels** has been shown to divide regularly to replace damaged or senescent cells.
   c. The smooth muscle of the **muscularis externa of the stomach and colon** regularly replicates and may slowly thicken throughout life.

Chapter 8

Connective Tissue

I. **INTRODUCTION.** Connective tissue comprises a diverse group of tissues with a variety of structures and functions. Connective tissues are characterized by a relatively **small number of cells** in a **large volume of extracellular matrix** that includes fibers, ground substance, and tissue fluid (Figure 8-1).

II. **FIBERS OF CONNECTIVE TISSUE.** Connective tissue contains three types of fibers, all synthesized and secreted by the fibroblasts.

A. **Collagen.** Collagen is a family of fibrous glycoproteins that constitutes the major fibrous component of connective tissue.

1. **Distribution.** Collagen forms the "white fibers" of loose connective tissue, and is the major component of tendons, ligaments, bone, and the stroma of the cornea.

2. **Composition and structure.** Collagen fibers, which have tensile strength equivalent to that of steel cables, are highly flexible bundles of collagen fibrils that are essentially unstretchable.

    a. **Collagen fibers.** Collagen fibers appear in the light microscope as eosinophilic (i.e., acidophilic), wavy structures of variable width and indeterminate length.

    b. **Collagen fibrils.** The electron microscope reveals collagen fibers as bundles of fine, thread-like subunits called collagen fibrils (Figure 8-2). Individual fibrils are of indeterminate length and may vary in diameter from as little as 7 nm in developing tissue to as much as 200 nm in some tendons.

       (1) Collagen fibrils have a **64 to 68 nm axial periodicity.** This banding pattern reflects the fibril subunit structure, and results from the arrangement of the tropocollagen molecules that **self-assemble** to form the fibril.

       (2) Collagen fibrils may appear as single units or may aggregate into reticular fibers, collagen fibers, and collagen lamellae.

    c. **Tropocollagen** is the basic structural unit of collagen. Tropocollagen molecules are approximately 280 nm long and 1.5 nm in diameter, with a distinct **axial polarity** (i.e., an identifiable head and tail).

       (1) **Molecular configuration.** Tropocollagen molecules are composed of three intertwined polypeptide α **chains** arranged in a right-handed **triple helix.**

          (a) **Every third amino acid** in the chain is a **glycine** molecule, except at the ends of the chains.

          (b) A **hydroxyproline** molecule frequently precedes each glycine and a **proline** frequently follows each glycine. The interaction of these three amino acids is essential for the triple-helix conformation.

          (c) **Hydroxylysine** molecules in the α chains are unique to collagen and are the sites at which sugar groups are joined to the chain, making collagen a **glycoprotein.**

          (d) Depending on the sequence of amino acids, the polypeptide chains are designated α1, α2, or α3.

       (2) **Fibril assembly.** Tropocollagen molecules aggregate longitudinally and laterally in a precise pattern during the self assembly of the collagen fibril.

          (a) The molecules align head to tail in a linear array, forming a row, and the rows align laterally in a **quarter-molecule stagger.** There is a gap between the molecules in each row. The characteristic 64 to 68 nm periodicity of collagen fibrils results from the deposition of osmium from fixative in these gaps.

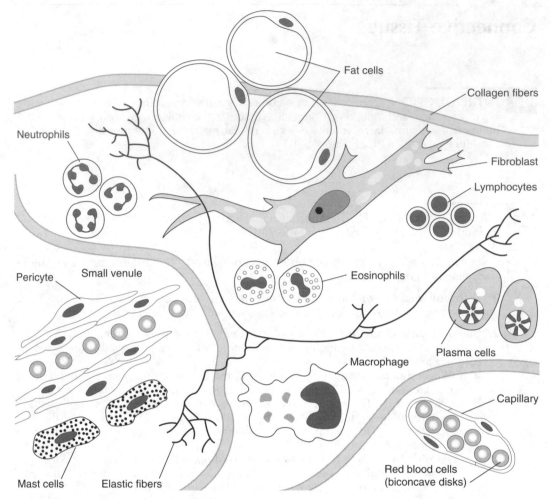

Fat cells

Collagen fibers

Neutrophils

Fibroblast

Lymphocytes

Pericyte

Small venule

Eosinophils

Plasma cells

Macrophage

Capillary

Mast cells

Elastic fibers

Red blood cells
(biconcave disks)

FIGURE 8-1. A schematic drawing of loose connective tissue illustrating some fundamental components of connective tissue: fibers, resident cells, and transient cells.

        (b) The strength of the fibril (and, hence, of the fiber) is due to covalent bonds between the tropocollagen molecules of adjacent rows.

   3. Collagen synthesis (Figure 8-3). Procollagen, the precursor molecule to collagen, is synthesized within the cell. As it is released to the extracellular matrix, procollagen is converted into tropocollagen.

     a. Cell types. The collagen of the connective tissue is synthesized and secreted primarily by **fibroblasts.** However, other cell types synthesize collagen, as well.

       (1) Epithelial cells and **Schwann cells** secrete both basal lamina (type IV) collagen and fibrillar banded collagens (see II A 4).

       (2) All **muscle cells** secrete type IV collagen; smooth muscle cells, especially those of the tunica media of blood vessels, also secrete fibrillar banded collagens.

     b. Procollagen synthesis

       (1) Polypeptide chains are produced by **polyribosomes** of the rough endoplasmic reticulum (rER). Newly synthesized polypeptides are discharged into the cisternae of the rER.

       (2) Post-translational modifications of the polypeptide chains (α chains) occur in the cisternae of both the rER and the Golgi complex.

          (a) The signal peptide is cleaved from the new α chain.

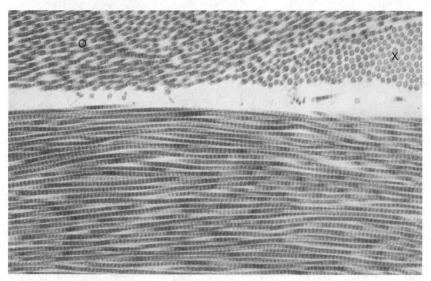

FIGURE 8-2. Electron micrograph showing portions of two collagen fibers. At the top, the collagen fibrils are sectioned transversely (X) and obliquely (O). At the bottom, the fibrils are sectioned longitudinally, and the 64 to 68 nm periodicity characteristic of fibrillar collagen is evident. In the living tissue, the clear spaces would be filled with glycosaminoglycans, proteoglycans, and glycoproteins other than collagen.

    (b) While the polypeptides are still in nonhelical form, proline and lysine residues are hydroxylated.
        (i) Vitamin C (ascorbate) is the essential **co-enzyme** for hydroxylation. Without hydroxylation, the hydrogen bonds essential to the triple-helical structure of collagen cannot form.
        (ii) In **scurvy** (i.e., severe vitamin C deficiency), the normal structure of the collagen molecule cannot be formed. Wounds fail to heal, bone formation is impaired, teeth become loose, and even old, healed wounds may open up.
    (c) O-linked sugar groups are added to some of the hydroxylysine residues (glycosylation) and N-linked sugars are added to the two terminal portions.
    (d) A triple helix is formed by the three polypeptide chains, except at the terminals, where the chains remain uncoiled.
    (e) Intrachain and interchain hydrogen bonds that determine the shape of the molecule and stabilize the interactions of the polypeptides are formed.
  (3) The procollagen leaves the cell by **exocytosis** of secretory vesicles.
 c. Tropocollagen synthesis. As the vesicle containing the procollagen fuses with the plasma membrane, a **procollagen peptidase** cleaves portions of the nonhelical ends of the molecule, converting it into tropocollagen.
 d. Collagen fibril assembly. The cell can control the orderly array of new collagen fibrils by directing the secretory vesicles to localized portions of the plasma membrane for exocytosis into **coves,** or indentations of its surface. These allow the newly secreted tropocollagen molecules to concentrate sufficiently to aggregate into parallel collagen fibrils.

4. Collagen types. The chains that make up the triple helix of collagen vary in their amino acid sequences, and in the manner in which they are combined, giving rise to more than 16 collagens that are presently characterized (Table 8-1). The collagens are classified by Roman numerals on the basis of the chronology of their discovery. Types I through IV are the most abundant.
 a. Type I collagen, the most prevalent type, occurs in loose and dense connective tissue. Two of its α chains are identical (α1) and one is different (α2); in collagen nomenclature this is designated $[\alpha 1(I)]_2 \alpha 2(I)$.

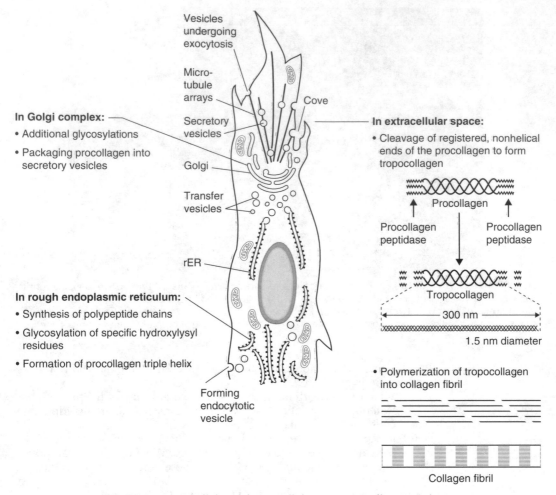

In Golgi complex:
- Additional glycosylations
- Packaging procollagen into secretory vesicles

In rough endoplasmic reticulum:
- Synthesis of polypeptide chains
- Glycosylation of specific hydroxylysyl residues
- Formation of procollagen triple helix

In extracellular space:
- Cleavage of registered, nonhelical ends of the procollagen to form tropocollagen

- Polymerization of tropocollagen into collagen fibril

Vesicles undergoing exocytosis

Micro-tubule arrays

Cove

Secretory vesicles

Golgi

Transfer vesicles

rER

Forming endocytotic vesicle

Procollagen

Procollagen peptidase

Procollagen peptidase

Tropocollagen

300 nm

1.5 nm diameter

Collagen fibril

FIGURE 8-3. Intracellular and extracellular events in collagen synthesis.

     (1) It is the major collagenous component of bone, tendon, dentin, and skin.
     (2) It generally occurs as large, banded fibrils aggregated into large fibers.
  b. Type II collagen occurs as very fine fibrils. Banding is not evident in routine electron micrograph preparations.
  c. Type III collagen consists of three identical α1 chains. Except for being scarce in bone and tendon, it has the same distribution as type I collagen.
  d. Type IV collagen does not form banded fibrils. It is a major constituent of the basal lamina, and forms a nonfibrillar network that gives structural cohesion to the basal and external laminae.
  e. Other nonfibrillar collagens, and collagens that form smaller fibrils, have been identified. Some of their roles have been elucidated, including regulation of the size of collagen type I and type III fibrils.

B. **Reticular fibers.** Reticular fibers provide a supporting framework for the cellular constituents of various tissues and organs.

  1. Distribution. Reticular fibers form a loose network around muscle fibers, nerves, blood vessels, and glandular and tubular organs, as well as under the basal lamina of epithelia. They also form the structural framework of hematopoietic and lymphatic organs, excluding the thymus.

TABLE 8-1. Major Collagen Types

Type	Composition*	Distribution	Functions
Fibrillar Collagens			
I	$[\alpha1(I)]_2\alpha2(I)$	Connective tissue of skin, bone, tendon, ligaments, dentin, cornea, sclera, fascia, organ capsules (90% of body collagen)	Resistance to force, tension, and stretch (64–68 nm periodicity)
II	$[\alpha1(II)]_3$	Hyaline and elastic cartilage, notochord, intervertebral disc, some ocular tissues	Resistance to pressure (64–68 nm periodicity)
III	$[\alpha1(III)]_3$	Connective tissue of organs, smooth muscle, endoneurium, blood vessels, fetal skin	Structural support, internal reticular framework of parenchyma (64–68 nm periodicity)
VI	$[\alpha1(VI)]_2\alpha2(VI)$ or $\alpha1(VI)\alpha2(VI)\alpha3(VI)$	Occurs as a microfibrillar component of connective tissues, similar to microfibrils found at the interface between elastic and collagen fibrils	Anchors cells, large collagen fibrils, and basal lamina to extracellular matrix. Can occur as banded fibrils with 100 nm periodicity
Nonfibrillar Collagens			
IV	$[\alpha1(IV)]_3$ or $[\alpha2(IV)]_3$	Basal laminae of epithelial and endothelial cells, kidney glomeruli, lens capsule, external laminae of muscle cells and Schwann cells	Physical support, filtration barrier
V	$[\alpha1(V)]_2\alpha2(V)$ or $\alpha1(V)\alpha2(V)\alpha3(V)$	Distributed uniformly throughout connective tissue stroma; may be related to reticular network	Physical support, coassembles with type I collagen in cornea to limit fibril diameter. Can form banded fibrils (64–68 nm periodicity)
VII	$[\alpha1(VII)]_3$	Isolated from human skin and amniotic epithelial cells; a major component of anchoring fibrils	Secures basal lamina to underlying connective tissue
VIII	$[\alpha1(VIII)]_3$	Synthesized by aortic and other vascular endothelial cells (initially called EC collagen), cells of neural crest origin, and various normal and tumor cell lines	Plays a role in induction and morphogenesis, particularly of vascular and ocular tissues
IX	$\alpha1(IX)\alpha2(IX)\alpha3(IX)$	Cartilage; associated with type II collagen in cartilage, primary corneal stroma, and adult vitreous humor	Stabilizes network of cartilage collagen fibrils and limits diameter of these fibrils; interacts directly with proteoglycans
X	$[\alpha1(X)]_3$	Synthesized by hypertrophic chondrocytes, particularly at endochondral growth plates	Facilitates chondroplasia at the growth plate; plays a role in calcification of cartilage

(continued)

TABLE 8-1. *(continued)*

Type	Composition*	Distribution	Functions
XI	$[\alpha 1(XI)]_3$	Cartilage	Fibril-associated; helps to stabilize type II collagen network
XII	$[\alpha 1(XII)]_3$	Isolated from a cDNA library from embryonic tendon	Fibril-associated with type I collagen in a manner similar to the association between types IX and II collagen

* The Roman numerals in parentheses indicate that each numbered chain has a distinctive peptide sequence that differs from the chains with other numerals. Thus, collagen type I has two identical $\alpha 1$ chains and one $\alpha 2$ chain; collagen type II has three identical $\alpha 1$ chains, etc. The Roman numerals indicating α chain designation are related to the Roman numerals indicating collagen type only in the fact that the original determination of structure of the α chain was made by analysis of the collagen type bearing the same Roman numeral. (Adapted with permission from Ross MH, Romrell LJ, Kaye GI: *Histology: A Text and Atlas,* 3rd ed. Baltimore, Williams & Wilkins, 1995, p 100.)

  2. **Composition and structure.** Reticular fibers are composed of type III collagen; they are the smallest diameter fibers in connective tissue.
     a. A typical reticular fiber may be formed by as few as 10 collagen fibrils, whereas a typical collagen fiber may contain hundreds or thousands of fibrils.
     b. The individual fibrils of the fiber are only about 20 nm in diameter and do not normally bundle to form thick fibers.
     c. **Staining characteristics.** Reticular fibers cannot be identified in routinely stained hematoxylin–eosin (H&E) preparations. If stains specific for reticular fibers are used, the fibers have a thread-like appearance.
        (1) Because they have a relatively greater amount of surface oligosaccharides than larger collagen fibers, reticular fibers are readily displayed by means of the **periodic acid–Schiff reaction.**
        (2) Reticular fibers are **argyrophilic.** Silver reduction staining procedures, such as the Gomori or Laidlaw methods, stain the fibers black.

  3. **Synthesis.** Reticular fibers are synthesized by several types of cells in the body.
     a. **Fibroblasts.** Most reticular fibers in the body are produced by the same fibroblasts that produce typical collagen fibers
     b. **Reticular cells.** In bone marrow, the spleen, and the lymph nodes, the collagenous reticular network is produced by a specialized fibroblast called a reticular cell.
        (1) Reticular cells maintain a unique relationship with the fibers, surrounding them with flattened cell processes.
        (2) The fiber is thus isolated physically from its environment.
     c. **Schwann cells** of peripheral nerves produce most of the reticular fibers of the endoneurium.
     d. **Smooth muscle cells** of the tunica media of blood vessels, and of the muscularis of the alimentary canal, secrete reticular fibers as well as other collagenous fibers.

C. **Elastic fibers.** Elastic fibers provide the structural mechanism that allows tissues to respond to stretch and distension.
  1. **Distribution.** Elastic fibers and elastic lamellae are major components of arterial walls, elastic ligaments, bronchioles, skin, and elastic cartilage. Elastic fibers are the highly refractile "yellow fibers" of loose connective tissue. Elastic lamellae are nonfibrous sheets of elastin.

  2. **Structure**
     a. Elastic fibers are typically **narrower than collagen fibers,** rarely reaching a size of 1.0 μm, and are of **indeterminate length.**
     b. They are arranged in a **branching pattern** to form a three dimensional network.

    c. Elastic fibers are usually interwoven with collagen fibers. This limits the distensibility of the tissue and prevents tearing caused by excessive stretching.

    d. Staining characteristics. Elastic fibers and elastic lamellae stain poorly with eosin and are not easily recognized in routine H&E preparations.

        (1) Elastic fibers and lamellae become **highly refractile** with certain fixatives and, thus, may become visible in H&E preparations, particularly in the skin and in the walls of the larger arteries.

        (2) Elastic fibers can be stained selectively with special dyes, including orcein and resorcin–fuchsin. They may also be demonstrated using fluorescent reagents for elastin-associated polysaccharides.

3. Composition. Elastic fibers are composed of two structural components, **elastin** and **microfibrils,** that change in relative proportions as the fibers grow. Elastin appears in the electron microscope as an amorphous material surounded by the microfibrils. Elastic lamellae lack the microfibrillar component.

    a. Elastin is a globular protein that, like collagen, is rich in proline and glycine. Unlike collagen, however, it is poor in hydroxyproline and completely lacks hydroxylysine.

    b. Microfibrils contain fibrillar glycoproteins and are relatively straight and thin, measuring 10 to 12 nm in diameter. They appear first and subsequently surround the elastin of the growing elastic fiber. Some of them become trapped in the fiber as it grows.

4. Synthesis. Elastic fibers and lamellae are produced by fibroblasts and smooth muscle cells.

    a. Elastin is synthesized by the same pathway as collagen. Both processes normally occur simultaneously in fibroblasts and other cells that secrete both molecules, along with the synthesis of many other proteins, glycoproteins, and carbohydrate components of the connective tissue.

    b. Tropoelastin. Elastin is secreted from the cell as single polypeptide chains of tropoelastin. In the adjacent extracellular matrix, tropoelastin molecules aggregate and crosslink to form elastic fibers.

        (1) The covalent crosslinks between the polypeptide chains of elastin are produced by **desmosine** and **isodesmosine,** two amino acids unique to elastin.

            (a) Desmosine and isodesmosine are derived from the oxidative deamination of lysine and subsequent reaction with nearby intact lysine residues.

            (b) This covalent crosslink is, therefore, much stronger than the hydrogen bond crosslinks of the collagen triple helix.

            (c) Crosslinking via desmosine and isodesmosine can involve up to four tropoelastin chains.

        (2) Crosslinking may serve as a nucleation process for additional elastin aggregation.

5. Elastic fiber system. Elastic fibers belong to the elastic fiber system, a larger family of fibers with related characteristics. The members of this family all contain elastin and microfibrils, each in specific proportions. Two other members of the family are:

    a. Oxytalin fibers. These are found in the dermis, in tooth sockets, and in the zonular fibers of the lens. They are formed of microfibrils with little or no elastin.

    b. Elaunin fibers. These are also found in the dermis. They are formed of microfibrils and a small amount of elastin.

    c. Because they contain a smaller proportion of elastin, oxytalin and elaunin fibers are less elastic than elastic fibers.

III. **GROUND SUBSTANCE OF CONNECTIVE TISSUE.** Ground substance is the component of connective tissue that fills the space not occupied by cells and fibers. In life, ground substance is a viscous, clear substance that has a slippery feel. It has a high water content that, combined with its apparently structureless nature (at least above the macromolecular level) provides little basis for morphologic characterization.

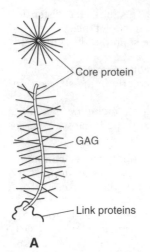

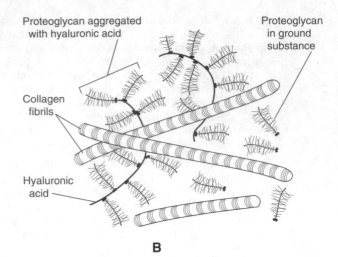

A

B

FIGURE 8-4. (*A*) Proteoglycan monomer (two views) formed by approximately 100 glycosaminoglycan (GAG) chains bound covalently to a core protein, as found in ground substance of cartilage. One end of the core protein contains link proteins that bind the proteoglycan monomer to hyaluronic acid. (*B*) Proteoglycan aggregate formed by many proteoglycan monomers bound to hyaluronic acid. Some proteoglycan monomers are free in the ground substance.

A. **Macromolecules of ground substance.** Chemically, ground substance consists of complexes of **glycosaminoglycans** (GAGs), **proteoglycans** (PGs), **hyaluronic acid,** and **glyco-proteins** (Figure 8-4).

1. **GAGs** are long-chained polysaccharides made up of repeating disaccharide units.
   a. One of the sugars in each disaccharide is glucosamine, which is a hexosamine. The hexosamine is linked through an O-glycosidic link to a uronic acid (glucuronic acid or iduronic acid).
   b. GAGs are highly negatively charged owing to the binding of sulfate and carboxyl groups to many of the sugars. The density of negative charges attracts water, forming a hydrated gel.
   c. A family of seven distinct GAGs is recognized based on differences in the sugar residues, the nature of the linkages, and the degree of sulfation (Table 8-2).

2. **PGs** are very large macromolecules composed of a core protein to which many GAG molecules are covalently bound. This structure has been described as resembling a bottle-brush, with the GAGs as the bristles and the protein core as the central stem.

3. **Hyaluronic acid,** although usually listed with the GAGs, differs from the others in several respects.
   a. It is an extremely long, rigid molecule consisting of several thousand sugars, compared with the several hundred or fewer that make up other GAGs.
   b. It does not bind to a protein to form a PG. Rather, by means of special linker proteins, PGs indirectly bind to hyaluronic acid, forming a giant macromolecule.
   c. These macromolecules can bind very large amounts of water and, thus, achieve a considerable degree of resistance to compression without inhibiting flexibility. Cartilage ground substance is rich in hyaluronic acid (see Chapter 10).

4. **Glycoproteins** in the ground substance are glycosylated molecules in which protein is the major component.
   a. **Collagen,** in both the unaggregated tropocollagen form and in the aggregated fibrillar form, is the most common glycoprotein.
   b. Other common glycoproteins include **unaggregated tropoelastin and elastin, microfibrillar protein** of elastic fibers, and **fibronectin.**

TABLE 8-2. Glycosaminoglycans

	Approximate Molecular Weight (Daltons)	Disaccharide Composition
Keratan sulfate	10,000	Galactose or galactose 6-sulfate + N-acetylglucosamine 6-sulfate
Heparan sulfate	15,000	Glucuronic acid or L-iduronic acid 2-sulfate + N-acetylglucosamine or N-sulfamylglucosamine
Chondroitin 4-sulfate	25,000	D-Glucuronic acid + N-acetylgalactosamine 4-sulfate
Chondroitin 6-sulfate	25,000	D-Glucuronic acid + N acetylgalactosamine 6-sulfate
Dermatan sulfate	35,000	L-Iduronic acid + N-acetylgalactosamine 4-sulfate
Heparin*	40,000	Glucuronic acid or L-iduronic acid 2-sulfate + N-sulfamylglucosamine or N-acetylglucosamine 6-sulfate
Hyaluronic acid	1,000,000	D-Glucuronic acid + N-acetylglucosamine

* Heparin, the most sulfated molecule in the body, is not a structural component of the connective tissue matrix. It is a vasoactive agent synthesized by mast cells and stored in the mast cell granules.

B. **Organization of ground substance.** Although not apparent even at the electron microscopic level, ground substance is highly organized, and that organization confers certain important properties.

1. **Organization of macromolecules**
   a. PGs often form large PG aggregates through noncovalent linkage to the end of the core protein of hyaluronic acid.
      (1) PG and PG aggregates may interact specifically with collagen to regulate collagen fibril size and spacing.
      (2) Because of their high anionic charge, PG and PG aggregates interact with cations, thereby regulating the diffusion of electrolytes and water.
   b. PG and PG aggregates form complex networks that regulate both the viscosity and lubricity of connective tissues.
      (1) PG and PG aggregates intertwine with one another, establishing molecular sieves in the connective tissue, particularly in layers underlying epithelia.
      (2) Because of the numerous interactions among the components of ground substance it is not inconceivable to think of ground substance as one gigantic macromolecular complex that has variable characteristics in different locations.

2. **Structural variation.** Among different types of connective tissue, ground substance can vary in both composition and density.
   a. The density of ground substance depends on the degree of supramolecular organization of macromolecules and the amount of fluid present in the tissue.
   b. Increase in the concentration of specific macromolecules in the ground substance, as well as mineralization, can change the density, rigidity, and permeability of connective tissues, as occurs in cartilage and bone.

C. **Histologic characteristics.** Routine histologic techniques do not preserve the ground substance. The result in H&E-stained sections is an empty-appearing background in which only the cells and some fibers of connective tissue are evident.

1. Ground substance may be preserved by freeze drying tissue or by preparing frozen sections. These techniques give it an amorphous appearance.

2. Freeze-dried or frozen ground substance stains with basic dyes, because of the anionic content of the GAGs, and with the periodic acid–Schiff reaction method, because of the sugar content.

D. **Tissue fluid.** Tissue fluid in ground substance provides the medium through which exchanges between blood, lymph, and tissue cells take place.

1. All metabolic substrates and wastes that move between the vascular system and the cells of tissues and organs must diffuse in the tissue fluid of the ground substance of the connective tissue.

2. Substances absorbed by the gastrointestinal epithelium must cross the ground substance of the connective tissue to enter the vascular system.

3. The movement of fluid from the vascular system to the ground substance of the connective tissue, and its retention therein, is responsible for **tissue swelling.**

IV. **CELLS OF CONNECTIVE TISSUE.** Cells found in connective tissue can be described as resident cells and transient cells (see Figure 8-1). The types of cells in connective tissue and their relative numbers reflect the functional state of the tissue.

A. **Resident cell population.** The resident cells of connective tissue are relatively stabile; except for some of the macrophages, they normally exhibit little movement and can be regarded as permanent residents of the tissue.

1. **Fibroblasts.** Fibroblasts are the type-specific cell of connective tissue and are derived from the **mesenchymal cells** of the embryo. The fibroblast secretes both the fibrous components and the ground substance of connective tissue.
   a. **Histologic characteristics**
      (1) **Light microscopy.** The fibroblast is difficult to discern in routine light microscopic preparations.
         (a) In routinely prepared H&E sections, only the basophilic nucleus of the fibroblast is clearly visible.
         (b) The extensive pale cytoplasm is usually not clearly defined.
      (2) **Electron microscopy.** The extent and content of the cytoplasmic compartment are discernable only when viewed with the electron microscope.
         (a) Although fibroblasts are often described as spindle-shaped or fusiform in sections, the fibroblast is actually a large flattened cell that resembles a fried egg in shape.
         (b) Although a fibroblast may cover large areas and touch adjacent fibroblasts, junctions are rarely seen between the fibroblasts in normal adult connective tissue.
         (c) The cytoplasm has a well-developed rER, one or more Golgi zones, and numerous mitochondria. Actively secreting fibroblasts have more rER than inactive ones.
         (d) The surfaces of active fibroblasts often exhibit the scalloping, or cove formation, indicative of collagen polymerization in the extracellular matrix adjacent to the plasma membrane.
   b. **Function of fibroblasts.** Fibroblasts are the major source of secreted collagen. The fibroblast is usually in close proximity to the collagen fibers it has secreted and is surrounded by the ground substance it has secreted.
   c. **Fibroblast replication and renewal.** Although all fibroblasts are able to divide and repair wounds, fibroblasts in some locations constitute **regularly replicating populations** of cells.
      (1) Fibroblasts of the endometrium of the uterus proliferate, differentiate, and degenerate in each menstrual cycle, all under the control of steroid hormones.
      (2) Fibroblasts immediately beneath the epithelium of the intestine replicate, migrate, and differentiate in parallel and in synchrony with the migrating epithelial cells.

(3) Fibroblasts immediately beneath the epidermis replicate and migrate into the deeper dermis.

d. **Morphologic heterogeneity of fibroblasts.** Fibroblasts occasionally contain fat droplets and prominent secondary lysosomes.

(1) In scurvy, fibroblasts develop large fat droplets as well as large vacuoles containing unsecreted, noncollagenous protein.

(2) In several hereditary connective tissue diseases (e.g., Hurler's syndrome), unsecreted PGs accumulate in large vacuoles in fibroblasts.

e. **Myofibroblasts.** Myofibroblasts display properties of both fibroblasts and smooth muscle cells. They contain bundles of **actin microfilaments** and **dense bodies** characteristic of smooth muscle cytoplasm, but do not have external laminae

(1) Myofibroblasts are commonly found in the granulation tissue, consisting of new connective tissue and blood vessels, that forms in large, healing wounds. Myofibroblasts are responsible for wound contraction.

(2) Myofibroblasts are also present in developing organs and organisms when morphogenetic events are occurring.

(3) Gap junctions are formed where processes of one myofibroblast contact those of another myofibroblast.

2. **Macrophages.** Macrophages are phagocytic cells and are the basic cell type of the **mononuclear phagocytic system.** The macrophages of the connective tissue are also called **histiocytes.** Macrophages of the mononuclear phagocytic system are listed in Table 8-3.

a. **Origin of macrophages.** Most macrophages derive from precursor cells in the bone marrow that differentiate initially into circulating **monocytes.**

(1) Monocytes leave the circulation and differentiate into macrophages in the loose connective tissue.

(2) Some histiocytic cells, such as those of the **lamina propria of the gut** and those of the **endometrium,** develop as the **terminal differentiation** of cells that previously had the morphologic and functional characteristics of fibroblasts.

(3) Some investigators contend that monocytes/macrophages can proliferate in the connective tissue.

b. **Histologic characteristics**

(1) **Light microscopy.** Most macrophages are difficult to distinguish from fibroblasts in routinely prepared H&E sections. However, they can be recognized if they display obvious evidence of **phagocytic activity,** such as visible ingested material in the cytoplasm.

(a) A vital dye (e.g., trypan blue) or a colloidal tracer (e.g., carbon) injected

TABLE 8-3. Cells of the Mononuclear Phagocytic System

Cell Type	Location
Macrophage (histiocyte)	Connective tissue
Perisinusoidal macrophage (Kupffer cell)	Liver
Alveolar macrophage	Lungs
Macrophage	Spleen, lymph nodes, bone marrow, and thymus
Pleural and peritoneal macrophage	Serous cavities
Osteoclast	Bone
Microglia	Central nervous system
Langerhans' cell	Epidermis
Fibroblast-derived macrophage	Lamina propria of intestine, endometrium of uterus

Reprinted with permission from Ross MH, Romrell LJ, Kaye GI: *Histology: A Text and Atlas,* 3rd ed. Baltimore, Williams & Wilkins, 1995, p 112.)

into an animal stimulates phagocytic activity by macrophages, making them easier to identify.

    (b) Macrophages contain **abundant lysosomes** that can be demonstrated using routine histochemical procedures for **phosphatases** and **esterases** at the light microscopic and electron microscopic levels.

  (2) Electron microscopy. Primary, secondary, and tertiary lysosomes; a large Golgi apparatus; significant amounts of both rER and smooth ER; and numerous mitochondria and small vesicles are visible with an electron microscope.

    (a) The surface of the macrophage is usually ruffled, with both finger-like and plate-like projections.

    (b) Large numbers of secondary and tertiary lysosomes typically fill the cytoplasm of active macrophages. Large numbers of primary lysosomes can be identified after histochemical staining of inactive or unstimulated macrophages.

    (c) Bundles of actin filaments are often arrayed under the plasma membrane and in the perinuclear region.

  c. Protective activities of macrophages. Macrophages are phagocytic cells. They respond to challenge by foreign organisms and materials and exposure to damaged tissue with **phagocytosis.** Materials too large to be phagocytized may be isolated by **giant cell formation** or **epithelioid modulation.**

    (1) Phagocytosis generally involves specific effector–receptor binding at the external surface of the macrophage plasma membrane. The material to be ingested is subsequently engulfed by a zipper-like closure of a macrophage plasma membrane process around the bound material.

      (a) Macrophages are coated with **antibody receptors.**

        (i) Antibody-coated foreign particles, organisms, and molecules bind to the surface of the macrophage and induce phagocytosis.

        (ii) Some particles, such as carbon, cellulose, and inorganic particulate materials, probably interact electrostatically with macrophages in a nonimmunologic phagocytic response.

      (b) Vacuoles containing material ingested by phagocytosis may fuse with primary lysosomes to form **phagolysosomes,** or may fuse with pre-existing functioning lysosomes, in which the material is digested by the lysosomal enzymes.

    (2) Giant cell formation. Some pathogenic organisms and other foreign bodies are ingested but cannot be digested by macrophages.

      (a) These include the bacilli of tuberculosis and leprosy, *Trypanosoma cruzi* (malaria), *Toxoplasma,* and *Leishmania*, as well as industrial particulate pollutants such as asbestos, coal dust, and cotton fibers.

      (b) In these instances, macrophages often fuse to form **multinucleate, foreign-body giant cells (Langhans giant cells).**

    (3) Epithelioid modulation. Macrophages can also form junctions and assemble in sheets of cells that resemble epithelia. Such **epithelioid cells** often wall off sites of chronic inflammation or infection.

    (4) Macrophages are essential in the recognition by an organism of **self, non-self,** and **modified self** (see IV A 2 e).

      (a) Recognition of non-self is essential in the removal of pathogenic organisms and noxious materials derived from the environment.

      (b) Recognition of modified self is essential in the removal of transformed (e.g., tumor) cells originating in the organism.

  d. Secretory activities of macrophages. Macrophages synthesize products (e.g., enzymes) that act intracellularly (in lysosomes) and extracellularly (by release of lysosomal contents and by the specific secretion of nonlysosomal materials).

    (1) Macrophages synthesize the following enzymes:

      (a) Lysosomal acid hydrolases, which degrade the contents of phagolysosomes

      (b) Lysozyme, which dissolves the cell wall of many microorganisms

      (c) Collagenase, elastase, and **PG-degrading enzymes,** which degrade connective tissue

(2) Macrophages secrete products that regulate other cells and extracellular systems.

    (a) These products include endothelial and fibroblast growth factors, macrophage and granulocyte colony-stimulating factors, and mitogenic factors, such as interleukin 1.

    (b) Also secreted are chemotactic factor for polymorphonuclear leukocytes (PMNs), proteins of the complement system, immunosuppressive factors, and enzyme inhibitors (e.g., α-2-macroglobulin).

(3) Macrophages also secrete products that participate in or mediate the inflammatory response. These include leukotriene-C, prostaglandins, and endogenous pyrogen.

e. Role of macrophages in the immune system. Macrophages participate in the immune response as antigen-presenting cells, as well as through direct and specific roles in the differentiation and functioning of lymphocytes. There are extensive and essential interactions between macrophages and lymphocytes in defense against foreign organisms and foreign cells (i.e., transplant tissue).

(1) **Antigen presentation.** Macrophages may bind (capture) antigens on their surface, or they may ingest, process, and resecrete antigens onto their surface. The antigens are then presented to lymphocytes, triggering proliferation of T and B lymphocytes by the process of **blastic transformation** (see Chapters 15 and 17).

(2) **Immunoregulation**

    (a) Macrophages secrete immunoregulatory agents (lymphokines) that stimulate the immune response. These include interleukin 1, a mitogen necessary for the proliferation and growth of T and B lymphocytes, and interleukin 6, which stimulates the differentiation of B lymphocytes into plasma cells.

    (b) Macrophages also secrete factors that may act as immunosuppressive agents.

(3) **Macrophage activation.** Macrophages may, in turn, be activated by secretory products of lymphocytes.

    (a) Activated macrophages exhibit increased microbicidal activity.

    (b) Activated macrophages exhibit increased cytotoxicity toward tumor cells.

f. Role of macrophages in wound healing. Macrophages are essential in the processes of inflammation and wound healing.

(1) Macrophages increase the inflammatory response to injury by secreting factors that attract PMNs and monocytes to the site of injury.

(2) Macrophages phagocytize and digest bacteria, damaged cells, exhausted PMNs, fibrin, and extracellular matrix.

(3) Macrophage activity is essential for the stimulation of proliferation and ingrowth of fibroblasts and endothelial cells at inflamed wound sites.

(4) If inflammation or macrophage activation is prevented, as occurs with the administration of corticosteroids, fibroblast and endothelial proliferation and ingrowth are slowed and wound healing is inhibited.

3. Mast cells. Mast cells are the third resident cell of the connective tissue and are usually found in close proximity to blood vessels. Mast cells are similar to—but not related to—basophils of the blood.

  a. Histologic characteristics. They are large, ovoid cells with a centrally located nucleus and numerous large, intensely basophilic granules. They are usually identifiable, however, only after special fixation methods are used that preserve the granules.

  b. Contents of mast cell granules. The mast cell granules contain several **vasoactive** and **immunoreactive** substances.

    (1) **Histamine** is a vasoactive agent. Its release from the cell, along with the release of **slow-reacting substance of anaphylaxis (SRS-A),** which is not stored in the granules, increases the permeability of nearby blood vessels, causing edema in the surrounding tissue.

(2) Heparin is a highly sulfated GAG that is structurally related to heparan sulfate, a GAG of the ground substance.

    (a) Heparin is an **anticoagulant** and an antilipemic agent; some investigators consider it a hemorrhagic agent.

    (b) Heparin is the most highly sulfated substance in the body. This concentration of anionic groups confers the basophilia of the granules, and also makes heparin the **most metachromatic substance in the body.**

        (i) Metachromasia describes the ability of a highly anionic substance to change the color (i.e., absorption spectrum) of a dye from blue toward red.

        (ii) Certain commonly used thiazin dyes, such as toluidine blue and cresyl violet, react metachromatically with the sulfate groups of GAGs and the phosphate groups of ribonucleic acids.

(3) Eosinophilic chemotactic factor of anaphylaxis (ECF-A) is also contained in the mast cell granules.

    (a) ECF-A stimulates eosinophils to migrate to the sites where mast cells have released their agents.

    (b) Secretions of the eosinophils counteract the acute inflammatory stimuli of histamine and SRS-A.

c. Mast cell degranulation. The release of mast cell granules is triggered by the binding of an antigen to its specific immunoglobulin-E antibody (IgE) on the mast cell surface.

    (1) Degranulation of mast cells occurs by fusion of granule membranes with the plasma membrane and with each other, producing intracellular channels that facilitate rapid extrusion of the granule contents into the connective tissue matrix.

    (2) Mast cells do not produce antibodies. The antibodies bound on their surface are produced by plasma cells that have been stimulated by the presence of an antigen to synthesize and release immunoglobulins into the connective tissue.

        (a) This is the process of **sensitization.** While several classes of antibodies are produced by the plasma cells, only immunoglobulins of the IgE class, specific to individual antigens, bind to receptors on the plasma membrane of the mast cells.

        (b) On subsequent exposure to the same antigen that triggered IgE production, an antigen--antibody reaction occurs that causes the **massive discharge of mast cell granules.**

d. Mast cell origin. Mast cells originate from stem cells in the bone marrow. They are transported to various connective tissue sites via the bloodstream. Mast cells concentrate and differentiate in the perivascular space of the subepithelial connective tissue of the skin, alimentary canal, respiratory system, and genitourinary tract (i.e., sites at which the individual interacts with the external environment).

e. Mast cells are very long lived. Although they originate in the bone marrow, they spend their long differentiated life in the loose connective tissue as permanent residents.

    (1) Mast cells do not divide in the connective tissue.

    (2) Degranulated mast cells synthesize and store new secretory product as granules.

4. Adipose cells. Adipose cells are the fourth major resident cell type of connective tissue. They are specialized for the **storage of neutral fats (triglycerides)** and can be present in large numbers in loose irregular connective tissue.

a. Origin of adipose cells. Adipose cells differentiate from fibroblasts and undifferentiated mesenchymal cells (see Chapter 9).

b. Histologic characteristics. Mature adipose cells consist of a thin shell of cytoplasm surrounding a large lipid droplet.

    (1) The nucleus is compressed into the thin shell of cytoplasm and is usually not visible because of the plane of section.

(2) The fat in adipose cells is usually extracted in routine histologic preparations, adding to the spongy appearance of loose connective tissue.

c. **Adipose tissue** is an accumulation of a large number of adipose cells.

5. **Undifferentiated mesenchymal cells.** Populations of undifferentiated mesenchymal cells persist in the connective tissue of adults. These cells are associated with the outermost layer (tunica adventitia) of small venules and with the less organized connective tissue surrounding venous capillaries and postcapillary venules.

   a. Autoradiographic and electron micrographic studies of healing skin wounds have demonstrated that new fibroblasts, endothelial cells, pericytes, and vascular smooth muscle derive from these undifferentiated mesenchymal cells.

   b. Fibroblasts, pericytes, and endothelial cells in the vicinity of a wound are stimulated to divide and give rise to new connective tissue and vascular cells.

B. **Transient cell population.** At sites of acute or chronic inflammation, several types of cells may leave the circulation and enter loose connective tissue, where they exist transiently, and sometimes semipermanently. These are primarily leukocytes (white blood cells), including lymphocytes, monocytes, neutrophils, eosinophils, and basophils. Plasma cells, which are derived from B lymphocytes, are also part of the transient cell population. These cells are discussed in more detail in the chapters describing blood (Chapter 12) and lymphatic tissues and the immune system (Chapters 15–17).

1. **Lymphocytes** (see Chapter 15). Lymphocytes are principally involved in immune responses. They are the smallest of the free cells in the connective tissue (6–8 μm in diameter) and exhibit a thin rim of lightly basophilic cytoplasm surrounding a deeply basophilic, heterochromatic nucleus.

   a. Small numbers of both T lymphocytes and B lymphocytes are found in the loose connective tissue throughout the body. Their number increases dramatically at sites of infection or inflammation.

   b. Lymphocytes are numerous in the lamina propria of the respiratory tract, alimentary canal, and genitourinary tract, where they are essential in **immunosurveillance** against pathogens and foreign substances that enter the body through these routes.

2. **Plasma cells** (see Chapter 15). Plasma cells are antibody-producing cells derived from B lymphocytes. They are found in loose connective tissue and in lymphatic organs. They are relatively large (20 μm in diameter) ovoid cells with a large amount of basophilic cytoplasm, an eccentric spherical nucleus with a characteristic distribution of chromatin, and a prominent juxtanuclear Golgi zone.

3. **Neutrophils, eosinophils, basophils,** and **monocytes** (see Chapter 12). These white blood cells are also commonly observed in loose connective tissue. Their presence generally reflects an acute inflammatory reaction.

   a. **Neutrophils.** Neutrophils (PMNs, neutrophilic granulocytes) are characterized by a nucleus that is multilobed and by cytoplasmic granules that have no special staining affinity (hence the name). They migrate from the circulation at sites of injury or infection.

   b. **Eosinophils.** Eosinophils are characterized by the presence of large, refractile eosinophilic granules in the cytoplasm and by a bilobed nucleus. They, too, leave the circulation at sites of injury or inflammation and are most commonly found at sites of allergic inflammation and chronic inflammation.

   c. **Basophils.** Basophils are circulating granulocytes that resemble mast cells in their function, granule content, and surface coating with IgE. In certain immune responses, basophils leave the circulation and function in the connective tissue.

   d. **Monocytes.** As described above, monocytes also leave the circulation and migrate into the connective tissue where they differentiate into macrophages.

V. **CLASSIFICATION OF CONNECTIVE TISSUE.** Connective tissue is classified on the basis of the kinds of cells present, the types of fibers present, and the character of the

TABLE 8-4. Connective Tissue Classification

Connective tissue proper
　　Loose connective tissue
　　Dense connective tissue
　　　Irregular
　　　Regular
Specialized connective tissues
　　Adipose tissue
　　Cartilage
　　Bone
　　Blood
　　Hemopoietic tissue
　　Lymphatic tissue
Embryonic connective tissue
　　Mesenchyme
　　Mucous connective tissue

ground substance. The specific properties of various connective tissues are determined by these features. Connective tissues are classified into connective tissue proper, specialized connective tissue, and embryonic connective tissue (Table 8-4). Connective tissue proper is divided into loose connective tissue and dense connective tissue.

A. **Loose connective tissue.** Loose connective tissue, also called **areolar tissue,** is characterized by relatively sparse loosely arranged fibers, by an abundance of ground substance, and by the presence of many different resident and transient cells. It is the most abundant and widely distributed type of connective tissue in the body (see Figure 8-1).

1. It is found in or forms the stroma of most organs; the core of the mesenteries; the superficial fascia; and the surrounding tissue for most blood vessels, nerves, and muscle cells.

2. Diffusion of oxygen, metabolic substrates and wastes, and regulatory agents between the vasculature and the cells of other tissues occurs through the ground substance of loose connective tissue.

3. Adipose (fat storing) cells are usually present to varying degrees. When these are the predominant cell population, the tissue is called adipose tissue.

4. Loose connective tissue underlies the epithelia covering the body surfaces. This is the primary site at which antigens and other foreign substances, such as bacteria, that have breached an epithelial surface can be challenged and destroyed by the immune system.

B. **Dense connective tissue.** Dense connective tissue is less cellular than loose connective tissue and has more and larger fibers. It may be described as either irregular or regular depending on the arrangement of its fibrous component (Figure 8-5).

1. **Dense irregular connective tissue** is usually arranged in sheets or layers. The fibers of dense irregular connective tissue are randomly interwoven, like the fibers in felt.
   a. It forms the deep dermis, periosteum and perichondrium, and the submucosa of the alimentary canal.
   b. It forms the connective tissue capsules of lymph nodes, spleen, testes, liver, and other organs.

2. **Dense regular connective tissue** is usually arranged in cords or bands of varying width. The fibers of dense regular connective tissue are arranged in parallel and are tightly packed and evenly spaced.
   a. It is found in or forms tendons, ligaments, aponeuroses, and the stroma of the cornea.

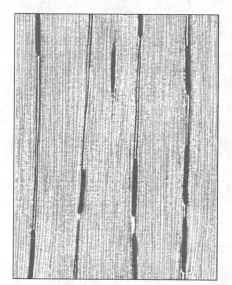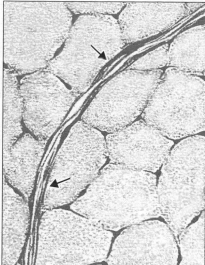

FIGURE 8-5. Drawings of human tendon. (Left) Longitudinal section showing rows of flattened, dense-staining nuclei of fibroblasts between bundles of regularly arranged collagen fibers. (Right) Cross-section showing fibroblasts between bundles of collagen fibers. A band of dense irregular connective tissue (arrows) separates the tendon bundles.

    b. Dense regular connective tissue may be collagenous or elastic, depending on the predominant fibrous component.

C. **Elastic and reticular tissue.** In the past, elastic tissue and reticular tissue were considered separate categories of specialized connective tissue. They are now included as varieties of connective tissue proper.

    1. Elastic tissue. This category includes the elastic ligaments associated with the spinal column, and the tunica media of the largest (elastic) arteries.

      a. The **elastic ligaments** are now considered a variety of dense regular connective tissue.

      b. The **elastic laminae** of the arteries are now known to be synthesized by **smooth muscle cells** rather than by fibroblasts.

    2. Reticular tissue

      a. The identifying feature of reticular tissue is the presence of **reticular fibers** and **reticular cells** forming a three-dimensional stroma.

      b. A reticular tissue stroma is a relatively loose connective tissue that is characteristic of hematopoietic tissue (red bone marrow) and of the spleen and lymph nodes and nodules.

D. **Specialized connective tissue** includes those forms of connective tissue that are distinct from connective tissue proper in either structure or function. These include adipose tissue, cartilage, bone, blood, and hematopoietic and lymphatic tissues.

VI. HISTOGENESIS OF CONNECTIVE TISSUE

A. **Embryonic origin.** Most connective tissue derives from mesoderm; some connective tissue derives from ectoderm.

    1. Mesoderm. The mesoderm gives rise to almost all of the connective tissues of the body. Mesoderm proliferates and differentiates into primary and secondary **mesen-**

chyme, from which various connective tissues develop, as does muscle, the vascular and urogenital systems, and the serous membranes of the body cavity.

2. **Ectoderm.** In the cranial region, mesenchymal cells are derived from neural crest cells that originate as neuroectoderm. Virtually all of the connective tissue, muscle, bone, and cartilage of the head region is derived from this **ectomesenchyme.**

B. **Embryonic development.** The manner in which the mesenchymal cells proliferate and organize sets parameters for the kind of connective tissue that will develop at any site.

1. As differentiation of mesenchymal cells begins, the cytoplasm increases in amount and becomes basophilic, a reflection of the synthesis of collagen and other matrix materials by the rER.

2. The pattern in which collagen is laid down, and the orientation of cells in relation to the fibers, reflects the type of connective tissue that is being formed.

Chapter 9

Adipose Tissue

I. **INTRODUCTION.** Adipose tissue is a specialized form of connective tissue consisting of **fat-storing cells (adipocytes)** associated with a rich blood supply. Individual fat-storing cells, adipocytes, are found throughout the loose connective tissue. When adipocytes are the primary cell type present in a tissue, it is designated **adipose tissue** (Figures 9-1, 9-2).

A. **Metabolic function of adipose tissue.** The body has a limited capacity to store carbohydrate and protein. The fat contained in the adipocytes represents the storage of nutritional calories in excess of what is normally utilized.

1. Fat is an efficient form of **calorie storage** because it has about twice the caloric density of carbohydrate and protein.

2. Fat metabolism can also be an **essential source of water** for the body under extreme conditions.

B. **Types of adipose tissue.** The two types of adipose tissue are named according to their color in the living state.

1. In **white,** or **unilocular, adipose tissue** each adipocyte is filled with a single large lipid droplet of neutral fat (see Figures 9-2, 9-3).

2. In **brown,** or **multilocular, adipose tissue** each adipocyte contains many small lipid droplets of neutral fat.

II. **WHITE ADIPOSE TISSUE.** White adipose tissue is the predominant type of adipose tissue in adult humans.

A. **Functions and distribution.** White adipose tissue provides **energy storage, insulation,** and **cushioning** of vital organs.

1. White adipose tissue forms an insulating layer called the **panniculus adiposus** deep to the dermis of the skin. It is thickest in individuals living in arctic and subarctic climates.

2. Concentrations of adipose tissue are located in the connective tissue under the skin of the abdomen, buttocks, axilla, thigh, and in the breasts of both males and females.
   a. The nonlactating female breast is composed of adipose tissue and fibrous connective tissue.
   b. In the abdomen, adipose tissue is preferentially located in the omentum, mesentery, and retroperitoneal space, especially around the kidneys.

3. White adipose tissue is also found in the bone marrow and between other tissues, such as between muscles and connective tissue, where it appears to fill in spaces.

4. White adipose tissue is also concentrated in the soles of the feet and the palms of the hands, beneath the visceral pericardium, and in the orbits, surrounding the eyeballs.
   a. In these sites it serves a structural function as a cushion.
   b. When adipose tissue elsewhere is depleted by reduced caloric intake, this structural adipose tissue remains undiminished.

B. **Histogenesis of white adipocytes** (Figure 9-3)

1. **Origin of adipocytes**

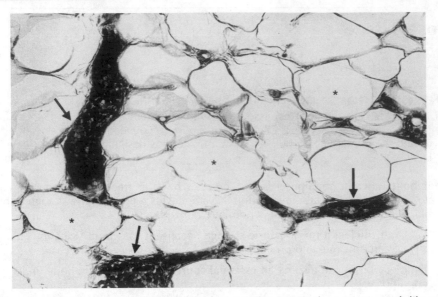

FIGURE 9-1. Photomicrograph of unilocular adipose tissue showing its characteristic mesh-like appearance in a routinely prepared hematoxylin–eosin (H&E) section. Each space (*) represents the site of the large lipid droplet that was present in each cell before the lipid was dissolved by organic solvents used in processing of the tissue. The surrounding material consists of the thin rim of cytoplasm of the adipocytes, some intervening loose connective tissue, and blood vessels (*arrows*).

    a. Most adipocytes derive directly from **undifferentiated mesenchymal cells** that are associated with the **adventitia of small venules.**
        (1) This is the same stem cell population from which fibroblasts and myofibroblasts in healing wounds originate.
        (2) Lipoblasts that have not begun to accumulate fat are morphologically indistinguishable from fibroblasts.

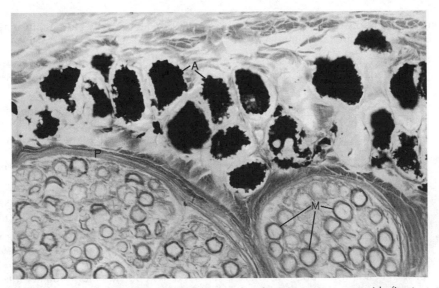

FIGURE 9-2. Adipose tissue in the epineurium of a peripheral nerve (osmium tetroxide fixation). The lipid of the unilocular adipocytes (*A*), as well as the myelin (*M*) of the nerve tissue, was preserved by the osmium tetroxide fixation and appears dark because of the density of the reduced osmium bound to the lipid components. The irregular surfaces of the lipid droplets of the adipocytes indicate partial extraction of the lipid during tissue processing. *P* = perineurium.

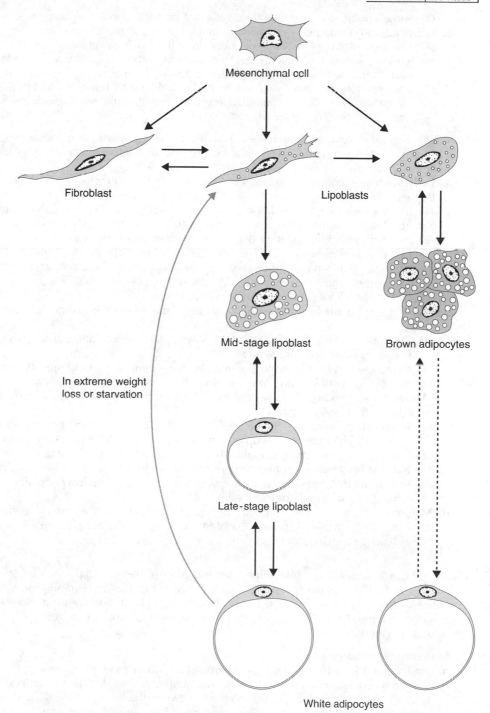

FIGURE 9-3. Summary diagram of the development of adipose tissue cells. Adipocytes, as all connective tissue cells, derive from mesenchymal cells (either mesodermally-derived mesenchyme or ectomesenchyme derived from neural crest). Mesenchymal cells give rise to fibroblasts and lipoblasts, fibroblast-like cells that are committed to become adipocytes. Lipoblasts develop an external (basal) lamina and begin to accumulate numerous lipid droplets in their cytoplasm. In white adipose tissue, these droplets fuse to form a single large lipid droplet that ultimately fills the cell, compressing the nucleus, cytoplasm and cytoplasmic organelles into a thin rim around the droplet. In brown adipose tissue, the individual droplets remain separate.

       (3) Some lipoblasts may derive from cells that pass through a fibroblast stage.
    b. White adipose tissue begins to develop in the embryo in miduterine life.
       (1) The groups of lipoblasts that develop along the small blood vessels in the fetus are free of fat. Nevertheless, they are committed to becoming fat cells even at this early stage and are called **primitive fat organs.**
       (2) The primitive fat organ is characterized by proliferating lipoblasts and proliferating capillaries. Lipid accumulation in the lipoblasts ultimately produces the typical morphology of the adipocytes.

  2. Morphology of developing adipocytes. The developing lipoblast undergoes a regular series of morphologic changes as it differentiates into an adipocyte and accumulates neutral fats into a single large lipid droplet (see Figure 9-3).
    a. Early lipoblasts look like fibroblasts but contain small lipid inclusions and have a thin external lamina.
       (1) In the earliest stages, the lipoblast is morphologically indistinguishable from a fibroblast except for the presence of a partially developed external lamina.
       (2) As lipoblastic differentiation begins, the number of smooth-surfaced vesicles in the cell increases (with a corresponding decrease in rough endoplasmic reticulum [rER]), small lipid droplets appear at one pole of the cell, and pinocytotic vesicles and an external lamina develop. Cells with these features are called early lipoblasts or **preadipocytes.**
    b. Mid-stage lipoblasts become ovoid as lipid accumulation changes the cell dimensions.
       (1) The most characteristic feature at this stage is the accumulation of smooth vesicles and small lipid droplets.
       (2) Glycogen particles begin to accumulate at the periphery of the lipid droplets.
       (3) Pinocytotic vesicles and the external lamina become more prominent.
    c. Mature adipocytes are characterized by a single, large lipid inclusion surrounded by a thin rim of cytoplasm.
       (1) In **late-stage lipoblasts,** the cells gradually increase in size and become more spherical. The large lipid droplet forms by the fusion of the smaller droplets.
       (2) Smooth vesicles remain abundant but rER becomes less prominent.
       (3) Eventually, the lipid droplet compresses the nucleus to an eccentric position within the thin rim of cytoplasm, giving the cells the **signet-ring** appearance typical of a mature lipocyte or adipocyte.
    d. Mature unilocular adipocytes that have depleted their stored lipid are morphologically indistinguishable from early lipoblasts. They gradually accumulate additional lipid and again pass through these developmental stages.

C. **Histologic characteristics of white adipocytes and adipose tissue.** Adipocytes are spherical when isolated but appear polyhedral when crowded together to form adipose tissue. In routine histologic preparations, the lipid is lost during dehydration with organic solvents, giving adipose tissue the appearance of a delicate meshwork of irregular polygonal profiles (see Figure 9-1).

  1. Structure of adipocytes
    a. Unilocular adipocytes are large, sometimes 100 μm or more in diameter.
    b. The lipid droplet in an adipocyte is not membrane bounded. When examined with an electron microscope, the interface between the lipid and the surrounding cytoplasm appears as a 5-nm–thick, condensed layer of lipid reinforced by parallel microfilaments that are 5 nm in diameter.
    c. Cytoplasmic organelles are concentrated primarily in the perinuclear cytoplasm.
       (1) There is a small Golgi complex, some free ribosomes, short profiles of rER, and microfilaments and intermediate filaments.
       (2) Long **filamentous mitochondria,** typical of adipose cells, may stretch from this zone into the thin rim of cytoplasm surrounding the lipid droplet.
       (3) Filaments, mitochondria, smooth ER, and glycogen particles are also found in the thin rim of cytoplasm surrounding the lipid droplet.

2. **Structure of adipose tissue**
   a. Adipose tissue is richly supplied with blood vessels. **Capillaries** are found at most of the angles of the meshwork where adipocytes abut one another.
   b. **Reticular fibers** secreted by the adipocytes surround the cells and are readily demonstrated with silver-reduction staining procedures.
   c. Special stains demonstrate numerous **unmyelinated nerve fibers** as well as numerous **mast cells** in adipose tissue.

D. **Physiologic regulation of adipose tissue.** The amount of adipose tissue in an individual is determined by **genetic factors** and by **caloric intake.**

1. Animal studies indicate that obesity is associated with an **increased efficiency** of food utilization.

2. Mobilization and deposition of lipid are influenced by **neural** and **hormonal** factors.
   a. In studies of induced starvation in rodents, adipose cells in a denervated fat pad continue to deposit fat, whereas adipose cells in the contralateral fat pad, with an intact nerve supply, mobilize fat.
   b. **Norepinephrine** is essential in the mobilization of lipid.
      (1) Norepinephrine, liberated by the nerve endings of the sympathetic nervous system, initiates a series of metabolic steps in adipocytes that leads to the activation of **lipase.**
      (2) Lipase splits **triglycerides,** which constitute over 90% of the neutral fat in the lipid droplets.
   c. **Insulin,** secreted by the B cells of the pancreas, enhances the conversion of glucose into the triglycerides of lipid by the adipocyte. **Thyroid hormone, glucocorticoids,** and **pituitary hormones** also affect steps in the metabolism of adipose tissue.

III. **BROWN ADIPOSE TISSUE.** Adipocytes of brown, multilocular adipose tissue are characterized by the presence of numerous fat droplets in the cytoplasm (see Figure 9-3). Brown adipose tissue has an extremely rich supply of blood capillaries that contribute to its color.

A. **Physiologic function of brown adipose tissue.** Large quantities of brown adipose tissue are present in hibernating animals and in newborn humans.

1. In **hibernating animals,** oxidation of the lipid in the multilocular adipocytes warms the blood on arousal from hibernation.

2. In **newborn humans,** the heat liberated by oxidation of the lipid in brown adipose tissue serves to compensate for some of the excessive heat loss due to the high surface-to-mass ratio in the infant.
   a. The amount of brown adipose tissue in the human decreases as the body grows, but remains widely distributed through the first decade of life.
   b. In the adult, it is found only around the kidney and aorta, and in regions of the neck and mediastinum.

B. **Histologic characteristics of brown adipocytes.** The cells of brown adipose tissue are smaller than those of white adipose tissue.
   1. The nucleus is usually eccentric but is not flattened, as is the nucleus of the unilocular adipocyte.
   2. In routine histologic preparations, the cytoplasm of multilocular fat cells consists largely of empty vacuoles because of the loss of lipid during tissue dehydration.
   3. The multilocular adipocyte contains numerous mitochondria, a small Golgi zone, and only small amounts of rER and smooth ER.
      a. The mitochondria of multilocular adipocytes are unique because they do not have the elementary particles that contain many of the enzymes for ATP production (i.e., oxidative phosphorylation).

    b. The energy produced by the mitochondria is dissipated as heat rather than utilized in the production of ATP.

    c. The mitochondria contain large amounts of cytochrome oxidase, which imparts the brown color to individual cells.

C. **Histogenesis of brown adipose tissue.** Until developing fat cells pass through the midstage lipoblast structure, it is not possible, except by location in the body, to determine if a particular group of cells will become white fat or brown fat. Some evidence exists that mature adipocytes can **interconvert** between unilocular (white) and multilocular (brown) states.

Chapter 10

Cartilage

I. INTRODUCTION. Cartilage is a type of **connective tissue** present in specific regions of the body. It often forms structures having characteristic shapes (e.g., external ear). In contrast, loose connective tissue is ubiquitous and generally lacks characteristic shapes.

A. Functions. In addition to giving form to certain structures, cartilage forms the articular surfaces of synovial joints, and provides a developmentally plastic scaffolding for endochondral ossification.

B. Organization. Cartilage is composed of a **cellular compartment** (chondroblasts and chondrocytes) and an extracellular **matrix compartment** (fibers and ground substance) that fills the space around chondrocytes.

C. Types. Three different types of cartilage exist: **hyaline, elastic,** and **fibrocartilage.** The morphologic characteristics of each type reflect the functional demands placed on it.

II. CARTILAGE CELLS. Cartilage cells constitute only a tiny fraction of the weight of cartilage. Four cell types are characteristic of developing and mature cartilage: perichondrial cells, chondroblasts, chondrocytes, and chondroclasts.

A. Perichondrial cells are stem cells that form the cellular part of the perichondrium.

1. Perichondrial cells are the germinative population of cells from which chondroblasts and, eventually, chondrocytes are derived. Perichondrial cells resemble fibroblasts of other connective tissues.

2. The **perichondrium** is the fibrous connective tissue sheath that surrounds most cartilage.

B. Chondroblasts are a replicating population of immature cartilage cells.

1. Chondroblasts form a layer of cells on the surface of cartilage.

2. Chondroblasts synthesize and secrete the matrix materials of cartilage.

3. When a chondroblast becomes completely surrounded by matrix, it is called a chondrocyte.

C. Chondrocytes (Figure 10-1). These are mature cartilage cells that retain mitotic activity.

1. Chondrocytes continue to secrete matrix, enlarging the extracellular compartment.

2. Chondrocytes are completely enclosed by the cartilage matrix and occupy compartments called **lacunae.**
   a. The chondrocyte completely fills the lacuna. This is well demonstrated in electron micrographs.
   b. In light microscopic sections, the space usually visible between the chondrocyte and the lacunar wall is a shrinkage artifact of sample preparation (Figure 10-2; see Figure 10-1).

3. Chondrocytes may be widely separated from each other or they may occur in groups.
   a. Groups of chondrocytes arise by division of preexisting chondrocytes. Such a group of chondrocytes is called an **isogenous group.**
   b. This is the first step in **interstitial growth** (see VI B) and is followed by secretion of additional matrix.

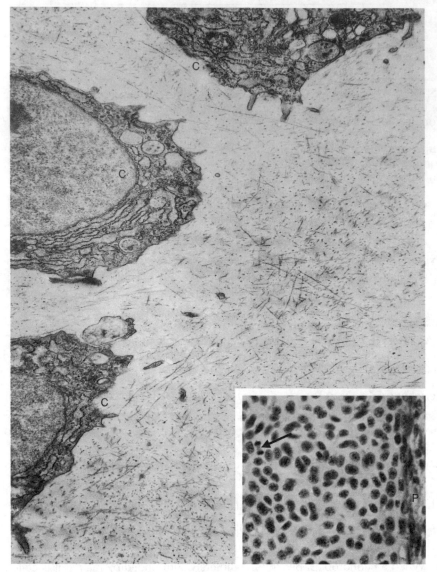

FIGURE 10-1. Electron micrograph of hyaline cartilage. Portions of three chondrocytes (*C*) completely filling their lacunae are visible. A loose feltwork of type II collagen fibrils is visible in the extracellular matrix. (*Inset*) Light micrograph of hyaline cartilage. Perichondrium (*P*), chondrocytes enclosed in lacunae, and a chondrocyte in anaphase (*arrow*) are present.

D. **Chondroclasts** are cells associated with cartilage resorption.

   1. During endochondral ossification, calcified cartilage is resorbed in one zone of the growth plate (see Chapter 11 VII F 5).

   2. Chondroclasts remove calcified cartilage, which is then replaced by bone. Chondroclasts are similar in structure and function to osteoclasts (see Chapter 11 II D).

III. **CARTILAGE MATRIX.** Matrix forms most of the mass of cartilage.

A. **Fibrous component of matrix**

   1. The fibrous components characteristic of cartilage types are as follows:

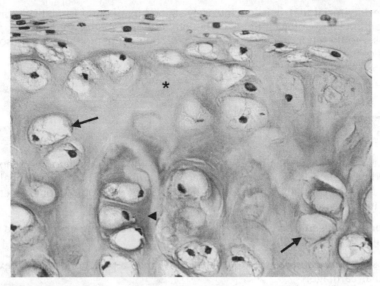

FIGURE 10-2. Hyaline cartilage. Several lacunae are visible (*arrows*). The territorial matrix (*arrowhead*) and interterritorial matrix (*) may also be discerned.

   a. Hyaline cartilage: type II collagen
   b. Elastic cartilage: elastic fibers and type II collagen
   c. Fibrocartilage: type I collagen

2. The fiber types laid down in the matrix by chondroblasts and chondrocytes determine the cartilage type.

B. **Ground substance component of matrix**

1. The ground substance of cartilage consists of sulfated glycosaminoglycans and proteoglycans.
   a. These macromolecules are organized primarily as large hyaluronic acid–proteoglycan aggregates.
   b. The water bound to these aggregates provides the resiliency characteristic of cartilage matrix.

2. Ground substance is the major organic component of the cartilage matrix; this contrasts with bone, in which collagen is the major organic component of the matrix.

3. The ground substance is responsible for the light microscopic staining characteristics of cartilage.
   a. Cartilage ground substance, especially that of hyaline cartilage, stains **basophilically** with hematoxylin and eosin (H&E) and **metachromatically** with thiazin dyes (e.g., toluidine blue).
   b. The staining reactions result from the **polyanionic nature of the ground substance,** produced by the high concentration of sulfate groups on ground substance macromolecules. This characteristic results in the ability of the ground substance to bind cationic dyes.

C. **Subcompartments of matrix.** Cartilage matrix contains chemically heterogeneous subcompartments. Territorial matrix and interterritorial matrix are evidence of this heterogeneity.

1. **Territorial matrix** is an intensely stained, basophilic zone of matrix close to chondrocytes or chondrocyte clusters. The staining reaction is probably due to a higher concentration of stainable sulfated glycosaminoglycans, or other ground substance macromolecules, closer to the chondrocytes.

2. **Interterritorial matrix** is less intensely stained matrix and is relatively distant from chondrocytes. Collagen fibrils in the interterritorial matrix are larger than those fibrils closer to the chondrocytes and may mask, by their acidophilia, the basophilic staining of the ground substance.

IV. TYPES OF CARTILAGE

A. **Hyaline cartilage** (see Figures 10-1,10-2). This is the most common and most widely distributed type of cartilage. Examples of hyaline cartilage include the tracheal rings, the articular surfaces of synovial joints, and the models of developing bones in endochondral ossification.

1. **Type II collagen** (see Chapter 8 II A 4 b; Table 8-2) is the characteristic fiber type of hyaline cartilage matrix.

2. Most hyaline cartilage structures are enclosed by a perichondrium; an exception is articular cartilage.

B. **Elastic cartilage** (Figure 10-3). This type of cartilage occurs in the external ear, in the wall of the auditory (eustachian) tube, and in the epiglottis.

1. **Elastic fibers** (see Chapter 8 II C) are prominent in the matrix, hence the name of the cartilage. Significant amounts of type II collagen are also present in the matrix of elastic cartilage.

2. Elastic cartilage cannot be distinguished readily from hyaline cartilage following H&E staining.
   a. Elastic tissue–specific stains (e.g., orcein, resorcin-fuchsin) may be used to demonstrate the elastic fibers.
   b. In the absence of histochemical staining, elastic cartilage may sometimes be recognized by the coarseness and refractility of its elastic fibers.

3. A perichondrium usually surrounds elastic cartilage.

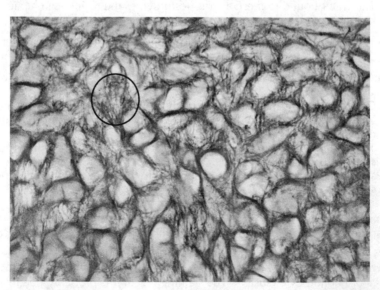

FIGURE 10-3. Elastic cartilage, resorcin stain. Lacunae are crowded together. Elastic fibers (*circled*) in the matrix are stained specifically by the resorcin.

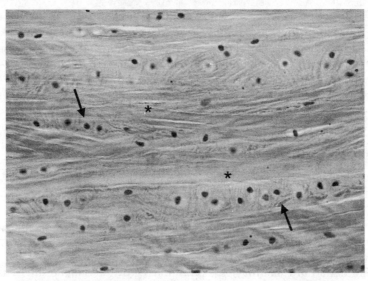

FIGURE 10-4. Fibrocartilage. Thick collagen fibers (*) predominate in the field. Chondrocytes (*arrows*) usually are restricted to the interfibrous spaces.

C. **Fibrocartilage** (Figure 10-4). This type of cartilage is present in the symphysis pubis, at the points of attachment of some tendons to bone, and it is part of each intervertebral disk.

   1. Fibrocartilage is characterized by **large amounts of collagen** and **minimal amounts of ground substance.** It does not have an obvious perichondrium.
      a. Collagen fibers are arranged in broad, parallel bands. Type I collagen (see Chapter 8 II A 4 a; Table 8-2) predominates in fibrocartilage.
      b. Chondrocytes are arranged in rows between the bands of collagen.
      c. Demonstrable amounts of ground substance are restricted to the space immediately surrounding the chondrocytes.

   2. While some histologists consider fibrocartilage a type of dense connective tissue, the presence of isogenous groups of chondrocytes argues for its classification as a cartilage.

V. **SUPPLY OF NUTRIENTS TO CHONDROCYTES**

A. Cartilage is an **avascular** tissue.

   1. Capillaries are not present in cartilage. (Bone, on the other hand, is a richly vascularized tissue.)

   2. Arterial and venous vessels may pass through the cartilage but do not form capillary beds in the cartilage.

   3. The perichondrium, however, is vascularized.

B. Nutrients diffuse through the cartilage matrix.

   1. Substances necessary to maintain the metabolism of chondrocytes diffuse from blood vessels in the perichondrium through the matrix to the chondrocytes. The gel-like nature of the cartilage matrix facilitates this diffusion.
      a. Cartilage matrix is a highly hydrated gel. Water is bound to the negatively charged proteoglycans (water of solvation).

b. This aqueous component of the matrix serves as an avenue for the diffusion of water-soluble nutrients from the vascularized perichondrium to the chondrocytes.

2. If the cartilage matrix calcifies, which occurs during endochondral ossification and also during aging, diffusion through the matrix is blocked and chondrocytes die.

VI. CARTILAGE GROWTH. Cartilage grows by two processes.

A. Appositional growth

1. Appositional growth, or **surface growth,** occurs at the cartilage surface, between the perichondrium and previously formed cartilage.
  a. Formation of chondroblasts
    (1) Stem cells of the perichondrium become partially surrounded by self-synthesized matrix. These partially surrounded cells are called chondroblasts.
    (2) Unlike osteoblasts in developing bone, chondroblasts do not form a distinct epithelioid layer on developing cartilage.
  b. Formation of chondrocytes. Appositional growth continues until the cells are completely surrounded by matrix (fibers and ground substance) that they have synthesized. The completely surrounded cells are called chondrocytes.

2. By this growth process, new cartilage—both cells and matrix—is added to the surface of preexisting cartilage.

B. Interstitial growth

1. Interstitial growth, or **internal growth,** occurs because chondrocytes, which are completely surrounded by matrix, retain the ability to divide and synthesize new matrix (see Figure 10-1, inset).

2. Evidence of interstitial growth. Groups, or "nests," of chondrocytes, also called **isogenous groups,** are derived from a single precursor chondrocyte.
  a. Initially, the chondrocytes of an isogenous group occupy one lacuna. Eventually, matrix partitions develop between chondrocytes, creating new lacunae, each containing a descendent of the original chondrocyte.
  b. The chondrocytes of an isogenous group remain relatively close together and are recognizable as an isogenous group for some time.
  c. A gradient may exist such that more chondrocytes are observed per nest at increasing distances from the perichondrium. Such isogenous groups are older than smaller groups that are closer to the perichondrium.

3. By interstitial growth, new cartilage—both cells and matrix—is added internally to the preexisting cartilage.

Chapter 11

Bone

I.   **INTRODUCTION.** Bone is a calcified connective tissue.

   A.   Bone has a **supportive** and a **protective** function. It also is a **storage site** for calcium and phosphate.

   B.   Like all connective tissues, bone is formed by **cells** and an extracellular compartment called the **matrix.**

   C.   Bone tissue forms bones, and bones are the **organs of the skeletal system.**

II.   **BONE CELLS.** Four cell types are characteristic of developing and mature bone: Osteoprogenitor cells, osteoblasts, osteocytes, and osteoclasts.

   A.   **Osteoprogenitor cells** are the least differentiated bone-forming cells.

     1. Osteoprogenitor cells are committed to form bone but have not yet synthesized recognizable deposits of bone matrix.

     2. The cells resemble fibroblasts and are morphologically indistinguishable from other undifferentiated mesenchymal cells.
       a. Osteoprogenitor cells on the outer surface of bone are part of the **periosteum** (see V A 1).
       b. Osteoprogenitor cells that line the marrow cavity are part of the **endosteum** (see V A 2).

   B.   **Osteoblasts** are germinative bone cells (Figure 11-1).

     1. Osteoblasts develop from osteoprogenitor cells and are found adjacent to the bone matrix that they have synthesized.

     2. Osteoblasts form an epithelial-like layer of cuboidal cells where bone deposition is occurring and form an inconspicuous layer of squamous cells on other bony surfaces where bone deposition is not occurring.

     3. Bone tissue is the calcified secretory product of osteoblasts.
       a. Type I collagen and the various components of the matrix are secreted by osteoblasts into the extracellular space.
       b. The secreting osteoblast may become engulfed by its own secretions. When this occurs, the cell is considered to be an osteocyte.

   C.   **Osteocytes** are mature bone cells (see Figure 11-1).

     1. An osteocyte has a large number of processes that radiate from the central, nucleus-containing region of the cell. Osteocytes are completely surrounded by bone matrix that they have synthesized.

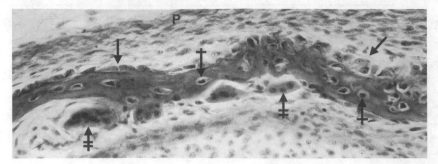

FIGURE 11-1. Spicule of bone from an area of intramembranous ossification. Osteoblasts (*arrow*), osteocytes (*crossed arrow*), and osteoclasts (*double-crossed arrow*) are functionally associated with the spicule. *P* = periosteum.

2. Bone matrix is permeated by an extensive and complex system of **lacunae** and **canaliculi.**
   a. Lacunae are the cavities in the bony matrix that are occupied by the **cell bodies of osteocytes.**
   b. Canaliculi are narrow channels that radiate from lacunae and contain the **processes of osteocytes.** Many canaliculi radiate from one lacuna.
   c. Blood vessels do not enter lacunae or canaliculi.

3. The processes of an osteocyte contact processes of nearby osteocytes.
   a. Contact occurs in the lumen of canaliculi and gap junctions are present at the points of contact.
   b. The coupling of osteocytes by gap junctions provides a cellular pathway for the transport of nutrients from the perivascular space to cells in lacunae.

4. Osteocytes are solitary cells and are not found in clusters, as are chondrocytes in cartilage matrix. This is evidence of the absence of interstitial growth in bone.

5. Osteocytes may participate in the resorption of bone matrix by a process called **osteocytic osteolysis.** This process, however, may be less important in bone resorption than osteoclasia by osteoclasts.

D. **Osteoclasts** are bone resorptive cells (Figure 11-2; see also Figure 11-1).

1. Osteoclasts are phagocytic, multinucleate giant cells located close to surfaces of bone where **osteoclasia,** or resorption of matrix, is occurring. The surface of the os-

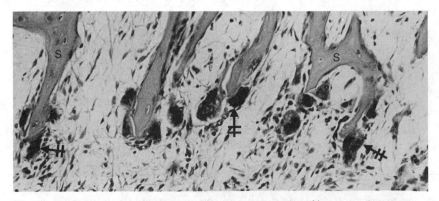

FIGURE 11-2. Spongy bone composed of multiple spicules (*S*). Areas of bone resorption on each spicule are indicated by the presence of numerous osteoclasts (*double-crossed arrow*). Loose connective tissue fills the complex and extensive interstices of the developing bone.

teoclast closest to the bony surface develops a microvillus-like border, or **ruffled border.**
  a. The multinucleate osteoclast is produced by repeated DNA replications and karyokinesis in a single cell, without subsequent cytokinesis.
  b. Osteoclasts are members of the **mononuclear phagocytic system** of cells because they are derived from monocytes of the peripheral blood.

2. Evidence of the bone resorptive function of osteoclasts includes the following:
  a. Lysosomal hydrolases are released from the osteoclast into the extracellular space between the cell and the bone surface.
    (1) These enzymes break down the organic matrix of the bone.
    (2) Calcium salts are dissolved in the extracellular space, probably by the establishment of a localized acidic environment.
  b. An osteoclast is often found in a depression, called a **Howship lacuna,** on the surface of the bone. This also is evidence of the absorptive, erosive function of the osteoclast.

3. Osteoclasts are sensitive to hormones produced by the parathyroid glands and by the parafollicular cells of the thyroid gland (see Chapter 31).

III. **BONE MATRIX.** Most of the mass of the bone is formed by matrix.

A. **Components.** Bone matrix has organic and inorganic components.

1. **Organic matrix.** Collagen and ground substance form the organic fraction of the matrix and account for about 25% of the bone mass.
  a. **Collagen** is the predominant organic component of bone matrix.
    (1) Type I collagen is secreted by osteoblasts and osteocytes. It accounts for about 90% of the organic part of the bone matrix.
    (2) The arrangement of collagen in the bone matrix determines whether a sample of bone tissue is **woven bone** or **lamellar bone** (see IV B)
    (3) The acidophilia (pink staining) visible in hematoxylin–eosin (H&E)-stained sections of decalcified bone is due to the large amount of collagen remaining in the matrix after removal of the hydroxyapatite (i.e., decalcification).
  b. **Ground substance** is the nonfibrillar component of the organic bone matrix. The ground substance fills the space around collagen fibrils and hydroxyapatite crystals.
    (1) This amorphous component of the matrix is also synthesized by osteoblasts and osteocytes. It accounts for a relatively small fraction of the organic bone matrix.
    (2) Ground substance of bone contains glycoproteins, proteoglycans, and glycosaminoglycans. Some of these molecules have been shown to bind calcium and may have a role in crystallization of the matrix.
    (3) The histochemical demonstration of bone matrix ground substance is difficult because of the masking effect of collagen, which is present in much larger amounts than ground substance.

2. **Inorganic matrix.** Calcium phosphate, as hydroxyapatite [$Ca_5(PO_4)_3(OH)$], forms the inorganic fraction of the matrix and accounts for about 75% of the bone mass.

B. **Maintenance of the bone matrix**

1. **Osteocytes** maintain the bony matrix. Death of an osteocyte results in resorption of the surrounding matrix.

2. This is evidence that bone is not an inert supporting material. Rather, it is a dynamic tissue in which cells constantly interact with matrix.

C. **Osteoid** is uncalcified matrix synthesized by osteoblasts.

1. Osteoid is newly formed matrix in which hydroxyapatite crystals have not yet developed. It is visible as a zone between a layer of osteoblasts and older, calcified matrix.

2. Osteoid usually stains differently than calcified matrix and is particularly obvious in areas of rapid bone growth.

D. **Calcification. Hydroxyapatite** crystallizes in association with matrix vesicles.

1. Calcification appears to be initiated by **matrix vesicles** (calcification vesicles), which are found in osteoid that is about to undergo calcification.
   a. The vesicles are probably derived from processes of nearby osteoblasts and osteocytes.
   b. The vesicles accumulate calcium and contain the necessary enzymes to promote precipitation of calcium salts.

2. Crystalline deposits of hydroxyapatite, which are visible by electron microscopy, are first observed within matrix vesicles.
   a. Later, crystallization spreads into the nonvesicular areas of the matrix.
   b. Some evidence suggests that the crystals may develop in register with the striations of collagen fibrils.

E. **Bone growth.** Bone is characterized by **appositional growth,** which is the addition of new matrix to a preexisting bony surface. Interstitial growth, which occurs in cartilage, does not occur in bone.

IV. TYPES OF BONE

A. **Compact bone** and **spongy bone** may be identified by visual inspection of a sawed section of dried bone (Figure 11-3).

1. Compact bone. This is the outer layer of solid bone that defines the shape of the bone and encloses an inner compartment of bony spicules.

2. Spongy bone. This is formed by the spicules. Spongy bone may also be called **cancellous bone.**

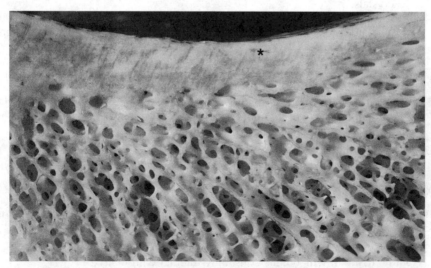

FIGURE 11-3. Sawed surface of a metaphysis of femur. The outer surface is compact bone (∗). Spongy (cancellous) bone is continuous with the compact bone and fills the interior of the bone.

a. Spongy bone forms much of the interior compartment of both developing and fully formed long bones.
b. Spongy bone develops during intramembranous bone formation.
c. Some fully developed bones (e.g., nasal chonchae) are formed completely by spongy bone.

B. Woven bone and lamellar bone may be identified by light microscopy.

1. **Woven bone.** This is immature bone. It is characterized by a **loose arrangement of collagen fibers and bundles** in the matrix.
   a. Probably all bone formed in the embryo and fetus is the woven type, and most is eventually replaced by lamellar bone.
   b. Woven bone persists in the adult in some widely scattered areas, such as tooth sockets and some tendinous insertions. Woven bone reappears in the adult during fracture repair and bone remodeling.

2. **Lamellar bone.** This is mature bone. It is characterized by a compact, **plywood-like arrangement of collagen** in the matrix. This appearance is due largely to the alternating orientations of collagen fibrils in adjacent bony lamellae. Bone may be studied histologically using ground sections of dried bone or embedded sections of decalcified bone.
   a. **Ground sections of bone.** The laminated appearance of lamellar bone is obvious in ground sections of bone (Figure 11-4A).
   b. **Decalcified sections of bone.** The laminated structure of bone is generally not observed in H&E-stained sections of decalcified bone (Figure 11-4B).

C. Comparison of bone types

1. **Compact bone** is composed almost entirely of lamellar bone.

2. **Spongy bone** may consist of either woven or lamellar bone.

V. BONE-ASSOCIATED FIBROUS CONNECTIVE TISSUE

A. Periosteum and endosteum are connective tissue sheaths of bone.

1. **Periosteum.** The periosteum is a layer of connective tissue covering the external surface of a bone. The periosteum may be divided into two components:
   a. An **outer fibrous layer** consists of dense irregular connective tissue.
   b. An **inner cellular layer** consists of osteoprogenitor (osteogenic) cells.

2. **Endosteum.** The endosteum is a less well-defined layer of connective tissue and osteogenic cells applied to the wall of a bony cavity.
   a. The endosteum lies between the bone tissue and the bone marrow.
   b. Unlike periosteum, endosteum lacks a distinct fibrous layer.

B. Tendons and ligaments attach to bone.

1. The collagenous fibers and bundles of tendons and ligaments merge with the connective tissue of the periosteum.

2. **Sharpey's fibers**
   a. At some points of attachment, the collagen fibers of a tendon are sometimes recognizable in the bone matrix. Such tendinous extensions are called Sharpey's fibers.
   b. Early in the development of a bone, the tendon attaches to the bone's surface. During growth of the bone the collagen of the tendon becomes embedded in the bone matrix, forming Sharpey's fibers. Sharpey's fibers are not always discernible, however.

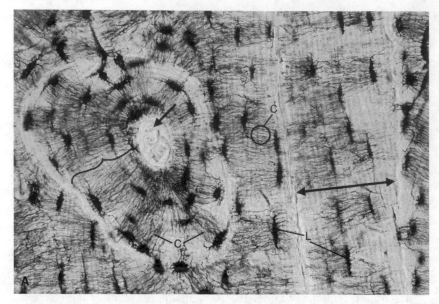

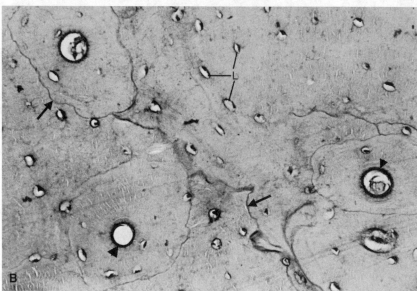

FIGURE 11-4. Histologic preparations of bone. (*A*) Ground section. Lacunae (*L*) and canaliculi (*C*) are clearly illustrated by this type of tissue preparation. The wall of an osteon (*bracket*), interstitial lamellae (*double-headed arrow*), and an osteonal canal (*single-headed arrow*) are indicated. (*B*) Decalcified section. Osteonal canals (*arrowheads*) and lacunae (*L*) are the only visible openings in the otherwise complete layer of bony matrix. Canaliculi are not visible in routinely stained sections of decalcified bone. Cement lines (*arrows*) are visible around osteons as well as in other areas of the matrix.

VI. OSTEOGENESIS: INTRAMEMBRANOUS OSSIFICATION. Intramembranous ossification is the mechanism of bone formation characterized by the absence of a cartilaginous model of the developing bone. The term *intramembranous* refers to the flat, membrane-like appearance of the developing bone.

A. The **flat bones** of the skull, the sternum, and the scapula are examples of bones that develop by intramembranous ossification.

B. **Stages in intramembranous ossification**

1. **Modulation of osteoprogenitor cells.** These fibroblast-like cells modulate to form osteoblasts in fibrous connective tissue.

2. **Secretion of matrix.** Osteoblasts secrete matrix and become osteocytes when surrounded by matrix.

3. **Formation of spicules.** Fine spicules of bone may be recognizable early in the intramembranous ossification of a particular bone (see Figure 11-1).
   a. A spicule may have a calcified interior and a covering of osteoid.
   b. Recently formed spicules are formed entirely of osteoid.

4. **Confluence of spicules.** As bone growth proceeds, isolated spicules become confluent, producing a three-dimensional meshwork of spongy bone.
   a. The three-dimensional nature of this network is often not appreciated because of the two-dimensional nature of a histologic section.
   b. At this stage, more of the bone is formed by fibrous connective tissue than by bone tissue.

5. **Transformation of spongy bone to compact bone**
   a. As bone synthesis continues, the irregular spaces in the mass of spongy bone filled with loose connective tissue are reduced.
   b. The spongy bone becomes compact bone when the volume of sample occupied by bone is greater than that occupied by loose connective tissue.

VII. **OSTEOGENESIS: ENDOCHONDRAL OSSIFICATION.** Endochondral ossification is a mechanism of bone formation characterized by the presence of a cartilaginous model of the developing bone. The term *endochondral* refers to the close association of the developing bone with the pre-existing hyaline cartilage model of that bone.

A. The **long bones** of the limbs (including the phalanges) and the ribs develop by endochondral ossification.

B. **Characteristics of endochondral ossification**

1. Endochondral ossification is distinguished from intramembranous ossification by the following characteristics:
   a. The presence of a hyaline cartilage model of the bone
   b. The presence of cartilage, along with bone, during the ossification process

2. Endochondral ossification occurs in the fetus, when the skeleton first starts to develop, and also during growth of bones in the infant and child.

C. **Stages in the initiation of endochondral ossification**

1. **Cartilage model development.** A miniature model of the future bone develops in the fetus.

2. **Bony collar formation.** A thin, tubular bony collar forms around the middle of the cartilage model of the developing bone. This is an indication that endochondral ossification is about to commence.

3. **Chondrocyte hypertrophy.** In the center of the cartilage model, chondrocytes increase in size and synthesize alkaline phosphatase, which is secreted into the extracellular matrix.

4. **Matrix calcification.** Calcification of the cartilage matrix occurs around the enlarged chondrocytes. Chondrocytes die because nutrients are unable to diffuse through the calcified matrix.

5. **Matrix erosion.** The calcified matrix and moribund chondrocytes break down and lacunae become confluent. An enlarging cavity is produced in the cartilage model.

6. Vascularization. Blood vessels penetrate the bony collar through channels in the spongy bone. The enlarging cavity in the middle of the cartilage model becomes vascularized and myeloid cells become established, forming the marrow cavity.

D. **Cartilage model growth and formation of growth plates**

1. The cartilage model enlarges as the fetus grows.

2. At either end of the enlarging marrow cavity, cartilage undergoes changes that resemble those that take place earlier in the center of the model. These developmental changes, which involve chondrocytes and matrix at either end of the cartilage model, produce the **growth plates** (epiphyseal plates).

3. A growth plate persists in a region of a developing long bone as long as growth is occurring in that region of the bone.

E. **Regions of developing long bone**

1. **Diaphysis.** The diaphysis is the shaft of the bone.
   a. Endochondral ossification commences in the region of the cartilage model that later becomes the diaphysis of the bone.
   b. After the early stages of ossification, no cartilage is present in the diaphysis of a developing long bone.

2. **Metaphysis.** A metaphysis is the funnel-shaped or flared region at either end of the diaphysis. The metaphysis encloses the part of the growth plate formed by mixed spicules (see VII F 6 a).

3. **Epiphysis.** An epiphysis is located at either end of a long bone.
   a. It is capped by a cartilaginous articular surface.
   b. A cartilaginous growth plate forms the metaphyseal border of the epiphysis.
   c. Secondary centers of ossification may also be found in an epiphysis, between the growth plate and the articular surface.

F. A **growth plate** indicates endochondral ossification. Several zones may be recognizable within a growth plate. Each zone extends laterally across the width of the plate (Figure 11-5).

1. **Zone of resting cartilage** (quiescent zone, reserve zone). This is the part of the growth plate closest to the articular surface.
   a. Lacunae and chondrocytes are small and appear not to be spatially organized.
   b. This zone is broad in rapidly growing cartilage and decreases in width as the end of growth approaches.

2. **Zone of proliferation.** This region of the growth plate is characterized by the presence of parallel stacks of chondrocytes that are perpendicular to the plane of the epiphyseal plate.
   a. A single epiphyseal plate contains a large number of such stacks.
   b. Growth in length of the developing bone occurs in this zone. This is an example of interstitial growth of cartilage (see Chapter 10 VI B).

3. **Zone of hypertrophy.** The lacunae and chondrocytes increase in volume and alkaline phosphatase is secreted into the extracellular matrix by the enlarged chondrocytes.

4. **Zone of calcification.** This is a relatively thin zone in which the cartilage matrix calcifies. Chondrocytes in this zone die because calcification of the surrounding matrix prevents diffusion of nutrients to the cells.

5. **Zone of cartilage breakdown.** The calcified matrix is partially broken down by the action of cells that have been called chondroclasts.
   a. Some of the calcified cartilage remains as thin, longitudinally oriented, irregular partitions on the diaphyseal side of the zone of calcification. This is visible in histologic section as spicules.

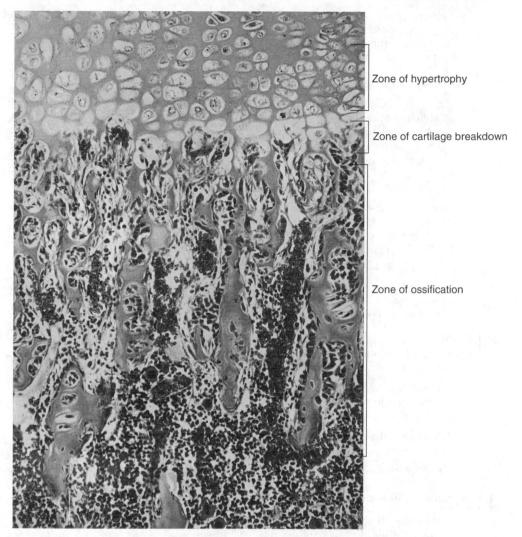

Zone of hypertrophy

Zone of cartilage breakdown

Zone of ossification

FIGURE 11-5. Part of a growth plate. Visible in this micrograph are enlarged chondrocytes and lacunae characteristic of the zone of hypertrophy, spicules of calcified cartilage characteristic of the zone of cartilage breakdown, and mixed spicules of calcified cartilage and woven bone (surrounded by hematopoietic tissue) characteristic of the zone of ossification.

    b. The remaining calcified cartilage forms a three-dimensional meshwork that becomes populated by red bone marrow (hematopoietic tissue).

6. Zone of ossification. Osteoid is deposited by osteoblasts on the surface of the remaining calcified cartilage.
    a. The structures formed, composed of a thin layer of woven bone covering calcified cartilage, are called **mixed spicules.** They are surrounded by red bone marrow.
    b. Mixed spicules are found only in endochondral ossification, never in intramembranous ossification. They are as characteristic of endochondral ossification as is the epiphyseal plate.
    c. The portion of a mixed spicule formed by newly synthesized woven bone contains osteocytes. The portion of a mixed spicule formed by calcified cartilage lacks chondrocytes.

7. Zone of resorption. Mixed spicules are resorbed by the action of osteoclasts.

a. Resorption occurs at the end of the spicule closest to the diaphysis of the developing bone.

b. Because mixed spicules are constantly being eroded, their lengths remain nearly constant as the marrow cavity gradually increases in volume.

G. **Secondary centers of ossification** shape the epiphyses of developing bones.

1. Loci of ossification develop in the ends (epiphyses) of growing long bones after the establishment of the primary ossification center and the initial formation of the two epiphyseal plates.
   a. A sequence of events occurs in each secondary center that is similar to the stages described in the formation of the growth plates.
   b. The distinct layering characteristic of the growth plate does not occur in secondary ossification centers.

2. Shaping of the ends of the long bone occurs by growth of the secondary centers.
   a. An epiphysis may have more than one center of ossification, in addition to that at its nearby growth plate.
   b. The human humerus, for example, has a total of eight ossification centers during its development.

3. Some bones that develop by endochondral ossification, such as carpal (wrist) bones, lack secondary centers. Other bones, such as phalangeal (finger) bones, have a secondary center only at one end.

H. **Closure of the epiphyses.** When growth ceases during adolescence, the growth plate is replaced by spongy bone; this is called closure of the epiphysis, and indicates cessation of growth.

1. The first indication of closure is penetration of the growth plate by vascular and marrow channels that join the diaphyseal marrow compartment with an epiphyseal marrow compartment.

2. At this time the rate of cartilage resorption appears to exceed the rate of cartilage proliferation.

3. Cartilage normally persists in adults only on the articular surface of the epiphysis.

I. **Significance of endochondral ossification**

1. Endochondral ossification is a mechanism that allows a growing bone to be a weight-bearing structure during its development.

2. The cartilage model—the hallmark structure of the endochondral process of ossification—provides a scaffolding on which a more rigid skeletal material (i.e., bone) is laid down.

3. Cartilage is a developmentally plastic tissue that accommodates growth.

VIII. OSTEONS AND LAMELLAR BONE

A. An **osteon,** or **haversian system,** is a unit of structure of lamellar bone (Figure 11-6; see also Figures 11-4, 11-7).

1. An osteon is a **columnar structure** with a maximum diameter of about 0.4 mm. It is formed by several concentrically arranged lamellae of bone.

2. The **osteonal (haversian) canal** is found in the center of the osteon and contains blood vessels, nerves, and loose connective tissue.

3. **Lacunae** (containing osteocytes) and **canaliculi** (containing processes of osteocytes) are visible in the wall of the osteon. A large number of lacunae and canaliculi are found in each osteon.

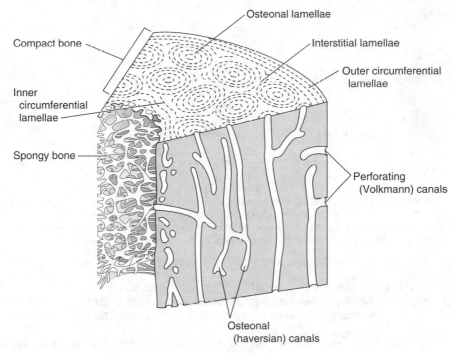

FIGURE 11-6. Segment of compact bone. Note the three types of lamellae (osteonal, circumferential, and interstitial), osteonal (haversian) canals, and perforating (Volkmann's) canals.

B. **Osteon development.** Osteons form on preexisting bony surfaces.

1. **Developmental prerequisite.** A **vascularized groove** on a bony surface or a vascularized bony tunnel is a necessary substrate for the development of an osteon.

2. **Steps in osteon development**
   a. The connective tissue adjacent to the bony surface is the source of osteogenic cells.
      (1) Osteoblasts line the groove or tunnel and synthesize a layer of matrix.
      (2) Some of the osteoblasts become completely surrounded by matrix, thus becoming osteocytes.
   b. More layers of matrix are laid down, decreasing the internal diameter of the osteon and, eventually, bridging the opening of the groove.
   c. Osteon formation is a self-limiting developmental process.
      (1) Development of the osteon proceeds, lamella by lamella, until a minimal internal diameter is reached.
      (2) This is the diameter of the osteonal canal.

3. Osteonal lamellae develop **centripetally** (Figure 11-7).
   a. The lamella of greatest diameter, which forms the outer limit of the osteon, is the oldest bone in that particular osteon.
   b. The lamella bordering the osteonal canal is the most recently formed layer of bone and is the final layer of bone to be laid down in that osteon.

C. **Relationship of osteons to ossification processes**

1. **Osteons and intramembranous ossification**
   a. Osteons develop in the interstices of the spongy bone produced early in intramembranous ossification.
   b. The gradual transformation of spongy bone to compact bone occurs by osteon development.

2. **Osteons and endochondral ossification**

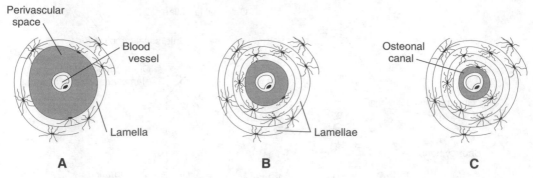

FIGURE 11-7. Centripetal deposition of bony lamellae in the formation of an osteon. (*A*) The first lamella of bone is deposited against the wall of a bony tunnel. Note the blood vessel and a relatively wide perivascular space. (*B*) Additional lamellae are laid down. (*C*) Osteogenesis continues until the osteon is fully developed. The final, most recently deposited lamella of bone forms the wall of the osteonal (haversian) canal containing the blood vessel. Note the narrow perivascular space.

     a. Osteons develop in association with the growth plate.
        (1) The diaphyseal side of the growth plate (zones of cartilage breakdown and ossification) is honeycombed with blindly ending tunnels of calcified cartilage.
        (2) The tunnels are the remains of the stacks of chondrocytes of the growth plate.
     b. Bone is deposited on the walls of the tunnels, producing mixed spicules.
     c. Some of the tunnels, especially those at the periphery of the growth plate, become filled in by bony lamellae, producing typical osteons. Such osteons would be incorporated into the wall of the growing metaphysis as it increases in diameter.
     d. Osteons may also develop in association with woven bone or in association with older lamellar bone during bone remodeling.

D. **Extraosteonal lamellae.** In addition to forming osteons, lamellae of bone also occur as circumferential lamellae and interstitial lamellae (see Figure 11-6).

   1 Circumferential lamellae
     a. Circumferential lamellae are layers of bone that follow the inner (endosteal) and outer (periosteal) circumferences of the diaphysis.
     b. Limits are placed on the thickness of circumferential lamellae by the maximum distance that an osteocyte can exist from a blood vessel.

   2. Interstitial lamellae
     a. Interstitial lamellae appear as irregular islands of bone filling in the spaces between osteons.
     b. Interstitial lamellae are derived from osteons and circumferential lamellae that have been partially removed by osteoclasia during growth and remodeling. The unresorbed bone persists as interstitial lamellae.

E. **Perforating (Volkmann's) canals.** These are nutrient channels that permeate lamellar bone.

   1. Volkmann's canals are channels in lamellar bone in which blood vessels and nerves travel from the periosteal and endosteal surfaces to reach osteons.

   2. The canals run at approximate right angles to the orientation of the osteonal canals.

   3. Unlike osteonal canals, Volkmann's canals are not surrounded by concentric lamellae of bone.

F. **Cement lines.** Junctions between new and old lamellar bone are marked by thin, basophilic surfaces called cement lines (see Figure 11-4B).

    1. Some cement lines outline osteons.

    2. Other cement lines wander through the bone matrix without an obvious relationship to osteons or other bony lamellae. This type of cement line is indicative of resorption and remodeling of bone that is completed in a particular region.

    3. The histochemistry of cement lines suggests that they contain less collagen than other areas of the bony matrix.

IX. GROWTH AND REMODELING OF A LONG BONE

A. The **diaphysis** increases both in length and in diameter during normal growth.

    1. The diaphysis of the bone increases in diameter by osteoblastic deposition of bone matrix on its periosteal surface and osteoclastic removal of bone from its endosteal surface.

    2. The length of the diaphysis increases as a result of growth, differentiation, and remodeling in the metaphysis and epiphysis.

B. The **metaphyses** are remodeled.

    1. The metaphyses contain mixed spicules that project toward the diaphysis from the growth plate.

    2. Peripherally located mixed spicules are incorporated into the endosteal wall of the metaphysis and bone is resorbed from the periosteal surface of the wall of the metaphysis.

    3. This mechanism accounts for the narrowing of the bone diameter as the relatively wide metaphysis becomes part of the narrower diaphysis.

C. The **epiphyses** increase in volume and acquire characteristic shapes.

    1. Growth of the epiphyseal cartilage accounts for the increase in length of the bone.

    2. Development of secondary centers of ossification, between the growth plate and the articular surface, produces the shape that is characteristic of the end of the bone.

X. GROWTH AND REMODELING OF A FLAT BONE

A. Flat bony plates are also remodeled to accommodate growth.

    1. Growing region
        a. A layer of cuboidal osteoblasts on the surface of a developing flat bone is evidence of a growing region.
        b. Such a layer of osteoblasts may resemble an epithelium.

    2. Quiescent (resorption) region
        a. Other regions of the same bone may be free of a cuboidal epithelioid layer of osteoblasts or may show osteoclasts.
        b. Such areas, usually on the opposite side of a bony plate from the growing surface, indicate regions of no bone growth or of bone resorption. For example, during growth of the skull, bone deposition occurs on the convex surface of the growing bone and at the sutures. Bone resorption occurs along the concave surface.

B. **Tables** and **diploe** develop in flat bones.

1. Flat bones of the skull initially are formed by a single layer of bone.

2. Later, two layers of bone develop and each layer of bone is called a table. The two bony tables enclose a compartment, called the diploe, that contains marrow and spongy bone.

XI. FRACTURE REPAIR

A. **Callus** develops at a fracture site.

1. Tissue debris and clotted blood at the fracture site are removed by invading neutrophils and macrophages.

2. Blood vessels enter the injured area and, together with newly formed connective tissue, form granulation tissue in the fracture gap.

3. Cartilage develops in the granulation tissue.

4. Callus is the fibrous connective tissue and cartilage collar that initially bridges and stabilizes the fracture gap. The callus may be palpated on physical examination.

B. **Bone** bridges the fracture gap.

1. Osteoblasts, derived from the population of osteoprogenitor cells of the periosteum and endosteum, form a layer of bone on the callus.

2. The cartilage of the callus is gradually replaced by bone in a process resembling endochondral ossification.

3. Some bone of the healing fracture develops by intramembranous ossification in the newly formed fibrous connective tissue.

4. The ends of the bone at the fracture site become joined by bone.
   a. Initially, the new bone is spongy bone. Over a period of several weeks it becomes transformed into compact bone.
   b. Gradually, evidence of the callus is reduced by the action of osteoclasts and the normal contours of the bone are regained by the remodeling process.

5. The healing process is facilitated by physical reapproximation (i.e., setting, reduction) of the broken ends of bone.

XII. BONE AND HORMONAL CONTROL OF CALCIUM

A. **Bone as calcium storage site.** Blood calcium levels are maintained by mobilization of calcium stored in bone and by the sequestration of excess blood calcium in bone.

1. Low blood calcium level may result in tetany and possibly death. Increased calcium levels may cause precipitation of calcium salts at various sites in the body.

2. Calcium is stored in bone matrix and may be removed from the matrix during episodes of hypocalcemia. Excess blood calcium may be removed from the blood and stored in bone.

B. **Parathyroid gland.** Parathyroid hormone (parathormone) raises blood calcium levels (see Chapter 31).

1. Parathyroid hormone stimulates osteoclasts and osteocytes to resorb bone and to release calcium into the blood. An indication of hormonal stimulation is the development of the ruffled border on osteoclasts.

2. Parathyroid hormone also functions outside of bone in regulating blood calcium levels. It raises blood calcium levels both by reducing calcium excretion by the kidney, and by increasing calcium absorption by the small intestine.

3. Parathyroid hormone also regulates blood phosphate levels by promoting loss of phosphate in the urine. Excess phosphate is generated by the breakdown of hydroxyapatite during the release of calcium.

C. **Thyroid gland.** Calcitonin secreted by the **parafollicular cells** of the thyroid gland reduces blood calcium levels (see Chapter 31). Calcitonin inhibits the resorptive capacity of osteoclasts and balances the effect of parathyroid hormone.

Chapter 12
Blood

INTRODUCTION

A. Blood is a specialized type of connective tissue in which the extracellular matrix is a fluid. Blood is contained in blood vessels.

B. Blood contains various types of cells and formed elements that are surrounded by a protein-rich fluid called plasma (Table 12-1). Like other types of connective tissue, blood consists of a relatively small number of cells in a large volume of extracellular material.

II. **ERYTHROCYTES**

A. **Cell size and quantity.** Erythrocytes, or red blood cells (RBCs), are the most numerous blood cell. They are about one thousand times more numerous than white blood cells.

1. RBCs are 7 to 8 μm in diameter.
   a. Normal RBCs are remarkably **constant in diameter.** They are therefore a useful gauge of the size of other biological structures in histologic sections.
   b. **Microcytes** are RBCs that are 5 μm or less in diameter; **macrocytes** are RBCs larger that 10 μm. Such RBCs are characteristic of microcytic and macrocytic anemias.

2. **Reticulocytes.** Immature RBCs are called reticulocytes (see Chapter 13 III E). They are released from the red bone marrow into circulation before erythropoiesis is completed.
   a. Reticulocytes are postnormoblast cells in which a reticulum of ribonucleoprotein may be demonstrated after supravital staining with brilliant cresyl blue.
   b. Reticulocytes comprise 1% to 2% of RBCs in peripheral blood. They exist as reticulocytes for less than one day before becoming mature RBCs.

B. **Cell structure and function.** RBCs are anucleate, biconcave, hemoglobin-containing disks.

1. **Shape**
   a. The unique **biconcave shape** of the red cell is produced when the nucleus of the normoblast is extruded during erythropoiesis (Chapter 13 III D 2). The shape is maintained in the mature red cell by **spectrin,** a filamentous protein that is attached to the cytoplasmic side of the plasma membrane.
   b. RBCs sometimes form **rouleaux.** A rouleau is a precise stack of RBCs that resembles a stack of coins.
      (1) The stacking is reversible and is of unknown significance.
      (2) Rouleau formation occurs in vitro and in vivo.

2. **Contents.** RBCs contain high concentrations of **hemoglobin;** approximately one third of the weight of an RBC is hemoglobin.

3. **Function.** Hemoglobin in RBCs **transports gases.**
   a. **Oxygen** is transported from the lungs to the tissues in association with the hemoglobin.
   b. **Carbon dioxide** is transported from the tissues to the lungs in association with hemoglobin. Some carbon dioxide is also transported in the plasma as bicarbonate ion.

TABLE 12-1. Cells and Formed Elements of Blood

Blood Component	Approximate Number/μl (mm^3)	
Erythrocytes (red blood cells, RBCs)		**Percent of Erythrocytes**
Mature erythrocytes	5,000,000	98%–99%
Reticulocytes	50,000	1%–2%
Leukocytes		**Percent of Leukocytes**
Granulocytes		
Neutrophils	4500	58%
Band cells	300	4%
Eosinophils	150	2%
Basophils	40	0.5%
Agranulocytes		
Lymphocytes	2300	29%
Monocytes	400	5%
Platelets	300,000	—

4. **Relationship of shape to function.** RBC shape is important to the transport of gases.
   a. The depressed central portion of the RBC places more molecules of hemoglobin closer to the plasma membrane than if the cell were a sphere.
   b. Gases have a shorter distance to diffuse intracellularly to a binding site on hemoglobin in the biconcave RBC.

C. **Hematocrit.** The percentage of volume of a blood sample occupied by red cells is the hematocrit. If a sample of blood is allowed to settle or if it is centrifuged (and clotting is prevented), **three layers** may be discerned: Supernatant plasma, buffy coat, and packed RBCs.

1. **RBC fraction.** Normally, the packed RBCs account for 45% of the original blood sample; this percentage is the hematocrit. A low hematocrit is an indication of an anemia.

2. **Buffy coat.** The buffy coat is a thin layer (about 1% of the total blood sample) between the packed RBCs and supernatant plasma. The buffy coat contains white blood cells and platelets.

D. **Alteration of RBC shape.** The characteristic biconcave disk shape of the RBC may be modified.

1. **Intravascular shape changes**
   a. RBCs are temporarily deformed by blood flow, contact with other blood cells, and by contact with the blood vessel wall. For example, an RBC may become cone-shaped with its apex oriented in the direction of flow.
   b. Deformation of an RBC is particularly obvious in a small capillary with an internal diameter that is less than the diameter of the RBC.

2. **Osmotically induced shape changes**
   a. A **hypotonic** environment causes the RBC to swell, producing a spheroidal, pale structure called a **ghost.**
      (1) Hemoglobin is lost from the RBC under hypotonic conditions.
      (2) This process is called **hemolysis.**
   b. A **hypertonic** environment causes the RBC to collapse, producing a **crenated cell.** A crenated RBC is characterized by the presence of numerous spine-like projections over its surface.
      (1) Water is lost from the RBC under hypertonic conditions.
      (2) The spiny appearance of a crenated cell may result from the draping of the

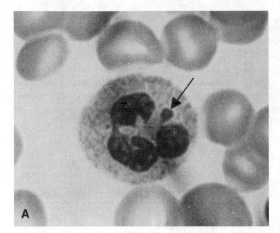

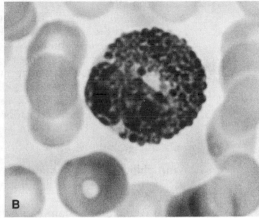

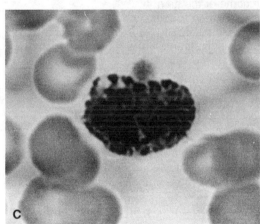

FIGURE 12-1. Granulocytes in blood smears. (*A*) Neutrophil. Note the Barr body (*arrow*). (*B*) Eosinophil. Note the two nuclear lobes, each with a distinct nucleolus. (*C*) Basophil. Intensely stained granules lie above the nucleus but do not totally obscure it.

plasma membrane over the cytoskeletal spectrin filaments that remain rigid in the osmotically collapsed RBC.

III. NEUTROPHILS (Figure 12-1A)

A. **Cell size and quantity.** Neutrophils are the most numerous leukocyte (see Table 12-1). The cytoplasmic granules of this cell are neither intensely acidophilic nor intensely basophilic, hence the origin of one of the names of this cell.

1. Neutrophils are 12 to 15 μm in diameter—larger than RBCs.

2. **Band cells.** Immature neutrophils, called band cells because of their incompletely segmented nuclei, are normally found in blood (see Chapter 13 IV E). Band cells account for approximately 4% of the total number of leukocytes.

B. **Nuclear characteristics.** There are two structural features of a neutrophil nucleus that distinguish it from nuclei of other blood cells.

1. **Multilobed nucleus**
   a. The nucleus of a neutrophil is constricted into 3 to 5 connected lobes. This gives the cell one of its names, **polymorphonuclear leukocyte** (PMN).
   b. The number of nuclear lobes does not increase with age of the cell.

    2. Sex chromatin
      a. The sex chromatin, or **Barr body** (see Chapter 4 II A 2 a, b) of a neutrophil appears as a **drumstick-like nuclear appendage,** rather than as a deposit of heterochromatin against the nuclear envelope, as in other cells. A Barr body is considerably smaller than a nuclear lobe.
      b. A Barr body is evident in about 3% of neutrophils from a female. Presumably, more neutrophil nuclei have drumstick-like Barr bodies, but their identification is impossible because of the angle of view (i.e., the Barr body is superimposed above or below a nuclear lobe).

C. **Cytoplasmic granules.** Two populations of granules characterize a neutrophil.

    1. Azurophilic (primary) granules
      a. These granules occur in all **granulocytes,** as well as in **lymphocytes** and **monocytes.**
        (1) The granules stain blue or purple by Romanovsky-type blood stains that contain azure dyes, hence the name of the granules.
        (2) Azurophilic granules develop earlier than specific granules (see III C 2) during granulopoiesis. Because of this, they are also called primary granules.
        (3) Fewer azurophilic granules than specific granules are found in a mature neutrophil.
      b. Azurophilic granules are **lysosomes.**
        (1) In addition to the expected lysosomal hydrolases, azurophilic granules also contain peroxidase.
        (2) Peroxidase activity is often used to demonstrate azurophilic granules cytochemically.

    2. Specific (secondary) granules
      a. The specific granules of human neutrophils do not stain intensely by routine blood stains. These granules are smaller and more numerous than the azurophilic granules.
      b. Substances with **bacteriostatic and bactericidal properties** have been identified in the specific granules of neutrophils.
        (1) Lysozyme, lactoferrin, and alkaline phosphatase are examples of substances found in specific granules.
        (2) Specific granules do not contain lysosomal hydrolases.

D. **Functions of neutrophils.** Neutrophils are amoeboid, phagocytic cells that function extravascularly. They are able to cross the endothelial wall of small venous blood vessels. Neutrophils leave the blood at sites of trauma or infection.

    1. Phagocytosis of bacteria. Bacteria at the infection site are phagocytized by the neutrophil. The vacuole that contains the bacterium is a **phagosome.**

    2. Role of cytoplasmic granules
      a. Specific granules fuse with the phagosome 30 to 60 seconds after formation of the phagosome. The bactericidal contents of the specific granule flow into the phagosome and affect the trapped microorganism.
      b. Azurophilic granules fuse with the phagosome–specific granule complex somewhat later. The hydrolytic enzymes of the lysosomal azurophilic granules digest the microorganism.

    3. Additional bactericidal agents. The bactericidal function of neutrophils is enhanced by the production of superoxide and hydrogen peroxide by the neutrophil, and by the effect of these oxidants on phagocytized bacteria.

    4. Acute phase of inflammation. The presence of large numbers of neutrophils in a tissue is evidence of the acute (i.e., early) aspects of inflammation, in which neutrophil granule contents may also be released extracellularly. Chronic inflammation is characterized by the presence of macrophages and lymphocytes.

IV. **EOSINOPHILS** (see Figure 12-1B)

A. **Cell size and quantity.** Eosinophils, which are about the same size as neutrophils, are the second most numerous granulocyte (see Table 12-1).

B. **Cytologic characteristics.** The usually **bilobed nucleus** and the presence of **acidophilic specific granules** are the two most important diagnostic characteristics of the eosinophil.

1. **Nucleus.** The connecting segment between the two nuclear lobes may not be included in the plane of section in electron micrographs. This results in the erroneous interpretation, frequently made by the student, of a binucleate eosinophil.

2. **Specific granules.** The specific granules of the eosinophil are unique (Figure 12-2).
   a. **Light microscopic characteristics**
      (1) The specific granules of eosinophils are **appreciably larger** than the specific granules of neutrophils. Eosinophils often can be identified in unstained preparations simply on the basis of the large size and **refractility** of their specific granules.
      (2) Eosinophilic specific granules are intensely acidophilic; that is, they are stained bright pink in routine blood smears.
   b. **Ultrastructural characteristics**
      (1) A large inclusion, in the form of an equatorial band, is visible in each granule. A crystalline substructure is visible in some of these inclusions. The presence of this **banded inclusion** is a distinctive characteristic of eosinophils.
      (2) By cytochemistry, some **lysosomal enzymes,** as well as peroxidase, have been localized in eosinophil specific granules.
      (3) The crystalloid inclusion of the eosinophil granule contains an arginine-rich protein called **major basic protein.** The characteristic staining of the granule is probably due to this protein.

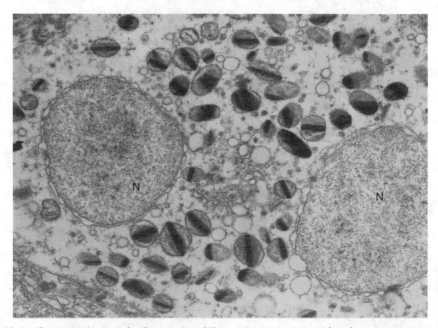

FIGURE 12-2. Electron micrograph of an eosinophil in connective tissue. The characteristic equatorial inclusions are visible in the specific granules of the cell. The connection between the two nuclear lobes (*N*) is not included in the plane of section.

C. **Role of eosinophils in immune reactions**

1. The quantity of eosinophils increases in peripheral blood during parasitic infections and allergic reactions. In addition, eosinophils leave the blood and accumulate in large numbers at sites of such reactions.

2. Eosinophils phagocytize antigen–antibody complexes.

V. BASOPHILS (see Figure 12-1C)

A. **Cell size and quantity.** Basophils, which are about the same size as neutrophils, are the least commonly encountered granulocyte (see Table 12-1).

B. **Specific granules of basophils**

1. **Light microscopic characteristics.** The specific granules of basophils are intensely basophilic.
   a. The granules are numerous, relatively large, and may have an irregular outline (i.e., they are not smooth surfaced).
   b. The nucleus of the basophil is usually obscured by the large number of darkly stained specific granules. Nuclear morphology is not a criterion of basophil identification.

2. **Granule contents.** Granules contain histamine and heparan sulfate.
   a. **Histamine** is a **vasoactive substance.**
      (1) Histamine has **variable effects on smooth muscle.** It causes contraction of bronchiolar smooth muscle and relaxation of arteriolar smooth muscle, and it promotes plasma leakage from capillaries and venules.
      (2) Approximately half the histamine found in blood is concentrated in the granules of basophils.
   b. **Heparan sulfate** is a **highly sulfated glycosaminoglycan.**
      (1) Heparan sulfate produces the **basophilia** and **metachromasia** that characterize the specific granules of basophils. Heparan sulfate is closely related chemically to heparin, which is contained in mast cell granules [see Chapter 8 IV A 3 b (2)].
      (2) The function of the heparan sulfate in basophils is not yet understood.

C. **Comparison of blood basophils and tissue mast cells.** Mast cells are resident cells of the connective tissue. Mast cells and basophils are similar in appearance and in the chemical nature of their contents.

1. **Secretions.** Both cell types contain histamine, but only mast cells contain heparin.

2. **Distribution.** Mast cells are connective tissue cells that tend to be concentrated along blood vessels and can be very numerous in some regions. Basophils are blood cells that are usually confined to the vascular space and are the least frequently encountered leukocyte.

3. **Developmental relationship.** There is no evidence that blood basophils may become tissue mast cells or vice versa. It is currently postulated that the two cells arose independently in evolution.

D. **Role of basophils in immune reactions.** Basophils leave the blood to function in connective tissue. Basophils may have a role in hypersensitivity and anaphylaxis.

1. Immunoglobulin E (IgE) attaches to basophils and the cells are then sensitized to the antigen.

2. A second exposure to that antigen may result in degranulation of the basophils, releasing their pharmacologically active substances.

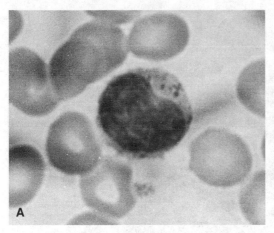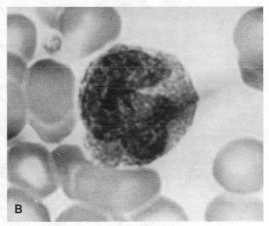

FIGURE 12-3. Agranulocytes in blood smears. (*A*) Lymphocyte with azurophilic granules. (*B*) Monocyte.

VI. LYMPHOCYTES (Figure 12-3A)

A. Cell size and quantity

1. **Quantity.** Lymphocytes are the most numerous agranular leukocyte (see Table 12-1).

2. **Size.** Small and medium lymphocytes occur in peripheral blood.
   a. **Small lymphocytes** are 7 to 8 μm in diameter. Over 90% of the lymphocytes in peripheral blood are small lymphocytes.
   b. **Medium lymphocytes** are 10 to 12 μm in diameter. Less than 10% of the lymphocytes in peripheral blood are medium lymphocytes. (Note: some authors call these cells the large lymphocytes of peripheral blood.)
   c. **Large lymphocytes (lymphoblasts)** are 15 μm or larger in diameter and do not normally enter peripheral blood. Large lymphocytes are mitotic cells found in lymphatic tissue.

B. Structural characteristics of lymphocytes

1. Lymphocytes have **minimal cytoplasm** (Figure 12-4).
   a. A distinct cytoplasmic compartment is often difficult to resolve with the light microscope. Medium lymphocytes have a slightly wider layer of cytoplasm than small lymphocytes.
   b. With the electron microscope, some small mitochondria, a few cisterns of the rough endoplasmic reticulum, some polyribosomes, and a small Golgi apparatus may be identified in the narrow cytoplasmic compartment.

2. Lymphocytes **lack specific granules.** A few azurophilic (lysosomal) granules may be encountered in lymphocytes, however.

C. Role of lymphocytes in immune reactions

1. **Lymphocyte types.** Lymphocytes in peripheral blood may be classified as **T-lymphocytes** (T-cells), B-lymphocytes (B-cells), or **natural killer** (NK) cells.
   a. **T-cells** and **B-cells** are indistinguishable in routinely stained blood smears or in histologic sections. Immunocytochemical staining, however, takes advantage of the different proteins in their plasma membranes (i.e., surface markers), and may be used to distinguish T- and B-cells.
   b. **NK cells** lack the characteristic surface markers of T-cells or B-cells.

2. **Effector cell types.** T- and B-cells **differentiate into effector cells** of the humoral and cell mediated immune responses.

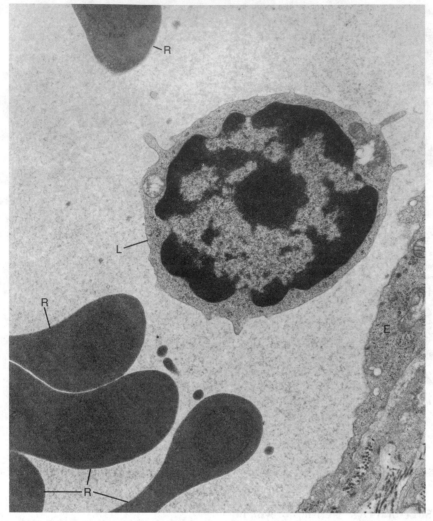

FIGURE 12-4. Electron micrograph of a lymphocyte (*L*) and red blood cells (*R*) in circulating blood. Note the characteristic narrow cytoplasmic compartment of the lymphocyte. Portions of five red blood cells are visible in the field. *E* = endothelium.

    a. In response to antigenic stimulation, T- and B-cells undergo **blastic transformation.**
        (1) **T-cells** divide and differentiate into **cytolytic killer cells** in the **cell-mediated immune response.**
        (2) **B-cells** divide and differentiate into immunoglobulin (antibody)-secreting **plasma cells** in the **humoral immune response.**
    b. The role of lymphocytes in immune responses is discussed in Chapters 15 to 20.

VII. MONOCYTES (see Figure 12-3B)

    A. **Cell size and quantity.** Monocytes, which are the largest cell type present in normal peripheral blood, are slightly more numerous than eosinophils (see Table 12-1). Monocytes may be as large as 20 μm in diameter.

B. Structural characteristics of monocytes

1. **Nuclear morphology.** Monocytes have **variable nuclear morphology.**
   a. **Shape.** Nuclei of monocytes vary in shape from spherical, to indented ovoids, to horseshoe-shaped structures. Distinct nuclear lobes comparable to those of neutrophils do not occur in monocytes.
   b. **Chromatin.** The chromatin of monocytes is less intensely stained than that of lymphocytes. The euchromatin–heterochromatin pattern of monocytes is sometimes described as lacy.

2. **Cytoplasmic granules.** Although monocytes are classified as agranulocytes, they contain some **azurophilic granules.**
   a. Azurophilic (lysosomal) granules in the cytoplasm portend the potential of monocytes to develop into macrophages.
   b. Specific granules do not occur in monocytes.

C. **Role of monocytes in the mononuclear phagocyte system.** Monocytes of peripheral blood serve as a source of cells that eventually will function extravascularly as macrophages.

1. Monocytes are the **precursor cell** of most phagocytic cells, such as perisinusoidal macrophages (Kupffer cells) of the liver, alveolar macrophages (dust cells) of the lung, osteoclasts of bone tissue, and connective tissue macrophages.

2. **Note on current terminology**
   a. Many of the cells of this system of phagocytic cells were once considered cells of the **reticuloendothelial system.**
   b. This term is **no longer appropriate** because the cells of the system are neither reticular cells nor are they endothelial cells, both of which are distinct cell types and are not phagocytic.

VIII. **PLATELETS** (Figure 12-5). Platelets are anucleate, membrane-bounded fragments of cells. They are shed from the surface of megakaryocytes in red bone marrow (see Chapter 13 V C).

A. Platelet size, shape, and quantity

1. Platelets are usually described as having a **biconvex discoidal** shape but they are less regular in shape than the remarkably uniform biconcave discoidal RBCs.

2. They are more numerous than any blood cell other than RBCs (see Table 12-1).

3. Platelets are much smaller than RBCs or any of the leukocytes. They are approximately 2 to 4 μm in diameter and often appear in clumps.

B. Structural characteristics of platelets

1. **Compartments.** A platelet is divided internally into **two concentric zones.**
   a. **Hyalomere.** This is the peripheral, ectoplasmic layer.
   b. **Granulomere.** This is the deeper, interior portion of the platelet. The granulomere compartment is characterized by at least two populations of granules.
      (1) **Alpha granules.** These granules, which are of variable size and shape, contain several proteins and coagulation factors, including fibrinogen and von Willebrand factor.
      (2) **Dense granules.** These granules, which are more electron dense than alpha granules, contain the vasoconstrictor serotonin.
      (3) **Lysosomes** may also be identified in the granulomere.

2. **Circumferential microtubule band.** Microtubules have an important cytoskeletal role in platelets.

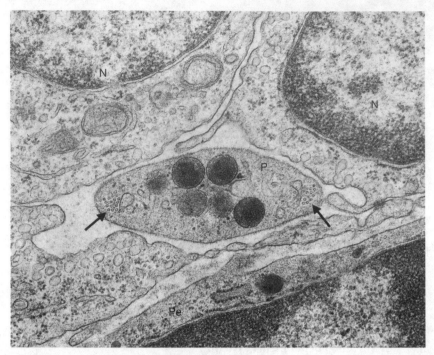

FIGURE 12-5. In this electron micrograph, a platelet (*P*) is visible in the lumen of a collapsed, fenestrated capillary. The biconvex shape of the platelet is evident as is its circumferential band of microtubules (*arrows*). *N* = endothelial cell nuclei; *Pe* = pericyte.

     a. Platelets have a circumferential band of microtubules in the hyalomere (see Figure 12-5).
     b. It is likely that the biconvex, lenticular shape of the platelet is to some extent maintained by the microtubules.

  3. Tubular systems. Two systems of membranous tubules have been described in platelets.
     a. Open canalicular system. These membranous tubules connect to the surface of the platelet and are invaginations of the plasma membrane. Platelet granules may release their contents into the channels provided by the open canalicular system.
     b. Dense tubular system. These membranous tubules appear to consist of smooth endoplasmic reticulum. They do not connect to the surface of the platelet.

  4. Absence of nuclei. Platelets lack nuclei and because of this are usually called one of the formed elements of blood. Human platelets should not be called thrombocytes and, strictly speaking, should not be called cells.

C. **Role of platelets in hemostasis.** Platelets have an important role in the maintenance of the cardiovascular system. They prevent loss of blood from vessels by promoting clotting. They also have an incompletely understood role in maintaining the integrity of the endothelial lining.

  1. Platelet aggregation. Platelets react to abnormal surfaces such as might be encountered in a bleeding wound. Such platelets are considered to be activated.
     a. Activated platelets adhere to the cut ends of blood vessels and especially to tissue components, such as collagen, that have been exposed by the traumatic event.
     b. As the mass of platelets increases, the open ends of the blood vessels become occluded by platelets. The mass of platelets is called a **thrombus.**

2. **Clot formation**
   a. The granules of platelets release their contents into the surface-connected tubular system. From here, the granule contents diffuse into the plasma and tissue spaces.
   b. Platelets release factors that participate in the clotting cascade and in **fibrin** formation. Fibrin is the main fibrous component of blood clots.

Chapter 13

Hematopoiesis

I.   **INTRODUCTION. Hematopoiesis** is the process by which specialized blood cells develop from less specialized precursor cells (Figure 13-1).

  A. **Site of hematopoiesis.** Hematopoiesis occurs in myeloid and lymphatic tissue.

    1. Myeloid tissue forms red bone marrow and is involved primarily with the formation of **erythrocytes, granulocytes, monocytes,** and **platelets.**

    2. Lymphatic tissue forms lymphatic organs (i.e., lymph nodes, spleen, and thymus gland) and is involved primarily with the formation of **lymphocytes** (see Chapter 15).

    3. Hematopoiesis is not a rigidly compartmentalized process; blood cells usually associated with myeloid tissue can arise in lymphoid tissue, and vice versa.

  B. **Tissue characterization.** Hematopoietic tissue is characterized microscopically by differentiating blood cells.

    1. A stained smear of bone marrow reveals a complex population comprising several types of blood cells and their precursors.

    2. These cell types can be sorted into several developmental sequences, each sequence culminating in one of the several types of mature blood cells (see Figure 13-1).

  C. **Morphologic criteria of blood cell development.** Changes in cell size and nuclear structure, plus the presence of differentiation products (e.g., cytoplasmic granules and hemoglobin), are indicators of cell development (Figure 13-2).

    1. Cell size. Less mature cells tend to be larger in overall diameter.

    2. Nuclear structure
      a. Chromatin configuration. Less mature cells have euchromatic (transcriptionally active) nuclei. Nuclei usually become heterochromatic (transcriptionally inactive) later in development.
      b. Nuclear lobulation. Granulocytes, during development, acquire characteristically lobed nuclei.
      c. Nuclear loss. Erythrocytes, during development, extrude the nucleus that is present in an immature cell.
      d. Nucleolar loss. This intranuclear organelle may be visible in immature blood cells but disappears from cells nearing completion of development.

    3. Differentiation products
      a. Cytoplasmic granules. In granulocytes, the presence and staining characteristics of azurophilic granules (see IV B 1 c) and specific granules (see IV C 1 c) are important developmental criteria.
      b. Hemoglobin. In erythrocytes, the gradual changes in cytoplasmic staining caused by accumulating hemoglobin are important developmental criteria (see III B 1 c, 2; C 1 c, 2).

II.   **HEMATOPOIETIC STEM CELLS.** The stem cell is a precursor cell type whose progeny give rise, eventually, to all of the definitive cell types of the blood. Stem cells are now known as **colony-forming cells** (CFCs), or **colony-forming units** (CFUs).

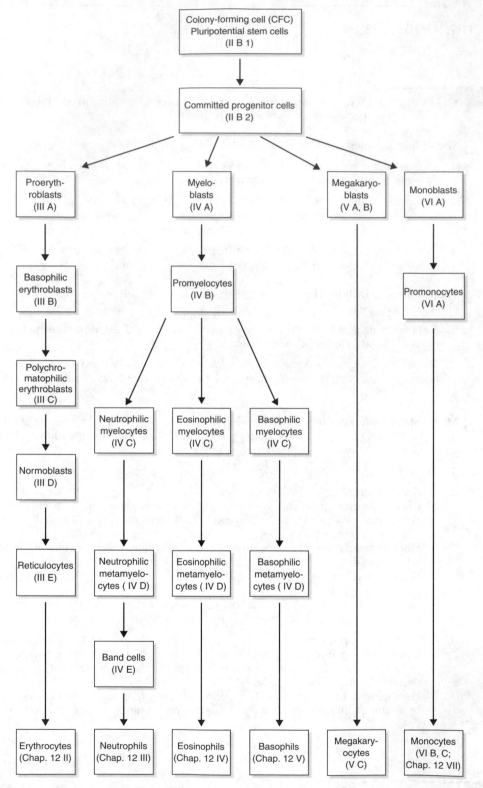

FIGURE 13-1. Some developmental relationships of hematopoietic cells of red bone marrow. (*Roman numerals* refer to text discussions.)

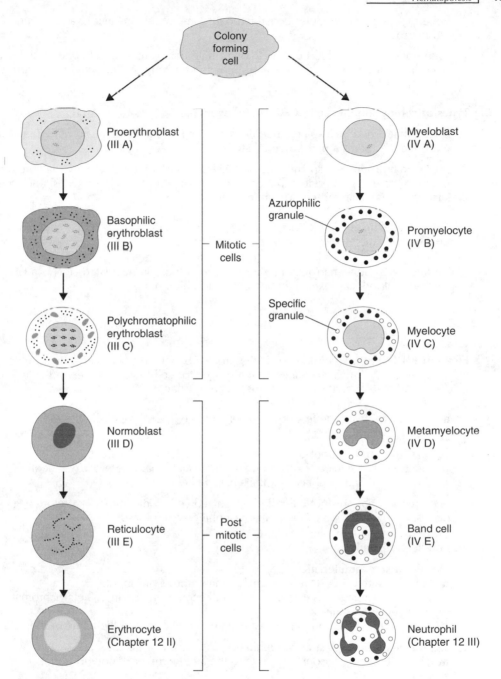

FIGURE 13-2. Stages in erythrocyte and neutrophil development, emphasizing major structural characteristics. (*Roman numerals* refer to text discussions.)

A. **Experimental identification of the stem cell.** In experiments that shed light on the nature of the stem cell, lethally irradiated mice were given transfusions of nonirradiated bone marrow cells. The transfused cells lodged in the spleens of the irradiated mice, where they produced nodules of hematopoietic tissue. (This is analogous to the growth of a colony of cells in culture after the seeding of the medium with one cell.)

1. Some of the splenic nodules contained all of the cell types found in normal red

bone marrow; other nodules contained only some of the lineages characteristic of red marrow.

  2. Each nodule appeared to be a clone of a single donor marrow cell, and all the cell types in a particular nodule appeared to be the progeny of that one donor marrow cell.

B. **Types of colony-forming cells.** CFCs are of two types:

  1. A CFC that produces a splenic nodule containing all the cell types usually found in red bone marrow is a **pluripotential stem cell.**

  2. A CFC that produces a splenic nodule lacking some of the cell types usually found in the marrow (e.g., a nodule that contains only neutrophils, erythrocytes, and megakaryocytes) is a **committed progenitor cell.**

C. **CFC structure.** Superficially, a CFC resembles a small lymphocyte. Functionally, however, CFCs and small lymphocytes are quite different.

D. **CFC numbers.** In bone marrow, one out of several thousand nucleated cells is a CFC. In peripheral blood, approximately one out of a million nucleated cells is a CFC.

III. **ERYTHROPOIESIS.** Erythropoiesis is the process by which red blood cells develop through several well-defined stages from a progenitor cell to a mature erythrocyte (see Figure 13-2). Mature erythrocytes are discussed in Chapter 12 II.

A. **Proerythroblast.** This is the first developmental stage in erythropoiesis.

  1. **Morphologic characteristics**
     a. **Size.** The proerythroblast is a large cell (18–25 μm in diameter).
     b. **Nucleus.** The nucleus is euchromatic and usually has one or two nucleoli.
     c. **Cytoplasm.** The cytoplasm exhibits basophilia.

  2. The proerythroblast is not an easily recognized cell. Some authors therefore begin discussion of erythropoiesis with the basophilic erythroblast.

B. **Basophilic erythroblast**

  1. **Morphologic characteristics**
     a. **Size.** This cell (15–18 μm) is smaller than a proerythroblast.
     b. **Nucleus.** The nucleus is spheroidal and becomes increasingly heterochromatic with successive mitoses.
     c. **Cytoplasm.** The cytoplasm is distinctly basophilic, hence the name of the cell.

  2. **Significance of cytoplasmic basophilia**
     a. The cytoplasmic basophilia is due to the large number of polyribosomes in the cell.
     b. The polyribosomes are assembled in preparation for the synthesis of hemoglobin.

  3. The experienced observer can distinguish between a proerythroblast and a basophilic erythroblast on the basis of subtle differences in cell size, amount of heterochromatin, and degree of basophilia.

C. **Polychromatophilic erythroblast.** This immature red cell (Figure 13-3) shows evidence of hemoglobin accumulation.

  1. **Morphologic characteristics**
     a. **Size.** This cell (12–15 μm) is slightly smaller than a basophilic erythroblast.

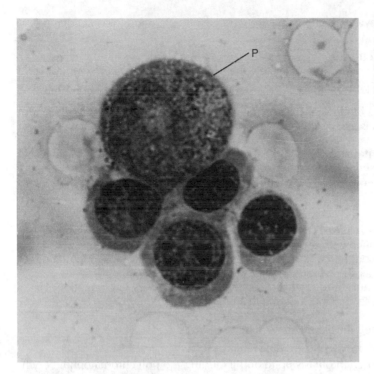

FIGURE 13-3. Promyelocyte (*P*) and cluster of four polychromatophilic erythroblasts. Note the granule-filled cytoplasm of the promyelocyte and the granule free cytoplasm of the erythroblasts.

   b. **Nucleus.** Coarse heterochromatin and alternating euchromatic regions form a characteristic "checkerboard" arrangement in a spherical nucleus, a useful identifying feature.
   c. **Cytoplasm.** The cytoplasm acquires a polychromatophilic staining character; that is, it is both acidophilic and basophilic. The staining reaction may combine to produce an overall gray or lilac color, or separate acidophilic (pink) and basophilic (blue) regions may be seen.

2. **Significance of cytoplasmic polychromatophilia**
   a. **Polyribosomes,** which appear earlier in erythropoiesis, are the **basophilic component** of the polychromatophilia.
   b. **Hemoglobin,** which accumulates in stainable amounts at this stage of erythropoiesis, is the **acidophilic component** of the polychromatophilia.
   c. The acidophilia of accumulating hemoglobin gradually dilutes the basophilia of the polyribosomes.

D. **Normoblast (orthochromatic erythroblast).** This cell is the last stage of erythropoiesis in which a nucleus can be identified.

1. **Morphologic characteristics**
   a. **Size.** The normoblast is smaller than a polychromatophilic erythroblast and slightly larger than a mature erythrocyte.
   b. **Nucleus.** The nucleus of the normoblast has become pyknotic and is intensely heterochromatic; little evidence of euchromatin is visible.
   c. **Cytoplasm.** The cytoplasm is acidophilic because of the high concentration of recently synthesized hemoglobin.

2. **Expulsion of the nucleus from the cell**
   a. The normoblast stage ends when the condensed, kernel-like nucleus is cast out of the cell.
   b. Even though a thin rim of cytoplasm and an enclosing membrane surround it, the expelled nucleus is not viable. It is phagocytized in the macrophage-rich hematopoietic compartment.

E. **Reticulocyte.** Reticulocytes are nearly mature red cells; they are found in circulating blood.

1. **Morphologic characteristics**
   a. **Size.** The reticulocyte is approximately the same size as the mature erythrocyte.
   b. **Nucleus.** The reticulocyte does not have a nucleus.
   c. **Cytoplasm**
      (1) After **routine blood stains,** the cytoplasm of the reticulocyte is strongly acidophilic and has essentially the same staining characteristics as the mature erythrocyte.
      (2) After **supravital staining** by brilliant cresyl blue, however, reticulocytes may be distinguished from mature erythrocytes. This procedure stains the remaining polyribosomes of the cell, producing the basophilic reticulum that names the cell.

2. **Circulating reticulocytes**
   a. Reticulocytes are released into the peripheral blood; therefore, developing red blood cells circulate before erythropoiesis is completed.
   b. In peripheral blood, reticulocytes comprise about 1% to 2% of the circulating red blood cells, as shown by supravital staining.
   c. Reticulocytes **mature into erythrocytes** after about 24 hours in circulation. Hemoglobin synthesis continues during this period.

F. **Kinetics of red blood cell development**

1. **Mitotic and postmitotic phases of erythropoiesis**
   a. Mitosis occurs in erythroblasts up to and including the polychromatophilic erythroblast.
   b. At each morphologically recognizable stage of development, an erythroblast divides several times.
   c. Normoblasts, reticulocytes, and mature erythrocytes are postmitotic cells. They do not divide.

2. **Distribution of the erythrocyte population**
   a. Virtually all erythrocytes are released into the circulation as soon as they are formed. Indeed, the cells that are normally released into circulation are reticulocytes, not fully mature cells, and erythropoiesis is completed as the cells circulate through the body.
   b. Bone marrow is not a site of red blood cell storage (compare this with neutrophils, IV F 2 b). The apparently mature erythrocytes observed in routinely stained bone marrow smears are either reticulocytes about to be released into the circulation or intravascular cells that were passing through the marrow at the time of biopsy.

3. **Duration of erythropoiesis and life-span of the mature erythrocyte**
   a. If an early basophilic erythroblast is tagged with a radioactive label, its progeny appear as mature erythrocytes in about 1 week.
   b. A mature erythrocyte functions in the peripheral blood for about 120 days before it is removed by macrophages in the spleen.

IV. **GRANULOPOIESIS.** The development of granulocytes (neutrophils, eosinophils, and basophils) passes through several well-defined stages. Emphasis is placed in this section on the development of **neutrophils** (see Figure 13-2).

A. **Myeloblast.** The myeloblast is the first developmental stage in granulopoiesis.

1. **Morphologic characteristics**
   a. **Size.** The myeloblast is a large cell (about 14–18 μm in diameter), approximately twice the diameter of an erythrocyte.

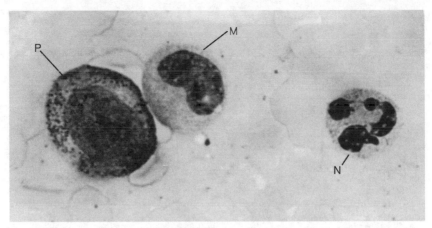

FIGURE 13-4. Promyelocyte (*P*), neutrophilic myelocyte or early metamyelocyte (*M*), and mature neutrophil (*N*). Note decreasing cell size and changes in nuclear structure.

      b. Nucleus. The nucleus is euchromatic and nucleoli are usually visible.
      c. Cytoplasm. The cytoplasm is agranular and slightly basophilic.
    2. The myeloblast is not an easily recognized cell. Discussions of granulopoiesis often begin, therefore, with the promyelocyte.

B. **Promyelocyte** (Figure 13-4; see also Figure 13-3)
    1. Morphologic characteristics
      a. Size. The promyelocyte (18–20 μm) is slightly larger than the myeloblast and is much larger than an erythrocyte.
      b. Nucleus. The nucleus is large and euchromatic, and nucleoli may be identified. No indentation of the nuclear surface is seen at this stage.
      c. Cytoplasmic granules
        (1) Azurophilic, or **primary, granules** are present in the cytoplasm of the promyelocyte and are an important indicator of this stage of granulopoiesis. These granules are stained by the azure dye that is one of the components of routinely used blood stains.
        (2) Specific granules are not present in promyelocytes.
    2. Characteristics of promyelocyte granules
      a. The azurophilic granules in promyelocytes (and in later granulocyte stages) are considered to be a type of **lysosome.**
      b. The granules contain both lysosomal enzymes and peroxidase. This peroxidase is often called **myeloperoxidase** to emphasize its presence in myeloid cells.
      c. Azurophilic granules are synthesized only by promyelocytes, and not by cells in later stages of granulopoiesis. Hence, the number of azurophilic granules per developing granulocyte diminishes with each cell division of the promyelocyte and its progeny.
    3. Multipotential nature of promyelocytes
      a. Promyelocytes cannot be divided into neutrophilic, eosinophilic, or basophilic subtypes.
      b. These subtypes of developing granulocytes become recognizable at the myelocyte stage, when specific granules appear in the cell.

C. **Myelocyte.** Myelocytes are a commonly encountered cell type in bone marrow. Neutrophilic myelocytes, eosinophilic myelocytes, and basophilic myelocytes may be recognized on the basis of the staining of their **specific granules.** These **secondary granules** are first seen at this stage of granulopoiesis.
    1. Morphologic characteristics

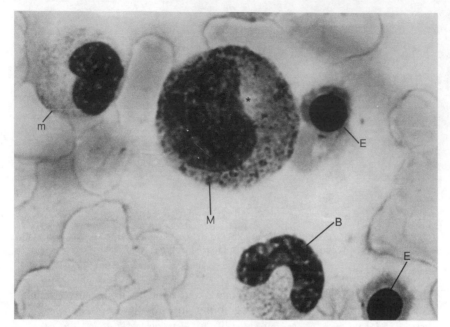

FIGURE 13-5. Neutrophilic myelocyte (*M*) showing an indented nucleus and a region from which the azurophilic granules are displaced by newly formed specific granules (∗), indicating the "dawn of neutrophilia." Also visible in the field are an older myelocyte (*m*), a band cell (*B*), and two late polychromatophilic erythroblasts (*E*).

    a. Size. The myelocyte is approximately the size of the mature granulocyte (12–15 μm).

    b. Nucleus

        (1) The nucleus acquires an indentation on its surface facing the interior of the cell (Figure 13-5).

        (2) The nucleus becomes more heterochromatic, and nucleoli are usually not visible.

    c. Cytoplasmic granules

        (1) Two populations of granules may be recognized in myelocytes.

            (a) Specific granules, with their characteristic staining reactions (neutrophilia, acidophilia, or basophilia), first appear in myelocytes.

            (b) Azurophilic granules form a decreasing fraction of the total number of granules in the developing granulocyte.

        (2) The azurophilic granules of eosinophils and basophils tend to be obscured by the larger, more numerous, more intensely stained, and more electron-opaque specific granules.

    d. The **"dawn of neutrophilia"** (see Figure 13-5) is a characteristic of the developing neutrophilic myelocyte.

        (1) This phenomenon is seen as a pale region in the center of the neutrophilic myelocyte, surrounded by stained azurophilic granules.

        (2) It occurs because an increasing number of very lightly stained (i.e., neutrophilic) specific granules in the region of the Golgi apparatus displaces the relatively intensely stained azurophilic granules.

  2. Specificity of secondary granules. Specific granules impart **functional specificity** as well as **morphologic specificity** to the developing granulocyte.

    a. Neutrophilic specific granules contain bacteriostatic and bactericidal substances such as lysozyme, lactoferrin, and alkaline phosphatase. These substances act in concert with the lysosomal azurophilic granules during the phagocytic function of neutrophils (see Chapter 12 III D 2).

    b. Eosinophilic specific granules are a specialized type of lysosome containing a paracrystalline, arginine-rich protein. This protein gives the granule its characteristic acidophilia, its refractility, and its unique fine structure (see Chapter 12 IV B 2).

  c. Basophilic specific granules contain histamine and heparan sulfate (see Chapter 12 V B 2).

D. **Metamyelocyte.** The metamyelocyte is the next developmental stage beyond the myelocyte.

  1. Nucleus
    a. The indentation of the nucleus deepens and the nucleus becomes **kidney-shaped.**
    b. The chromatin is slightly more condensed (heterochromatic) than in the myelocyte stage.

  2. Cytoplasmic granules
    a. A few hundred granules are found in the cytoplasm of a metamyelocyte, with **specific granules** outnumbering **azurophilic granules** by 3 or 4 to 1.
    b. No new azurophilic or specific granules are formed in the metamyelocyte or in later granulopoietic stages.

E. **Band cell.** The band cell (Figure 13-6) is developmentally closest to the mature neutrophil. There is no comparable stage for developing eosinophils and basophils.

  1. Morphologic characteristics
    a. Nuclear shape. The nucleus is a band-like, horseshoe-shaped structure. The

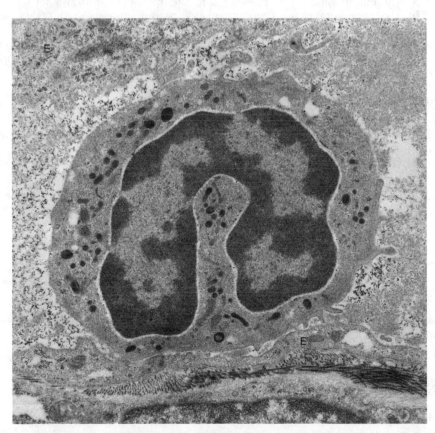

FIGURE 13-6. Electron micrograph of a band cell in peripheral circulation. Note the horseshoe-shaped nucleus and the cytoplasmic granules (azurophilic granules and specific granules cannot readily be differentiated from each other in the absence of a cytochemical reaction). *E* = endothelium.

band cell is also called a **stab cell** (fr. German, bar or rod) in recognition of the shape of its nucleus.

    b. Nuclear lobulation

        (1) The first indications of nuclear lobe formation are seen in the band cell.

        (2) Only when nuclear lobulation is complete and when, typically, 3–5 distinct segmented lobes are apparent is the cell considered a mature **polymorphonuclear leukocyte (PMN, neutrophil)** [see Chapter 12 III].

2. Circulating band cells. A small number of band cells may be found in normal blood smears. The number of band cells in peripheral blood is elevated under conditions that place demands on the neutrophil population.

F. | **Kinetics of neutrophil development**

1. Mitotic and postmitotic phases of granulopoiesis

    a. Cell divisions cease by the late myelocyte stage.

    b. Metamyelocytes, band cells, and mature neutrophils are postmitotic cells. They do not divide.

2. Distribution of the neutrophil population

    a. Approximately 15 times more mature neutrophils and nearly mature neutrophils (band cells) are found in the marrow than in the peripheral blood.

    b. Large numbers of neutrophils are stored in the marrow and enter the circulation in response to injury and infection.

    c. Neutrophils leave the circulation to enter the perivascular connective tissue.

3. Duration of granulopoiesis and life-span of a mature peripheral neutrophil

    a. The mitotic phase, from myeloblast to late myelocyte, lasts about 1 week.

    b. The postmitotic phase, from late myelocyte to mature neutrophil, also lasts about 1 week.

    c. Neutrophils circulate for 6 to 12 hours in peripheral blood before they enter the perivascular connective tissue. After 1 to 2 days in the perivascular compartment, neutrophils are phagocytized and destroyed by macrophages.

G. | **Numbers of neutrophils and erythropoietic cells in bone marrow**

1. Neutrophils are the predominant cell type in bone marrow (Table 13-1).

    a. Immature neutrophils (metamyelocytes and band cells) and mature neutrophils account for approximately 50% of the cells in a bone marrow smear.

    b. Erythropoietic cells, from early basophilic erythroblasts to normoblasts, account for only about 18% of the cells in a marrow smear.

2. Therefore, while erythrocytes vastly outnumber granulocytes in circulating blood, their immature forms are a distinct minority in the marrow compartment.

V. **MEGAKARYOCYTOPOIESIS. Megakaryocytes** are the bone marrow cells that give rise to **platelets** (see Chapter 12 VIII).

A. | **Megakaryoblast.** The megakaryoblast is an immature cell derived from the pluripotential CFC.

1. Morphologic characteristics. The megakaryoblast is a large cell (about 30 μm in diameter) with a nonlobulated nucleus.

2. No evidence is seen of platelet formation by the megakaryoblast.

B. | **Megakaryoblast–megakaryocyte transition**

1. Successive endomitoses occur in the megakaryoblast.

    a. DNA replicates and the number of chromosomes increases.

    b. Neither karyokinesis nor cytokinesis takes place, however, so that the chromo-

TABLE 13-1. Approximate Frequency of Hematopoietic
Cells in Normal Bone Marrow

Cells	Frequency (Range)
Erythropoietic cells	
Basophilic erythroblasts (including proerythroblasts)	3% (0.2%–4%)
Polychromatophilic erythroblasts	12% (6%–18%)
Normoblasts (orthochromatic erythroblasts)	3% (1%–5%)
Granulopoietic cells	
Promyelocytes (including myeloblasts)	3% (0.4%–5%)
Myelocytes	
Neutrophilic myelocytes	12% (5%–19%)
Eosinophilic myelocytes	1.5% (0.5%–3%)
Basophilic myelocytes	0.3% (0–0.5%)
Metamyelocytes (all types)	8% (4%–15%)
Band cells	24% (12%–34%)
Mature cells	
Neutrophils	18% (13%–20%)
Eosinophils	2% (0–6%)
Basophils	0.2% (0–5%)
Lymphocytes	10% (10%–16%)
Monocytes	2% (0–6%)
Plasma cells	0.3% (0–2%)

Modified from Beutler E, Lichtman MA, Coller BS, et al (eds): *Williams Hematology,* 5th ed. New York, McGraw Hill, 1995, p 18.

somes remain within one enlarging nucleus and ploidy increases from 2N to 32N or 64N.

2. Once the cell becomes large and polyploid, it is considered a megakaryocyte.

C. **Megakaryocyte.** This cell is the mature, platelet-forming cell (Figure 13-7). Chromosome replication does not occur in the megakaryocyte; it is a postendomitotic cell.

1. **Morphologic characteristics**
   a. **Size**
      (1) Megakaryocytes vary in size from 50 to 100 μm in diameter. The megakaryocyte is the largest cell in normal marrow (see Figure 13-7).
      (2) Both the cell and its nucleus have increased in size over the megakaryoblast, in proportion to the ploidy of the cell.
   b. **Cytoplasm.** As seen with the electron microscope, the superficial cytoplasm of the megakaryocyte is divided into small compartments by multiple invaginations of the plasma membrane. These invaginations are called **platelet demarcation channels** and they define future platelets.
   c. **Cell surface.** In smears of bone marrow examined by light microscopy, clusters of platelets, about to be released, are often seen at the surface of megakaryocytes.

2. **Platelet formation and release**
   a. Each cytoplasmic compartment, defined by platelet demarcation channels in the megakaryocyte, corresponds to a developing platelet.
   b. A platelet is released from the megakaryocyte when its surrounding demarcation channels become continuous with one another.
   c. Platelets are shed from the surface of the megakaryocyte as small, membrane-bounded cytoplasmic packets.

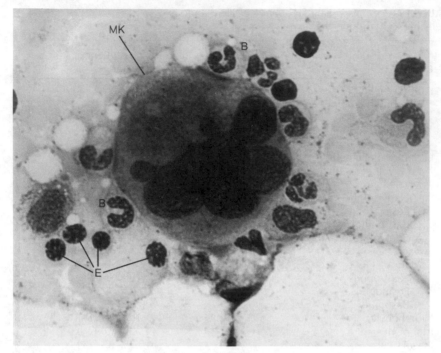

FIGURE 13-7. Megakaryocyte (*MK*) and several developing blood cells [erythroblasts (*E*) and band cells (*B*)]. Note the conspicuous size difference between the megakaryocyte and the other hematopoietic cells.

VI. MONOCYTOPOIESIS. Development of the monocyte–macrophage cell line takes place in three sites.

A. In **bone marrow,** the monocyte develops from the CFC through intermediate stages. These intermediates, called **monoblasts** and **promonocytes,** are not easily recognized.

B. In **peripheral blood,** monocytes can be recognized (see Chapter 12 VII A, B); in this location, however, they are not fully differentiated cells.

C. In **perivascular connective tissue,** final differentiation occurs.

   1. Monocytes leave the blood by crossing the vessel wall to enter the connective tissue around the blood vessel.

   2. In this environment, monocytes differentiate into several types of **mononuclear phagocytic cells** (e.g., connective tissue macrophages, Kupffer cells, osteoclasts).

   3. A macrophage is the final stage of development of a monocyte.

VII. MICROSCOPIC ANATOMY OF THE MARROW COMPARTMENT

A. **Red and yellow bone marrow.** Red marrow is hematopoietic, blood-forming marrow. Yellow marrow is largely adipose connective tissue.

   1. During the **neonatal period,** all bone marrow is red marrow.

   2. During **childhood,** yellow marrow gradually replaces red marrow in some sites (e.g., in the diaphyses of many bones). Red marrow persists in other areas (e.g., in the epiphyses of these same bones).

3. In the **adult,** distribution of red marrow is largely restricted to the sternum, to areas of the skull and vertebrae, and to certain regions of the pelvic bones.

4. Yellow marrow may transform to red marrow in times of stress to the hematopoietic system (e.g., post-hemorrhage).

B. **Blood vessels of the marrow compartment**

1. **Nutrient arteries** from the periosteum pass through the compact bone to enter the marrow space. The foramina through which they pass may be identified by eye on the surface of a bone.

2. **Longitudinal arteries** are formed by the division of a nutrient artery; they run parallel to the long axis of a bone.

3. **Radial arteries** are spoke-like branches that arise from longitudinal arteries to form thin-walled **sinusoids** in the hematopoietic tissue. Radial arteries also enter perforating (Volkmann) canals and, eventually, osteonal (haversian) canals to supply the bone tissue.

C. **Cell associations in red bone marrow**

1. Histologic sections of bone marrow show the following relationships.
   a. **Nests of erythroblasts and myelocytes.** These developing blood cells are often seen clumped into nests or islets. The cells clump when mitotic events increase their numbers and the daughter cells remain restricted to the immediate vicinity.
   b. **Normoblasts (orthochromatic erythroblasts) and macrophages.** Macrophages are found in close association with nests of normoblasts, where they phagocytize nuclei expelled by the normoblasts during erythropoiesis.
   c. **Megakaryocytes and the sinusoidal wall.** Megakaryocytes are found in close proximity to the walls of marrow blood capillaries (i.e., sinusoids); this facilitates the release of platelets into the blood stream.

2. During preparation of a bone marrow smear, these normal cellular relationships are demolished.

Chapter 14

Cardiovascular System

I. **INTRODUCTION.** The cardiovascular system transports gases, nutrients, and waste products. Pressure is maintained in the system largely by the pumping of the heart. Materials being transported are contained in blood vessels and lymphatic vessels.

II. **THE HEART**

A. **Anatomy.** The heart is a **four-chambered muscular pump** that is functionally connected to the major blood vessels (Figure 14-1).

1. **Chambers of the heart.** The chambers of the heart and their associated vessels are as follows:
   a. The **right atrium** receives systemic venous blood from the two venae cavae.
   b. The **right ventricle** receives blood from the right atrium and pumps blood to the lungs via the pulmonary trunk and arteries.
   c. The **left atrium** receives oxygenated blood from the lungs via the four pulmonary veins.
   d. The **left ventricle** receives blood from the left atrium and pumps blood into the aorta for systemic circulation.

2. **Cardiac valves.** Certain cardiac orifices are guarded by valves—**flap-like extensions of the endocardium** that prevent backflow of blood.
   a. There are **four major cardiac valves.**
      (1) **Atrioventricular (AV) valves**
         (a) The **tricuspid valve** is between the right atrium and right ventricle.
         (b) The **mitral (bicuspid) valve** is between the left atrium and left ventricle.
      (2) **Semilunar valves**
         (a) The **aortic valve** is located at the origin of the aorta from the left ventricle.
         (b) The **pulmonary valve** is located at the origin of the pulmonary trunk from the right ventricle.
   b. A slight, **valve-like modification** of the endocardium occurs at the **entrance of the inferior vena cava into the right atrium.** This "valve" is physiologically incompetent. No comparable valve-like modification occurs at the entrance of the superior vena cava into the right atrium.
   c. There are no valves where the four pulmonary veins enter the left atrium.

B. **Cardiac tissues**

1. **Heart wall.** The wall of the heart is composed of **three layers.**
   a. **Endocardium.** The endocardium is the innermost layer of the wall of the heart. The thickness of the endocardium varies inversely with the thickness of the adjacent myocardium. The endocardium is thinnest in the left ventricle and thickest in the atria. The layers of the endocardium are:
      (1) **Endothelium.** The endothelial layer is a simple squamous epithelium that is continuous with the endothelium of blood vessels and is in contact with the blood.
      (2) **Fibroelastic tissue.** A fibroelastic layer composed of collagen fibers, elastic tissue, and some smooth muscle subtends the endothelium. The fibroelastic layer is usually thicker in atria than in ventricles.
      (3) **Subendocardial connective tissue.** The subendocardial connective tissue layer is the deepest part of the endocardium and it merges with the perimy-

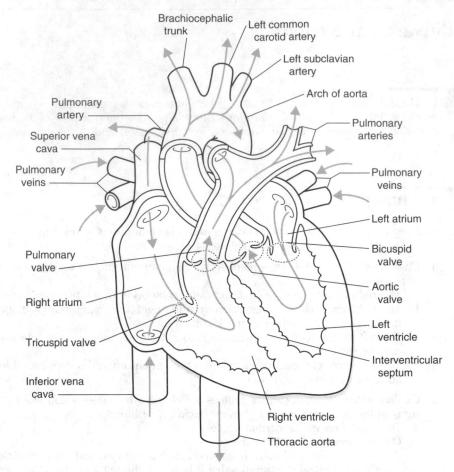

FIGURE 14-1. Mammalian heart, diagram. Chambers of the heart, major blood vessels, valves, and direction of blood flow are labeled. (Adapted with permission from Abeloff D: Medical Illustration Library. General Anatomy Collection 1 & 2. Baltimore, Williams & Wilkins, 1994.)

sial and endomysial connective tissue of the myocardium. The impulse conducting system of the heart is located in the subendocardium (see II C 4 b).

  b. **Myocardium.** The myocardium is the **contractile layer** of the heart wall and is formed by cardiac muscle, connective tissue, and an extensive vasculature.

   (1) The myocardium varies considerably in thickness. It is thinnest in the atria, much thicker in the right ventricle, and thickest in the left ventricle.

   (2) Cardiac muscle is **striated muscle.**

   (a) The individual muscle cells, with their centrally placed nuclei, are joined end-to-end by intercalated disks into long, branching fibers (see Chapter 7).

   (b) A typical histologic section of the myocardium shows layers and bundles of interlaced fibers oriented in all planes.

   (3) Atrial muscle cells also have an endocrine function that is usually not shared by ventricular muscle cells. **Atrial natriuretic factor (ANF)** is a polypeptide hormone synthesized by cells of the atrial myocardium.

   (a) ANF is a diuretic that inhibits the secretion of renin and aldosterone.

   (b) ANF is also synthesized by ventricular cells in states of cardiac hypertrophy and during embryonic development of the heart.

  c. **Epicardium.** The epicardium is the **outermost layer** of the wall of the heart and is the **visceral layer of the pericardium.**

      (1) Histologically, the epicardium is formed by a simple squamous epithelium (mesothelium) and a layer of connective tissue.

      (2) The connective tissue space of the epicardium may be expanded considerably by the deposition of **adipose tissue.**

        (a) Fat provides a protective cushion for the heart.

        (b) Maximum thickness of the epicardium is seen in the fat-filled coronary sulcus, between the atria and ventricles.

2. Cardiac skeleton. This part of the heart is formed by **dense irregular connective tissue.**

    a. Structure

      (1) The connective tissue skeleton encircles and supports the four cardiac valves.

        (a) These four circular openings in the fibrous cardiac skeleton are the **annuli fibrosi.**

        (b) The connective tissue stroma that forms most of the interior of the cardiac valves is continuous with the connective tissue of the cardiac skeleton.

      (2) The cardiac skeleton separates the atrial level of the heart from the ventricular level.

        (a) The myocardium of the atria and the myocardium of the ventricles are distinct and separate muscular compartments (i.e., muscle fibers of the working myocardium are not shared between atria and ventricles).

        (b) The connective tissue of the skeleton is penetrated, however, by the common AV bundle (bundle of His) of the impulse conduction system.

    b. Function

      (1) The cardiac skeleton supports the patency of the AV orifices and the major arterial points of outflow. Deformation of these openings would jeopardize the competency of the cardiac valves.

      (2) The connective tissue skeleton also provides attachment points for cardiac muscle.

C. **Impulse-generation and impulse-conduction system.** Modified cardiac muscle cells generate the stimulus for each heartbeat and conduct the stimulus to various regions of the myocardium. The components of the system are as follows:

1. Sinoatrial (SA) node. The SA node, located near the junction of the superior vena cava and right atrium, is the **pacemaker of the heart.** It is a mass of small (approximately 5 μm in diameter), fusiform-shaped cardiac muscle cells, partially isolated from the working myocardium by a connective tissue sheath.

    a. The **electrical events that initiate the heartbeat originate in the SA node.**

    b. The impulse sweeps from the SA node, across the atrial wall (by way of regular muscle fibers of the working myocardium), to the AV node.

2. Atrioventricular (AV) node. The AV node is located in the lower part of the interatrial septum and **receives impulses originating from the SA node.** The cells of the AV node resemble the cells of the SA node.

3. The AV bundle (bundle of His). The AV bundle originates from the AV node and penetrates the cardiac skeleton to enter the ventricular compartment of the heart. The bundle divides into right and left branches that travel through the subendocardium on either side of the interventricular septum.

    a. Proximally, the AV bundle is formed by cells that resemble the modified cardiac muscle cells of the SA and AV nodes.

    b. Distally, the bundle is formed by Purkinje fibers.

4. Purkinje fibers

    a. Purkinje fibers are also modified cardiac muscle cells but are conspicuously larger than the fibers of the working myocardium (Figure 14-2).

      (1) Purkinje fibers contain relatively few myofibrils but large amounts of glycogen.

      (2) These characteristics give Purkinje fibers a pale appearance by hematoxylin-

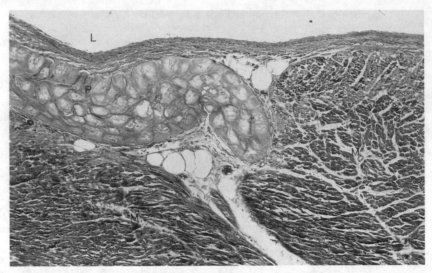

FIGURE 14-2. Endocardium and myocardium, light micrograph. Iron hematoxylin stain. Purkinje fibers (*P*) are visible in the subendocardium. The large size and pale appearance of the Purkinje fibers contrast with the nearby muscle fibers of the working myocardium (*M*). *L* = ventricular lumen.

eosin (H&E) staining, compared with working myocardial cells that are smaller and stain more darkly.

b. The conduction system of Purkinje fibers ramifies in the subendocardium. At its most distal point, the fibers leave the subendocardium to terminate in close association with regular cardiac muscle cells.

D. **Regulation of the heart by the nervous system**

1. The **autonomic nervous system** influences the **heart rate.** Both parasympathetic and sympathetic fibers end near the SA and AV nodes.
   a. Autonomic stimulation modifies—but does not initiate—the heartbeat. The heartbeat is initiated by the cells of the SA node and is transmitted to the myocardium by the impulse conduction system.
   b. Parasympathetic (vagal) stimulation decreases the heart rate and sympathetic stimulation increases the heart rate.
   c. Cardiac muscle cells have an intrinsic beat that appears during embryonic development. This intrinsic beat is coordinated by the impulse-generating and impulse-conducting system.

2. **Autonomic sensory receptors**
   a. The **carotid sinus** is a **baroreceptor** (pressure receptor) that affects cardiac function.
      (1) Structure
         (a) The carotid sinus is a dilation in each internal carotid artery, close to its origin from the common carotid artery.
         (b) Histologically, the sinus is characterized by an unusually thin tunica media and a correspondingly thick, extensively innervated tunica adventitia.
      (2) Function. A carotid sinus is sensitive to blood pressure changes and the associated sensory nerve fibers convey information to the central nervous system.
   b. The **carotid body** is a **chemoreceptor** that affects cardiac function.
      (1) Structure. The carotid body is a mass of ovoid cells, sinusoidal blood vessels, and nerve fibers in the wall of the internal carotid artery, close to its origin from the common carotid artery. Its histologic structure resembles that of an endocrine organ.

(2) **Function.** The carotid body is a sensory receptor that conveys information to the central nervous system concerning blood pH and concentrations of oxygen and carbon dioxide.

III. **GENERAL STRUCTURE OF BLOOD VESSELS.** Three layers are identifiable in the walls of most blood vessels: the **tunica intima,** the **tunica media,** and the **tunica adventitia** (Figure 14-3). The layers, or tunics, tend to be more obvious in arteries than in veins. The three layers are not present in capillaries.

A. **Tunica intima.** The tunica intima is the luminal, or innermost, layer of a blood vessel.

1. **Endothelium** forms the **luminal boundary of the vessel wall** and is continuous with the endothelium found throughout the cardiovascular system. The endothelium is in contact with the blood.
   a. **Structure.** The endothelium is a **simple squamous epithelium.** Very rarely, the endothelium is formed by cuboidal or columnar cells.
      (1) The squamous endothelial cells are usually elongated in the direction of blood flow.
      (2) A basal lamina is found along the deep surface of the endothelial cell and loose connective tissue fills the subendothelial space.
   b. **Functions.** In addition to forming the physical interior wall of the blood vessel, endothelial cells are also **secretory cells.**
      (1) Various components of the extracellular matrix, such as **collagens** (types II, IV, and V) and **laminin** are synthesized and secreted by endothelial cells. Other substances are synthesized and secreted intravascularly, including **von Willebrand factor,** which functions in platelet aggregation at the site of vascular injury, and **endothelin I,** which is a potent hypertensive agent.
      (2) Most synthetic and secretory activity of endothelial cells appears to be **constitutive** (i.e., secretions are not stored in the cytoplasm but are secreted continuously). An exception is the storage of von Willebrand factor in the **Weibel-Palade bodies** of arterial endothelial cells.

2. An **internal elastic lamina** (elastica interna, internal elastic membrane) is the deepest component of the tunica intima and forms the boundary between the tunica intima and the tunica media.

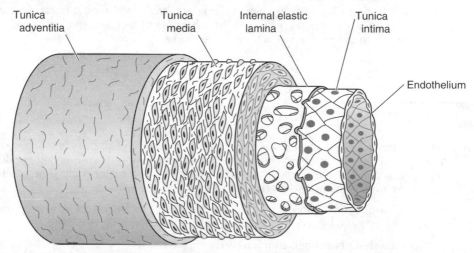

FIGURE 14-3. Muscular artery, diagram. The three tunics of the arterial wall and the characteristic internal elastic lamina are shown. (Adapted with permission from Junqueira LC, Carneiro J, Kelley RO: *Basic Histology,* 8th ed. Norwalk, CT, Appleton & Lange, 1995, p 203.)

    a. This layer of elastic tissue varies considerably among blood vessel types. The internal elastic lamina is distinct in muscular arteries, it is less obvious in elastic arteries, and usually it is indistinct in veins.

    b. The internal elastic lamina of a muscular artery is seen as a **wavy, hyaline layer** and is an important histologic characteristic of muscular arteries.

B. **Tunica media.** The tunica media is prominent in arteries and indistinct in veins.

  1. Arteries. The tunica media of an artery is the **thickest layer of the vessel wall** and is formed mainly by smooth muscle cells and the elastic tissue components secreted by them.

    a. In elastic arteries, fenestrated lamellae of elastic tissue are the most obvious component of the tunica media. The smooth muscle cells are visible in the interlamellar space.

    b. In muscular arteries, the smooth muscle cells are the predominant component of the tunica media. Some elastic tissue is visible as well.

  2. Veins. The media of a vein generally is **thin and inconspicuous,** and is formed by varying amounts of connective tissue and smooth muscle.

C. **Tunica adventitia.** The tunica adventitia is the outermost layer in the wall of a blood vessel.

  1. This is primarily a **connective tissue** layer but smooth muscle may also be present, especially in the tunica adventitia of veins.

  2. In **veins,** the tunica adventitia is the **thickest and most prominent layer.**

  3. In **arteries,** the tunica adventitia is **inconspicuous** in comparison with the relatively thick tunica media. The arterial tunica adventitia merges with perivascular connective tissue (i.e., fascia).

  4. An **external elastic lamina** may be noted in some **arterial vessels** and, when present, forms a distinct boundary between the media and adventitia. An external lamina usually is much less distinct than its internal counterpart.

  5. The **vasa vasorum** are the blood vasculature of the vessel wall and are most obvious in the tunica adventitia.

    a. These are the small arterial or venous vessels commonly observed in sections of large veins and less frequently in large arteries.

    b. Because the blood vessel itself is an organ, it has its own blood supply, in addition to receiving some oxygen and nutrients from the blood it contains. The largest vasa vasorum are seen in the adventitia of a vessel; smaller branches penetrate the media and approach the intima.

IV. THE ARTERIAL VESSELS

A. **Elastic arteries.** The **largest diameter** arteries in the body (e.g., the aorta and common carotid arteries) are elastic arteries. These large vessels are also called **conducting arteries** because they conduct blood from the heart to major body regions. Elastic arteries in adult humans vary from 0.5 to 5 cm in diameter.

  1. The elasticity of the arterial wall enables the vessel to absorb the systolic pressure and to maintain, by recoil, a relatively high pressure during diastole.

  2. Distinguishing histologic characteristics

    a. Fifty or more **fenestrated lamellae,** or sheets, of **elastic tissue** are concentrically arranged in the tunica media. Adjacent lamellae are connected by septa and strands of elastic tissue.

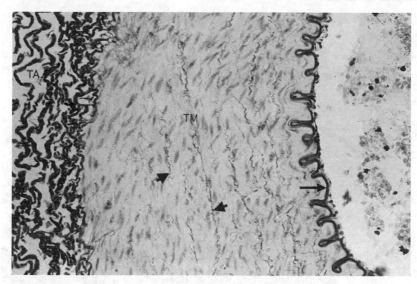

FIGURE 14-4. Muscular artery, light micrograph, elastic tissue stain. The internal elastic lamina (*arrow*) is distinct and is folded because of contraction of the smooth muscle in the vessel wall. The tunica media (*TM*) is formed mainly by smooth muscle but some delicate fibrils and lamellae of elastic tissue may also be identified (*arrowheads*). The abundant elastic tissue of the tunica adventitia (*TA*) contrasts with the sparse elastic tissue of the tunica media.

      b. Fibroblasts, smooth muscle cells, and extracellular matrix occupy the spaces between elastic lamellae in the tunica media.

B. **Muscular arteries** (Figure 14-4). The arterial vessels that **vary most widely in diameter** are muscular arteries. Muscular arteries are also called **distributing arteries** because they distribute blood from the elastic (conducting) artery to specific body regions.

  1. Muscular arteries encompass a family of blood vessels ranging from approximately 0.3 mm to 1 cm in diameter.
    a. Larger muscular arteries are named (e.g., radial artery), but smaller ones are unnamed.
    b. Muscular arteries usually travel in connective tissue accompanied by a corresponding vein, a nerve, and often a lymphatic vessel.

  2. Muscular arteries control the distribution of blood to different body regions by contracting or relaxing the smooth muscle that is the predominant tissue in the vessel wall.

  3. **Distinguishing histologic characteristics**
    a. An **internal elastic lamina** usually is conspicuous, and is identifiable in even the smallest muscular arteries.
    b. Varying numbers of **layers of smooth muscle** form the tunica media.
      (1) Larger muscular arteries have 30–40 layers of smooth muscle forming the tunica media. The smallest muscular arteries have only 3–4 layers of smooth muscle.
      (2) Small amounts of elastic tissue may be demonstrated between the muscle cells of the media by the use of elastin-specific stains.
    c. The fusiform smooth muscle cells are generally oriented in a tight spiral perpendicular to the long axis of the vessel.

C. **Arterioles** (Figure 14-5). These are the **terminal vessels** of the arterial system. Arterioles are **resistance and regulating vessels.** They are the site of **greatest resistance to blood flow,** and they **regulate blood flow to capillary beds.**

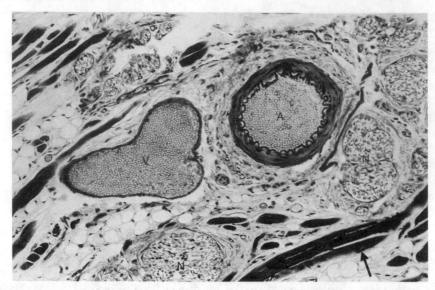

FIGURE 14-5. An arteriole and a venule, light micrograph, Mallory trichrome stain. Both the arteriole (*A*) and the venule (*V*) are filled with blood cells. Note the internal elastic lamina of the arteriole, the arteriolar tunica media formed by just two layers of smooth muscle, and the relatively thin wall of the venule. Nearby are bundles of nerve fibers (*N*) and skeletal muscle fibers (*arrow*).

1. The larger arterioles are 0.2–0.4 mm (200–400 μm) in diameter; the smallest arterioles are approximately 50 μm in diameter.

2. No clear demarcation is seen between a very small muscular artery and a large arteriole. Structurally, they merge imperceptibly.

3. At this level, also, arterioles are usually in close association with a venule, a nerve, and a lymphatic vessel.

4. **Distinguishing histologic characteristics**
   a. The tunica media of an arteriole is formed by one or two layers of smooth muscle.
   b. An internal elastic lamina is seen in larger arterioles.
   c. The lumen of the arteriole generally is open (i.e., the vessel is not collapsed). The patent arteriole contrasts with the venule, which is generally collapsed, unless filled with blood.

5. **Metarterioles** are the smallest diameter arterioles (Figure 14-6).
   a. Distinguishing histologic characteristics of these very small arterioles are **small size** and a **discontinuous layer of smooth muscle.**
      (1) Any single smooth muscle cell usually completely encircles the vessel.
      (2) Gaps exist between adjacent muscle cells along the length of the metarteriole, thus producing a discontinuous layer of smooth muscle.
   b. Metarterioles are the smallest diameter arterial vessels immediately proximal to a capillary bed. They are **precapillary sphincters** and regulate blood flow to the capillaries.

V. CAPILLARIES

A. **Distribution.** Capillaries are the **smallest diameter vessels** in the cardiovascular system (Figure 14-7). Cumulatively, however, capillaries are the longest segment of the system.

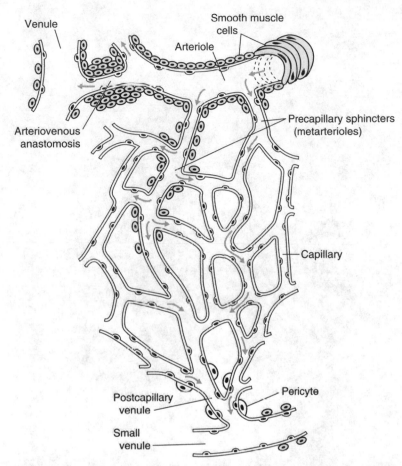

FIGURE 14-6. Diagram illustrating the relationships between arterioles, metarterioles, arteriovenous anastomoses, capillaries, and venules. Note the arrangement and density of smooth muscle and pericytes. (Adapted with permission from Kelly DE, Wood RL, Enders AC: *Bailey's Textbook of Microscopic Anatomy*, 18th ed. Baltimore, Williams & Wilkins, 1984, p. 388.)

1. The luminal diameter of a capillary varies from 4–10 μm. The elasticity of red blood cells, which average 7–8 μm in diameter, enables them to pass through even the smallest capillaries.

2. The human body contains approximately 50,000 miles of capillaries. Any one capillary, however, is only 0.5–1.0 mm long between its metarteriole supply and its postcapillary venule drainage.

3. The concentration of capillaries per square millimeter reflects the metabolic activity of the tissue. Capillary concentrations range from 2000/mm² in myocardium to 50/mm² in dermis.

B. **Function.** Capillaries are well suited for the exchange of gases and metabolites between cells and the blood stream. Capillaries, and postcapillary venules, are also called **exchange vessels.** Exchange is facilitated by:

1. Their thin walls, often perforated by fenestrae (fenestrated capillaries) or by relatively wide clefts (discontinuous capillaries)

2. Their close proximity to metabolically active cells and tissue spaces

3. Their high ratio of capillary volume to endothelial surface area, which favors the movement of materials across the vessel wall

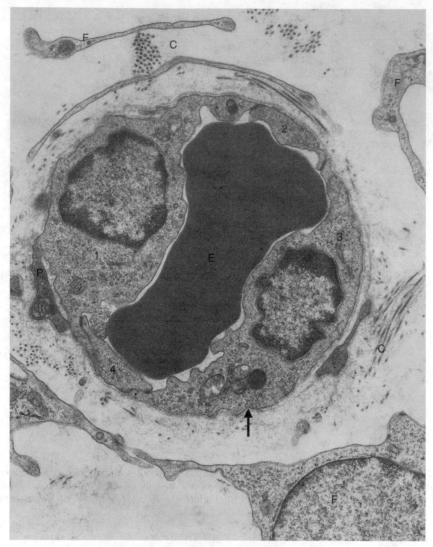

FIGURE 14-7. Capillary, transmission electron micrograph. An example of a continuous (non-fenestrated), thick-walled capillary. The circumference of the vessel is formed by portions of four endothelial cells (*1–4*). Nuclei are seen in two of the endothelial cells (*1* and *3*). An erythrocyte (*E*) conforms to and nearly completely fills the irregular lumen of the capillary. Note the fibroblast and fibroblast processes (*F*), part of a pericyte (*P*), basal lamina (*arrow*), and some small bundles of collagen fibrils (*C*).

C. **Components of the capillary wall.** The "tunics" characteristic of the walls of larger blood vessels are not found in the thin walls of capillaries.

1. **Endothelial cells** are the main cellular component of the capillary wall.
    a. One squamous endothelial cell may form the entire circumference of the capillary (and form a junction with itself). Alternatively, more than one endothelial cell may be visible in a transverse or oblique section of the vessel, forming the wall of the capillary (see Figure 14-7).
    b. A basal lamina subtends the adluminal surface of the endothelial cells.

2. **Pericytes** are often closely associated with capillaries.
    a. **Distribution**
        (1) Pericytes are most frequently found at the venous end of the capillary bed, and also extend onto the postcapillary venules (see Figure 14-6).

(2) Pericytes do not form a continuous layer around a capillary. Most capillaries show no evidence of an associated pericyte.

b. Histologic characteristics. Pericytes have characteristics of both smooth muscle cells and endothelial cells.

(1) Scanning electron microscopy reveals that the long processes of the pericyte grasp the vessel in an octopus-like manner. This contrasts with the precise, parallel arrangement of smooth muscle in the tunica media of larger vessels.

(2) The basal lamina of the pericyte usually fuses with the basal lamina of its associated capillary (or venule).

(3) In some longitudinal sections of a vessel, a single perivascular cell may show the characteristics of both a pericyte and a typical smooth muscle cell.

c. Function

(1) Pericytes may be contractile cells that affect blood flow through the capillary.

(2) There is evidence that pericytes differentiate to smooth muscle cells during blood vessel growth and during repair after injury to a vessel.

D. **Classification of capillaries.** The structure of capillaries varies from tissue to tissue, and from organ to organ. Indeed, a capillary may vary in structure from its arterial to its venous end.

1. Continuous capillaries are found principally in tissues and organs in which gases, electrolytes, and small soluble metabolites are exchanged (e.g., central nervous system, muscle, lung). These are capillaries in which the endothelium is not perforated by fenestrae (pores).

a. The capillary wall appears as two cell membranes enclosing a thin layer of cytoplasm and, if included in the plane of section, a nucleus and other organelles.

b. At least one junctional area is visible around the circumference of a capillary; at this site, the vessel wall is sealed by a tight junction.

c. The squamous endothelial cells forming the capillary wall may range from exceedingly thin (0.1 μm) to relatively thick (0.3 μm). This group of capillaries can therefore be subdivided into **continuous thin** and **continuous thick** capillaries.

2. Fenestrated capillaries are found principally in organs in which large volumes of fluids and electrolytes, as well as large molecules, are exchanged (e.g., endocrine glands, kidney, gastrointestinal mucosa). In these capillaries, the endothelial wall is pierced by fenestrae that provide a channel across the vessel wall.

a. Fenestrae may originate when a pinocytotic vesicle spans the narrow cytoplasmic layer of the squamous endothelial cell and simultaneously opens on both surfaces of the endothelial wall.

b. A thin, nonmembranous diaphragm may span a fenestra. This may be a remnant of the glycocalyx enclosed when the vesicle formed.

3. Sinusoids, or **discontinuous capillaries** are found principally in organs in which very large molecules, such as plasma proteins (e.g., the liver) and cells (e.g., hematopoietic tissue and the spleen), are exchanged.

a. Histologic characteristics. Sinusoids have a much wider luminal diameter than the other capillary types. The endothelial wall of a sinusoid is punctuated by wide gaps, or clefts, and offers little impediment to the exchange of materials between the blood vessel lumen and the perivascular space.

b. Hepatic sinusoids (see Chapter 26)

(1) In the liver, the basal lamina is indistinct at the subendothelial surface and the lamina is absent from the wide gaps in the sinusoidal wall.

(2) Blood cells are contained within the discontinuous endothelium-delimited vascular space of hepatic sinusoids.

c. Splenic sinusoids (see Chapter 18)

(1) In the spleen, reticular fibers form hoop-like rings around the discontinuous endothelium. The ring, however, is continuous across the wide gaps in the sinusoidal wall.

(2) Blood cells appear to move with ease from the lumen of splenic sinusoids, across the discontinuous sinusoidal endothelium, into the splenic cords.

VI. THE VENOUS VESSELS

A. **Venules** are small diameter, thin-walled vessels (see Figure 14-5).

1. **Classification**
   a. **Postcapillary venules** drain capillary beds.
      (1) No abrupt transition in structure occurs between a capillary and a venule.
         (a) Larger capillaries are not easily distinguished from smaller, postcapillary venules.
         (b) Some histologists therefore refer to the larger, capillary-like vessels as **venous capillaries.**
      (2) The diameter of the capillary gradually increases to about 10–30 μm.
      (3) The number of pericytes associated with the vessel increases, as well.
   b. **Collecting venules** are larger diameter (30–50 μm) venules.
      (1) A collecting venule joins postcapillary venules to a muscular venule.
      (2) A collecting venule is invested by a complete layer of pericytes. Postcapillary venules and collecting venules are also termed **pericytic venules.**
   c. **Muscular venules** are the largest diameter (50–200 μm) venules.
      (1) Pericytes are replaced by one or two layers of smooth muscle cells.
      (2) A muscular venule generally is accompanied by an arteriole and a nerve.

2. **Venule function**
   a. Physiologically, postcapillary venules and capillaries appear to have similar functions in the normal exchange of fluid, solutes, and cells between the vascular and perivascular compartments.
   b. In inflammation, however, the postcapillary venules are the major site of vascular leakage. During the inflammatory response, initiated by the release of vasoactive agents from mast cells, plasma and leukocytes move rapidly from the venule lumen to the perivascular space.

B. **General characteristics of postvenule veins** (i.e., small, medium, and large veins). Much variation is encountered in the histologic structure of veins, depending on size of the vein and location in the body.

1. Generally, veins have larger diameters and thinner walls than accompanying arterial vessels.

2. Like venules, veins are often collapsed, to varying degrees, compared with the patent accompanying artery.

3. The three tunics—the intima, media, and adventitia—become evident in small veins but are less distinct than in the wall of a small artery.
   a. The tunica adventitia of a vein is the thickest layer in the vessel wall.
   b. The tunica media may be difficult to discern as a separate layer in the walls of some veins.

4. Some veins have valves (see VI E); arterial vessels do not have valves.

C. **Small and medium veins**

1. **Small veins** are less than 1 mm in diameter and are continuous with muscular venules, which they closely resemble, except for size.

2. **Medium veins** range in diameter from 1 to 10 mm. Most named veins of all regions of the body fall into this category (e.g., basilic vein).

    a. The **tunica media** of a medium vein is formed by a few layers of smooth muscle, usually oriented perpendicular to the long axis of the vessel.

    b. The **tunica adventitia** of a medium vein contains longitudinally oriented smooth muscle, generally arranged not as a complete layer but as separate bundles of muscle cells.

    c. The **adventitia is thicker than the media.** Often, the junction between the two tunics is not obvious.

D. **Large veins**

    1. This category of vessel includes veins larger than 1 cm in diameter (e.g., the venae cavae).

    2. The **tunica intima** and the **tunica media** of large veins are **thin and not sharply delineated** from one another.

        a. A **fragmented internal elastic lamina** sometimes can be identified between the intima and media. More often, however, there is no clear evidence of this lamina.

        b. The media contains only a small amount of connective tissue and circularly oriented smooth muscle. Cardiac muscle may extend into the media of the venae cavae and pulmonary veins.

    3. The **tunica adventitia** of large veins is thick and forms most of the mass of the wall of the vein.

        a. Bundles of longitudinally oriented smooth muscle cells, collagen, and elastic fibers form the adventitia.

        b. The smooth muscle does not form a continuous layer in the adventitia. The smooth muscle bundles are separated by connective tissue.

        c. **Vasa vasorum** are most commonly encountered in the tunica adventitia of large veins.

E. **Valves.** Valves are characteristic of veins in which **blood moves against gravity.**

    1. **Function and distribution.** Valves **allow flow of blood toward the heart and prevent flow in the opposite direction.**

        a. Veins of the lower extremity have well-developed valves.

        b. Valves are generally lacking in cerebral and visceral veins.

    2. **Histologic characteristics.** Valves are derived from the **intima** of the vein.

        a. A valve is seen in a histologic section as **two thin semilunar flaps,** or cusps, each covered by endothelium and enclosing a thin connective tissue stroma.

        b. The valve extends into the lumen of the vein and its free edges project toward the heart.

VII. **PORTAL BLOOD VESSELS.** A portal system of circulation **begins and ends in capillaries.** Either an artery or a vein may join the two capillary beds.

A. **Function.** Portal systems are specialized for the **efficient absorption, transport, and release of materials.**

B. **Specific portal systems.** Portal systems are found in the following locations:

    1. The **hepatic portal vein** functions between the intestine and the liver.

    2. The **hypothalamic–hypophyseal portal system** functions between the hypothalamus and pars distalis.

    3. The **glomerulus–cortical tubule portal system** functions between the renal corpuscle and tubules of some nephrons.

C. The **cascading blood flow in most endocrine organs,** involving only capillaries and postcapillary venules, functions as a portal system that carries hormones from one region of the organ to another region.

VIII. ARTERIOVENOUS ANASTOMOSIS (AVA)

A. An arteriovenous anastomosis is an arrangement of blood vessels and modifications of the vessel wall that allows the **shunting of arteriolar blood directly to venules,** thus **bypassing capillaries.**

  1. Function and distribution. AVAs are commonly found in areas of the skin, such as the fingertips and tip of the nose. This vascular arrangement assists thermoregulation by shunting blood away from cool surfaces to prevent heat loss. AVAs are also found in erectile tissue.

  2. Structure. The arteriole of an AVA is highly coiled and is enclosed by a connective tissue capsule. The tunica media of the arteriole has an unusually thick layer of smooth muscle and is richly innervated.

B. AVA shunt mechanism

  1. The smooth muscle of the arteriole's tunica media has a sphincter-like function. **Contraction** of this smooth muscle directs blood to a capillary bed, causing subsequent **heat loss.** This is the "normal" state of the vasculature.

  2. Relaxation of this smooth muscle allows arteriolar blood to flow directly to a venule, bypassing the capillary bed, with subsequent **conservation of body heat.**

IX. LYMPHATIC VESSELS.
The lymphatic vessels are the part of the circulatory system that convey lymph, an ultrafiltrate of blood plasma, back to the blood.

A. Functions of the lymphatic vessels

  1. In the general circulation:
    a. Lymphatic vessels return to the blood vascular system fluid and plasma proteins that have leaked from small-diameter blood vessels into the perivascular connective tissue.
    b. Lymphatic vessels transport absorbed molecules, usually proteins and lipids, that are too large to enter the blood capillaries of the intestinal mucosa.

  2. In the immune system:
    a. The lymphatic vessels convey antigens to lymph nodes, stimulating an immune response in the nodes. Immunoglobins (antibodies) synthesized in the nodes are then transported into the blood vascular system.
    b. The lymphatic vascular system provides avenues of transit for lymphocytes that move between various body compartments during immune surveillance.

B. **Lymphatic capillaries,** the smallest vessels of the lymph vascular system, function as a **drainage system** for the removal of fluids from tissue spaces.

  1. They originate in connective tissue spaces as delicate, endothelium-lined tubules.

  2. Lymphatic capillaries are structurally similar to blood capillaries. However, **a fragmented, indistinct basal lamina** distinguishes lymphatic capillaries from blood capillaries, which are completely enclosed by a basal lamina.

  3. Anchoring filaments have been described in lymphatic capillaries.

    a. These are fine filaments that extend from the basal surface of the endothelial cell of the lymphatic capillary into the perivascular connective tissue.

    b. Anchoring filaments may **ensure patency of the vessel** during periods of mildly elevated tissue pressure (e.g., inflammation, exercise).

C. **Larger lymphatic vessels** of the lymph vascular system **resemble veins** of the blood vascular system.

  1. A tunica intima, tunica media, and tunica adventitia form the wall of the lymphatic vessel. These layers are even less distinct in lymphatics than in veins.

  2. In a histologic section, one or more lymphatic vessels are often seen accompanying a small muscular artery (or arteriole) and a small vein (or venule).

  3. The following criteria may be used to **distinguish between lymphatic vessels and veins:**

    a. Lymphatic vessels would be expected to be **free of cells** or might **contain lymphocytes;** veins would be expected to contain peripheral blood. Some red blood cells, however, may enter a lymphatic after death, at autopsy, or after trauma.

    b. Lymph contained in a lymphatic vessel tends to be more **darkly stained** than the plasma of a vein, if both are retained by their respective vessels in the histologic specimen.

    c. **Valves are more numerous** in lymphatic vessels than in veins.

D. **Transport of lymph**

  1. **Lymph moves sluggishly** through the lymphatic vessel.

    a. **Compression of the vessel** by adjacent skeletal or smooth muscle has an important role in the movement of lymph through the lymphatic vessel.

    b. In larger lymphatic vessels, **contraction of smooth muscle** in the media and adventitia of the vessel wall also appears to aid in the movement of lymph.

  2. **Backflow of lymph is prevented by valves.**

    a. The valves are similar in structure but more numerous than the valves of veins.

    b. A lymphatic vessel may have a **beaded appearance** when viewed grossly, because of its numerous valves.

  3. **Lymph enters the venous system** at the root of the neck where the largest lymphatic vessels, the **thoracic duct** and the **right lymphatic duct,** empty into the great veins.

Chapter 15

Lymphatic Cells and Tissues

I. **INTRODUCTION.** Lymphatic cells and tissues are the morphologic basis of the immune system of the body.

A. **Components.** The lymphatic system is composed of cells, tissues, and organs that monitor body surfaces and internal fluid compartments, and react to the presence of antigens.

1. **Cells.** Lymphocytes are the predominant cells found in lymphatic tissues and organs (see II; see also Chapter 12 VI). Macrophages, plasma cells, antigen-presenting cells, and reticular cells are also found in lymphatic tissues and organs.

2. **Tissues.** Lymphatic tissues exist throughout the body as diffuse deposits (see VII) or as more sharply defined nodules (see VIII).

3. **Organs.** Lymphatic cells and tissues are assembled into organs that are discussed in subsequent chapters.
   a. **Central (primary) lymphatic organs.** The bone marrow (Chapter 13) and thymus gland (Chapter 19) are sites of lymphocyte differentiation, but are not normally sites of immune reactions.
   b. **Peripheral (secondary) lymphatic organs.** Lymph nodes (Chapter 17), spleen (Chapter 18), and tonsils and Peyer patches (Chapter 16) are sites of immune reactions.

B. **Function.** The lymphatic system **produces immune responses** against potentially harmful antigenic substances. In performing this function, the lymphatic system normally distinguishes **self** from **non-self.**

II. **LYMPHOCYTES.** Lymphocytes encompass a **spectrum of cell sizes.**

A. **Small lymphocytes** (Figure 15-1) are 7 to 8 μm in diameter.

1. Small lymphocytes are the most commonly encountered lymphocyte type in peripheral blood and in lymphatic tissues.

2. The heterochromatic nucleus of a small lymphocyte is surrounded by an exceedingly thin rim of cytoplasm.

B. **Medium lymphocytes** are 10 to 11 μm in diameter.

1. Medium lymphocytes are also encountered in peripheral blood and in lymphatic tissues but are less numerous than small lymphocytes.

2. They are considered a developmentally intermediate form between small and large lymphocytes.

C. **Large lymphocytes** are 12 μm or larger in diameter.

1. Large lymphocytes normally are not found in peripheral blood but do occur in lymphatic tissue.

2. They are also called **activated lymphocytes** or **lymphoblasts** because they are mi-

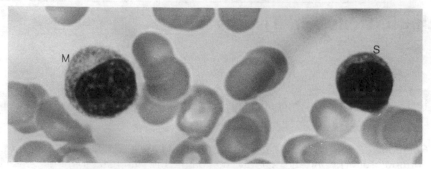

FIGURE 15-1. Small lymphocyte (*S*) and medium-sized lymphocyte (*M*) in peripheral blood.

totically active cells. The nuclei of large lymphocytes are less heterochromatic than the nuclei of smaller lymphocytes; this is consistent with their mitotic activity.

III. B LYMPHOCYTES AND HUMORAL IMMUNITY

A. Origin of B lymphocytes and nomenclature in humoral immunity

1. In humans, **B lymphocytes** (**B cells**) originate from the colony-forming cells of hematopoietic tissue in red bone marrow.

2. The designation *B* derives from the fact that in birds this population of lymphocytes develops in the **b**ursa of Fabricius, an evagination of the cloaca.

3. The immune reaction produced by the stimulation of B cells is referred to as the **humoral immune response** because of the central role played by **immunoglobulins** (**antibodies**) circulating in the blood.

B. Recognition of antigen by B cells

1. **Surface receptors.** B cells synthesize immunoglobulin molecules that are inserted in their plasma membranes. These molecules serve as **receptors,** or **recognition sites,** that enable a B cell to react with an antigen.

2. **Specificity of the immune reaction.** The reaction between a B cell and an antigen is highly specific; that is, a particular B cell can recognize and react with only a particular antigen or antigenic site on a large molecule or microorganism.
   a. The **clonal selection theory** states that there are B cells, somewhere in the body, that are programmed to react against a particular antigen without ever having had prior exposure to that antigen. (Such unstimulated B cells are known as **virgin** B cells.)
      (1) An immune reaction is initiated by the chance encounter of a B cell with the antigen to which it is genetically programmed to react.
      (2) Thus, the antigen **selects** a clone of lymphocytes that are programmed to react against it.
   b. The selected cells will go on to produce an immune response. This initial response to antigen is the **primary immune response.**
   c. A lymphocyte and its clonal progeny are **committed** to respond only to the antigen that selected them.

C. Blastic transformation of B cells

1. **Developmental process.** The recognition of an antigen by a B cell stimulates the lymphocyte to undergo **blastic transformation,** in which the B cell, which is a small lymphocyte, develops into a **lymphoblast,** which is a large lymphocyte.

2. **Products of blastic transformation.** The lymphoblast divides repeatedly, producing a clonal population of cells that differentiate into either **plasma cells** or **memory cells.**

3. **Helper T cells.** The differentiation of B cells into plasma cells and, indeed, most aspects of B cell function, are dependent upon helper T cells (see IV F).

D. **Plasma cells.** These cells appear in tissues as the result of the antigenic stimulation of B cells.

1. **Plasma cells as effector cells**
   a. Plasma cells are able to **effect,** or produce, a **humoral immune reaction,** characterized by the synthesis and release of large amounts of **antibodies.**
      (1) Antibodies bind to antigenic sites on a bacterium or particle.
      (2) The presence of antigen–antibody complexes enhances the phagocytosis of the bacterium or particle by a neutrophil or macrophage.
   b. A particular clone of plasma cells synthesizes and releases the same antibody that was present as receptors in the cell membrane of the virgin B cell before antigenic stimulation.

2. **Structural characteristics of plasma cells** (Figures 15-2, 15-3)
   a. **Nucleus and its clockface chromatin pattern**
      (1) The nucleus of a plasma cell is often located eccentrically in the cell.
      (2) Heterochromatin is dispersed around the edge of the nucleus in a manner vaguely reminiscent of the numerals of an analog clockface.
   b. **Rough endoplasmic reticulum and cytoplasmic basophilia**
      (1) Plasma cells contain a large amount of rough endoplasmic reticulum (rER), befitting their prodigious output of protein (immunoglobulin, or antibody).

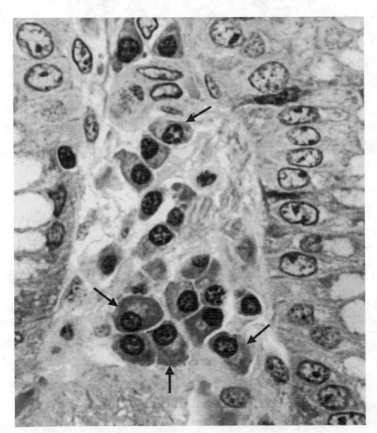

FIGURE 15-2. Plasma cells of the gastric lamina propria (light micrograph). Several plasma cells are indicated (*arrows*). Note the cytoplasmic staining that is evidence of the rough endoplasmic reticulum, the pale region closer to the nucleus that is the negative image of the Golgi apparatus (the "Golgi ghost"), and the prominent heterochromatin in the nucleus.

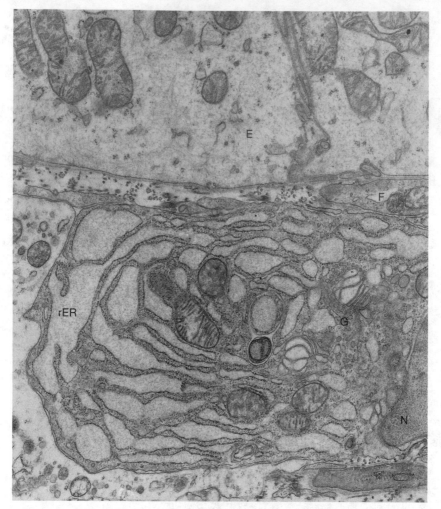

FIGURE 15-3. Plasma cell of the colonic lamina propria (electron micrograph). Note the rough endo-plasmic reticulum (*rER*), with its dilated cisterns, and the membrane stacks of the Golgi apparatus (*G*). The basal surface of the colonic epithelium (*E*) is close to the plasma cell, and a process of a pericryptal fibro-blast (*F*) is insinuated between the plasma cell and the basal lamina of the epithelium. *N* = nucleus of the plasma cell.

        (2) The rER, probably because of its concentration of negatively charged phos-phate groups, imparts characteristic **cytoplasmic basophilia** to the plasma cell when examined by light microscopy (see Figure 15-2).

    c. Golgi apparatus and its negative image

        (1) A Golgi apparatus is found in a plasma cell, usually occupying the center of the cell between the nucleus and the rER.

        (2) Most routine light microscopic stains fail to stain the Golgi apparatus. This unstained region, surrounded by stained structures, is referred to as a **nega-tive image** of the **Golgi apparatus,** or **"Golgi ghost"** (see Figure 15-2).

E. **B Memory cells.** These are the second cell type produced by the antigenic stimulation of B cells.

    1. Memory cells are programmed to react against the same antigen that stimulated the initial blastic transformation.

    2. Memory cells greatly increase the number of small lymphocytes that can react on re-exposure to a particular antigen.

a. Subsequent exposures to that antigen will result in a faster immune response because of the larger pool of committed cells capable of responding.

b. This subsequent, faster response to an antigen is the **secondary immune response.** It is the cellular basis of immunization.

IV. T LYMPHOCYTES AND CELL-MEDIATED IMMUNITY

A. Origin of T lymphocytes and nomenclature in cell-mediated immunity

1. **T lymphocytes (T cells),** like B lymphocytes, originate from the colony-forming cells of hematopoietic tissue. T cells, however, complete their development in the thymus gland—hence the name.

2. The immune reaction produced by the stimulation of T cells is referred to as the **cell-mediated immune response,** or **cellular immunity,** because of the role played by cytotoxic (killer) T lymphocytes.

B. Graft rejection illustrates the T cell–mediated immune response.

1. **First-set rejection**
   a. Skin grafted onto an experimental animal or human being from an unrelated, genetically distinct donor will be rejected in about 10 days. This is the **first-set rejection,** also called first-set reaction.
   b. The experimental animal or human being that rejected the graft is now **sensitized** to antigens of the graft.

2. **Second-set rejection**
   a. A second graft from the same donor to the same, sensitized recipient will be rejected in about 6 days. This is the **second-set rejection,** or reaction.
   b. The faster second-set rejection occurs because the first-set rejection created T memory cells, thereby increasing the numbers of specific T lymphocytes capable of reacting to antigens of the graft.

C. Blastic transformation of T cells

1. **Cell response.** T cells recognize a graft as foreign, and this stimulates the cells to undergo **blastic transformation,** in which the T cells, which are small lymphocytes, enlarge into lymphoblasts.

2. **Products of blastic transformation.** The lymphoblasts divide repeatedly and differentiate into a number of **T cell subsets:** cytotoxic (killer) T cells, helper T cells, T memory cells, and suppressor T cells.

D. Cytotoxic T cells. These cells appear at the site of graft rejection as the result of the antigenic stimulation of T cells.

1. **Structural characteristics.** Cytotoxic T cells closely resemble the T lymphocytes from which they were derived by blastic transformation.

2. **Cytotoxic T cells as effector cells.** Cytotoxic T lymphocytes are the cells that effect, or produce, the cell-mediated immune response.
   a. Microscopic examination of either a first- or second-set graft site shows the infiltration of the area by small lymphocytes; these are the cytotoxic T cells.
   b. The cytotoxic T cells invade the graft and establish physical contact with the graft.
   c. The **interactions** that occur between the **cytotoxic T cells** and their **target cells** include the following:
      (1) Cytotoxic T cells synthesize and secrete the protein **perforin,** which is inserted into the plasma membrane of the target cell.
         (a) Perforin forms **transmembrane channels** in the target cell.

          (b) The channels disrupt the osmotic and ionic balance of the cell. Death of the cell ensues.

     (2) Proteases called **fragmentins** are also passed to the target cell, possibly via the transmembrane channels. The proteases are thought to induce **apoptosis** (programmed cell death) of the target cell.

E. **T memory cells.** These cells are also produced during the blastic transformation of T cells.

    1. As with B cells, T memory cells increase the available supply of immunologically competent lymphocytes, and thus allow a more rapid immune reaction on subsequent exposure to an antigen.

    2. T memory cells are morphologically identical to the T lymphocytes from which they were derived during blastic transformation.

F. **Helper T cells.** These cells appear to have an effect on most aspects of B cell function.

    1. Helper T cells promote the differentiation of B cells to plasma cells.

    2. The critical role of helper T cells in the humoral immune response is apparent in AIDS.
        a. The human immunodeficiency virus (HIV) that causes AIDS depletes the number of helper T cells.
        b. This severely compromises the ability of the immune system to respond to antigens, and opportunistic infections occur.

G. **Suppressor T cells.** This T cell subtype inhibits the activity of cytotoxic T cells and helper T cells.

V. OTHER FEATURES OF HUMORAL AND CELL-MEDIATED IMMUNE RESPONSES

A. **Cellular similarity.** Morphologically similar cells have different roles in immune responses.

    1. Virgin B lymphocytes, virgin T lymphocytes, memory cells of either origin, helper T cells, and cytotoxic T cells are histologically indistinguishable from one another; in a blood smear, they would all be called small lymphocytes.

    2. However, the different kinds of cells have distinctive surface marker proteins that are identifiable immunocytochemically.

B. **Concurrent immune responses.** Humoral responses and cell-mediated responses occur simultaneously.

    1. An antigenic substance generally will produce both humoral and cell-mediated responses.

    2. Many different clones of effector cells and memory cells will be produced by the response to an antigenic substance because the substance usually will have many antigenic sites over its surface. Each site will provoke its own immune response.

C. **Antigen-presenting cells.** These are needed by both B and T lymphocytes.

    1. Antigen-presenting cells form a heterogeneous group of cells that ingest antigen, process it, and then present fragments of the antigen to lymphocytes.

    2. Examples of antigen-presenting cells are Langerhans cells of the epidermis, dendritic cells of lymphatic organs, and macrophages.

3. Antigen-presenting cells may be encountered in peripheral blood and in afferent lymph. In blood, they are called veiled or dendritic cells and account for less than 0.1% of white cells.

VI. STRUCTURAL FRAMEWORK OF LYMPHATIC TISSUES. The stroma of lymphatic tissues is formed by a cellular reticulum and a fibrous reticulum, which usually are masked by the presence of large numbers of lymphocytes.

A. Cellular reticulum

1. **Fibroblast-like cells.** Reticular cells form a complex cellular framework throughout lymphatic tissues.
   a. Reticular cells, except those of the thymus gland (see Chapter 19), are morphologically and functionally **similar to fibroblasts.**
   b. Reticular cells were once thought to be phagocytic cells, but studies with the electron microscope demonstrate that the fibroblast-like reticular cells and the monocyte-derived macrophages are distinct cell types.
   c. Reticular cells synthesize the fibrous reticulum.

2. **Absence of cellular junctions.** Processes of reticular cells end close to the processes of other reticular cells but there are **no cell–cell junctions formed between the apposed cells.** An exception is the epithelial reticular cells of the thymus gland that are connected by desmosomes (see Chapter 19).

B. Fibrous reticulum

1. **System of collagen fibrils.** Reticular fibers are **fine type III collagen fibrils** with a large amount of bound proteoglycans.

2. **Staining characteristics.** The bound proteoglycans are responsible for the **argyrophilia** of the reticular fibers, as well as their staining with the **periodic acid–Schiff (PAS) reaction.**

C. Cellular reticulum–fibrous reticulum relationships

1. The reticular cells of the cellular reticulum synthesize the reticular fibers and their associated ground substance molecules of the fibrous reticulum.

2. The reticular fibers are ensheathed by processes of the reticular cells, which isolate the fibers from their environment.

3. The fibrous reticulum, therefore, follows the contours of the cellular reticulum.

VII. DIFFUSE LYMPHATIC TISSUE

A. Accumulation of lymphocytes (Figure 15-4)

1. Diffuse lymphatic tissue is found in many regions of the body, especially in connective tissue beneath moist mucosal surfaces (e.g., trachea and intestine).

2. A limiting capsule is not present; the lymphatic tissue merges with the surrounding connective tissue.

B. Chronic inflammation

1. An accumulation of **lymphocytes** deep to a mucosal surface is evidence of **chronic inflammation.**
   a. Those mucosal surfaces normally have a bacterial flora that is prevented from entering the body by the mucosal epithelium.

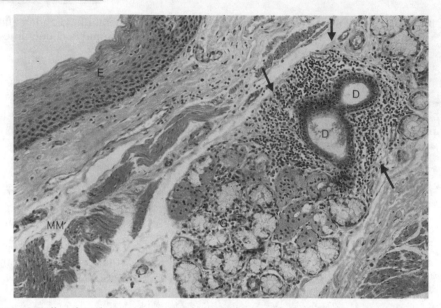

FIGURE 15-4. Diffuse lymphatic tissue in a submucosal esophageal gland (light micrograph). The lymphatic tissue (*arrows*) surrounds ducts (*D*) of the gland (*G*). This is an example of chronic inflammation and is evidence of an immune response to antigens that have invaded the submucosa by penetrating the duct wall. *E* = esophageal epithelium, *MM* = muscularis mucosae.

       b. The development of diffuse lymphatic tissue deep to the mucosal epithelium indicates that the mucosal barrier has been breached.

   2. A concentration of **neutrophils** in a similar location, however, is evidence of **acute inflammation** (see Chapter 12 III D 4).

VIII. LYMPHATIC NODULES AND GERMINAL CENTERS

A. **Nodules (follicles)** are a unit of structure of lymphatic tissues and organs.

   1. Appearance. Nodules are unencapsulated, ovoid masses of lymphatic tissue (Figure 15-5).

   2. Size. Nodules range widely in size and may reach a maximum diameter of 1.5 to 2.0 mm.

   3. Distribution. Nodules are found in large numbers throughout the body. They occur either as solitary structures associated with diffuse lymphatic tissue, or as components of a much larger lymphatic organ. For example:
      a. Thousands of solitary nodules exist in the wall of the normal gastrointestinal tract.
      b. The cortex of lymph nodes is formed largely by nodules.

B. **Germinal centers** indicate a humoral immune response.

   1. Appearance. A germinal center is a pale, central region in a lymphatic nodule (see Figure 17-2). The pale appearance is due to the presence of many lightly staining **lymphoblasts.**

   2. Origin. The germinal center is produced by **antigenic stimulation** of the immunoreactive cells of a nodule.
      a. The germinal center is a site of blastic transformation of B lymphocytes.

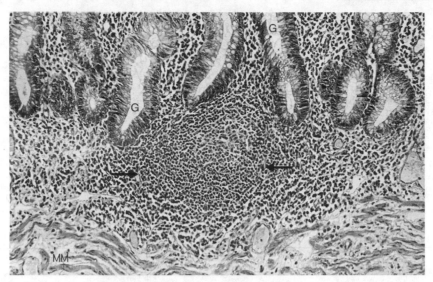

FIGURE 15-5. Lymphatic nodule (*arrows*) in the lamina propria of the colon (light micrograph). The nodule is unencapsulated and it merges with the connective tissue of the lamina propria. *G* = colonic glands; *MM* = muscularis mucosae.

    b. Germinal centers are rarely encountered in germ-free and fetal animals. Germinal centers are absent from the thymus gland, an organ in which immune reactions normally do not occur (see Chapter 19).

3. Primary and secondary lymphatic nodules. These designations are used by some authors.

    a. A **primary nodule** is a homogeneous mass of small lymphocytes.

    b. A **secondary nodule** is a nodule with a germinal center.

4. Cells present in germinal centers

    a. **B lymphocytes,** especially B lymphoblasts, are numerous in a germinal center.

    b. Some **T lymphocytes** are present in the center, where they function as helper T cells in the blastic transformation of B cells.

    c. Mature **plasma cells** are seldom encountered in a germinal center, because most **plasma cells** migrate out of the germinal center as they differentiate from stimulated B cells.

C. **Subregions of a lymphatic nodule–germinal center complex** (see Figure 17-2). These regions may not be visible in a particular section of a nodule because of the plane of section.

1. Lymphocyte cap. A crescent-shaped layer of small lymphocytes, probably memory cells, caps one pole of the nodule. The cap is oriented toward the source of antigen.

2. Pale pole. This is the concentration of lightly staining lymphoblasts immediately deep to the lymphocyte cap. It corresponds to the germinal center.

3. Dense pole. This is the pole of the nodule–germinal center complex that is opposite the lymphocyte cap. The pale pole, or germinal center, separates the dense pole from the lymphocyte cap.

4. Mantle layer. Some histologists refer to the entire rim of dense lymphatic tissue that surrounds a germinal center (i.e., the lymphocyte cap and dense pole) as the **nodular** or **follicular mantle.**

Chapter 16

Tonsils, Peyer Patches, and Appendix

I. INTRODUCTION

A. **Nodule aggregation.** The **tonsils** of the pharynx, the **Peyer patches** of the ileum, and the **appendix** of the cecum are characterized by aggregations of lymphatic nodules.

B. **Gut-associated lymphatic tissue (GALT).** Tonsils, Peyer patches, and the appendix are included in the category of lymphatic tissue called gut-associated lymphatic tissue, or GALT (see Chapter 21 III A 2).

II. TONSILS. The tonsils are part of a ring-like arrangement of lymphatic tissue around the entrances to the digestive and respiratory systems. The tonsils are three named enlargements in this continuous ring.

A. **Types of tonsils**

1. **Palatine tonsils**
   a. **Location.** These are paired masses of lymphatic tissue, one on either side of the pharynx. Each palatine tonsil is in the fossa between the glossopalatine and pharyngopalatine arches.
   b. In common usage, the term *tonsils* refers to the palatine tonsils.

2. **Lingual tonsil**
   a. **Location.** This is a single mass of lymphatic tissue on the dorsal median surface of the posterior one-third of the tongue.
   b. The lingual tonsil is posterior to the row of circumvallate papillae.

3. **Pharyngeal tonsil**
   a. **Location.** This is a single mass of lymphatic tissue in the posterior wall of the nasopharynx.
   b. The enlarged and inflamed pharyngeal tonsil constitutes the **adenoids.**

B. **Histologic characteristics of tonsils** (Figure 16-1)

1. **Relationship to pharyngeal wall.** Tonsils are immediately deep to antigen-laden mucosal surfaces. The tonsils bulge into the lumen of the pharynx.

2. **Tonsillar epithelium.** The epithelium covering a tonsil is characteristic of that particular region of the pharynx.
   a. The **palatine and lingual tonsils** are covered by a **stratified squamous epithelium.** The **pharyngeal tonsil** is covered by a **pseudostratified ciliated epithelium.**
   b. The structure of the epithelium, however, is **often obscured by infiltration of lymphocytes** from the nearby lymphatic tissue.

3. **Tonsillar lymphatic tissue.** Tonsils are found in the loose connective tissue beneath the mucosal epithelium.
   a. **Lymphatic nodules,** usually with **germinal centers** (see Chapter 15 VIII B), form much of the tonsillar mass.
   b. Such **secondary nodules** are especially numerous in pathologic, surgically removed palatine tonsils.

4. **Mucosal invaginations.** The mucosa of the pharynx invaginates to form **tubular crypts** in the palatine and lingual tonsils and **folds** in the pharyngeal tonsil. Crypts and folds provide a **larger area of contact** between the bacteria-covered mucosal surface and the immunoreactive cells of the tonsils.

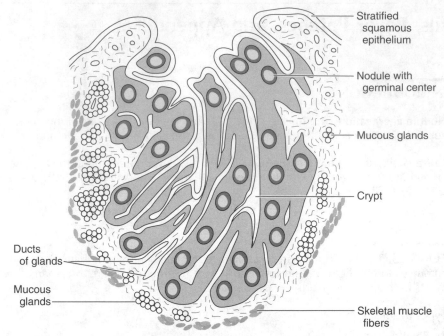

FIGURE 16-1. Palatine tonsil.

a. **Lingual tonsillar crypts**
   (1) Small salivary glands empty into the crypts of lingual tonsils and flush the crypts with their secretions.
   (2) Debris, therefore, generally does not accumulate in the crypts of lingual tonsils.

b. **Palatine tonsillar crypts**
   (1) The salivary glands near the palatine tonsils do not empty into the crypts but open directly onto the pharyngeal surface.
   (2) Debris and bacteria tend to accumulate in the crypts of palatine tonsils. Possibly because of this, the palatine tonsils are more subject to chronic infection.

5. **Capsule and trabeculae.** An indistinct connective tissue capsule and some trabeculae may be identifiable.

6. **Peritonsillar tissues.** Most histologic sections of tonsils include some **skeletal muscle** and **secretory tubuloacini of minor salivary glands.** The presence of muscle and gland tissue aids in the identification of the organ.

C. Function of tonsils

1. Tonsils probably have no function that is not shared by lymphatic tissue located elsewhere in the body.

2. Because of their location, tonsils are part of the defense mechanism against antigens attempting to enter the body via the pharynx.

III. PEYER PATCHES. Peyer patches are aggregations of lymphatic nodules in the small intestine.

A. Location

1. Peyer patches are found in the wall of the distal small intestine (ileum) and are useful in identifying this region of the small intestine.

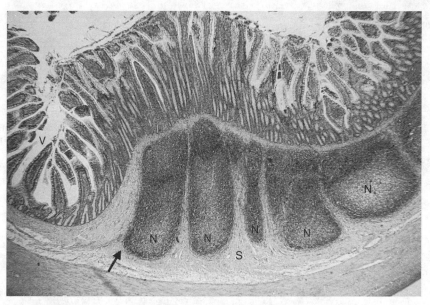

FIGURE 16-2. Peyer patch, ileum. Several lymphatic nodules (*N*) of one Peyer patch are visible in this light micrograph. The junction between the Peyer patch and the Peyer patch–free portion of the circumference of the ileum is indicated with an *arrow. V* = villi, *S* = submucosa.

   2. Some authors, however, loosely refer to any nodules anywhere in the wall of the alimentary canal as Peyer patches.

   3. Peyer patches tend to be more obvious in younger individuals.

B. **Histologic characteristics of Peyer patches** (Figure 16-2)

   1. One patch is a multinodular aggregate.
      a. Each Peyer patch is a macroscopic accumulation of as many as a few hundred lymphatic nodules (see Chapter 15 VIII). A patch may have a diameter of 1 to 3 centimeters.
      b. 20 to 30 such patches, comprising thousands of lymphatic nodules, are found throughout the length of the ileum (approximately 3.5 meters).
      c. Peyer patches are restricted to the antimesenteric surface of the ileum. Thus, part of the circumference of the ileum does not contain Peyer patches.

   2. Nodules originate in the lamina propria of the mucosa.
      a. The nodules of the patch enlarge and may **distort overlying villi and crypts.**
      b. The nodules **protrude through the muscularis mucosae into the submucosa.** Indeed, fully developed nodules are mostly submucosal in location.

C. **Function of Peyer patches**

   1. This localized concentration of lymphatic tissue probably develops in response to the microbial flora of the intestine.

   2. Peyer patches are not prominent in the ileum of germ-free animals, indicating that their development is stimulated by the antigen-rich luminal contents of the conventional (i.e., non–germ-free) gut.

IV. **APPENDIX.** The vermiform appendix is a thin, worm-shaped diverticulum of the cecum. It varies from 2 cm to 20 cm in length. Considerable lymphatic tissue is found in its wall.

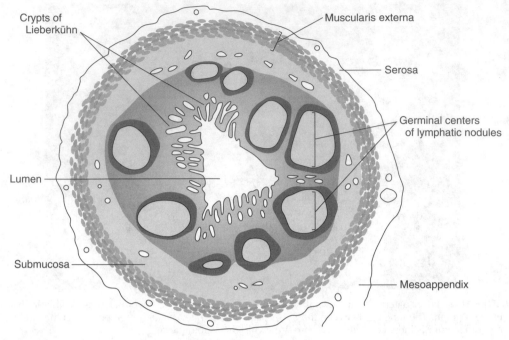

FIGURE 16-3. Appendix.

A. **Histologic characteristics of the vermiform appendix** (Figure 16-3)

1. **The appendix is part of the colon.**
   a. Most of the appendix wall resembles the wall of the colon.
   b. The muscularis externa of the appendix differs histologically from the rest of the colon, however.
      (1) The **teniae coli** (see Chapter 25 II D) converge at the base of the appendix and merge into a thin, continuous layer of smooth muscle in the appendix wall.
      (2) The appendix, therefore, lacks teniae coli.

2. **Nodular and diffuse lymphatic tissue** is found throughout the appendix wall (see Chapter 15 VII, VIII).
   a. The large amount of lymphatic tissue probably is the result of **stagnation of the luminal contents** in this blindly ending tube and **subsequent immune stimulation** of the GALT of the mucosa.
   b. By midlife or later, much of the colonic mucosal structure of the appendix is obscured or replaced by **fibrous connective tissue** that forms in response to chronic, subclinical appendicitis.

B. **Function of the vermiform appendix.** The appendix is a vestigial structure in humans. It has no known significant function.

V. **M CELLS.** M cells (*M* for membranelike, microfold), also called follicular epithelial cells, are found in close association with Peyer patches. Similar cells may also be associated with tonsils, the appendix, and solitary mucosal lymphatic nodules.

A. **Location and structure of M cells**

1. M cells are thin cells that are part of the mucosal epithelium covering lymphatic tissue.

2. The luminal surface of the M cell is covered by a honeycomb-like arrangement of the plasma membrane; hence the name *microfold.* Other M cells appear to be covered by scattered microvilli.

B. **Significance of M cells.** M cells separate antigen-covered mucosal surfaces from immunoreactive cells.

1. M cells sample the extracellular environment by taking up material in clathrin-coated vesicles and transporting the material to the basal surface of the cell.

2. The sampled material is then released from the M cell into the immediate vicinity of lymphocytes and macrophages, where it may initiate immune responses.

Chapter 17

Lymph Nodes

I. **INTRODUCTION.** Lymph nodes, which are lymphatic organs, are sites of immune reactions to lymph-borne antigens.

A. **Distribution.** Lymph nodes are widely found in the body but tend to be concentrated in certain regions (e.g., axilla, groin, mesenteries).

B. **Lymph drainage.** Nodes, which appear as gross enlargements along the lymphatic vessels, intercept the flow of lymph through those vessels.

    1. **Lymph is filtered** through lymph nodes as it flows from tissue spaces back to the venous system.

    2. All lymph **passes through at least one lymph node** before returning to the blood.

II. **SURFACE LANDMARKS OF LYMPH NODES**

A. **Shape and size** (Figure 17-1)

    1. Lymph nodes are **irregularly rounded structures** with much variation in shape. Many nodes are **kidney-shaped.**

    2. Usually, **concave and convex surfaces** of a lymph node can be recognized. The **hilum** of the node is located on the concave surface.

    3. Nodes vary in size from a few millimeters to a few centimeters.

B. **Lymphatic vessels** (see Figure 17-1). Valves present in the lymphatic vessels assure the unidirectional flow of lymph from the afferent vessels, through the node, to the efferent vessels.

    1. Afferent lymphatic vessels
        a. Afferent vessels convey lymph to nodes.
        b. Usually, **several afferent vessels** enter a node over its convex surface.

    2. Efferent lymphatic vessels
        a. Efferent vessels drain lymph from nodes.
        b. Usually, **a single efferent vessel** (or sometimes two) leaves a node at the hilum.

C. **Blood vessels.** The arterial vessels supplying a node, and the veins draining it, are both found at the hilum.

D. **Capsule.** A connective tissue capsule envelops a node, and trabeculae extend from the capsule into the node. The capsule is perforated at several points by afferent lymphatic vessels.

III. **LYMPH NODE COMPARTMENTS: CORTEX AND MEDULLA**

A. **Cortex** (Figure 17-2). The cortex is **superficial to the medulla.** Two arrangements of lymphatic tissue form the cortex of a lymph node: the nodular, or outer, cortex and the non-nodular, or inner, cortex.

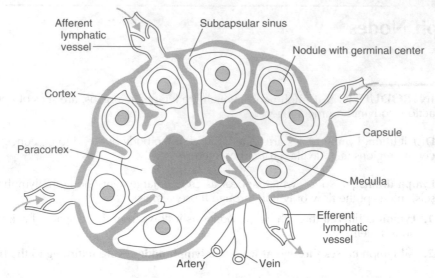

FIGURE 17-1. Schematic representation of a sagittal section of a lymph node, showing the three major subcompartments (cortex, paracortex, medulla). *Arrows* indicate direction of lymph flow. (Modified from Hyde RM: *Immunology,* 3rd ed. Baltimore, Williams & Wilkins, 1995, page 94.]

1. **Nodular (outer) cortex.** The outermost layer of lymphatic tissue in the node, the nodular (or superficial) cortex, is usually one nodule thick.
   a. Most of the nodules in this layer contain germinal centers.
   b. The nodular cortex is rich in B cells. Macrophages, T helper cells, and antigen-presenting cells, such as dendritic reticular cells, are also found in the nodular cortex.
2. **Non-nodular (inner) cortex.** This region of the cortex, also called the **paracortex** (or deep cortex), lies between the nodular cortex and the medulla.

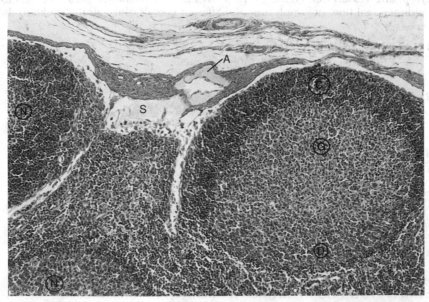

FIGURE 17-2. Cortex of lymph node, light micrograph. The lymphocyte cap (*C*), germinal center (*G*), and dense pole (*D*) of a lymphatic nodule are visible. Portions of two additional nodules (*N*) are also included in the field. An afferent lymphatic vessel (*A*) is shown passing through the capsule (transverse section, including cusps of the valve). *S* = subcapsular sinus.

  a. The non-nodular cortex varies in thickness, is densely cellular, and lacks nodules.
  b. Lymphocytes in this region are mainly T cells.
    (1) Development of this region of the cortex is dependent on an adequate supply of T cells.
    (2) Animals thymectomized during the perinatal period will have poorly developed non-nodular cortical regions in their lymph nodes because they are deficient in T cells.
  c. Because of the relationship of the thymus gland to the paracortex, this region of the lymph node is also called the **thymus-dependent area.**

B. **Medulla**

  1. Location. The medulla of a lymph node is found between the cortex and the hilum.

  2. Composition. The medulla is formed by cords of dense lymphatic tissue separated by lymphatic sinuses (Figure 17-3). **Nodules are not present in the medulla.** Medullary tissues converge at the hilum.

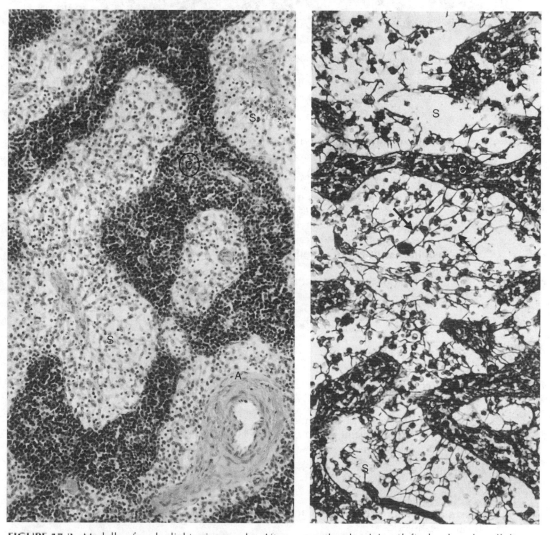

FIGURE 17-3. Medulla of node, light micrographs. After conventional staining (*left*), the densely cellular cords (*C*) of lymphatic tissue and the sinuses (*S*), which are characteristic of the medulla, are clearly demonstrated. *A* − arteriole. After silver staining (*right*),the reticular fibers (*arrows*) that form a meshwork in the medullary sinuses can be identified.

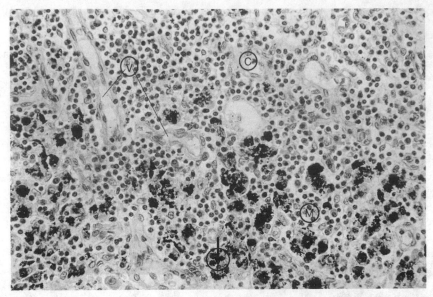

FIGURE 17-4. Light micrograph of the junction between the non-nodular cortex (*C*) and medulla (*M*) of a lymph node. Note the numerous high endothelial venules (*V*) of the non-nodular cortex. Macrophages can be recognized by the presence of intracellular deposits of dense particles; each granular deposit is one engorged macrophage (*arrow*). Macrophages are more numerous in the medulla than in the cortex.

    a. Medullary cords are formed by reticular cells and reticular fibers, small lymphocytes, plasma cells, and macrophages.

        (1) The cords of medullary tissue are continuous with the lymphatic tissue of the deep cortex.

        (2) Immature plasma cells migrate to the medullary cords, where they develop into mature, immunoglobulin-secreting plasma cells.

        (3) Phagocytosis is more evident in the medulla than in the cortical compartment (Figure 17-4).

    b. Medullary sinuses are channels for the flow of lymph and tend to be more obvious than cortical sinuses (see Figure 17-3). Medullary sinuses empty into the efferent lymphatic vessels at the hilum.

IV. LYMPHATIC SINUSES

A. System of channels. Lymphatic sinuses are **channels that branch and anastomose,** permeating all subcompartments of the lymph node.

    1. Unlike blood vessels, lymph node sinuses are not sharply defined tubules. The sinuses are often indistinct because of the large number of lymphocytes retained in the lumen of the sinus.

    2. Endothelial cells line the sinuses. In most areas of the node the endothelium is discontinuous.

B. Sinuses are crisscrossed by cells and fibers. Lymphatic sinuses resemble a cellular and fibrous meshwork.

    1. Lymphatic sinuses do not have an open lumen as do blood vessels. They are spanned in an apparently haphazard manner by reticular fibers ensheathed by cell processes (see Figure 17-3).

2. Lymph flows slowly through a lymph node, and cells are slowed down by the meshwork that crisscrosses the sinus.

3. Recognition of foreign materials and subsequent phagocytosis is facilitated by the sluggish circulation of lymph through the node.

C. **Sinuses and phagocytosis.** Extensive phagocytosis of lymph-borne foreign material occurs in the medulla (see Figure 17-4).

1. Some of the macrophages are located in the medullary sinuses.

2. Other macrophages are located in the medullary cords and only a portion of the macrophage extends into the sinus.

V. LYMPH PATHWAY THROUGH A LYMPH NODE

A. **Afferent lymphatic vessel.** Lymph enters a node through an afferent vessel (see Figure 17-1).

1. Many afferent lymphatic vessels pierce the capsule along its convex surface.

2. Valves often are present in the afferent vessels.

B. **Subcapsular (marginal) sinus**

1. The subcapsular sinus is an extensive but narrow space over the entire convex surface of the node. The sinus separates the capsule from the nodular cortex.

2. The subcapsular sinus receives lymph from the afferent vessels (see Figure 17-2).

C. **Cortical sinuses**

1. These sinuses are radially arranged channels that receive lymph from the subcapsular sinus.

2. Cortical sinuses are found between adjacent nodules and often are less obvious than the subcapsular sinus and the medullary sinuses.

D. **Medullary sinuses**

1. These channels are found between the cords of lymphatic tissue. They are continuous with the cortical sinuses.

2. Lymph flows from the cortical sinuses to the medullary sinuses.

E. **Efferent lymphatic vessels.** Lymph flows through the medullary sinuses and empties into the efferent lymphatic vessels. Lymph leaves the node through the efferent vessels (Figure 17-5; see also Figure 17-1).

1. The efferent vessels are continuous with the medullary sinuses at the hilum of the node.

2. Efferent vessels also contain valves, which restrict the backflow of lymph to the node.

VI. BLOOD PATHWAY THROUGH A NODE AND LYMPHOCYTE RECIRCULATION

A. **Vascular pattern of a lymph node**

1. **Arteries (or arterioles)** enter the node at the hilum and pass through the medullary compartment (see Figure 17-3).

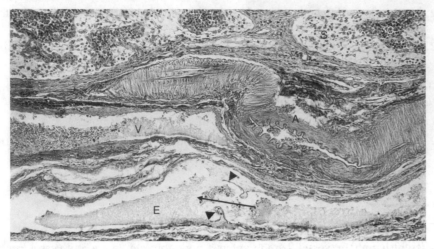

FIGURE 17-5. Hilum of a lymph node, light micrograph. *S* = medullary sinus; *C* = medullary cord; *A* = arteriole; *V* = venule containing blood cells; *E* = efferent lymphatic vessel containing precipitated lymph and a few cells. The *arrow* indicates direction of lymph flow. *Arrowheads* = cusps of valve. The continuity of medullary sinuses and the efferent lymphatic vessel is not illustrated.

    2. Capillaries are given off by arterioles in the medulla. The arterioles end in capillary beds in the cortex.

    3. Postcapillary venules form in the deep cortex (see Figure 17-4). Larger venules appear in the medulla.

    4. Veins (or large venules) exit the node at the hilum.

B. **Immune surveillance.** Movement of lymphocytes between the blood compartment and the lymphatic tissue compartment is an essential aspect of immune surveillance.

    1. Site of lymphocyte exit from the blood. High endothelial venules (HEVs), which are postcapillary venules with a **cuboidal or columnar endothelium,** are found in the non-nodular, thymus-dependent cortex (see Figure 17-4).

      a. T lymphocytes and B lymphocytes leave the blood stream by diapedesis in this non-nodular region of the cortex.

      b. T cells remain in the thymus-dependent region and B cells migrate to the nodular cortex.

    2. Reentry of lymphocytes into the blood stream

      a. After a period of time, lymphocytes leave the node to recirculate systemically.

      b. The cells enter a nearby lymphatic sinus and leave the node by the efferent lymphatic vessel.

    3. Significance of lymphocyte recirculation

      a. Lymphocytes are programmed to react with foreign, antigenic materials. Those antigens may enter the body at various points and become localized to specific regions of the body.

      b. The movement of lymphocytes from one region of the body to another, and from peripheral blood to lymphatic tissue, increases the likelihood of a lymphocyte encountering the antigens to which it is programmed to react.

VII. FUNCTIONS OF LYMPH NODES

A. Mechanical filters of lymph

    1. Reticular cell processes ensheathing reticular fibers and endothelial cell processes crisscross sinuses within a lymph node to produce a complex, coarse meshwork through which lymph is filtered.

    2. Substances filtered from lymph in this way (i.e., retained by the cellular and fibrous meshwork) include microorganisms, colloidal particles, and metastatic (cancer) cells.

B. **Cellular filters of lymph**

    1. Cells and other substances retained by mechanical filtration may be removed from the lymph by cellular filtration (i.e., phagocytosis) by macrophages (see Figure 17-4). Resident macrophages project processes into the lymph sinuses. Other macrophages are free in the sinuses.

    2. The phagocytosis of material in a lymph node is remarkably efficient. Nearly all phagocytizable material is removed from the lymph in one pass through a node.

C. **Sites of immune responses**

    1. Antigens in lymph elicit immune responses in lymph nodes.

    2. Germinal centers in cortical nodules are evidence of immune responses.
        a. Germinal centers are sites of blastic transformation of B lymphocytes.
        b. Blastic transformation increases the populations of memory cells and plasma cells (see Chapter 15 III C).

Chapter 18

Spleen

I. INTRODUCTION. The spleen is a distinctly compartmentalized organ. Splenic red pulp functions as a filter of aging blood cells. Splenic white pulp functions as an immunologic reaction site to blood-borne antigens.

A. Location. The spleen is in the left side of the abdominal cavity beneath the diaphragm.

B. Size and shape. The spleen is the largest lymphatic organ in the body. It is approximately the size of a clenched fist, and the hilum of the organ resembles the line of fingernails of a fist.

C. Functions. Splenic white pulp is lymphatic tissue that responds to blood-borne antigen. Splenic red pulp is a complex arrangement of blood sinuses and reticular connective tissue that processes aging blood cells.

II. HISTOLOGIC LANDMARKS OF THE SPLEEN (Figure 18-1)

A. Capsule and trabeculae

1. The **capsule** is a thick layer of dense irregular connective tissue, and some smooth muscle, that encloses the spleen.

2. **Trabeculae** of connective tissue extend from the capsule into the parenchyma of the organ.

B. Interior of the spleen. The spleen has white pulp and red pulp compartments.

1. **White pulp** appears as greyish islands of tissue. On microscopic examination, these can be recognized as areas of dense lymphatic tissue.

2. **Red pulp** appears as reddish material around the white pulp. Microscopic examination reveals that the red pulp consists of vast numbers of blood cells contained in blood sinuses and in reticular connective tissue.

3. **Absence of a cortex and medulla.** The terms cortex and medulla are not used when describing the structure of the spleen. Cortex and medulla imply the existence of outer and inner compartments, which do not occur in the spleen.

III. WHITE PULP. The white pulp is the **lymphatic tissue** that surrounds central arterioles.

A. Periarteriolar lymphatic sheath. The white pulp forms the periarteriolar lymphatic sheath (PALS), closely investing post-trabecular arterial vessels.

1. **T-lymphocytes** are numerous in the non-nodular areas of the PALS. These non-nodular regions are the **thymus-dependent areas** of the white pulp (comparable to the deep cortex of a lymph node).

2. **Lymphatic nodules,** many with **germinal centers,** develop in the PALS (Figure 18-2).
   a. A large number of nodules develop in the white pulp of a spleen (see Figure 18-2).
   b. Germinal centers are regularly encountered in nodules, especially in the antigenically stimulated spleen.

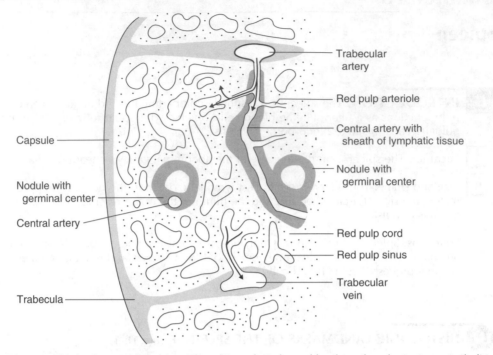

FIGURE 18-1. Spleen, low magnification. The white pulp is formed by dense lymphatic tissue, including nodules and germinal centers, that encloses the post-trabecular arterial tree of the organ. The red pulp is formed by a reticular meshwork, called the splenic cords, and by anastomosing vascular channels, called splenic sinuses. The red pulp surrounds the white pulp; conversely, the red pulp is permeated by the white pulp. *Arrows* indicate direction of blood flow.

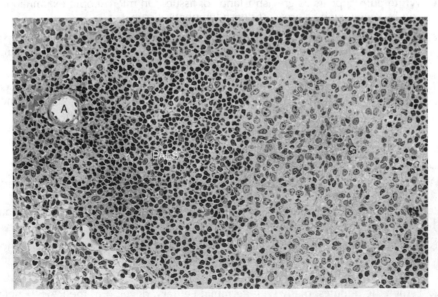

FIGURE 18-2. White pulp of the spleen. *A* = central artery, *PALS* = periarteriolar lymphatic sheath, *G* = germinal center.

B. Functions of white pulp

1. Proliferation of lymphocytes occurs in the PALS.

2. Nodules in the PALS are evidence of lymphocyte proliferation and are sites of immune reactions to antigens contained in the blood.

IV. **MARGINAL ZONE.** The marginal zone is the region of splenic parenchyma between the white pulp and the red pulp.

A. **Structure.** The marginal zone follows the complex, branching contour of the white pulp.

1. The junction of the marginal zone with the white pulp is more sharply defined than its junction with the red pulp.

2. Some branches of central arterioles terminate in the marginal zone.

B. **Function.** The marginal zone is the region of **initial immune reactions.**

1. This is the subcompartment of the spleen in which blood-borne antigens first encounter immunologically competent cells.

2. Lymphocytes leave the blood in the marginal zone to enter the white pulp and to reside there temporarily before re-entering the blood to continue the process of immune surveillance.

V. **RED PULP.** This is the compartment of splenic parenchyma that fills the volume of the organ not already occupied by the white pulp, the marginal zone, or the trabeculae. **Two vascular compartments,** sinuses and cords, form the red pulp.

A. **Sinuses.** Sinuses are blood vessel–like channels that branch and anastomose irregularly (Figure 18-3).

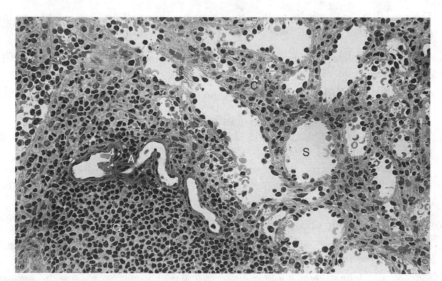

FIGURE 18-3. Junction between white pulp and red pulp of the spleen. The central artery (*A*) of the white pulp is sectioned longitudinally. A small germinal center (*G*) is associated with the artery. The red pulp sinuses (*S*) and red pulp cords (*C*) are clearly differentiated from one another because of the paucity of erythrocytes in the specimen.

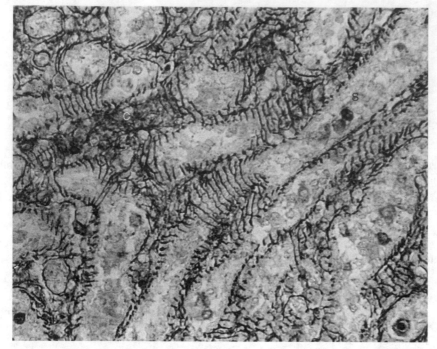

FIGURE 18-4. Red pulp of the spleen (high magnification, silver stain for reticular fibers). Sinuses (S) and cords (C) are visible. Note the wrapping of reticular fibers around the walls of sinuses.

1. **Endothelium.** The wall of the sinus is formed by spindle-shaped endothelial cells oriented parallel to the long axis of the sinus.
   a. A narrow, slit-like intercellular space separates adjacent endothelial cells.
   b. Junctional complexes are found between endothelial cells.

2. **Subendothelial support.** Reticular fibers wrap around the outside of the sinus (Figure 18-4).

3. **Sinuses often are indistinct** on histologic examination. Blood is generally found in a sinus, often to an extent that obscures the structure of the sinus.

B. **Cords** (cords of Billroth). Cords are the splenic tissue that fills in the space around the sinuses in the red pulp (see Figure 18-3).

1. **Reticular meshwork.** A three-dimensional meshwork of reticular cells and reticular fibers forms the structural framework of the red pulp cords.
   a. Macrophages occupy the intertices of the meshwork.
   b. A large fraction of the volume of the cords is extracellular space (i.e., the reticular cells and macrophages are not compactly arranged).

2. **Vascular space.** A cord is a vascular space in the sense that blood cells may fill the extensive extracellular space of the cord, like blood filling the lumen of a blood vessel.

C. **Comparison of splenic sinuses and cords**

1. The lumina of sinuses and the extracellular spaces of cords are the blood-containing regions of the red pulp.

2. Sinuses are defined, endothelium-lined vascular channels; cords are the perivascular, reticular connective tissue.

3. Both sinuses and cords contain all the cell types, erythrocytes and leukocytes, found in circulating blood.

D. **Functions of red pulp**

1. Senescent red and white blood cells are removed from the circulation by macrophages of the red pulp. The targeted cells are broken down by lysosomal enzymes of the macrophages.
   a. The iron of hemoglobin is retrieved and stored as ferritin for eventual recycling.
   b. The heme portion of hemoglobin is broken down into bilirubin. Bilirubin is transported to the liver, where it becomes a component of bile.

2. The spleen of some mammals, but not humans, serves as a reservoir for healthy erythrocytes and other blood cells, which may be added rapidly to the circulation in response to sudden blood loss (i.e., hemorrhage).

VI. BLOOD VESSELS OF THE SPLEEN

A. **Arterial tree of the spleen**

1. **Splenic artery.** Several branches of the splenic artery enter the organ along its broad hilum.

2. **Trabecular arteries.** Small arteries are found in the connective tissue trabeculae that penetrate the organ from the capsule.

3. **Central arteries.** Arteries leave trabeculae and acquire a sheath of dense lymphatic tissue, which is the white pulp.
   a. The largest central arteries are small muscular arteries. Most central arteries are actually **arterioles** (see Chapter 14 IV C).
   b. As a result of nodule development, the central artery is often **located eccentrically** in its sheath of lymphatic tissue.
   c. The presence of a small arterial vessel surrounded by dense, nodular lymphatic tissue with a germinal center is a useful characteristic for the identification of the spleen in the histology laboratory.

4. **Branches of central arteries.** Branches of central arteries may end in either the white pulp or the marginal zone. The fine, terminal portion of the central artery loses its lymphatic tissue sheath and enters the red pulp. The terminal central artery then branches and gives rise, in the red pulp, to the following sequence of vessels.
   a. **Penicillar arterioles** are straight, non-branching vessels, also referred to as **arterioles of the red pulp.** Penicillar refers to the straight, bristle-like appearance of these vessels.
   b. **Sheathed arterioles** acquire a sheath of phagocytic cells, which has been referred to as the **periarterial macrophage sheath.** These arterioles are not prominent in the human spleen.
   c. **Arterial capillaries** are typical capillaries and lack both smooth muscle and macrophages in their walls. Most arterial capillaries end in the cords of the red pulp. Some arterial capillaries may end in venous sinuses (see VII).

B. **Venous drainage of the red pulp**

1. **Blood collects in red pulp sinuses.**
   a. Blood cells are often seen in fixed tissue in the wall of the sinus between endothelial cells.
   b. This is evidence of blood cell movement across the sinus endothelial wall.

2. **Sinuses are drained by veins.**
   a. Red pulp sinuses drain into **pulp veins,** which are typical venules. Blood cells do not cross the wall of a pulp vein.
   b. Pulp veins collect into **trabecular veins,** which lie within the connective tissue trabeculae of the spleen.
   c. Trabecular veins drain into the **splenic vein.**

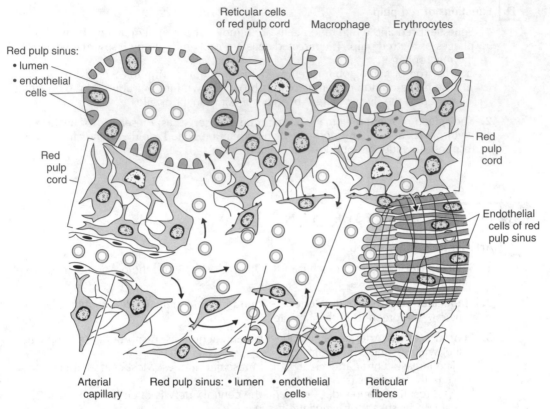

FIGURE 18-5. Drawing of the open type of blood circulation in the red pulp of the spleen. Blood cells leave arterial capillaries to enter the reticular meshwork of the red pulp cords. Blood cells also have access to red pulp sinuses by crossing the porous walls of the sinuses. Sinuses eventually empty into pulp veins and blood cells leave the red pulp compartment.

VII. BLOOD CIRCULATION THROUGH THE RED PULP: CLOSED VERSUS OPEN. Disagreement existed for decades over the pathway taken by blood as it passed through the red pulp of the spleen.

A. Closed circulation

1. **Definition.** Closed circulation refers to the emptying of the arterial capillaries directly into endothelium-lined sinuses of the red pulp. The endothelium of an arterial capillary and the endothelium of a red pulp sinus would be a continuous epithelial surface.

2. **Significance.** Blood would be confined to a closed, continuous, uninterrupted vascular space in the red pulp and, thus, would not be exposed to any connective tissue elements.

B. Open circulation

1. **Definition.** Open circulation refers to the ending of arterial capillaries directly into the reticular meshwork of the red pulp cords, rather than into endothelium-lined sinuses (Figure 18-5).

2. **Significance.** Blood entering the red pulp by this route would percolate through the cords, where it would be exposed to a macrophage-rich environment. Eventually, the blood would enter a sinus and exit the organ via a trabecular vein.

C. Evidence supports open circulation. An open pathway results in more efficient exposure of blood to the macrophages of the red pulp.

Chapter 19

Thymus

I.   **INTRODUCTION.** The thymus is a lymphatic organ that has a central role in the immune response because it provides an environment for the differentiation of **thymic lymphocytes (T lymphocytes).** Under normal conditions, however, the thymus is not a site of either humoral or cell-mediated immune responses.

A.   **Location.** The thymus is located in the **superior mediastinum** posterior to the sternum and anterior to the arch of the aorta.

B.   **Origin.** Unlike purely lymphatic organs such as lymph nodes, the thymus is considered a **lymphoepithelial organ** because of its **dual embryologic origin;** it develops from both **endoderm and mesoderm. Ectoderm** may also contribute to the thymus.

II.   **HISTOLOGIC LANDMARKS OF THE THYMUS**

A.   **Cortex and medulla**

1. Cortex and medulla are the terms used to describe the **parenchyma** of the thymus (cf. the red and white pulp of the spleen).

2. **Thymic (Hassall) corpuscles** are characteristic configurations of epithelial reticular cells found only in the medulla.

B.   **Thymic lobule.** A lobule is a **unit of structure** of thymic tissue. It is a spheroidal arrangement of lymphatic tissue approximately 1 mm in diameter (Figure 19-1).

1. A lobule is formed by a **cortical cap** of dense lymphatic tissue covering a less dense **medullary core.**

2. This lobular arrangement of cortex and medulla **superficially resembles a lymphatic nodule** with a germinal center (see Chapter 15 VIII). The thymic lobule, however, is not a site of immune response.

C.   **Thymic vessels**

1. **Blood vessels**
   a. **Cortex.** Capillaries are the only blood vessels in the cortical compartment. Arterioles and venules are not present in the cortical parenchyma.
   b. **Medulla.** Arterioles, capillaries, and venules are present in the medulla.

2. **Lymphatic vessels.** The thymus has efferent lymphatic drainage but lacks afferent vessels.

D.   **Capsule.** A thin connective tissue capsule encloses the thymus, and **trabeculae** extend from the capsule to the interior of the organ.

III.   **THYMIC EPITHELIAL RETICULAR CELLS.** These cells form the cellular framework of the thymus and share some of the characteristics of reticular cells of other lymphatic organs.

A.   **Embryonic origin and cellular characteristics**

1. Thymic reticular cells are **endodermal** in origin, whereas reticular cells of other

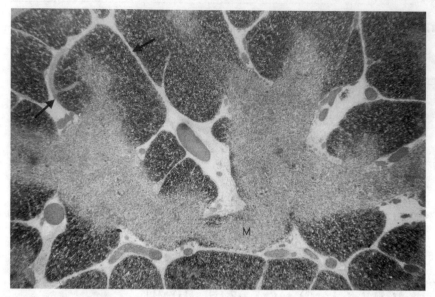

FIGURE 19-1. Thymus, human, non-involuted. The medulla (*M*) is continuous from lobule to lobule. A lobule (*arrows*) is formed by a central core of medullary tissue and a cap of denser cortical lymphatic tissue.

lymphatic organs are mesodermal. This embryonic origin gives the reticular cells of the thymus some epithelial characteristics (e.g., numerous desmosomes and keratin intermediate filaments), hence they are called **epithelial reticular cells.**

2. The thymus has a **cellular reticulum** formed by the epithelial reticular cells. Unlike other lymphatic organs, however, it **has no fibrous reticulum.** The thymus does not contain the fibroblast-like reticular cells that synthesize a fibrous reticulum.

B. **Proximity to thymic lymphocytes**

1. Lymphocytes are packed into the interstices of the cellular reticulum.

2. Lymphocytes vastly outnumber and obscure the epithelial reticular cells.

C. **Secretory function.** Epithelial reticular cells secrete hormones that are necessary for the normal functioning of the thymus, such as **thymosin** and **thymopoietin.**

IV. **CORTEX OF THE THYMUS.** The cortex is the **peripheral compartment** of lymphatic tissue. This is the site of T-cell production.

A. The cortex appears as a discontinuous layer of dense lymphatic tissue. Each lobule is capped by a layer of cortex.

1. The superficial cortex (i.e., close to the capsule) contains a mixture of large lymphocytes (lymphoblasts) and small lymphocytes.

2. The remainder of the cortex contains exclusively small lymphocytes.

B. The cortical epithelial reticular cells are partially masked by the more numerous lymphocytes.

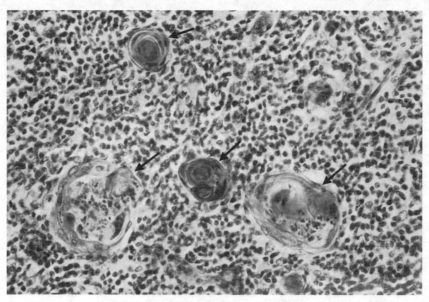

FIGURE 19-2. Thymic (Hassall) corpuscles. Four corpuscles (*arrows*) are surrounded by the lymphatic tissue of the medulla.

V. **MEDULLA OF THE THYMUS.** The medulla is an extensive, branched arrangement of lymphatic tissue that is continuous from lobule to lobule (see Figure 19-1). It is the **inner compartment** of lymphatic tissue.

A. **Lymphocyte packing**

   1. Lymphocytes are less densely concentrated in the medulla than in the cortex. This results in the **paler appearance of the medulla** in histologic sections.

   2. Epithelial reticular cells are more easily identified in the medulla than in the cortex because of the lower concentration of lymphocytes. Some of the medullary epithelial reticular cells form thymic corpuscles.

B. **Thymic (Hassall) corpuscles.** These structures are unique to the medulla of the thymus.

   1. A thymic corpuscle is a **cyst-like, concentric arrangement of epithelial reticular cells** (Figure 19-2). Thymic corpuscles range in size from about 30 to 150 μm.
      a. The squamous, centrally located cells of a thymic corpuscle lack nuclei and resemble keratinized epidermal cells.
      b. Larger Hassall corpuscles may enclose other cell types (e.g., macrophages) and cell debris.

   2. The presence and concentration of thymic corpuscles are variable, but they appear to reach their largest size and are most numerous in the fully developed thymus at puberty.

   3. The function of thymic corpuscles, if any, is unknown.

VI. **BLOOD–THYMUS BARRIER**

A. The blood–thymus barrier **shields T lymphocytes from antigens.**

   1. Even though the thymus has a critical role in the establishment of immune competence, the thymus does not normally react to blood-borne or lymph-borne antigens.

2. Antigens may circulate through the thymus but they do not provoke immune responses in the organ.

B. **Location of the blood–thymus barrier.** Use of molecular probes such as horseradish peroxidase has demonstrated a barrier between blood vessels and parenchymal cells of the **thymic cortex.** The barrier is less effective, however, in the medulla.

C. **Components** of the cortical blood–thymus barrier include the following:

1. **Tight junctions** of capillary endothelial cells

2. Perivascular **macrophages** that phagocytize the small amounts of material that cross vessel walls

3. Wrapping of **epithelial reticular cell processes** around capillaries and perivascular tissue

D. **Experimental bypass of the blood–thymus barrier.** Injection of antigen directly into the thymus will produce an immune response. Such a procedure bypasses the barrier and exposes the normally shielded immunocompetent cells to antigen.

VII. INVOLUTION OF THE THYMUS

A. **Developmental sequence.** The thymus is an unusual organ because it is **fully developed at birth** and, at this time, is approximately the size of the heart. At **puberty,** the thymus has attained its largest absolute size and then undergoes involution.

B. **Characteristics of thymic involution**

1. **Size.** The thymus gradually decreases in weight and loses its definition as a distinct organ.

2. **Tissue alteration.** The lobulated structure of the pubertal thymus is replaced by adipose connective tissue and isolated clumps of lymphatic tissue (Figure 19-3).

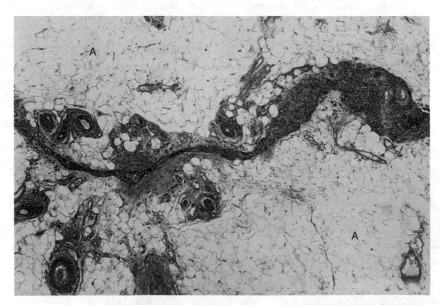

FIGURE 19-3. Thymus, involuted. The adult, involuted thymus is characterized by a large amount of adipose connective tissue (*A*) and irregular clumps of vascularized lymphatic tissue.

C. **Continued function.** The involuted thymus remains a functioning lymphatic organ.

    1. The emphasis once placed on involution and what was thought to be complete loss of function is unjustified.

    2. Evidence indicates that the thymus continues to be a source of T lymphocytes even after involution.

D. **Stress involution.** The process of involution may be accelerated in ill or injured infants or children. The stress-involuted thymus will regenerate to its former size if the stress is eliminated.

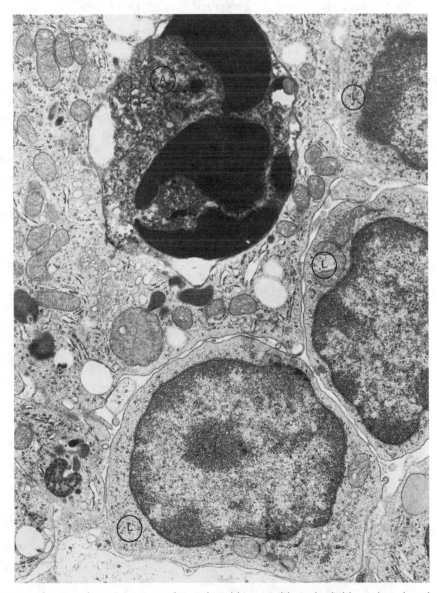

FIGURE 19-4. Thymus, electron micrograph, 42-day-old rat. Visible in the field are three lymphocytes (*L*) and an apoptotic cell (*A*). The apoptotic cell exhibits characteristic nuclear fragmentation and condensation. (Courtesy of B. C. Basaca, Stratton V.A. Medical Center and Albany Medical College, Albany, NY.)

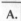 **ROLE OF THYMUS IN IMMUNE RESPONSE**

A. The thymus provides an **environment for the differentiation of T lymphocytes.**

1. The thymus is "seeded" by stem cells from the bone marrow during fetal life. Cells that develop in the thymus acquire the characteristics that define their role in both the cell-mediated immune response and the humoral immune response.

2. The blood–thymus barrier establishes and maintains an isolated environment for T lymphocyte development.

B. The thymus is a site of **extensive cell selection and cell destruction.**

1. Large numbers of lymphocytes that are produced in the thymus die by apoptosis in the thymus because they are recognized as being programmed to react immunologically against self (Figure 19-4).

2. T lymphocytes that are not programmed to react with self survive the selection process and are released into the circulation.

C. **Effects of thymectomy.** The critical role of the thymus in the immune response is demonstrated by the effects of neonatal and adult thymectomy.

1. **Neonatal thymectomy** results in **severe impairment of the cell-mediated immune response.**
   a. Thymectomy deprives the young animal of its normal complement of T lymphocytes, which are the cells that effect the cell-mediated response. The humoral immune response is also affected because of the loss of helper T cells.
   b. The thymectomized neonate can **tolerate grafts** because of the absence of cytotoxic killer cells.
   c. The **thymus-dependent areas of lymph nodes and spleen fail to develop,** reducing the overall size of the lymph nodes and spleen.

2. **Adult thymectomy** results in **less severe impairment of immune responses** because peripheral tissues are already well-stocked with T lymphocytes at the time of thymectomy. T cells are **long-lived** and this also delays observable effects of adult thymectomy.

Chapter 20

Skin

I. **INTRODUCTION.** The skin is the largest organ of the body. It covers the entire body surface and accounts for 15% to 20% of the body weight. It is formed by the epidermis, which is an epithelial compartment; the dermis, which is a connective tissue compartment; and several types of epidermally derived appendages.

A. **Functions**

1. **Protection.** The skin protects the individual from the generally hostile external environment.

2. **Homeostasis.** The skin preserves the constancy of the life-sustaining internal environment.

3. **Sensation.** The skin enables the individual to obtain sensory information from the external environment.

B. **Components.** All four basic tissues are represented in skin.

1. The epidermis is an **epithelial** compartment that forms the actual interface with the environment.

2. The dermis is a **connective tissue** compartment that forms most of the mass of the skin.

3. **Nerve** fibers and nerve endings are numerous in the dermis.

4. Smooth **muscle** is associated with hair follicles as the arrector pili muscles, and is present in the walls of dermal blood vessels.

C. **Epidermal appendages.** During embryonic and fetal development, the epidermis gives rise to **hair follicles, sebaceous glands, eccrine sweat glands,** and **apocrine glands.** During adult life, the epidermis remains continuous with these skin adnexa.

II. **EPIDERMIS.** The epidermis is a **stratified squamous keratinizing epithelium** that encloses the entire surface of the body and forms a protective interface with the environment.

A. **General characteristics of the epidermis**

1. **Thickness of the epidermis varies considerably,** from approximately 0.1 mm in protected areas such as the anterior surface of the forearm, to about 1.0 mm in areas subject to abrasion, such as the plantar or palmar surfaces (Figure 20-1).

2. **Epidermis is continuous** with the epithelial lining of the alimentary canal and of the urogenital system. The epidermis is also continuous with the conjunctiva of the eye and with the epithelial covering of the tympanic membrane of the ear.

3. **Epidermis is avascular,** as are epithelia in general.

4. **Four epidermal strata** can be distinguished in the epidermis. These layers consist primarily of keratin-producing cells, **keratinocytes,** in various stages of differentiation.
   a. The strata can be grouped into two regions:
      (1) **Nonkeratinized cells.** The **malpighian layer** is the deeper of the two regions, and consists of living, nonkeratinized cells. It can be further subdivided into the basal (germinative), spinous, and granular layers.

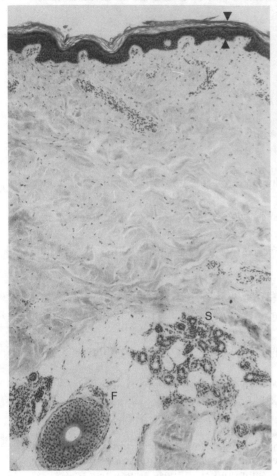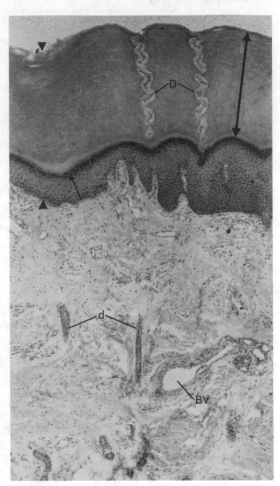

FIGURE 20-1. Light micrographs of two types of skin. (*Left*) Thin epidermis is denoted by *arrowheads.* The structure of the stratum corneum is characteristically frayed. Dense irregular connective tissue of the dermis fills most of the field. A transverse section of a hair follicle (*F*) and the coiled portion of an eccrine sweat gland (*S*) are visible in the deep dermis, surrounded by adipose tissue. (*Right*) Thick epidermis is denoted by *arrowheads*, and the compact stratum corneum is denoted by a *double-headed arrow*. The stratum granulosum is indicated (*single-headed arrow*) but individual keratohyalin granules are not resolved at this magnification. A pale-staining stratum lucidum is visible between the stratum granulosum and stratum corneum. The helical pathways of the intraepidermal portions of two eccrine sweat gland ducts (*D*) contrast with the straight pathways of the intradermal portions (*d*) of the sweat gland ducts. *BV* = blood vessel.

        (2) Keratinized cells. The superficial layer of the epidermis consists of dead, keratinized, squamous cells.

    b. The **process of keratinocyte differentiation** begins deep in the epidermis in the cells of the basal layer (Figure 20-2).

        (1) As they differentiate, keratinocytes rise through successive epidermal layers, finally emerging at the free surface of the tissue as fully differentiated keratinized cells.

        (2) It takes 3 to 4 weeks for a cell to move from the basal layer to the superficial stratum corneum.

    c. The epidermis also contains a small number of cells other than keratinocytes (see II F).

B. **Basal cells.** The **stratum germinativum,** or basal layer, is the deepest layer of the epidermis. It ranges in thickness from one cell in thin epidermis, to a few cells in thick epidermis.

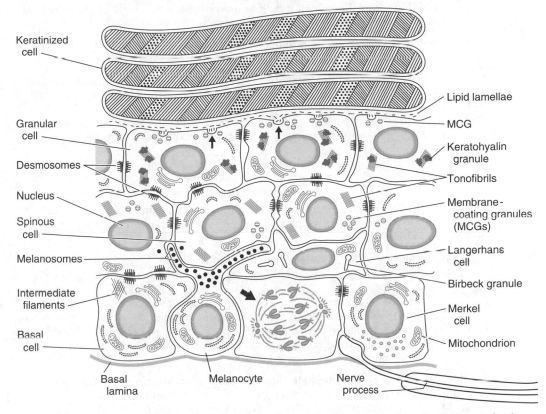

Keratinized cell

Granular cell

Desmosomes

Nucleus

Spinous cell

Melanosomes

Intermediate filaments

Basal cell

Basal lamina

Melanocyte

Nerve process

Lipid lamellae

MCG

Keratohyalin granule

Tonofibrils

Membrane-coating granules (MCGs)

Langerhans cell

Birbeck granule

Merkel cell

Mitochondrion

FIGURE 20-2. Diagram illustrating cells of the epidermis and major aspects of keratinization. A dividing germinative cell is depicted in anaphase (*thick arrow*). Keratin intermediate filaments are synthesized in basal cells. Filaments aggregate into tonofibrils in spinous cells, and tonofibrils associate with keratohyalin granules in granular cells. Membrane-coating granules (MCGs) are synthesized in spinous cells and release their lipid lamellae by exocytosis (*thin arrows*) at the granular cell–keratinized cell interface. Melanosomes are illustrated within both melanocytes and adjacent keratinocytes. Keratinized cells are squamous cells that are enclosed by a thickened cell membrane and are filled with a compact arrangement of intermediate filaments and filaggrin.

1. **Epidermal cell generation.** Basal cells are **germinative cells.**
   a. The basal cell layer contains the stem cells from which all keratinocytes derive.
   b. Mitotic division of these cells replaces the epidermal cells that are continuously being lost from the skin.
2. **Intermediate filaments.** Basal cells contain keratin intermediate filaments.
   a. Keratin intermediate filaments, or **tonofilaments,** are approximately 10 nm in diameter and of indeterminate length. They are present in high concentration in all epidermal cells.
   b. The intermediate filaments of epidermal cells are not formed of a single, homogeneous protein. Several different filament proteins (40 kD to 70 kD in size) are expressed at different epidermal strata.

C. **Spinous cells.** The **stratum spinosum,** or spinous layer, can be several cell layers thick in thick epidermis but may be inconspicuous in thin epidermis. It is formed primarily of **postmitotic keratinocytes** that have **migrated from the basal layer.**

1. **Cell shape.** Their numerous processes give the cells a characteristic spiny appearance. This appearance may result from selective effects of fixation on the cells at this stage in their differentiation in combination with persistence of the numerous cell–cell junctions.
   a. The processes of adjacent cells contact one another; **desmosomes** are found at the points of contact.

    b. These desmosomal cell–cell junctions are present at all levels of the epidermis, but are most obvious in the stratum spinosum.

  2. Intermediate filaments. Keratin filaments tend to aggregate laterally in spinous cells and granular cells to form **tonofibrils,** which are visible by light microscopy.

  3. Membrane-coating granules. Spinous cells synthesize membrane-coating granules (MCGs), which have an integral role in the formation of the epidermal water barrier (see II E 1 b).

    a. MCGs are small, ovoid structures visible only with the electron microscope. The granule is membrane-bounded and is filled with closely packed lipid lamellae.

    b. MCGs first become apparent close to the Golgi apparatus of the spinous cells. MCGs increase in number as differentiation progresses.

D. **Granular cells.** The **stratum granulosum,** or granular layer, is the most superficial level of the nonkeratinized, living part of the epidermis. Granular cells are characterized by the following:

  1. Keratohyalin granules. Granular cells contain intracellular keratohyalin granules.

    a. Keratohyalin granules are variable in size and shape but are readily visible by light microscopy.

      (1) Tonofibrils are often visible passing through keratohyalin granules.

      (2) Ribosomes cluster around the keratohyalin granules.

    b. The granules contain proteins that are rich in cystine and phosphorylated histidine. The characteristic basophilia of keratohyalin granules is the result of the high concentration of phosphate groups.

  2. Filaggrin. This is an **intermediate filament–associated protein** contained in keratohyalin granules. It is integral to the process of keratinization.

    a. As keratinization proceeds, filaggrin becomes more dispersed in the cell.

    b. Filaggrin ultimately aggregates keratin intermediate filaments into a compact mass that fills the keratinized cell.

  3. Membrane-coating granules. MCGs appear to be more numerous in granular cells than in spinous cells. They may account for up to 15% of the volume of a granular cell.

    a. MCGs congregate beneath the apical plasma membrane of the granular cell.

    b. Exocytosis of the MCG contents at the granular cell–keratinized cell junction is regularly observed.

E. **Keratinized cells.** The **stratum corneum** is formed by keratinized cells, also called cornified or horny cells, and is the most superficial portion of the epidermis. It provides a barrier against dehydration, mechanical abrasion, and entry into the body of potentially harmful materials.

  1. Cellular and intercellular components of the stratum corneum

    a. Keratinized cells. The stratum corneum is composed of shingle-like layers of **anucleate, desiccated, squamous cells.**

    b. Intercellular material. A lipid-rich material derived from the contents of MCGs contributes to the water-barrier function of the stratum corneum.

      (1) The lipid lamellae of MCGs are released from granular cells by exocytosis into the intercellular space between the granular layer and the keratinized layer.

      (2) Lamellae may remain recognizable as disks in the intercellular space or they may coalesce into broad sheets that appear to fill the intercellular space of the stratum corneum.

      (3) Intercellular lamellae or sheets are more evident deep in the stratum corneum, closer to the stratum granulosum. This may partially explain the greater effectiveness of the dehydration barrier at progressively deeper levels of the stratum corneum.

2. **Thickness and organization of the stratum corneum**
   a. **Thickness.** The stratum corneum from different areas of the body falls into two categories (see Figure 20-1):
      (1) **Thin stratum corneum,** 5 to 7 cells thick, is characteristic of surfaces not subject to frequent friction.
      (2) **Thick stratum corneum,** 25 to 30 cells thick, is characteristic of the volar surfaces that are subject to frequent friction.
   b. **Organization.** In regions of the body characterized by a thin stratum corneum, the keratinized cells are arranged in **precise columnar stacks** and adjacent stacks slightly overlap each other.
      (1) Sections routinely processed for light microscopy do not show stacking clearly.
      (2) Exposure of frozen sections of skin to a dilute alkali solution rehydrates the keratinized cells, which become slightly less squamous, making cell–cell boundaries and columnar stacking more obvious.

3. **Transformation to keratinized cells.** The transformation of a granular cell to a keratinized cell takes only a few hours.
   a. An **abrupt change in cell shape** is apparent between the cuboidal, living cells of the granular layer and the squamous, dead cells of the cornified layer.
   b. An additional cell layer called the **stratum lucidum** is generally present at this transition in thick epidermis. This unstained layer, usually only a few cells thick, is a **transitional zone** formed by cells in the terminal stages of differentiation from non-keratinized granular cells to keratinized cells of the horny layer.
   c. In thin epidermis, transitional cells (i.e., a stratum lucidum) are usually not apparent.

4. **Characteristics of keratinized (cornified) cells**
   a. **Filaments and matrix.** The cell is filled with closely packed keratin intermediate filaments that are surrounded by an electron-opaque (i.e., darker) matrix.
      (1) The matrix is derived from the filaggrin of keratohyalin granules.
      (2) The compact arrangement of filaments and matrix, visible in thin sections using a transmission electron microscope, is called the **keratin pattern.**
   b. **Cell membrane.** The cell membrane thickens during keratinization from 8–9 nm to as much as 20–25 nm by the deposition of the protein **involucrin** on the cytoplasmic side of the membrane.
      (1) The thickened plasma membrane of the keratinized cell is a remarkably resilient structure.
      (2) For example, the cell membrane of the keratinized cell is not dissolved by 0.1 N NaOH, which normally hydrolyzes other animal proteins such as collagen.
   c. **Organelles.** Mitochondria, Golgi bodies, and other organelles are **not visible** in cornified cells, and their fate is unclear.
      (1) Organelles may be degraded and released from the cell.
      (2) Possibly, components of organelles are retained in the keratinized cell in an unrecognizable form.
      (3) However, membrane specializations such as desmosomes do remain recognizable in the stratum corneum.

5. **Epidermal barrier to dehydration.** The prime epidermal barrier to water loss is in the **stratum corneum** and consists of keratinized squamous cells and intercellular material derived from membrane-coating granules.
   a. Small, but measurable amounts of water (approximately 0.2 mg/cm^2/hr) are lost to the environment by diffusion through the epidermis.
   b. Complete removal of the stratum corneum, exposing the stratum granulosum, results in the loss of the barrier to water diffusion across the epidermis. Such a denuded region, as in a common abrasion, is freely permeable to water.

F. **Nonkeratinocytes present in the epidermis.** These cells are much less numerous than keratinocytes.

1. **Melanocytes** are highly branched, pigment-producing cells of neural crest origin present in the basal level of the epidermis. Approximately 2% to 10% of cells in the basal layer are melanocytes. **Melanin** is the pigment produced by melanocytes.
   a. Melanin is produced by the **oxidation of tyrosine** in melanocytes. Melanin granules, or **melanosomes,** are transferred by an endocytic process to adjacent keratinocytes (see Figure 20-2).
      (1) Skin coloration is due largely to the secretory activity of melanocytes.
      (2) Two types of melanin are produced by human melanocytes: **eumelanin,** a black-brown pigment, and **pheomelanin,** a red-yellow pigment.
   b. **Ultraviolet radiation** (e.g., unfiltered sunlight) stimulates synthesis of melanin, which manifests as tanning.
      (1) A keratinocyte from a tanned region contains more melanin granules than a keratinocyte from an untanned region.
      (2) Increased amounts of pigment in the epidermis shield the more deeply located nucleic acids and proteins in the germinative cells from the harmful effects of ultraviolet radiation.
   c. An **epidermal-melanin unit** is a melanocyte and the several keratinocytes that receive melanin from it.

2. **Langerhans cells** are branched cells that are widely scattered in the nonkeratinized level of the epidermis.
   a. Langerhans cells were once thought to be effete melanocytes of neural crest origin, but are now believed to be mesenchymal cells derived from a precursor in the bone marrow.
   b. The presence of characteristic rod- or tennis-racket–shaped granules seen with the electron microscope (sometimes called Birbeck granules) may be used to identify Langerhans cells in the epidermis.
   c. Langerhans cells function as antigen-presenting cells, particularly in cutaneous hypersensitivity reactions.

3. **Merkel cells** are present in the basal level of the epidermis and are closely associated with nerve processes that enter the epidermis from the dermis (see Figure 20-2).
   a. Merkel cells contain small, electron-opaque granules that resemble the granules of neuroendocrine cells.
   b. The complex formed by a Merkel cell and a nerve process is called a **Merkel corpuscle.**

III.   DERMIS. The dermis is formed by loose irregular (areolar) and dense irregular connective tissues and it accounts for most of the mass of the skin.

A.   General characteristics

1. **Thickness.** The thickness of the dermis is variable and may reach 5 mm in some areas of the body.
2. **Boundaries.** The dermis is sharply defined superficially at the dermoepidermal junction. Its deep boundary is less well defined as it merges with subcutaneous connective tissues (see Figure 20-1).

B.   Dermal components. The dermis can be divided into two layers.

1. **Papillary layer.** This is a layer of **loose (areolar) connective tissue** that is subjacent to the epidermis.
   a. It is often a relatively thin layer.
   b. It is named for the papillary interdigitations at the dermal–epidermal junction.
   c. A **basal lamina** separates the basal surface of the epidermis from the papillary layer (see Figures 20-2, 5-5).

2. **Reticular layer.** This a layer of **dense irregular connective tissue** deep to the papillary layer.
   a. The reticular layer is usually much thicker than the papillary layer.
   b. The term "reticular layer" is somewhat of a misnomer. The reticular layer consists primarily of large, thick collagen fibers, rather than delicate, thin reticular fibers.
   c. The reticular and papillary layers merge, often imperceptibly.

C. **Dermal fibroblasts.** Fibroblasts are the predominant cell type of the dermis. They synthesize most of its extracellular matrix materials, both collagen and ground substance.

   1. A population of fibroblast **stem cells** resides in the superficial dermis, close to the stratum germinativum.

   2. These fibroblasts replicate and most daughter cells **migrate** to deeper levels of the dermis. Some daughter cells remain as stem cells.

D. **Langer lines.** Collagen and elastic fibers are not randomly arranged in the dermis. Langer lines are **lines of tension** in the skin produced by the orientation of the fibers.

   1. **Evidence of Langer lines**
      a. A circular hole in the skin gradually becomes elongated into a narrow oval, the long axis of which is parallel to Langer lines in that region.
      b. Conversely, a linear incision made at a right angle to Langer lines will form an oval-shaped, open wound if left unsutured.

   2. **Implications in wound healing and scar formation**
      a. Linear wounds oriented parallel to Langer lines tend to close and heal with minimal scarring, even if left unsutured.
      b. Linear wounds oriented perpendicular to Langer lines tend to gape and heal slowly with conspicuous scarring, if left unsutured.

E. **Dermoepidermal junction.** The dermoepidermal junction is remarkably variable in structure.

   1. In some areas of the body, the junction between epidermis and dermis is relatively flat, whereas in other areas the junction shows a complex, interdigitated arrangement of papillae, ridges, and furrows.
      a. Generally, a **flat junction is associated with thin epidermis** and a **complex junction is associated with thick epidermis.**
      b. Where the junction is complex, the surface area of the basal layer of the epidermis is several times that of the free surface.
      c. The two types of dermoepidermal junctions can be compared in a sagittal section of a digit, where the dorsal epidermis is thin and the volar epidermis is thick.

   2. **Functional significance of a complex dermoepidermal junction**
      a. The increased surface area of the complex dermoepidermal junction produces **greater adhesion between epidermis and dermis.** This is particularly important on surfaces subject to frictional and shearing stress.
      b. Because of the increased surface area of the stratum germinativum, **many more kerantinocytes enter the more superficial levels of the epidermis per unit time** (assuming a constant rate of mitosis in the stratum germinativum). This may partially account for the thickened epidermis that is characteristically found on surfaces exposed to nearly constant friction.

   3. **Dermatoglyphics**
      a. A superficial relationship is occasionally noted between dermatoglyphic ridges and grooves (fingerprints) and the ridges and grooves of the dermoepidermal junction.
      b. Skin surface ridges that form dermatoglyphics are in register with certain, but not all, epidermal ridges that project into the dermis at the dermoepidermal

junction. Therefore, dermatoglyphic patterns are not duplicated at the dermo-epidermal junction.

F. **Hypodermis.** The **panniculus adiposus** and **panniculus carnosus** are subcutaneous layers that make up the hypodermis, which is often grouped with skin.

1. The **panniculus adiposus** is a layer of adipose connective tissue subjacent to the reticular layer of the dermis.
   a. It is variable in thickness and may be absent from some sites or from some individuals.
   b. The panniculus adiposus functions as an insulating compartment and as a storage site for energy.

2. The **panniculus carnosus** is a thin layer of skeletal muscle that is subjacent to the panniculus adiposus. In humans, most of this layer is vestigial, but portions persist as the platysma muscle and the muscles of facial expression.

IV. **HAIR FOLLICLES.** Hair follicles are appendages of the epidermis that produce hairs, which are columns of keratinized cells (Figure 20-3). Hair follicles may project several millimeters into the dermis. Except for size, the basic structure of all follicles is the same.

A. **Follicle size.** Hairs and hair follicles vary considerably in size.

1. Hairs vary from long, coarse **terminal hairs** to short, fine **vellus hairs.** Hairs from different regions of the body have characteristic lengths and diameters (e.g., the fine vellus hairs of the forehead and the coarse terminal hairs of the beard).

2. There is a correlation between the size of the hair produced by a follicle and the size of the follicle itself. Terminal hairs are produced by large-diameter, long follicles and vellus hairs are produced by much smaller follicles.

B. **Germinative region.** The germinative region of the hair follicle is localized in the follicle bulb.

1. **Follicle bulb.** The follicle is of nearly constant diameter except at its deepest point where it expands to form the bulb.

2. **Dermal papilla.** The bulb is deeply indented by a tuft of vascularized connective tissue called the dermal papilla (not to be confused with dermal papillae of the dermoepidermal junction).

3. **Follicle matrix.** The matrix of the hair follicle is adjacent to the dermal papilla and is the **germinative compartment** of the follicle.
   a. Mitoses occur in this compartment and account for **growth of the hair.** The mitotic activity is supported by the nearby richly vascularized dermal papilla. Destruction of the papilla causes atrophy of the hair follicle.
   b. Melanocytes are also present in this region of the follicle, close to the dermal papilla, and contribute pigment to the differentiating cells of the hair shaft.
      (1) These melanocytes produce both eumelanin (black–brown) and pheomelanin (yellow–red) pigments.
      (2) The ratio of these pigments determines hair color.

C. **Differentiating region.** The differentiating region of the hair follicle is located between the bulb and the middle of the follicle. Cells in the upper bulb differentiate into the several layers of the hair follicle and hair shaft, producing a column of concentrically arranged layers of cells. The following layers may be identified:

1. **Outer root sheath.** This is the outermost epithelial cell layer of the follicle. It is continuous with the basal layer of the epidermis.
   a. A connective tissue layer surrounds the outer root sheath.

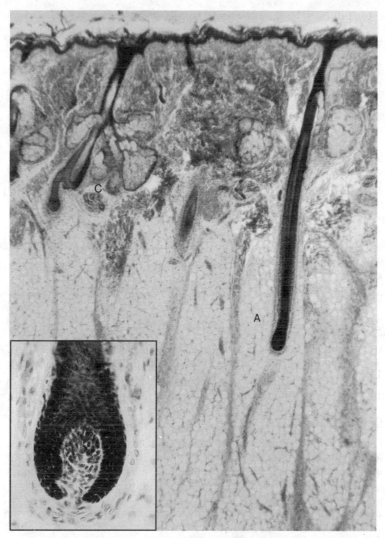

FIGURE 20-3. Light micrograph of skin showing an anagen hair follicle (*A*) and a catagen hair follicle (*C*). Both follicles are associated with large sebaceous glands. (*Inset*) Anagen hair follicle bulb with distinct dermal papilla.

    b. The connective tissue is separated from the outer root sheath by the **glassy membrane,** which is a thickened basement membrane.

2. Inner root sheath. This lies between the outer root sheath and the hair shaft.
    a. The cells of the inner root sheath keratinize and the keratinized cells desquamate into the pilosebaceous canal at the level of the sebaceous gland.
    b. The inner root sheath comprises three layers: **cuticle** (adjacent to the hair shaft), **Huxley layer,** and **Henle layer** (adjacent to the outer root sheath).

3. Hair shaft. This is composed of three types of cells:
    a. Cuticle cells are squamous cells that form the outermost layer of the hair shaft and interdigitate with the cuticular cells of the inner root sheath.
    b. Cortical cells are cuboidal cells and contain intermediate filaments densely packed in the keratin pattern.
    c. Medullary cells form a central column of vacuolated cells. They are stacked, producing a ladder-like appearance.

D. **Arrector pili muscles** are bundles of smooth muscle that extend between the connective tissue sheath of the follicles and the superficial dermis. Contraction of this muscle causes the hair follicle to stand erect, producing "goose flesh."

E. **Sebaceous glands** (see V). These glands develop from the outer root sheaths of the follicles.

1. The duct of the gland empties into the hair follicle in the space around the hair shaft.
   a. The **pilosebaceous canal** begins at the point of entry of the sebaceous gland duct and opens on to the surface of the epidermis.
   b. The canal contains the hair shaft, desquamating cells, and the secretions of the sebaceous gland.

2. A roughly triangular space is formed by the hair follicle, the arrector pili muscle, and the basal surface of the epidermis. The sebaceous gland occupies part of this triangular space.

F. **Follicle Growth Cycle.** A hair follicle exhibits cycles of development characterized by distinct **growing and resting phases.**

1. **Anagen** is the **growing stage** of the follicle.
   a. During anagen the follicle reaches its maximum length. Some anagen follicles may be 4–5 mm long.
   b. A hair shaft is being produced by a follicle during this stage at a rate of 0.3 to 0.4 mm per day.
   c. A human hair follicle can remain in anagen for several years, but considerable variation is encountered in follicles from different body regions.

2. **Catagen** is a **transitional stage** between anagen and telogen and is characterized by **atrophy** of the follicle.
   a. The lower half of the follicle is reduced to an epithelial strand.
   b. The dermal papilla, however, remains recognizable.

3. **Telogen** is a **quiescent stage.** No hair growth occurs during telogen.
   a. The atrophied, telogen follicle is reduced to half of its original length or less.
   b. The hair remains attached to the atrophied follicle and is called a club hair because of the appearance of its proximal end. Hairs are easily lost from telogen follicles during grooming.
   c. Telogen may last for a few months in humans, at the end of which the quiescent follicle re-enters anagen for another cycle of follicle regeneration and hair growth.

G. **Baldness.** In androgenic alopecia, hair follicles remain identifiable.

1. After several growth cycles, large terminal follicles gradually become converted to small vellus follicles. During this gradual reduction in size, the diameter of the hair being produced also decreases.
   a. The mechanism controlling this change is unknown but may be related to levels of androgens and to increased metabolism of androgens by hair follicles.
   b. Vellus follicles of the bald scalp remain in telogen for relatively long periods.

2. The completely bald scalp is not hairless but is populated by vellus follicles. The concentration of vellus follicles in the "bald" scalp approximates the concentration of terminal follicles of the hirsute scalp.

V. **SEBACEOUS GLANDS** (Figure 20-4). These are holocrine glands that secrete onto the surface of the skin. The secretions give skin its oily characteristic.

A. **Structure**

1. Sebaceous glands are **associated with hair follicles.**

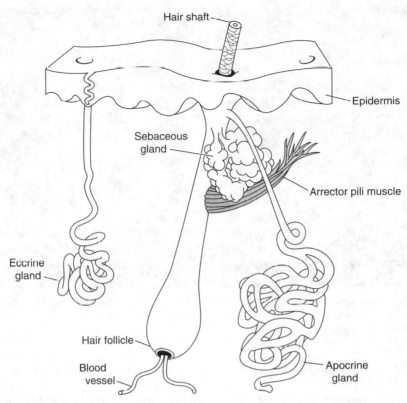

FIGURE 20-4. Drawing depicting the relationships of the three cutaneous glands to epidermis and hair follicle. (Adapted with permission from Montagna W, Parakkal PF: *The Structure and Function of Skin,* 3rd ed. New York, Academic Press, 1974, p 334.)

  a. All hair follicles have sebaceous glands. Conversely, most—but not all—sebaceous glands are associated with hair follicles.
  b. There is an inverse relationship in size between a hair follicle and its associated sebaceous gland.
    (1) Large, terminal hair follicles usually have relatively small sebaceous glands.
    (2) Smaller, vellus follicles generally have relatively large sebaceous glands.

 2. The **acinus** is the unit of structure of the sebaceous gland.
   a. An acinus is a round or ovoid, lobule-like group of cells.
   b. A sebaceous gland is formed by several acini bound loosely by connective tissue into a lobe (Figure 20-5).

B. **Sebaceous transformation.** This is the developmental process undergone by sebaceous cells. The cell is transformed from a cell similar to an epidermal germinative cell to a fully differentiated, moribund cell filled with lipid droplets.

 1. **Immature cells.** Peripheral cells in the acinus are immature and mitotically active. As differentiation proceeds, the sebaceous cells are displaced from the periphery toward the center of the acinus.
 2. **Differentiating cells.** The differentiating sebaceous cells rapidly synthesize lipid and their cytoplasm becomes filled with lipid droplets.
 3. **Mature cells.** Near the center of the acinus the sebaceous cells, filled with lipid droplets, disintegrate.
 4. An interval of about 8 days occurs between incorporation of a radioactive label into an immature sebaceous cell and appearance of the label in sebum on the skin surface.

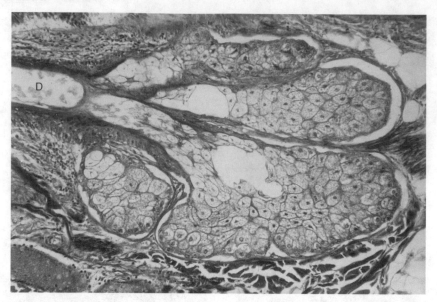

FIGURE 20-5. Sebaceous gland showing several lobules converging on the gland duct (*D*). Sebaceous cells are filled with lipid droplets. Evidence of cell breakdown (i.e., holocrine secretion) is visible deep in the lobule close to the beginning of the duct.

C. **Sebaceous secretion.** Sebaceous glands secrete by a holocrine mechanism (see Chapter 23 II D 2).

1. **Holocrine secretion** in sebaceous glands is characterized by the death of the secreting cell.
   a. This process is an example of **programmed cell death,** or **apoptosis.**
   b. The remains of the cell together with its recently synthesized lipids form the sebaceous secretion, called sebum.

2. **Sebum** is composed of lipids and cell debris.
   a. Sebum contains triglycerides, wax esters, squalene, cholesterol, and cholesterol esters.
   b. Sebum flows from the center of the acinus into the sebaceous duct and then into the pilosebaceous canal. In the canal, sebum coats the hair shaft and, eventually, reaches the skin surface.

D. **Function of sebum.** The role of the sebaceous gland secretion is not well understood.

1. Speculation regarding the function of sebum has involved its possible role as a bacteriostatic agent, as an emollient, as a component of the transepidermal barrier, and as a pheromone. The subtle scent of the clean, unperfumed human body is due to sebum.

2. Sebaceous gland activity is under endocrine control, evidenced by the stimulation of glandular activity by androgens and its suppression by estrogens.

3. Sebum has a role in the development of **acne.**
   a. Triglycerides are a component of sebum and are broken down to free fatty acids by microorganisms of the skin flora.
   b. Such fatty acids may be an irritant in formation of acne lesions.

VI. **ECCRINE SWEAT GLANDS** (see Figure 20-4). These are cutaneous glands that produce sweat and are important in **thermoregulation.**

A. **Eccrine gland distribution**

1. The eccrine glands are widely distributed over the body surface.

2. The concentration of eccrine sweat glands differs among regions of the body. Lips are free of eccrine glands, whereas the volar surfaces (palms and soles) have the highest concentration of glands (approximately 600/cm^2).

B. **Eccrine gland structure.** Eccrine glands are **simple, coiled, tubular glands.**

1. The glands develop embryologically from the epidermis, and connection to the epidermis is maintained in the adult by the duct of the gland.

2. An eccrine sweat gland has three distinct regions.
   a. The **coiled region** lies in the dermis, sometimes very deeply, and is formed by a coiled tubule (Figure 20-6).
      (1) The **secretory region** of the gland accounts for approximately half of the coiled portion. This portion is formed by pseudostratified epithelium of **clear (serous) cells, dark (mucous) cells,** and **myoepithelial cells.**
      (2) The remainder of the coiled tubule is gland duct.
   b. The **straight region** of the duct rises through the dermis to connect the coiled portion of the gland to the epidermis.
      (1) The duct of the gland, both straight and coiled portions, is formed by two layers of cuboidal epithelial cells. This is an example of the infrequently encountered **stratified cuboidal epithelium.**
      (2) The duct is a transporting epithelium, and the electrolyte composition of sweat is significantly modified as it flows through the duct.
   c. The **spiral region** of the duct follows a helical pathway through the epidermis before ending as an orifice at the epidermal surface.
      (1) The helical nature of the duct is most obvious in a section through thick epidermis where the duct is visible in several profiles as it turns through the epidermis (see Figure 20-1, *right*).
      (2) Orifices of sweat glands may be seen on the fingertips using a hand lens or dissecting microscope.

C. **Eccrine gland function.** Eccrine sweat glands function in the **maintenance of body temperature.**

1. **Composition of sweat.** Sweat is a dilute watery solution containing sodium, chlo-

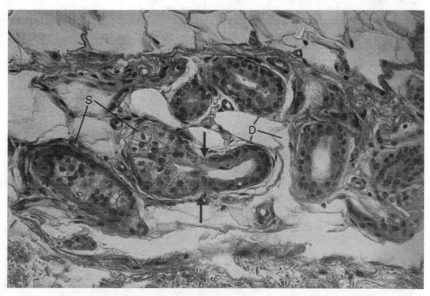

FIGURE 20-6. Eccrine sweat gland showing the coiled region of the gland surrounded by adipose tissue. The junction between the secretory region (*S*) and the coiled duct (*D*) is indicated (*arrows*).

ride, potassium, and smaller amounts of other substances, such as urea and ammonia.

    a. Electrolytes are transported out of sweat as it moves through the duct. Sweat is iso-osmotic in the coiled secretory region of the tubule, but is hypo-osmotic by the time it reaches the skin surface.

    b. Excessive sweating can deplete the body of electrolytes and water.

  2. Thermoregulatory sweating. Sweat secreted onto the body surface evaporates, thereby cooling the body. Thermoregulatory sweating is controlled by postganglionic cholinergic sympathetic fibers of the autonomic nervous system.

  3. Emotional sweating. This type of sweating is controlled by postganglionic adrenergic sympathetic fibers of the autonomic nervous system.

VII.   **APOCRINE GLANDS** (see Figure 20-4). These are large cutaneous glands that produce a chemically complex secretion. Apocrine glands are derived from epidermis or hair follicles.

A.   **Apocrine gland distribution.** The glands are found in the axilla, in the perianal region, and in the external auditory canal (i.e., the ceruminous glands). Unlike eccrine sweat glands, apocrine glands are not found over the general body surface.

B.   **Apocrine gland structure.** Apocrine glands are simple, coiled, tubular glands.

  1. Connection to the epidermis or to a hair follicle is maintained in the adult by the gland duct. The gland may extend into the subdermal connective tissue.

  2. The secretory part of the gland is a large, often macroscopic, tangle of anastomosing tubules.

    a. The wall of the secretory tubule is formed by a simple epithelium that varies in height with functional state and accumulation of a granular secretory product.

    b. Myoepithelial cells are found between the base of the columnar secretory cells and the basal lamina.

C.   **Apocrine gland function**

  1. Secretory mechanisms. Release of secretion from the apocrine gland is an **apocrine and merocrine** process.

    a. The gland was originally thought to secrete solely by an apocrine process, in which the cell apex is pinched off, resulting in the loss of cell membrane and cytoplasm.

    b. More recent research indicates that the secretory process also involves a merocrine (exocytotic) process.

  2. Secretory product. The apocrine gland secretion is a chemically complex, viscous substance.

    a. The secretion of the apocrine gland is initially odorless. It becomes malodorous through the action of cutaneous microorganisms (e.g., the odor of the unwashed axilla). Some investigators believe that apocrine secretions may function as **pheromones** in human beings, as they do in other mammals.

    b. Apocrine glands are a secondary sex characteristic. The glands develop under the influence of gonadal hormones at the same time that axillary hair and pubic hair follicles develop.

  3. Although sometimes called apocrine sweat glands, these glands do not respond to the same stimuli that produce sweat from eccrine glands.

    a. The secretion of apocrine glands differs chemically from the secretion of eccrine glands.

    b. Apocrine glands do not function in thermoregulation.

VIII. **NAIL.** The nail is a highly differentiated epidermal structure in which the stratum corneum is thickened, hardened, and coherent.

A. **Structure.** Fingernail and toenail are formed by a **compact layer of keratinized cells.** The components of the nail and surrounding structures are:

1. **Nail plate.** The nail plate is a flattened, compact layer of squamous keratinized cells found on the terminal phalanges of the fingers and toes.

2. **Nail root.** The nail root is the most proximal part of the nail plate and is covered by the eponychium and the proximal nail wall.

3. **Nail wall, eponychium, and cuticle.** The proximal and lateral nail walls (or folds) define the visible margins of the nail plate. The **eponychium** is the forward extension of the proximal nail wall. The stratum corneum of the eponychium extends onto the surface of the nail plate as the **cuticle.**

4. **Nail bed and nail matrix.** The nail bed is the **stratified epithelium** that lies subjacent to the nail plate. Proximally, this stratified epithelium is thicker and is called the nail matrix. The **hyponychium** is the thickened epidermis distal to the nail bed and covered by the free edge of the nail.

B. **Nail Growth.** The nail plate grows by cell divisions in the nail matrix.

1. Cell divisions in the matrix, and to a lesser extent in the nail bed, are reflected as growth of the nail plate.
   a. Growth rate of nail varies considerably, but rates in the range of a few tenths of a millimeter per day are generally accepted.
   b. Nail regeneration time, after surgical or traumatic removal of the nail plate, is about 150 days for fingernail and 1 year for toenail.

2. Evidence of the nail matrix is seen as the **lunula,** the light-colored, crescent-shaped region visible through the proximal nail plate and extending under the eponychium.
   a. The light color of the lunula is the result of the thick layer of matrix cells that masks underlying blood vessels.
   b. The nail bed is thinner than the matrix, and underlying dermal blood vessels produce the characteristic pink color that is visible through the translucent nail plate.

IX. **SKIN INJURY, CUTANEOUS APPENDAGES, AND WOUND HEALING**

A. **Epithelial repair.** Surviving parts of epidermal appendages contribute cells to healing of skin wounds.

1. If the full thickness of the epidermis is removed, either surgically or by trauma, the superficial portions of the appendages are lost. Only the deepest parts of hair follicles and glands remain as islands of epithelial cells in the exposed dermal connective tissue.

2. These surviving epithelial cells divide and migrate over the wounded surface and, eventually, re-establish a complete epidermal layer.

B. **Total epithelial destruction.** Destruction of all epithelial cells—epidermal, follicular, and glandular—such as in a third-degree burn or full-thickness abrasion, severely retards re-epithelialization.

1. In such cases, the bare dermis would be re-epithelialized very slowly by cells from

the periphery of the wound, with resulting complications of infection, dehydration, and scarring.

2. To prevent the risks of infection and scarring, skin grafts are used to cover such wounds.

C. **Dermal repair.** Dermal healing in skin wounds occurs through division of fibroblasts and differentiation of new fibroblasts from vascular adventitial cells. These fibroblasts then secrete extracellular matrix to restore the dermal structures.

Chapter 21

General Plan of the Alimentary Tract

I. INTRODUCTION

A. Components of the alimentary tract (digestive system)

1. The **alimentary canal** is a hollow tube of varying diameter. It is longitudinally divided into the **esophagus,** the **stomach,** the **small intestine,** the **colon** (large intestine), and the **rectum.**

2. The **associated organs** of the alimentary tract include:
   a. The **tongue, teeth,** and **salivary glands** of the oral cavity
   b. The extramural digestive organs, specifically, the **liver** and **gallbladder,** and the **exocrine pancreas**

B. Phylogenetic and general functional considerations

1. The alimentary tract is the representation in humans of the tube-within-a-tube plan of animal structure typical of the phylum Chordata.

2. The lumen of the digestive tract is continuous with the external environment. Hence, it is both physically and functionally external to the body.

3. The epithelial lining of the alimentary canal is the surface across which most substances enter the body.
   a. As the principal interface between the body and the environment, the epithelium has three major functions: **protection, absorption,** and **secretion.**
   b. Different regions of the epithelial lining are structurally specialized to augment these various functions.

II. BASIC PLAN OF THE WALL OF THE ALIMENTARY CANAL (Figure 21-1). From the cranial end of the esophagus to the caudal end of the rectum, the wall of the alimentary canal is formed by four distinctive layers. Starting at the lumen, these layers are the **mucosa,** the **submucosa,** the **muscularis externa,** and the **serosa** (or adventitia).

A. **Mucosa.** The mucosa consists of three concentric layers. From the lumen outward, these layers are a lining epithelium, an underlying connective tissue called the lamina propria, and a smooth muscle layer called the muscularis mucosae.

1. **Epithelium.** The epithelial lining of the alimentary canal is in direct contact with its contents, namely ingested and partially or wholly digested foods, the secretions of the digestive system, and the waste products of digestion.
   a. Different regions of the alimentary canal have different types of epithelium.
      (1) The **esophagus** has a **nonkeratinized, stratified squamous epithelium** that provides protection from the friction of undigested food passing along its length.
      (2) The **stomach, small intestine,** and **colon** have a **simple columnar epithelium** that contains several cell types.
         (a) **Mucous secretory cells** are found in all three regions. Mucus-secreting cells occur as sheets of cells in the stomach and as individual goblet cells in the small intestine and colon. Other secretory cells produce hydrochloric acid (stomach), digestive enzymes (stomach), and bactericidal enzymes (small intestine).
         (b) **Absorptive cells** that take up metabolites, electrolytes, and water predominate in the small intestine and colon.

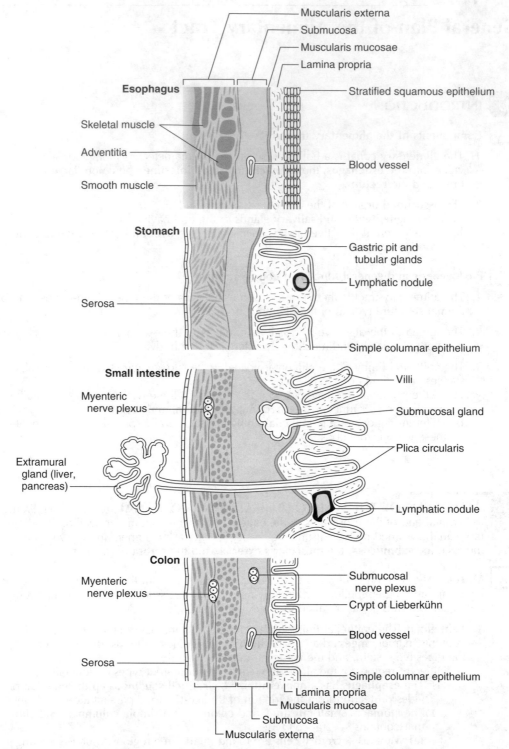

FIGURE 21-1. Diagram of the structure of the wall of the alimentary canal showing variation in the basic four layers of the wall in different areas of the canal. *A* = esophagus; *B* = stomach; *C* = small intestine; *D* = colon.

(c) **Enteroendocrine cells,** present from the stomach to the rectum, secrete peptide hormones that regulate digestive functions.
b. The epithelium of the alimentary canal is a **regularly replicating** tissue.
  (1) The epithelium in each portion of the alimentary canal has a characteristic **turnover rate,** ranging from 2 to 3 days in the small intestine to as much as a year in the gastric glands.
  (2) Each portion of the alimentary canal has a morphologically localized stem cell population from which all of the epithelial cells of that portion of the digestive tract derive.

2. **Lamina propria.** This layer of loose connective tissue lies immediately beneath the epithelium. It contains:
  a. Blood vessels and, except in the colon, lymphatic vessels
  b. Mucosal glands that invaginate from the surface and contain the secretory and replicative cell populations (see IV A 2)
  c. Lymphatic tissue and other elements of the immune system
  d. Scattered smooth muscle cells

3. **Muscularis mucosae.** This layer of smooth muscle cells is part of the mucosa, hence its name. It separates the rest of the mucosa from the submucosa.
  a. The cells of the muscularis mucosae are arranged as an **inner circular layer** and an **outer longitudinal layer.** This is not always obvious because of the thinness of the muscularis mucosae, which may be only two cells thick in some parts of the gastrointestinal tract.
  b. This muscle layer can produce movement of the mucosa independent of movement of the entire wall of the digestive tract.
  c. The muscle also serves to inhibit neoplastic cells that arise in the epithelium from invading the deeper parts of the gastrointestinal tract wall.

B. **Submucosa.** This is a moderately dense, irregular connective tissue layer located between the muscularis mucosae and the muscularis externa. A number of structures lie in the submucosa.

1. **Blood vessels.** The submucosa contains the larger blood vessels that send branches to the mucosa, to the muscularis externa, and to the serosa.

2. **Lymphatic vessels.** The lymphatic vessels of the submucosa drain the lymphatic vascular networks that surround the muscularis mucosae and the muscularis externa.

3. **Nerve tissue.** The **submucosal plexus** (**Meissner plexus**) consists of sensory fibers, motor fibers, and ganglion cells of the enteric nervous system (ENS). The enteric system is the third, and largest, division of the autonomic nervous system (ANS), which includes the parasympathetic and sympathetic divisions.

4. **Glands.** Submucosal glands are found in some locations, such as the esophagus and the proximal small intestine (see IV A 3). The presence of these glands in histologic sections often aids in identifying the specific segment or region of the digestive tract.

C. Muscularis externa (muscularis propria)

1. **Layers.** In most parts of the digestive tract, the muscularis externa is formed by two concentric and relatively thick layers of smooth muscle.
  a. **Inner circular layer**
    (1) The inner circular layer is so named because its cells are arranged in a tight spiral at nearly right angles to the long axis of the digestive tract.
    (2) Contraction of the inner circular layer compresses and mixes the contents of the digestive tract by constricting the lumen.
  b. **Outer longitudinal layer**
    (1) The outer longitudinal layer is so named because its cells are arranged in a loose spiral that is nearly parallel to the long axis of the digestive tract.
    (2) Contraction of the outer longitudinal layer propels the contents of the lumen caudally by shortening the tube.

2. Peristalsis
a. The slow, rhythmic, wave-like contractions of the muscularis externa, called peristalsis, move the luminal contents along the intestinal tract.
b. Peristalsis is under the control of the enteric nervous system.

3. Structures within the muscularis externa
a. The **myenteric plexus** (**Auerbach plexus**) is the other major component of the ENS and lies in the loose connective tissue layer between the two muscle layers.
b. **Blood vessels** and **lymphatic vessels** are also found in this connective tissue.

4. Sphincters and valves. Thickenings of the inner circular layer form sphincters at several points along the digestive tract.
a. The **pyloric sphincter** (**gastroduodenal sphincter**) regulates emptying of the stomach into the proximal small intestine.
b. The **ileocecal valve** regulates emptying of the small intestine into the colon.
c. The **internal anal sphincter** regulates the emptying of the colon to the exterior.

5. Variations. The usual pattern of two layers of smooth muscle varies in some regions of the muscularis externa.
a. In the proximal portion of the **esophagus,** striated muscle forms the muscularis externa. The **pharyngoesophageal sphincter** is the striated cricopharyngeus muscle.
b. In the **stomach,** a third, obliquely oriented layer is often described as internal to the inner circular layer.
   (1) However, the smooth muscle is not usually so clearly organized into layers in the stomach.
   (2) A more random orientation facilitates both mixing in the lumen and irregular movement of small boluses of partially digested material into the small intestine.
c. In the **colon,** parts of the outer longitudinal layer are thickened to form three distinct, equally spaced longitudinal bands, the **teniae coli.**
   (1) Contractions of the teniae facilitate the rapid, violent shortening of the digestive tube in defecation.
   (2) Between the teniae, the outer longitudinal layer is thin but, nonetheless, forms a continuous layer.
d. In the anal canal, the **external anal sphincter** is striated muscle.

D. **Serosa and adventitia.** The serosa is the most superficial layer of those portions of the digestive tract that are suspended in the peritoneal cavity. Adventitia covers those portions that are fixed in position (i.e., retroperitoneal).

1. Serosa. The serosa consists of a loose connective tissue covered with a simple squamous epithelium, the **mesothelium** (visceral peritoneum).
a. The connective tissue contains large blood and lymphatic vessels, nerve trunks, and a considerable amount of adipose tissue.
b. The serosa is continuous with the mesentery by which the viscera are suspended.
c. The mesothelium of the serosa is the visceral epithelium of the abdominal cavity.

2. Adventitia. Those portions of the digestive tract that do not possess a serosa are attached to surrounding structures by a loose connective tissue, the adventitia, that blends with the general connective tissue of the region.
a. Adventitia covers the esophagus and those portions of the digestive tract in the abdominal cavity that are fixed to the posterior wall; that is, the duodenum, the ascending colon, and the descending colon.
b. The mesothelium that covers the posterior wall in the abdominal cavity is the parietal epithelium (parietal peritoneum).

III. **FUNCTIONS OF THE ALIMENTARY MUCOSA.** The alimentary mucosa has numerous important functions in its role as the principal interface between the body and the environment (Figure 21-2).

A **Secretion**

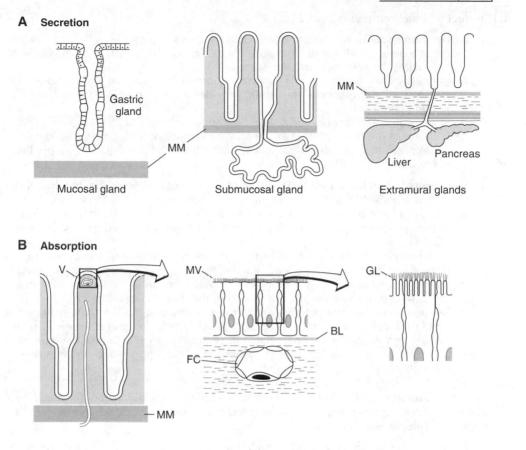

B **Absorption**

C **Protection**

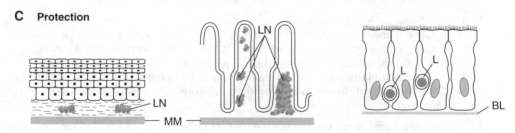

FIGURE 21-2. Morphologic specializations related to the major functions of the digestive tube. (*Part A*) Increased surface for secretion of digestive enzymes is provided by mucosal glands (e.g., gastric glands), submucosal glands (e.g., Brunner glands), and extramural digestive glands (i.e., pancreas and liver). (*Part B*) In areas particularly engaged in absorption (i.e., small intestine, colon, gallbladder), surface area is increased at several levels. Gross submucosal folds (plicae circulares) are shown in Figure 21-1C. Villi (*V*) are covered with absorptive epithelial cells that, in turn, have microvilli (*MV*) that project from the apical plasma membrane. Glycoproteins of the glycocalyx (*GL*) extend from the plasma membrane of the microvilli. Fenestrated capillaries (*FC*) underlie the absorptive epithelium. (*Part C*) Protective functions of the alimentary canal are exemplified by the stratified squamous epithelium of the esophagus and by components of the gut-associated lymphatic tissue (GALT), present along the entire alimentary canal, namely lymphatic nodules (*LN*) in the lamina propria and lymphocytes (*L*) in the epithelial intercellular spaces.

A. **Protective functions** (see Figure 21-2C)

1. **Barrier function.** The epithelium of the mucosa serves as a barrier to the entry of antigens, pathogens, and other noxious substances. The epithelial barrier of the intestine also regulates the entry of metabolic substrates into the body.
   a. In the proximal portions of the alimentary tract, that is, the oral cavity and esophagus, a **stratified squamous epithelium** provides protection from abrasion by ingested materials.
   b. In the stomach, intestine, and colon, **tight junctions** between the columnar epithelial cells of the mucosa serve as the primary exclusion barrier; they also serve as a component of the system that allows active transport of substances across the epithelium.

2. **Immunologic functions. Lymphatic tissue** in the mucosa provides the first line of defense of the body carried out by the immune system.
   a. This lymphatic tissue includes the tonsils and the many lymphatic nodules in the lamina propria of the mucosa that constitute the **gut-associated lymphatic tissue (GALT).**
   b. Free lymphocytes in the intercellular spaces of the gastrointestinal epithelium serve as an early warning system, reacting to antigens that enter the epithelium.
   c. Macrophages, as well as granulocytes that leave the circulation, also function in the lamina propria of the mucosa as part of the immunologic barrier.
   d. **Immune exclusion** is a process that involves immunoglublulin A (IgA) synthesized by plasma cells in the lamina propria. The IgA is taken up and resecreted, as **secretory IgA (sIgA)**, by the epithelial cells of the salivary glands and the intestine. The sIgA then binds to antigens in the gastrointestinal lumen and prevents their absorption.

B. **Secretory function.** In addition to antibodies, the lining of the alimentary tract secretes, at specific sites, digestive enzymes, hydrochloric acid, mucin, bactericidal enzymes, and peptide hormones (see Figure 21-2A).

1. In the **oral cavity, salivary glands** secrete mucin, carbohydrate-digesting enzymes, a bactericidal enzyme (lysozyme), electrolytes, and metabolic wastes.

2. In the **stomach,** secretions come from several sites.
   a. **Gastric glands** (mucosal glands) secrete hydrochloric acid, a proteolytic proenzyme (pepsinogen), and intrinsic factor (needed for absorption of cyanocobalamin) into the stomach lumen and peptide hormones into the lamina propria.
   b. The **surface epithelium** and the epithelium of the **gastric pits** (which lead from the gastric glands to the surface epithelium) consist of sheets of cells that secrete mucins.

3. In the epithelium of the **small intestine, goblet cells** secrete mucins, **enteroendocrine cells** secrete peptide hormones, and **Paneth cells** secrete lysozyme.

4. In the **large intestine** (colon), goblet cells and enteroendocrine cells are the only secretory cells normally found in the epithelium that forms the mucosal glands and surface lining.

5. **Liver and pancreas.** Both of these extramural glands have exocrine and endocrine secretions. The ducts that convey the exocrine secretions of these glands end in the duodenum.
   a. **Liver.** The same cell synthesizes and secretes both the exocrine and the endocrine products.
      (1) The **exocrine secretion** of the liver is bile. Bile is stored and concentrated in the gallbladder before delivery to the lumen of the proximal small intestine.
      (2) The **endocrine secretions** (far more voluminous) include albumin, the non-immune globulins, and other blood proteins; cholesterol; and lipoproteins.
   b. **Pancreas**
      (1) The **exocrine secretions** of the pancreas include trypsinogen, chymotrypsinogen, and other peptidase proenzymes; lipases; and HCO_3^-.

(2) The **endocrine secretions** of the pancreas include insulin, glucagon, and somatostatin, hormones that regulate glucose, lipid, and protein metabolism throughout the body.

C. **Absorptive function.** The epithelium of the alimentary mucosa, particularly in the small intestine, absorbs metabolic substrates, the products of digestion (see Figure 21-2B).

1. **Sites of absorption**
   a. In the **small intestine,** these substrates include sugars and amino acids, as well as fatty acids and glycerol. Also absorbed here are vitamins, water, electrolytes, recyclable materials such as bile components and cholesterol, and most other substances essential to the functions of the body.
   b. The **colon** absorbs primarily water and electrolytes to concentrate the solid wastes produced by the digestive system.

2. **Methods of absorption.** Materials are absorbed in the intestine by all the known methods by which substances can cross cell membranes and epithelial cell layers. These methods include all the following passive and active transport mechanisms, alone and in various combinations.
   a. **Simple diffusion.** A substance enters a cell or crosses the epithelium by moving down its concentration (electrochemical) gradient, that is, the concentration in the alimentary lumen is greater than that in the epithelial cell or in the connective tissue.
   b. **Facilitated diffusion.** The cells of an epithelium contain in their plasma membrane carrier proteins or channel proteins that facilitate the crossing of the membrane by the substrate, albeit still moving down its electrochemical gradient.
   c. **Active transport.** Membrane carrier proteins (pumps) are coupled with energy sources in the cell and, usually, with a unique geometry in the arrangement of epithelial cells, to effect movement of a substance against its electrochemical gradient.

IV. **FUNCTIONAL SPECIALIZATIONS IN THE WALL OF THE ALIMENTARY CANAL.** Several morphologic specializations increase the surface area of the alimentary canal to facilitate the principal digestive functions of secretion (see Figure 21-2A) and absorption (see Figure 21-2B).

A. **Secretion.** There are four levels of secretory gland development in the alimentary tract. Each successively more complex level significantly increases the surface across which secretion may occur.

1. **Intraepithelial glands** are usually unicellular and may be either exocrine or endocrine.
   a. **Goblet cells,** found throughout the intestinal epithelium, are unicellular exocrine glands that secrete mucins. Goblet cells may also be found in clusters in some sites.
   b. **Enteroendocrine cells,** found at all levels of the gastrointestinal tract, secrete peptide hormones. They, too, may appear singly or in small groups.

2. **Mucosal glands** develop as invaginations of the luminal epithelium into the lamina propria of the stomach, small intestine, and colon.
   a. Mucosal glands may secrete mucins, enzymes, electrolytes, antibodies, or any combination thereof.
   b. Mucosal glands deliver their secretions directly onto the luminal epithelial surface.
   c. Individual cells of mucosal glands may develop increased surface area for secretion by several methods.
      (1) Invagination of the apical plasma membrane forms **intracellular canaliculi,** as in the acid-secreting cells of the gastric glands

      (2) Invagination of the basal and basal-lateral plasma membranes forms **membrane folds,** as in the ducts of the salivary glands.

3. Submucosal glands also develop as invaginations of the epithelial surface of the fetal alimentary canal. They are found primarily in the esophagus (esophageal glands and esophageal cardiac glands), the proximal duodenum (Brunner glands), and the anal canal (circumanal apocrine glands).

   a. Submucosal glands may secrete similar substances as mucosal glands but significantly increase the surface available for secretion by virtue of being large glands.

   b. Their secretory portions reside in the submucosa of the canal wall, and their secretory products are delivered to the lumen of the alimentary canal by ducts that pass through the mucosa.

4. Extramural digestive glands, the **liver** and the **pancreas,** also form during development of the alimentary canal by invagination of the surface epithelium. In this instance, the invaginating gland primordium passes completely through the wall of the alimentary canal.

   a. The secretions of the liver and pancreas are briefly described above, and their structure and functions are presented in Chapters 26 and 27, respectively.

   b. The hepatic and pancreatic exocrine secretions are delivered to the lumen of the proximal small intestine by **ducts** that pass through the wall of the intestine. These ducts are adult representations of the original invaginations that formed the organ primordia.

B. **Absorption.** Projections of the submucosa, the mucosa, and the mucosal epithelium into the lumen of the digestive tract increase the surface available for digestion and absorption.

1. Rugae are longitudinally oriented mucosal and submucosal folds in the stomach that flatten out when the stomach is fully distended. Rugae do not increase the surface area of the gastric mucosa but, rather, allow the stomach to accommodate to expansion and filling.

2. Plicae circulares (circular folds, **valves of Kerckring**) are circumferentially oriented submucosal folds that are present throughout the length of the small intestine (see Chapter 25 I B 1).

3. Villi are unique to the small intestine. They are finger-like and leaf-like mucosal projections that cover the entire surface of the small intestine and extend into the intestinal lumen (see Chapter 25 I B 2).

4. Microvilli of the intestinal epithelial cells provide the major amplification of the luminal surface [see Chapter 25 I C 1 d (1)].

5. Glycocalyx. The glycocalyx consists of glycoproteins of the plasma membrane that project externally. It is well developed on the apical surface of the absorptive epithelial cells of the intestine, where it provides additional surface for the adsorption of materials and contains enzymes that are essential for the final steps of digestion of proteins, sugars, and fats [see Chapter 25 I C 1 d (2)].

Chapter 22

Oral Cavity

I. **INTRODUCTION.** The oral cavity consists of the mouth and its contents, specifically, the tongue, the teeth, the salivary glands, and the tonsils.

A. **Mouth.** The mouth, at the cranial end of the alimentary canal, is the orifice through which substances enter the canal.

B. **Structural and functional components**

1. The **tongue,** a muscular organ, is essential in chewing, swallowing, taste, speech, and gathering sensory information about the mouth and its contents.

2. The **teeth** grind and macerate foods.

3. The **salivary glands** provide lubricants (mucin) for the oral cavity, some digestive enzymes (chiefly amylase), electrolytes essential to tooth maintenance, a bactericidal enzyme (lysozyme), and secretory immunoglobulin A (sIgA) (see Chapter 23 VI A 4 b).

4. The **tonsils** are diffuse lymphatic tissue and lymphatic nodules that form an immuno-protective ''ring'' around the junction of the oral cavity with the pharynx (see Chapter 16 II).

II. **MUCOSA OF THE ORAL CAVITY.** The oral cavity is lined by three types of mucosa: masticatory, lining, and specialized mucosa.

A. **Masticatory mucosa** is the mucosa of the gingiva (gums) and the hard palate.

1. **Epithelium.** Masticatory mucosa has a keratinized or parakeratinized stratified squamous epithelium.
   a. The **keratinized epithelium** resembles that of the skin.
   b. The **parakeratinized epithelium** is similar to keratinized epithelium, but the cells of the stratum corneum retain their nuclei and stain less intensely with eosin.

2. **Lamina propria.** The lamina propria of the masticatory mucosa has two layers: a **thick papillary layer** of loose connective tissue and a **deep reticular layer** of dense connective tissue.
   a. The many deep **papillae** firmly anchor the masticatory epithelium, helping it to resist frictional and shearing stresses.
   b. The lamina propria is continuous with the periosteum of the underlying bone, except in some areas on the hard palate, where a **submucosa** containing adipose tissue and glands is found.

B. **Lining mucosa** covers the lips, the inside of the cheeks, the floor of the mouth, the mucosal surface of the alveolar bone not covered by gingiva, the inferior surfaces of the tongue, and the soft palate.

1. **Epithelium**
   a. Generally, the epithelium of the lining mucosa is **nonkeratinized.** On the vermilion border of the lip, however, it is **keratinized.** If subject to unusual frictional stress, the epithelium may become **parakeratinized,** or even keratinized.
   b. Other cells found in the epithelium of the lining mucosa are Langerhans cells, melanocytes, and Merkel cells.

2. **Subepithelial relationships.** The lining mucosa covers various types of tissues.
   a. On the lips, cheeks, and tongue, it covers striated muscle.

      b. On the surface of the mandible and maxilla, it is called **alveolar mucosa** and covers the alveolar bone in which the teeth are anchored.

      c. On the soft palate, cheeks, inferior surface of the tongue, and floor of the mouth, lining mucosa covers glands and loose connective tissue.

  3. Lamina propria. Under the epithelium of the lining mucosa, a loose connective tissue with thin collagen fibers forms a **papillary lamina propria** that carries blood vessels, lymphatic vessels, and nerves.

      a. The papillae are not as numerous, nor as deep, as those in the masticatory mucosa.

      b. Some nerves send bare axons into the basal layers of the epithelium as free sensory endings. Other nerves form encapsulated sensory endings in the papillae.

  4. Submucosa. A distinct submucosa underlies the lining mucosa, except on the inferior surface of the tongue.

      a. The submucosa contains large bands of collagen and elastic fibers that bind the mucosa to the underlying muscle.

      b. The submucosa also contains the larger nerves, blood vessels, and lymphatic vessels that supply the neurovascular networks of the lamina propria throughout the oral cavity.

      c. In the lips, tongue, and cheeks, the submucosa contains many minor salivary glands.

C. **Specialized mucosa** is restricted to the dorsal surface of the tongue, and is characterized by the presence of surface papillae of several types (see III C) and by taste buds in the epithelium (see III D).

III. **TONGUE.** The tongue is a muscular organ projecting into the oral cavity.

A. **Muscles of the tongue**

  1. The muscles of the tongue are both extrinsic and intrinsic.

      a. Extrinsic muscles have one attachment, the origin, outside the tongue.

      b. Intrinsic muscles are confined entirely to the tongue.

  2. The muscles of the tongue are arranged in bundles that course through the organ in approximately three planes, each at right angles to the other two.

      a. This arrangement of striated muscle imparts enormous precision and flexibility in the movements of the tongue that are essential to its functions in speech, digestion, and swallowing.

      b. The arrangement is unique to the tongue and facilitates identification of this tissue as lingual muscle.

  3. Variable amounts of adipose tissue are found among the muscle fiber groups.

B. **Gross appearance of the dorsal surface of the tongue** (Figure 22-1)

  1. The dorsal surface of the tongue is divided into a posterior one-third and an anterior two-thirds by the **sulcus terminalis,** a V-shaped depression whose apex points posteriorly. The apex of the sulcus, the **foramen cecum,** is the site of the evagination of the developing thyroid gland from the embryonic pharynx.

  2. The velvety appearance of the anterior two-thirds reflects the presence of several types of **lingual papillae.**

  3. Uneven bulges in the dorsal surface of the tongue's posterior one-third indicate the presence of the **lingual tonsils** in the lamina propria (see Chapter 16 II A 2). (The **palatine tonsils** underlie the surface of the fauces between the oral cavity and the oropharynx. See Chapter 16 II A 1.)

Apex

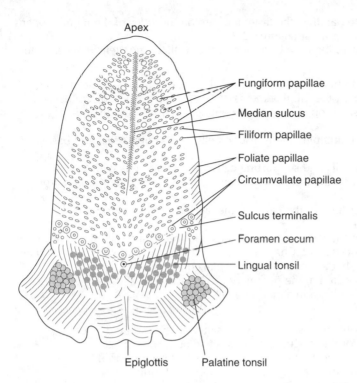

FIGURE 22-1. Dorsal surface of the human tongue.

- Fungiform papillae
- Median sulcus
- Filiform papillae
- Foliate papillae
- Circumvallate papillae
- Sulcus terminalis
- Foramen cecum
- Lingual tonsil

Epiglottis   Palatine tonsil

C. **Lingual papillae.** Four types of papillae cover the anterior two-thirds of the tongue's dorsal surface: filiform, fungiform, circumvallate, and foliate, each with different morphology and functions. Fungiform, circumvallate, and foliate papillae carry taste buds.

1. **Filiform papillae,** the most numerous of the lingual papillae, are conical, elongated projections distributed over the entire anterior dorsal surface of the tongue. Filiform papillae are covered with keratinized epithelium that does not contain taste buds.

2. **Fungiform papillae,** as the name indicates, are mushroom-shaped. They, too, are covered with keratinized epithelium. They project above the filiform papillae on the anterior portion of the dorsal tongue surface and are most numerous near the tip.

3. **Circumvallate papillae** are large, dome-shaped structures that project from the dorsal surface of the tongue just anterior to the sulcus terminalis. They are covered with keratinized epithelium. Usually, 8 to 14 are found in humans.
   a. Each circumvallate papilla is surrounded by a moat-like mucosal invagination that is lined with stratified squamous epithelium containing numerous taste buds (see Figure 22-2A).
   b. Ducts of numerous small salivary glands (von Ebner's glands) empty into the moats. Their secretions flush material from the moat, enabling the taste buds to respond rapidly to new stimuli.

4. **Foliate papillae** are parallel low ridges that are most prominent on the posterior lateral surfaces of the tongue. They are easily seen in children but are more difficult to recognize in adult humans.

D. **Taste buds**

1. **Location.** Taste buds are concentrated in the epithelium of the oral mucosa that covers the fungiform, foliate, and circumvallate papillae. They are also found on the soft palate, the epiglottis, and the posterior wall of the pharynx.
   a. On the **fungiform papillae,** the taste buds are on the dorsal surface.

b. On the **circumvallate papillae,** the taste buds are on the sides of the papilla, opening into the surrounding moat (Figure 22-2A).
c. On the **foliate papillae,** the taste buds are on the walls of the clefts that separate the ridges.

2. **Structural features.** Taste buds appear in histologic sections as oval, pale-staining bodies that extend through the full thickness of the stratified squamous epithelium.
   a. The **taste pore** is a small opening onto the epithelial surface at the apex of the taste bud.
   b. Taste buds contain neuroepithelial (sensory) cells, supporting cells, and basal cells (Figure 22-2B).
      (1) **Neuroepithelial cells** and **supporting cells** are mature cells with microvilli that extend through the taste pore to sample the surrounding fluid environment.
         (a) The turnover time of the neuroepithelial cells and supporting cells is about 10 days.
         (b) The neuroepithelial cells of taste buds and the neuroepithelial cells of the olfactory mucosa [see Chapter 28 II C 1 a (3)] are examples of nerve cells in the adult that are continuously replaced.
      (2) **Basal cells** are located at the periphery of the taste bud and are the stem cells for the neuroepithelial and supporting cells.

3. **Taste perception**
   a. Taste buds react to only four stimuli: sweet, salty, bitter, and acid (sour).
      (1) Those at the tip of the tongue detect sweet stimuli.
      (2) Those immediately posterolateral to the tip detect salty stimuli.
      (3) Those on the circumvallate papillae detect bitter stimuli.
      (4) Those on the anterior two-thirds of the dorsal surface and along the lateral margin detect sour stimuli.
   b. Most sensory information that is colloquially called "taste" is actually olfactory sensation subserved by the olfactory mucosa of the nasal cavity (see Chapter 28 II C 1 a).

IV. **TEETH.** The teeth are a major organ of the oral cavity and are an essential component of the digestive process. They are embedded in and attached to the maxilla and the mandible. The adult tooth has four histologically distinct structural components: enamel, cementum, dentin, and pulp cavity (Figure 22-3).

A. **Enamel**

1. **Location.** Enamel covers the exposed, visible portion (the **crown**) of the tooth. The enamel layer ends at the **neck (cervix)** of the tooth, at the **cementoenamel junction.**

2. **Characteristics.** Enamel is the hardest substance in the body.
   a. It varies in thickness over the crown and may be as thick as 2.5 mm on some tooth cusps (the biting and grinding surfaces).
   b. Enamel is much more highly mineralized than bone; nearly 98% of enamel is inorganic material, mostly **hydroxyapatite.**
   c. Enamel can be damaged by acid-producing bacteria living on the tooth surface; this is the basis of **dental caries** (i.e., cavities).
   d. **Enamel rods** are the units of enamel **structure.**
      (1) Enamel rods are long prisms of hydroxyapatite, 4 to 8 μm in diameter, that span the thickness of the enamel layer. Hydroxyapatite also fills the spaces between rods.
      (2) Cross-striations on enamel rods have a periodicity of about 5 μm and are evidence of rhythmic growth of developing enamel.

3. **Enamel formation (amelogenesis).** Enamel is produced by ameloblasts with the close

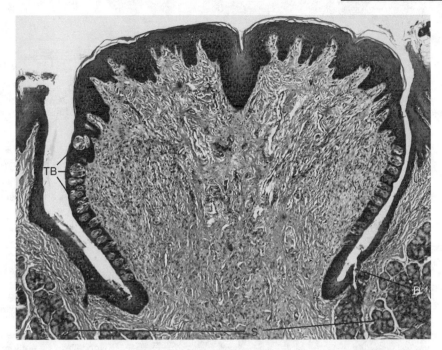

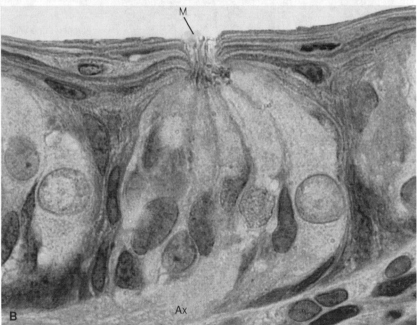

FIGURE 22-2. (*A*) Light micrograph of a circumvallate papilla. Taste buds (*TB*) are located on the side of the papilla, opening into the moat that surrounds it. Portions of several salivary glands, or von Ebner glands (*S*) are visible, and a salivary duct (*D*) is clearly seen opening into the bottom of the moat. (*B*) High-magnification light micrograph of a taste bud from the papilla shown in A. Microvilli (*M*) from the neuroepithelial (sensory) and supporting cells of the taste bud are visible protruding through a taste pore to sample the surrounding fluid environment. The axons (*Ax*) of the sensory cells can be discerned leaving the taste bud. (Courtesy of Michael H. Ross.)

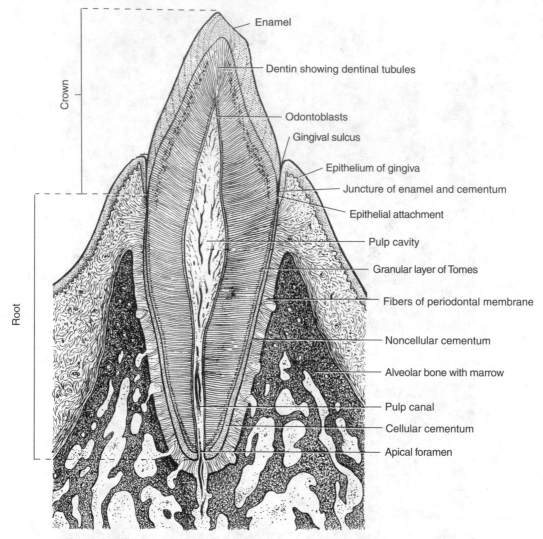

Crown

Root

Enamel

Dentin showing dentinal tubules

Odontoblasts

Gingival sulcus

Epithelium of gingiva

Juncture of enamel and cementum

Epithelial attachment

Pulp cavity

Granular layer of Tomes

Fibers of periodontal membrane

Noncellular cementum

Alveolar bone with marrow

Pulp canal

Cellular cementum

Apical foramen

FIGURE 22-3. Sagittal section through an incisor tooth and its bony and mucosal supporting structures. (Adapted from Ross MH, Romrell LJ, Kaye GI: *Histology: A Text and Atlas,* 3rd ed. Baltimore, Williams & Wilkins, 1995, p 411.)

cooperation of other cells in a specialized structure called an enamel organ. Mature enamel is acellular and nonreplaceable; it neither grows nor repairs after it is formed.

a. Overview

(1) In the formation of the mineralized tissues of the tooth, dentin production (see IV C) precedes production of enamel.

(2) In enamel formation, **secretory ameloblasts** first deposit a partially mineralized **enamel matrix** on the dentin; **maturation ameloblasts** then complete the change to mature, **mineralized enamel.** One ameloblast produces one enamel rod; inter-rod material is also secreted by ameloblasts.

(3) The ameloblasts degenerate after the enamel layer is fully formed, about the time when the tooth erupts from the gum.

b. Secretory ameloblasts are tall, narrow, highly polarized columnar cells with junctional complexes at both the apical and basal ends.

(1) Tomes process, an apical process, is surrounded by the developing enamel.

(2) Actin filaments joined to the junctional complexes may help to move the secretory ameloblast over the surface of the developing enamel, leaving the growing enamel rod in its wake.

c. **Maturation ameloblasts.** Maturation ameloblasts differentiate from secretory ameloblasts. They function primarily as a transport epithelium, moving material into and out of the maturing enamel.

   (1) Maturation ameloblasts transport calcium and phosphate, depositing the minerals on the organic enamel matrix as hydroxyapatite.

   (2) Maturation of the partially mineralized enamel matrix requires the removal of organic components by the maturation ameloblasts, as well as the continued influx of calcium and phosphate.

4. **Enamel matrix proteins**

   a. **Developing enamel matrix** contains three characteristic major proteins: **amelogenins, enamelins,** and **tuft protein.**

   b. **Mature enamel** contains only enamelins and tuft protein. Amelogenins are removed by the maturation ameloblasts during enamel maturation.

   (1) Enamelins are distributed throughout the enamel layer.

   (2) Tuft protein is concentrated near the **dentinoenamel junction,** in **enamel tufts** that are hypomineralized.

B. Cementum

1. **Location.** Cementum covers the **root** of the tooth, the part of the tooth that fits into its socket, or alveolus, in the maxilla or mandible. Cementum is contiguous with the enamel at the **cementoenamel junction,** which normally lies beneath the gingiva.

2. **Characteristics**

   a. Cementum is a relatively thin layer of bone-like material. It is less mineralized than enamel, having, like bone, a content of 45% to 50% hydroxyapatite.

   b. Cementum is secreted by **cementoblasts.**

   (1) Cementoblasts lie on the outer surface of the cementum, adjacent to the periodontal ligament.

   (2) When surrounded by cementum, these cells are called cementocytes and, like osteocytes of bone, lie in lacunae and extend processes into canaliculi.

   c. The periodontal ligament attaches the cementum to the adjacent bone.

C. Dentin

1. **Location.** Dentin encloses the pulp cavity. It is covered by enamel at the crown of the tooth, and by cementum at the root of the tooth.

2. **Characteristics.** Dentin is a calcified material that forms most of the substance of the tooth. It contains about 70% hydroxyapatite—less than enamel but more than bone and cementum.

3. **Dentin formation.** Dentin is secreted slowly throughout life.

   a. **Overview. Odontoblasts,** located at the periphery of the pulp cavity, secrete **predentin,** which is subsequently mineralized to form **dentin.** Like enamel, dentin thickens by rhythmic growth.

   b. **Odontoblasts,** like ameloblasts, are tall, columnar cells. They develop from typical mesenchymal cells to form an epithelial layer over the innermost surface of the dentin, which faces the pulp cavity.

   (1) The apical surface of the odontoblast is in contact with the forming dentin.

   (2) Apical junctional complexes between odontoblasts separate the dentinal compartment from the pulp compartment.

   (3) Odontoblasts contain all of the organelles associated with the secretion of large amounts of protein.

      (a) The odontoblasts first secrete **predentin,** the organic matrix of dentin, at their apical pole.

      (b) As the predentin layer thickens, the odontoblasts are displaced centrally, toward the pulp cavity.

      (c) A wave of mineralization follows, converting the predentin into **dentin.**

4. Odontoblast processes and dentinal tubules
   a. As the odontoblasts retreat toward the pulp, **apical processes** of the odontoblasts remain embedded in the dentin, forming long narrow channels called **dentinal tubules.** Dentinal tubules are more regularly arranged than the canaliculi of bone or cementum.
   b. The odontoblast processes and dentinal tubules continue to elongate as the dentin layer thickens by rhythmic growth.
   c. The rhythmic growth also produces **growth lines** in the dentin. These can identify developmental events (e.g., a neonatal line represents birth), and can be useful in forensic medicine.

D. **Pulp cavity.** This vascularized and innervated connective tissue compartment lies in the center of the tooth, bounded by the dentin; it has the general shape of the tooth (see Figure 22-3).

   1. Blood vessels and nerves enter the pulp cavity through the **apical foramen,** an opening at the tip of the root distal to the crown of the tooth.
      a. The blood vessels and nerves distribute in the connective tissue of the pulp cavity, forming vascular and neural networks beneath and within the odontoblast layer.
      b. Some bare nerve endings enter the proximal portions of dentinal tubules and contact the odontoblast processes therein. Stimuli at the tooth surface are transmitted through the tooth substance by the odontoblast processes to reach the nerve endings of the pulp nerves.

   2. The pulp cavity decreases in volume with age because dentin continues to be secreted throughout life.

V. **SUPPORTING TISSUES OF THE TEETH.** These include the alveolar bone of the alveolar processes of the mandible and maxilla, the periodontal ligament, and the gingiva (see Figure 22-3).

A. Alveolar processes and alveolar bone

   1. The **alveolar processes** of the maxilla and the mandible contain the **alveoli** (**sockets**) for the roots of the teeth.

   2. **Alveolar bone proper** is a thin layer of compact bone that forms the wall of the tooth socket.
      a. Sharpey fibers are collagen fibers that attach the alveolar bone proper to the periodontal ligament by penetrating from the thick, parallel fibers of the ligament into the substance of the bone. They are equivalent to the Sharpey fibers that attach tendons and ligaments to other bones.
      b. The surface of the alveolar bone proper usually shows areas of bone resorption and deposition. This is particularly evident when teeth are moved, as in the orthodontic procedures used to straighten teeth and reduce malocclusion.

   3. **Supporting alveolar bone** makes up the balance of the maxillary and mandibular alveolar processes; it is much less labile than is alveolar bone proper.

   4. Loss of both types of alveolar bone, with subsequent loosening and loss of teeth, can result from periodontal disease (chronic inflammation of the gingiva and periodontal ligaments), severe malocclusion, or the loss of an opposing tooth.

B. Periodontal ligament

   1. Components
      a. The periodontal ligament consists of thick, parallel, dense collagen fibers and loose connective tissue.
         (1) The **thick collagen fibers** and associated **fibroblasts** project from the matrix of

the cementum and give rise to the Sharpey fibers that insert in the matrix of the alveolar bone proper.

(a) The thick, dense collagen fibers are believed to form by the movement of fibroblasts back and forth along parallel collagen fibrils, leaving trails of newly synthesized collagen fibrils that gradually build up into fibers.

(b) Periodontal fibroblasts often contain ingested mineralized collagen fibrils that are subsequently digested by collagenases in the lysosomes of the fibroblasts. Thus, periodontal fibroblasts are an example of fibroblasts that both synthesize and resorb collagen.

(2) The areas of loose connective tissue contain blood vessels and nerves along with thin, randomly arrayed collagen fibers and cells.

b. The periodontal ligament also contains longitudinally disposed **oxytalin fibers,** which resemble developing elastic fibers and may give some elastic properties to the ligament.

2. **Functions.** The periodontal ligament has numerous functions.

a. It provides attachment and support for the tooth.

b. It exerts the tension needed for bone remodeling during movement of a tooth.

c. It also provides nutrition to adjacent structures, acts as a transducer in tooth proprioception, and aids in tooth eruption.

C. **Gingiva.** The gingiva (commonly called the **gum**) is an example of the masticatory mucosa (see II A).

1. The gingiva is firmly attached to the teeth at the level of the cementoenamel junction and covers the surfaces of the alveolar processes that are exposed to the oral cavity.

2. The **junctional,** or **attachment, epithelium** is firmly bound to the tooth surface by hemidesmosomes and a basal lamina–like material.

a. In young individuals, the attachment is to the enamel.

b. In older individuals, passive tooth eruption and normal gingival recession can expose the roots; the attachment is then to the cementum.

3. Above this epithelial attachment is the **gingival sulcus,** a shallow crevice that is lined with **crevicular epithelium,** which is continuous with the attachment epithelium.

D. **Periodontium.** This is a collective name for all of the tissues involved in the attachment of a tooth to the jaw. These include the crevicular and junctional epithelium, the cementum, the periodontal ligament, and the alveolar bone proper.

Chapter 23

Exocrine Glands—Salivary Glands

I. INTRODUCTION

A. **Exocrine glands.** All salivary glands are included in a larger category of structures called exocrine glands. The single unifying characteristic of exocrine glands is the presence of ducts that convey recently synthesized secretions from the secretory cells to a site of release onto a body surface.

  1. In addition to the salivary glands, exocrine glands include the **exocrine pancreas** and **liver,** whose secretions are essential to digestion in the small intestine; **sweat glands** in the dermis, whose secretions function in body temperature regulation; and the **lacrimal glands,** whose secretion (tears) lubricates and protects the corneal and conjunctival epithelium.

  2. This chapter presents a description of the general characteristics of exocrine glands, followed by a detailed description of the major salivary glands as typical exocrine glands.

B. **Major salivary glands.** The major salivary glands are the paired **parotid, submandibular,** and **sublingual** glands.

  1. The parotid and submandibular glands are located outside the oral cavity and their secretions are carried to the cavity by long ducts.

  2. The sublingual glands are located in the floor of the oral cavity and relatively short ducts connect the glands to the cavity.

C. **Minor salivary glands.** The minor salivary glands are found in the submucosa throughout the oral cavity and are named for their location. They are the **buccal, labial, lingual, molar,** and **palatine** glands.

II. GENERAL CHARACTERISTICS OF EXOCRINE GLANDS.
Exocrine glands originate as tubular invaginations of an epithelial surface. Their secretory portions may be **tubular** or **acinar,** or some combination of the two. Secretory acini and tubules in an exocrine gland are organized by connective tissue septa into **lobules** and **lobes.** A dense connective tissue capsule surrounds large exocrine glands such as the major salivary glands.

A. **Secretory acini and tubules.** The secretory portion of an exocrine gland, whether acinar or tubular, is formed by a simple cuboidal or simple columnar epithelium of secretory cells. The secretory cells of most exocrine glands may be classified into two types:

  1. **Serous cells** are protein-secreting cells (Figure 23-1).
     a. Serous cells have a pyramidal shape, with a relatively broad basal surface facing the connective tissue and a smaller apical surface facing the lumen of the acinus or tubule. The nucleus is usually clearly visible and is in the middle region of the cell.
     b. Cytoplasmic basophilia is characteristic of the basal portion of the cell and may extend into the perinuclear region. This represents the localization of the rough endoplasmic reticulum in the cell.
     c. Secretory (zymogen) granules are found in the supranuclear cytoplasm, often filling the apical region of the cell. The number of granules varies with the functional state of the cell.

  2. **Mucous cells** are mucin-secreting cells (Figure 23-2).

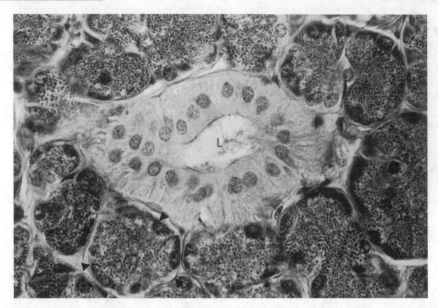

FIGURE 23-1. Light micrograph of a section of submandibular gland. In this specimen, a striated duct is clearly demonstrated, as are its characteristic radial striations. The striated duct, which is an intralobular duct, is surrounded by serous acini in which zymogen granules are numerous and conspicuous. *L* = lumen of the striated duct; *arrowheads* = an acinus.

    a. Mucous cells are also pyramidal, with clearly visible basal, lateral, and apical margins. The nucleus is compressed against the lateral or basal plasma membrane, and may be difficult to recognize because its basophilia is masked by the intensely basophilic rough endoplasmic reticulum that surrounds it.

    b. Mucigen droplets fill much of the cytoplasm.

        (1) In histologic section, the droplets usually appear as clear vacuoles because the mucin dissolves in routine tissue preparation.

        (2) In specially fixed specimens, mucigen droplets stain intensely with the periodic acid-Schiff reaction and other stains that bind to the oligosaccharides of the mucigen.

  3. Secretory acini or tubules may be pure serous, pure mucous, or mixed. **Mixed acini** are made up primarily of mucous cells, with a cap of serous cells (Figure 23-3).

    a. The serous cells secrete into the convoluted intercellular space between the mucous cells.

    b. The serous cap is called a **serous demilune** because it appears as a half-moon shape in histologic sections.

B. **Myoepithelial cells**

  1. Myoepithelial cells are contractile cells that lie between the basal lamina and the basal plasma membrane of the acinar cells. They may also underlie the proximal portion of the duct system.

  2. Myoepithelial cells play an important role in moving the secretory products of an exocrine gland toward its excretory duct.

C. **Duct system of exocrine glands.** The lumen of the secretory acinus or tubule is continuous with that of a duct system.

  1. **Duct location.** Ducts may be intralobular or interlobular.

    a. **Intralobular ducts**

        (1) These are contained in the parenchyma of the gland and include the **intercalated ducts** and **striated ducts.**

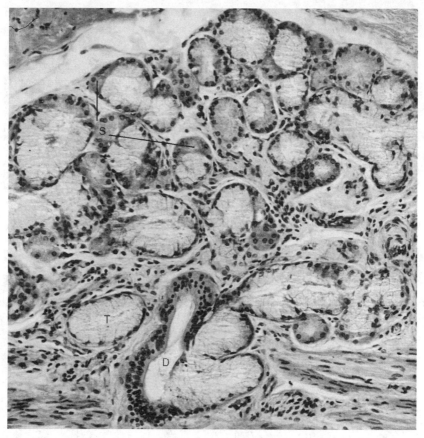

FIGURE 23-2. Light micrograph of a typical mixed exocrine gland from the tracheal mucosa. The secretory portion contains primarily mucous tubules (*T*), many of which are capped by serous demilunes (*S*). Two mucous tubules empty into the duct (*D*), which is formed by a stratified cuboidal epithelium.

       (2) These parenchymal ducts modify the serous secretion by **absorption** of specific components from the acinar secretion, and by **secretion** of additional components.

   b. Interlobular ducts. These travel in the interlobular and interlobar connective tissue septa and are also called the **excretory ducts.**

2. Duct segments. A duct system may have some or all of three sequential segments: intercalated duct, striated duct, and excretory duct (Figure 23-4).

   a. Intercalated ducts. Intercalated ducts connect the lumen of the secretory acinus to a larger intralobular duct (see Figure 27-4).

       (1) Serous glands often have well-developed intercalated ducts.

       (2) In serous and mixed glands, intercalated ducts **secrete bicarbonate** into the acinar product and **absorb chloride** from the acinar product.

   b. Striated ducts. Striated ducts are large intralobular ducts found only in some salivary glands. They are formed by a confluence of intercalated ducts, and are characterized by **radial striations** around the circumference of the duct.

       (1) The striations are produced by **infoldings of the basal plasma membrane** that partially surround longitudinally oriented **elongated mitochondria** in the base of the cuboidal duct epithelial cells.

       (2) This association of basal infoldings and mitochondria is a characteristic feature of many types of epithelial cells that reabsorb fluid and electrolytes. In glands that have prominent striated ducts, such as the parotid and submandib-

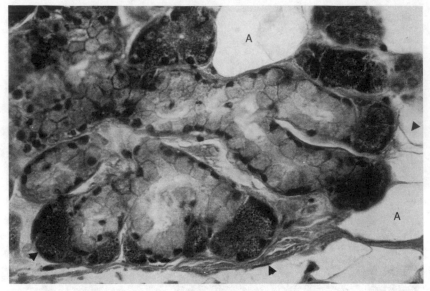

FIGURE 23-3. Light micrograph of a section of submandibular gland. Branching tubuloacinar secretory units are visible. The tubules are primarily mucus-secreting and most are capped by serous demilunes (*arrowheads*). Zymogen granules nearly fill the cytoplasm of the serous cells. *A* = adipocyte.

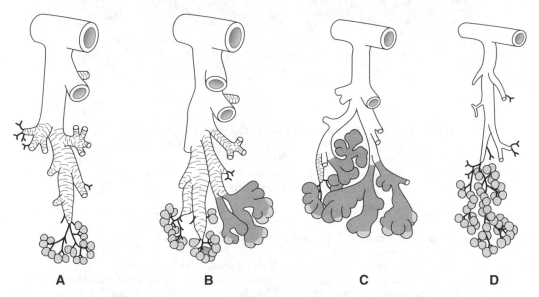

FIGURE 23-4. A schematic drawing illustrating the variations in the basic structure of exocrine glands, as exemplified by the three major salivary glands and the exocrine pancreas. (*A*) Parotid gland showing small intercalated ducts (*black*) leading to larger striated ducts (*striped*) and, finally, to excretory ducts (*white*). (*B*) Submandibular gland showing the same three ductal components. (*C*) Sublingual gland showing a paucity of both intercalated and striated ducts. (*D*) Exocrine pancreas showing intercalated ducts leading directly to excretory ducts. The serous secretory units (*light shading*) are acinar; the mucous secretory units (*dark shading*) are tubular and tubuloacinar. (Modified from Copenhaver W (ed): *Bailey's Textbook of Histology*, 16th ed. Baltimore, Williams & Wilkins, 1971, p 466.)

ular glands, these ducts have been shown to **reabsorb sodium** from the primary secretion and to **add potassium** to the secretion.

    c. Excretory ducts. Excretory ducts connect with the epithelial surface onto which the gland secretes, either directly or by emptying into a major named duct.

        (1) Small excretory ducts have a simple cuboidal epithelium that gradually becomes columnar as the ducts enlarge.

        (2) This may become stratified columnar or stratified squamous epithelium.

3. Major named ducts. The major named ducts leave the gland and travel in the surrounding connective tissue to reach the surface onto which they release the secretion.

    a. The submandibular duct (Wharton duct) and the parotid duct (Stensen duct) travel in the connective tissue of the neck and face, respectively, for a considerable distance from the gland before reaching the oral mucosa.

    b. The pancreatic duct travels in the connective tissue of the pancreas before joining the common bile duct to empty into the duodenum.

4. Variations in duct systems. Characteristic variation in the duct system structure is one criterion used in the identification and classification of exocrine glands.

    a. The sublingual gland has few, if any, intercalated or striated ducts, but has numerous large excretory ducts.

    b. The parotid and submandibular glands are characterized by numerous large striated ducts.

    c. The exocrine pancreas (see Chapter 27) has an extensive system of intercalated ducts that lead directly to interlobular and interlobar excretory ducts. It completely lacks striated ducts.

D. **Secretion mechanisms**

1. Merocrine secretion is characterized by the **exocytosis of stored secretory (zymogen) granules.**

    a. In this mechanism, the membrane of the secretory granule fuses with the apical plasma membrane of the secretory cell, releasing the secretion into the acinar or tubular lumen.

    b. The membrane added to the plasma membrane is conserved and recycled.

    c. Merocrine secretion is the most commonly encountered secretory mechanism in the body and is typical of salivary glands and the exocrine pancreas (see Chapter 27).

2. Holocrine secretion is characterized by the **secretion of whole cells,** live or dead.

    a. In sebaceous glands (see Chapter 20), secretory droplets accumulate in the cells until they become engorged and die. The secretion, along with cell fragments, then flows into the duct.

    b. Secretion of spermatozoa by the seminiferous tubules (see Chapter 36) is also considered holocrine secretion. In this case, live, whole cells are the secretory product.

3. Apocrine secretion is characterized by the **loss of apical cytoplasm** from the secretory cells, along with the secretory droplets.

    a. Mammary glands (see Chapter 35) are modified sweat glands. They secrete the lipid component of milk by an apocrine mechanism, and the protein component of milk by a merocrine mechanism.

    b. Apocrine sweat glands of the skin (see Chapter 20) are also reported to secrete by both apocrine and merocrine mechanisms.

III. **PAROTID GLANDS.** The paired parotid glands are the largest of the major salivary glands.

A. **Location and morphology.** The glands are located subcutaneously, below and in front of each ear, lateral and posterior to the masseter muscle.

1. The **parotid duct** (Stensen duct) runs forward along the masseter muscle and then turns medially to penetrate the buccinator muscle and enter the oral cavity opposite the second upper molar tooth.

2. Branches of the **facial nerve (cranial nerve VII)** pass through the parotid gland.
   a. Large sections of this nerve, usually found in routine histologic sections of the gland, are helpful in identifying the gland.
   b. **Mumps,** a viral infection of the parotid gland that was epidemic before development of an effective vaccine, often caused transient or permanent damage to the facial nerve.

3. Large amounts of adipose tissue are usually present in the parotid gland and may be one of its distinguishing characteristics.

B. **Secretory units and ducts.** The parotid gland is a **compound tubuloacinar gland.** All of its secretory units are serous.

1. Intercalated ducts are numerous, but are inconspicuous because of their narrow diameter.

2. Striated ducts, however, are conspicuous because of their large size and large number.
   a. The diameter of the striated ducts may exceed that of the secretory tubuloacinus.
   b. The striated ducts (intralobular) lead to excretory ducts (interlobular) that lead to the main parotid duct.

IV. **SUBMANDIBULAR GLAND.** The paired submandibular glands are **mixed seromucous glands** that are mostly serous in humans.

A. **Location and morphology.** The submandibular glands are located on either side of the floor of the mouth, close to the mandible.

1. The **submandibular duct** (Wharton duct) runs forward and medially to a papilla on the floor of the mouth, just lateral to the frenulum of the tongue.

2. Many of the short excretory ducts of the sublingual gland empty into the submandibular duct.

3. The submandibular gland and duct are sometimes called submaxillary gland and duct in older texts. This derives from British usage, in which the mandible was called the submaxilla.

B. **Secretory units and ducts.** The submandibular gland, like the parotid gland, is a **compound tubuloacinar gland.** Most of its secretory units are purely serous, although some mucous tubuloacini may be encountered.

1. The mucous tubuloacini are usually capped by serous demilunes.

2. Intercalated ducts are present but inconspicuous. Striated ducts are numerous and obvious.

3. The striated ducts connect to excretory ducts that lead to the main submandibular duct.

V. **SUBLINGUAL GLAND.** The paired sublingual glands are the smallest of the major salivary glands.

A. **Location and morphology.** Sublingual glands are located in the floor of the mouth and are anterior to the submandibular glands.

    1. The sublingual gland is not drained by a single large duct.

    2. Many short excretory ducts lead directly to the floor of the mouth or to the larger submandibular duct.

B. **Secretory units and ducts.** The sublingual glands are **compound tubular glands.** They are mixed glands that are mostly mucus secreting in humans.

    1. Most of the tubular secretory units are purely mucus secreting.
       a. Some mucus-secreting tubules may be capped with serous demilunes.
       b. Purely serous acini are rarely encountered.

    2. Most tubular secretory units appear to drain directly into interlobular (excretory) ducts.
       a. The tubular secretory units are long and assume a ductal function in addition to a secretory function.
       b. Intercalated ducts and striated ducts are rarely seen in sections and may be absent from the gland.

VI. **SALIVA.** Saliva consists of the combined secretions of all of the major and minor salivary glands, together with other fluids derived from the oral mucosa. About 1200 ml of saliva are produced per day.

A. **Functions of saliva.** Saliva has numerous functions, only some of which are related to digestion.

    1. **Moistening.** Saliva moistens the oral mucosa and adds moisture to dry foods as an aid to swallowing.

    2. **Aid in tasting.** Saliva provides a medium for the **solution or suspension of food materials** that chemically stimulate taste buds.

    3. **Initial digestion and buffering.** Saliva contains enzymes that begin the digestion of carbohydrates and some other foodstuffs, and contains **bicarbonate ion,** which helps buffer the contents of the oral cavity.

    4. **Protection.** Saliva also plays an important role in the protection of the body.
       a. The presence of the bactericidal enzyme **lysozyme** helps control the bacterial flora of the oral cavity.
       b. **Immunoglobulin A** (IgA), synthesized by plasma cells in the connective tissue surrounding salivary acini, is endocytosed, modified, and resecreted by salivary acinar cells as **secretory IgA** (sIgA), which participates in the **immune exclusion process** (see Chapter 21 III A 2 d).
       c. Proteins in saliva also provide a protective coat for the teeth called the **acquired pellicle.**

    5. **Tooth mineralization.** Saliva is a major source of **calcium** and **phosphate** essential for normal tooth development and maintenance. Calcium and phosphate ions in saliva are needed for mineralization of newly erupted teeth and for normal repair of precarious lesions in erupted teeth.

B. **Control of salivation.** Salivation is part of a reflex arc that is normally stimulated by **ingestion of food.** Sight, smell, and thoughts of food can also stimulate salivation.

    1. Salivary glands are innervated by the **sympathetic** and **parasympathetic** divisions of the autonomic nervous system. Nerves from both divisions end adjacent to salivary acini.
       a. **Sympathetic stimulation** causes secretion of a **viscous saliva** rich in enzymes.

    b. Parasympathetic stimulation causes secretion of large amounts of a **watery saliva** that serves as a lubricant and buffer.

2. Salivary secretion and content can be modified by hormonal stimulation. **Aldosterone,** an adrenal hormone that regulates sodium and potassium content of the urine (see Chapters 29 and 32), significantly **increases sodium reabsorption** and **potassium secretion** by the striated ducts.

Chapter 24

Esophagus and Stomach

I. ESOPHAGUS. The esophagus is a **muscular tube** that extends about 25 cm from the oropharynx to the stomach. It is a **conduit for food and fluids.**

A. Layers of the esophageal wall. The esophagus has the same four basic layers as the rest of the digestive tract (see Chapter 21). There are, however, important specific differences.

1. **Mucosa.** The mucosa consists of the three concentric layers typical of the digestive tract: epithelium, lamina propria, and muscularis mucosae.
   a. **Epithelium.** The esophagus is lined throughout with **nonkeratinized stratified squamous epithelium** (Figure 24-1).
      (1) The surface epithelial cells in the human esophagus may contain some keratohyalin granules, but keratinization does not normally occur.
      (2) In some animals, notably carnivores who swallow large chunks of unchewed food, the epithelium is keratinized.
   b. **Lamina propria.** The lamina propria is not distinctive in the esophagus.
      (1) **Diffuse lymphatic tissue** is present in this layer throughout its length.
      (2) **Lymphatic nodules** are located in proximity to the ducts of esophageal glands (see I B).
   c. **Muscularis mucosae**
      (1) This deep layer of the mucosa consists of longitudinally arranged smooth muscle that begins at the level of the cricoid cartilage.
      (2) The muscularis mucosae is unusually thick in the upper portion of the esophagus. This is believed to **aid in swallowing** once the reflex portion of that act begins.

2. **Submucosa.** The submucosa forms a number of **longitudinal folds** that include the muscularis mucosae.
   a. These folds give the collapsed tube a highly irregular surface profile in cross section.
   b. As a bolus of food passes down the esophagus, however, the folds flatten, allowing dilation of the lumen to accommodate the food.

3. **Muscularis externa.** The esophageal muscularis externa differs significantly from that of the rest of the digestive tract in humans.
   a. **Striated muscle** constitutes both layers of the muscularis externa in the **upper one-third** of the esophagus.
      (1) These muscles are continuations of the muscles of the laryngopharynx.
      (2) They are important at the beginning of the act of swallowing, which is a voluntary action.
   b. **Striated muscle and smooth muscle are interwoven** in the muscularis externa in the **middle one-third** of the esophagus (Figure 24-2).
   c. **Smooth muscle** forms both layers of the muscularis externa in the **distal one-third** of the esophagus, as in the rest of the digestive tract.

B. Esophageal glands. The esophagus has both **mucosal** and **submucosal glands.** Both are **mucus-secreting,** but their locations and specific secretions differ.

1. **Mucosal glands.** Mucosal glands are concentrated in the lamina propria of the terminal portion of the esophagus, near the junction with the stomach. They are present in the proximal portion of the esophagus, as well.
   a. The mucosal glands secrete a **neutral mucus** that **protects the distal esophagus** from regurgitated gastric contents.
   b. They are sometimes called **esophageal cardiac glands** because of their resemblance to the cardiac glands of the stomach.

FIGURE 24-1. Esophagus, light micrograph. The mucosa and part of the submucosa are shown. The duct (D) of a submucosal mucus-secreting gland (G) is visible crossing the muscularis mucosae (MM). L = lumen of esophagus, E = stratified squamous nonkeratinized epithelium, LP = lamina propria.

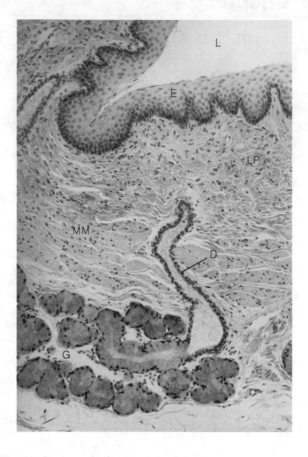

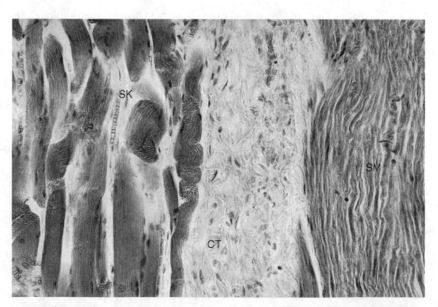

FIGURE 24-2. Esophagus, light micrograph. Muscularis externa fills the field. This layer is formed by a mixture of skeletal muscle (SK) and smooth muscle (SM) that is characteristic of the middle portion of the esophagus. CT = loose irregular connective tissue.

2. **Submucosal glands.** Submucosal glands are found throughout the esophagus, but tend to be more concentrated in the upper half (see Figure 24-1).

   a. The submucosal glands are small, simple tubuloalveolar glands that secrete a **slightly acidic mucus** that serves to **lubricate the lumen.**

   b. The ducts of these glands pass through the full thickness of the mucosa to reach the lumen.

      (1) These large excretory ducts are lined with stratified cuboidal epithelium. They are conspicuous when found in a section because they are usually dilated by the relatively viscous secretion.

      (2) Lymphatic tissue often surrounds the ducts as they pass through the muscularis mucosae and lamina propria (see Figure 15-4).

II. **STOMACH.** The stomach is an expanded portion of the digestive tract in which the bolus of food received from the esophagus is further **macerated** and **partially digested.** The addition of fluids from the gastric secretions gradually converts the bolus of food to a viscous pulp, called **chyme.**

A. **Functions.** Secretion of fluids, electrolytes, and enzymes is the primary function of the gastric mucosa. Nearly 2 liters of fluid secretion are produced by the gastric glands daily. Absorption is not normally an important function.

   1. **Secretion**

      a. **Hydrochloric acid.** The mucosal glands of the stomach secrete 0.16N hydrochloric acid into the lumen to mix with the chyme.

      b. **Pepsin.** The mucosal glands secrete **pepsinogen,** which is converted into the potent proteolytic enzyme pepsin in the acid environment of the gastric lumen.

      c. **Intrinsic factor.** In addition to water, electrolytes, acid, and enzymes, the gastric glands secrete intrinsic factor, a glycoprotein essential for **absorption of vitamin B_{12}** in distal parts of the digestive tract.

      d. **Hormones. Enteroendocrine cells** in the gastric epithelium secrete **gastrin** and other hormones and hormone-like secretions. These secretions regulate **acid secretion** in the gastric mucosa locally, and regulate **intestinal motility** and other digestive functions distally.

   2. **Absorption.** The stomach epithelium does not normally function as an absorptive tissue.

      a. Some water, salts, and lipid-soluble drugs pass across this layer.

      b. Alcohol, aspirin, and other drugs reach the vascular system of the stomach by damaging the surface epithelium and diffusing into the lamina propria.

B. **Morphologic specializations.** Grossly, the stomach may be divided into four regions: **cardia, fundus, body,** and **pylorus.** Histologically, however, the body and fundus are identical and contiguous. The wall contains the four layers characteristic of the digestive system (see Chapter 21 II), with regional and functional specializations.

   1. **Regions of the stomach**

      a. **Cardia.** The cardia (cardiac region) consists of the first 10 to 40 mm distal to the **esophagogastric junction.** It contains the gastric cardiac glands.

      b. **Fundus and body.** The fundus and body, situated between the cardia and pylorus, form the largest part of the organ. They contain the fundic, or gastric, glands.

      c. **Pylorus.** The pylorus is the narrowed portion of the stomach immediately proximal to the **gastroduodenal (pyloric) sphincter.** It contains pyloric glands.

   2. **Rugae.** Longitudinal folds or ridges, called rugae, are prominent in the narrower regions of the stomach.

      a. The rugae are composed of the mucosa and the underlying submucosa.

      b. The rugae flatten to accommodate expansion and filling of the stomach.

   3. **Gastric pits.** Examination of the surface of the mucosa with a hand lens, dissecting

microscope, or scanning electron microscope shows numerous openings in all regions of the mucosal surface. These are the **gastric pits,** or **foveolae.**

    a. The mucosal glands empty into the bottom of the gastric pits.

    b. The gastric pits, therefore, serve as short ducts that convey gastric secretions from the mucosal glands to the lumen of the stomach.

C. **Gastric mucosa.** The gastric mucosa consists of a **columnar epithelium,** the **mucosal glands,** the **lamina propria,** and the **muscularis mucosae.** The mucosa ranges in thickness from 0.3 mm at the cardiac end to more than 1.5 mm in the body of the stomach (Figure 24-3).

    1. Surface epithelium

        a. Surface mucous cells. These are the simple columnar epithelial cells that line the surface and the gastric pits throughout the stomach.

            (1) This columnar epithelium is continuous with the basal layer of the esophageal epithelium at the esophagogastric junction.

            (2) These cells form a glandular sheet, with each cell containing a large **apical cup of mucinogen granules,** called a **mucin droplet.** Mucin droplets stain intensely with toluidine blue and with the periodic acid–Schiff (PAS) procedure.

                (a) PAS staining emphasizes the **glycoprotein** nature of the secretion.

                (b) Toluidine blue staining indicates the presence of the many **strongly anionic groups** of the glycoproteins.

            (3) The secreted mucus, called **visible mucus,** forms a thick, viscous, gel-like coat that adheres to and **protects** the epithelial surface.

                (a) The most important function of the mucus is to protect the epithelium from the **acidic environment of the lumen.** This is accomplished by the buffering effect of the high concentration of bicarbonate ion in the mucus.

                (b) The mucus layer also provides protection from **abrasion** by rough components of the chyme.

        b. Epithelial cell renewal. Stem cells in the stomach are localized in the mucous neck and the base of the gastric pit. Division of these cells gives rise to all of the epithelial cells of the stomach, including the next generation of stem cells.

            (1) Most of the newly replicated cells migrate toward the surface to become sur-

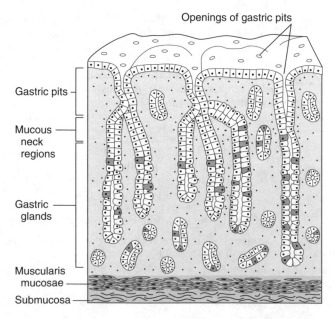

FIGURE 24-3. Gastric mucosa. The surface is generally smooth, but is broken up into irregular, slightly elevated areas described as mamillated. Tubular invaginations of the surface form the gastric pits. The gastric glands empty into the bottoms of the gastric pits. The gastric glands are restricted to the mucosa, descending from the mucous neck toward the muscularis mucosae.

Openings of gastric pits

Gastric pits

Mucous neck regions

Gastric glands

Muscularis mucosae

Submucosa

face mucous cells, but some of them remain in the mucous neck and differentiate into mucous neck cells.

    (a) Surface mucous cells turn over rapidly, having a life span of only 5 days in humans.

    (b) They are constantly being shed from the surface and trapped in the visible mucus.

  (2) Other newly replicated cells migrate in the opposite direction, into the glands, where they differentiate into parietal cells, chief cells, and enteroendocrine cells (see III A).

    (a) Gland cells have a relatively long life span of approximately 1 year.

    (b) Senescent gland cells are shed into the gland lumen, from which they are carried in the gastric secretions to the stomach lumen.

2. Mucosal glands

  a. Cardiac glands. Cardiac glands are coiled tubular glands that sometimes branch. They are found only in the cardia, the narrow region surrounding the esophageal orifice.

    (1) Cardiac glands consist of **mucus-secreting cells** with some interspersed **enteroendocrine** cells. The composition of the mucus is similar to that secreted by the esophageal cardiac glands, and different from that secreted by the surface mucous cells.

    (2) The **gastric pits** of the cardia are relatively shallow, occupying less than one-fourth the thickness of the mucosa.

    (3) A short duct-like segment, the **mucous neck,** is interposed between the secretory portion of the gland and the gastric pit into which it secretes.

      (a) The mucous neck is the site of the **stem cells** that give rise to both the surface mucous cells and the gland cells (see II C 1 b).

      (b) Mucous neck cells secrete only small amounts of a **soluble mucus.**

  b. Gastric (fundic) glands. These glands are the principal mucosal glands of the stomach and produce **gastric juice.** They are present throughout the mucosa, except in the relatively small regions where cardiac glands and pyloric glands are found.

    (1) The gastric glands are simple branched tubular glands (Figure 24-4). Several gastric glands normally empty into a single gastric pit.

    (2) The glands are closely packed and extend through the full thickness of the mucosa, from the bottom of the gastric pits to the muscularis mucosae.

      (a) The gastric pit occupies only about 20% to 30% of the length of the gland.

      (b) The **mucous neck segment** is relatively long.

      (c) The base of the gland may divide into two or three branches that become coiled as they reach the muscularis mucosae.

  c. Pyloric glands. Pyloric glands are located in the pylorus and in the portion of the stomach nearest the pylorus.

    (1) They, too, are branched tubular glands that are coiled in their deep portion. The lumen of the gland is relatively wide.

    (2) Most pyloric secretory cells resemble surface mucous cells.

      (a) Enteroendocrine cells are present at all levels of the gland.

      (b) Occasional parietal cells are also found in the pyloric glands.

    (3) The pyloric glands drain through a short mucous neck into relatively deep gastric pits, which occupy nearly half the thickness of the mucosa.

3. Lamina propria. The lamina is relatively scant because the gastric pits and glands are so closely packed.

  a. The stroma consists of reticular fibers, fibroblasts, and some smooth muscle cells.

  b. Components of the immune system, namely, lymphocytes, plasma cells, macrophages, and eosinophils, are well represented and widely distributed.

    (1) Neutrophils may be found when there is any inflammatory condition present, such as gastric ulcers.

    (2) Lymphatic nodules are also present in the mucosa, close to the muscularis mucosae.

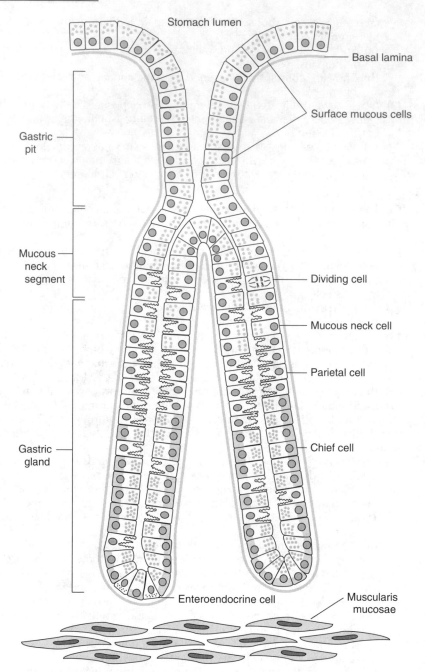

FIGURE 24-4. Gastric glands of a human stomach. Two tubular glands emptying into one gastric pit are shown. Parietal cells are large, ovoid, acidophilic cells found in the mucous neck and throughout the gland, being most concentrated in the upper portion. Chief cells and enteroendocrine cells are found at all levels of the gland, but are most concentrated in the basal portion.

4. **Muscularis mucosae.** The muscularis mucosae is composed of two relatively thin layers of smooth muscle. The inner layer encircles the organ, and the outer layer is oriented roughly parallel to the long axis of the organ. The layering of this smooth muscle is usually indistinct.

    a. Strands of smooth muscle extend into the lamina propria from the inner layer of smooth muscle toward the surface. They accompany loops of lymphatic vessels that arise from the network around the muscularis mucosae.

    b. This smooth muscle may aid in the emptying of the gastric glands into the stomach lumen.

D. **Submucosa.** The submucosa is a dense connective tissue that contains blood vessels, nerves, and adipose tissue. The ganglia and nerve fibers of the submucosal (Meissner) plexus innervate the blood vessels of the submucosa and the mucosa, and the smooth muscle of the muscularis mucosae.

E. **Muscularis externa.** The muscularis externa has traditionally been described as having three layers, consisting of the circular and longitudinal layers characteristic of the alimentary canal (see Figure 21-1), and an innermost oblique layer. This description, however, is more imaginative than accurate.

1. **Random orientation.** As with most hollow spheroidal organs that must empty through a narrow orifice, the smooth muscle of the muscularis externa is more randomly oriented than in tubular organs. (Compare with the distinct layers of the muscularis externa of the intestine; see Chapter 25.)

    a. The longitudinal layer is absent from large portions of the anterior and posterior surfaces of the stomach, and the circular layer is poorly developed in the cardiac region.

    b. The circular layer is thickened at the pyloric end, contributing to the sphincter function at that level.

2. **Peristalsis and gastric emptying.** Peristaltic waves in the randomly arranged smooth muscle of the body and fundus mix the chyme with acid and enzymes by compressing the luminal contents from all directions.

    a. The peristaltic wave moves faster than the chyme. Thus, the propulsion of the contents is greater toward the expanded portions of the stomach than toward the narrowed pyloric portion.

    b. Because of this differential propulsion, and the sphincter actions of the thickened circular muscle at the pylorus, only a small bolus of chyme enters the small intestine with each contraction wave.

3. **Innervation.** The muscularis externa is locally innervated by the ganglia and nerves of the myenteric (Auerbach) plexus.

    a. These ganglia are located between the ill-defined layers of muscle.

    b. Gross emptying of the stomach is regulated by the vagus nerve (cranial nerve X), which can also influence the rate of acid secretion.

III. **CELLS OF THE GASTRIC GLANDS.** The glands are composed of four functionally and morphologically distinct cell types, and the single stem cell population that gives rise to them.

A. **Cell types** (Figure 24-5; see also Figure 24-4)

1. **Mucous neck cells.** These are **mucus-secreting** cells. These cells are localized in the mucous neck segments of the mucosal glands, just deep to the gastric pits.

    a. They are shorter than surface mucous cells and contain fewer mucinogen droplets.

    b. The stem cells of the gastric epithelium and some differentiated parietal cells are interspersed among the mucus-secreting cells.

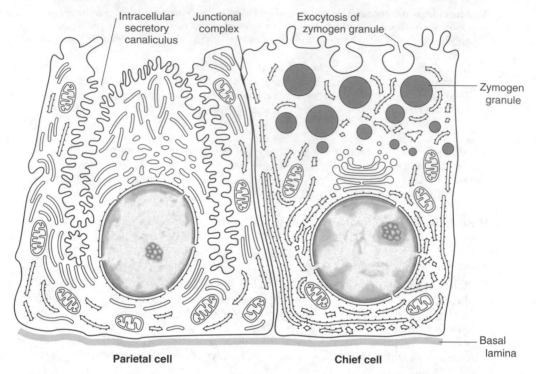

FIGURE 24-5. Parietal cell and chief cell, gastric mucosa. In the parietal cell, the complex intracellular canaliculus increases the surface area of plasma membrane across which the cell can secrete hydrochloric acid. The large number of mitochondria provide energy for the active transport process that is the basis of this secretory mechanism. The chief cell contains an extensive rough endoplasmic reticulum, a prominent Golgi apparatus, and numerous zymogen granules, which are characteristic of a protein-secreting cell.

2. **Parietal (oxyntic) cells.** These are **acid-secreting** cells. They secrete 0.l6N hydrochloric acid into the gastric juice (see III B), as well as **intrinsic factor.**
   a. Parietal cells are located principally in the upper and middle portions of the gastric glands. They are also found in the mucous neck portion of the gland, interspersed among the mucous neck cells, and to a lesser extent, in the base of the glands, among the chief cells.
   b. Parietal cells are very large, acidophilic cells that are sometimes binucleate. They have a roughly triangular shape, with the base resting on the basal lamina.
   c. With transmission electron microscopy (TEM), parietal cells are seen to contain **numerous mitochondria,** with complex cristae and many matrix granules, as well as an elaborate **canalicular system,** derived from and continuous with the apical plasma membrane, thus connecting it to the gland lumen.
      (1) Numerous microvilli project from the membranes of the canaliculi.
      (2) An elaborate cytoplasmic **tubulovesicular system** is found adjacent to the canaliculi in parietal cells that are not actively secreting.

3. **Chief cells.** These are **protein-secreting** cells. Chief cells are the predominant cell type in the **lower half of the gastric glands** (Figure 24-6).
   a. They have the morphology of typical zymogen-secreting cells; that is, they resemble pancreatic acinar cells (see Figure 27-3).
   b. An extensive rough endoplasmic reticulum fills the basal cytoplasm, making that part of the cell intensely basophilic. This permits easy identification in hematoxylin–eosin (H&E) sections.
   c. Chief cells secrete pepsinogens and lipase.
      (1) **Pepsinogens** are converted to **pepsins,** potent proteolytic enzymes, by the

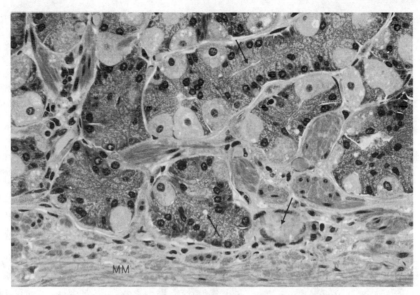

FIGURE 24-6. Light micrograph showing the convoluted lower portions of several gastric glands. Chief cells stain darkly, have basal nuclei, and exhibit numerous, lightly staining stored zymogen granules. Parietal cells are large pale cells with a centrally located nucleus. A small blood vessel (*arrow*) is visible in the lamina propria just above the muscularis mucosae (*MM*). *Crossed arrows* indicate the lumens of gastric glands.

acidic gastric juice. Pepsins hydrolyze proteins to smaller peptides, which are further digested to amino acids by enzymes in the small intestine.

(2) Gastric **lipase** is a weak enzyme that may not be significant in humans.

4. **Enteroendocrine cells.** These are **hormone-secreting** cells.
   a. **Distribution**
      (1) Enteroendocrine cells are **widely distributed.** They are present in the digestive tract from the level of the esophageal cardiac glands to the rectum, as well as in the ducts of the pancreas and liver. They are also found in the respiratory system (see Chapter 28 V B 1 e), which is also derived from the embryonic gut.
      (2) Enteroendocrine cells are present at all levels of the mucosal glands, but they are more numerous in the base of the glands, close to the muscularis mucosae (see Figure 25-8).
   b. **Enteroendocrine cell types**
      (1) Enteroendocrine cells are named for the more than 20 hormones and putative hormones they secrete into the lamina propria (e.g., gastrin-secreting cells, somatostatin-secreting cells), and are characterized by immunocytochemistry.
      (2) The names given to these cells in the older literature reflect their staining properties with salts of heavy metals, hence the names **argentaffin, enterochromaffin,** and **argyrophil** cells.
   c. **Structural characeristics**
      (1) TEM reveals that each type of enteroendocrine cell contains granules of a particular density and size in the basal portion of the cell.
      (2) Most enteroendocrine cells only contact the basal lamina of the epithelium. Some cells, however, have thin apical cytoplasmic extensions with microvilli that are exposed to the gland lumen. These cells are believed to sample the luminal contents and release their hormones into the lamina propria in response to that sensory activity.
   d. **Hormonal secretion.** The polypeptide secretions of the enteroendocrine cells include well defined hormones known to have specific roles in regulation of the digestive tract.

    (1) Gastrin promotes secretion of acid by the parietal cells in response to filling of the stomach.

    (2) Secretin promotes secretion of enzyme precursors and bicarbonate by the exocrine pancreas.

    (3) Cholecystokinin promotes emptying of the gallbladder, as well as enzyme and bicarbonate secretion by the pancreas.

e. Gastroenteropancreatic (GEP) endocrine system. The enteroendocrine cells of the digestive and respiratory systems, including the endocrine islets (of Langerhans) of the pancreas, collectively constitute the largest purely endocrine organ in the body, the GEP endocrine system.

    (1) Enteroendocrine cells are also described as constituting part of the **diffuse neuroendocrine system.** This is because they closely resemble neurosecretory cells in the central nervous system that secrete many of the same hormones and regulatory peptides.

    (2) Some enteroendocrine cells may be **functionally classified as APUD cells** (amine precursor uptake and decarboxylation) because they produce biogenic amines and have the appropriate enzyme systems.

        (a) These cells should not, however, be confused with APUD cells that derive from the neural crest and migrate to other sites in the body during development.

        (b) Rather, all the cells of the GEP in the embryo and in the adult differentiate from progeny of the same stem cells as do all of the other epithelial cells of the digestive and respiratory tracts.

B. **Mechanism and regulation of acid secretion.** Hydrochloric acid is secreted across the parietal cell plasma membrane into the lumen of the canaliculus, and then into the lumen of the fundic and pyloric glands.

1. Mechanism

    a. Acid pump. The secretion is driven by the active transport of H^+ from the cytoplasm by an **H^+, K^+-activated membrane ATPase** coupled to an Na^+-driven Cl^-–HCO_3^- exchange.

    b. Increased surface area for secretion. In an actively secreting parietal cell, the tubulovesicular system is significantly reduced and the number of microvilli in the canaliculi is significantly increased.

        (1) The tubulovesicular system is a membrane reserve that can be mobilized by stimulation of acid secretion.

        (2) The number of microvilli is reduced and the tubulovesicular system is restored when the parietal cell is no longer actively secreting acid.

2. Regulation

    a. Stimulation of secretion

        (1) Gastrin, a polypeptide hormone secreted by enteroendrocrine cells of the cardiac and fundic glands, stimulates secretion of hydrochloric acid by the parietal cells. Gastrin receptors present on the parietal cell membrane can react to gastrin presented as an endocrine or as a paracrine stimulus.

        (2) Histamine and **acetylcholine** also stimulate acid secretion.

    b. Role of immune system. Recent studies suggest a regulatory relationship between plasma cells and macrophages in the lamina propria and the parietal cells.

        (a) Gastrin receptor messenger RNA has been localized immunochemically in plasma cells but not in parietal cells.

        (b) Anti-ulcer drugs that block attachment of histamine to receptors in the gastric mucosa may act on these plasma cells, rather than directly on the parietal cells to block acid secretion.

Chapter 25

Small Intestine and Colon

I. **SMALL INTESTINE.** The small intestine is the principal site for the **digestion of food-stuffs** and for the **absorption of nutrients** derived from digestion. **Enzymes** and **bile** act in the lumen of the small intestine to break down the chyme delivered from the stomach into molecules small enough to be absorbed by the intestinal cells.

A. **Anatomic segments.** The small intestine is the longest portion of the alimentary canal, measuring more than 6 meters in length. Its wall contains the layers characteristic of the gastrointestinal tract (see Chapter 21 II; Figure 21-1) It is divided along its length into three segments, the **duodenum,** the **jejunum,** and the **ileum,** each with particular specializations relating to its roles in digestion and absorption.

1. **Duodenum.** The duodenum is the proximal portion of the small intestine and extends for approximately 25 cm from the gastroduodenal junction at the pyloric sphincter.
   a. Enzymes from the **pancreas** and bile from the **liver** are delivered to the duodenum, in which the chyme is broken down to molecules that can be absorbed by intestinal cells.
   b. **Duodenal submucosal glands** called **Brunner glands** secrete an alkaline mucin that helps to neutralize the chyme and establish a slightly alkaline pH that is optimal for pancreatic enzyme activity.
   c. Terminal digestion of disaccharides and dipeptides also occurs in the duodenum, catalyzed by enzymes in the glycocalyx of the luminal plasma membrane of the intestinal absorptive cells (enterocytes).

2. **Jejunum.** The jejunum is the next segment of the small intestine, measuring about 2.5 meters in length.
   a. The jejunum is the primary site of absorption of nutrients in the intestine.
   b. In diarrheic diseases such as acute infant diarrhea and cholera, fluids and electrolytes lost in the stool can be replaced and nutrition maintained by absorption of sugared electrolyte solutions in the jejunum.

3. **Ileum.** The ileum is the terminal, and longest, portion of the small intestine, measuring approximately 3.5 meters.
   a. Water and electrolytes that reach the small intestine with the chyme and with the pancreatic and hepatic secretions are reabsorbed in the ileum.
   b. Vitamin B_{12} is absorbed in the ileum, as are bile components that will be recycled to the duodenum via the liver.
   c. The ileum is characteized by **aggregated lymphatic nodules** called **Peyer patches** that are visible, even to the unaided eye, in the lamina propria of the antimesenteric side of the tube.
   d. The organisms that cause diarrheic diseases affect primarily the absorptive cells of the ileum, preventing reabsorption of electrolytes and water.

B. **Morphologic specializations of the mucosa.** The small intestine exhibits several levels of morphologic adaptations designed to increase the surface area available for terminal digestion and absorption (Figure 25-1).

1. **Plicae circulares.** Plicae circulares (valves of Kerckring) are permanent transverse folds that involve both the submucosa and the mucosa.
   a. Each semilunar fold extends around one-half to two-thirds of the circumference of the lumen.
   b. They are most prominent in the distal duodenum and the jejunum. They become reduced in size distally, and end about 1 meter proximal to the ileocecal valve.

2. **Villi.** Villi are finger-like and leaf-like projections of the lamina propria that extend the mucosal surface into the lumen.

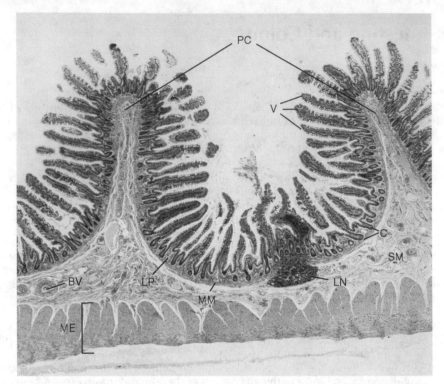

FIGURE 25-1. Small intestine, light micrograph (low power). Portion of a longitudinal section showing the full thickness of the intestinal wall. The two large folds, which include the submucosa (*SM*), are examples of the numerous plicae circulares (*PC*) that characterize this portion of the gastrointestinal tract. Villi (*V*) cover the plicae and the surface between them. Note the shortness of the crypts of Lieberkühn (*C*) compared to the length of the villi. Blood vessels (*BV*) are visible in the submucosa and a lymphatic nodule (*LN*) extends from the lamina propria (*LP*) of the mucosa, through the muscularis mucosae (*MM*), into the submucosa. The inner, circular layer and the outer, longitudinal layer of the muscularis externa (*ME*) are visible.

   a. Villi are unique to the small intestine, covering its entire surface and creating a velvety appearance.

   b. The simple columnar epithelium that covers the villi contains primarily absorptive cells, with some interspersed goblet cells and enteroendocrine cells (Figure 25-2).

   c. The lamina propria that forms the core of a villus consists of a loose connective tissue containing numerous fibroblasts and smooth muscle cells, as well as macrophages, lymphocytes, plasma cells, eosinophils, and other elements of the immune system.

      (1) The lymphocytes, together with lymphatic nodules of various sizes, are part of the **gut-associated lymphatic tissue (GALT),** probably the largest accumulation of lymphatic tissue in the body (see I E).

      (2) Each villus has a network of fenestrated capillaries immediately beneath the epithelial surface, and a blind-ending lymphatic capillary called a **lacteal** (Figure 25-3). Lacteals, accompanied by smooth muscle cells, extend into the villi from the network of lymphatic vessels that surrounds the muscularis mucosae.

   d. Villi have been observed to contract intermittently.

      (1) This action may help to force lymph from the lacteal into the perimuscular lymphatic network.

      (2) Contraction of the strands of smooth muscle that extend from the muscularis mucosae, as well as of myofibroblasts that have been described as extending across the diameter of the villus, may account for the changes in dimension of the villi.

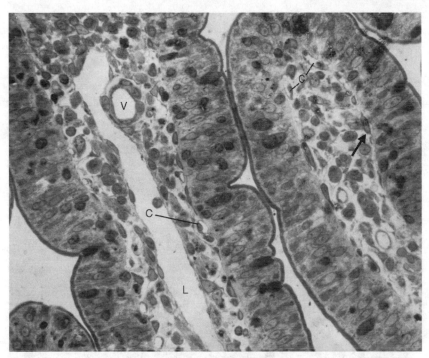

FIGURE 25-2. Intestinal villi. Photomicrograph showing sagittal sections through two adjacent villi. The epithelium surrounds a very cellular lamina propria. The villus on the left shows both a small venule (V) and the lacteal (L) in the core of the lamina propria. Both villi show capillaries (C) immediately subtending the basement membrane of the epithelium. The dark line at the apical surface of the epithelium is the brush border, the light microscopic representation of the microvilli that cover the epithelial cells. Subepithelial fibroblast of the pericryptal sheath indicated by *arrow*.

3. **Microvilli.** Microvilli are regular, finger-like projections of the apical cell surface (see Chapter 1 V B 1). They are found on all the mature cells of the intestinal epithelium except some enteroendocrine cells [see I C 1 d (1)].

4. **Crypts of Lieberkühn (mucosal glands).** The intestinal glands, or crypts, are simple tubular invaginations of the mucosal surface that extend to the level of the muscularis mucosae (Figure 25-4).
   a. **Crypt–villus relationship.** The crypts open onto the luminal surface at the base of the villi. The simple columnar epithelium of the crypts is continuous with that covering the villi (Figure 25-5).
      (1) In the three-dimensional sheet that constitutes the intestinal epithelium, each crypt contributes cells to 3 to 6 villi.
      (2) Also, each villus may have on its surface epithelial cells from 3 to 6 crypts.
   b. **Replicative zone.** The lower half of the crypts is the replicative zone of the intestinal epithelium.
      (1) The **stem cells** from which all of the cells of the intestinal epithelium derive are located in the base of each crypt.
      (2) The progeny of the stem cells give rise primarily to **immature goblet** and **absorptive cells** that undergo 2 to 3 additional divisions before final maturation.
      (3) Also present in the replicative zone are a few mature goblet cells, mature enteroendocrine cells, and mature Paneth cells (see I C).
   c. **Pericryptal fibroblast sheath.** The intestinal crypt is surrounded by pericryptal fibroblasts, a special population of stellate fibroblasts that lie just beneath the epithelial basal lamina.
      (1) The pericryptal fibroblasts secrete a circumferentially oriented layer of reticular fibers and proteoglycans that, together with the fibroblasts, forms the pericryptal fibroblast sheath (see Figure 25-4).

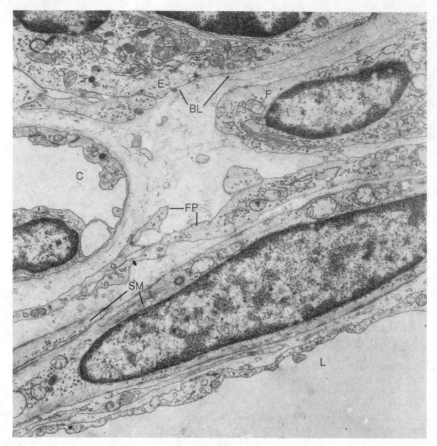

FIGURE 25-3. Jejunal villus, electron micrograph. The epithelium (*E*) rests on its basal lamina (*BL*). Immediately subtending this are fine collagen fibrils of the reticular layer of the basement membrane and a portion of a subepithelial fibroblast (*F*). A fenestrated absorptive capillary (*C*) is also visible immediately beneath the absorptive epithelium. Fibroblast processes (*FP*) and smooth muscle cells (*SM*) accompany the lacteal (*L*) in the core of the lamina propria.

    (2) The sheath continues as a layer under the absorptive epithelium of the villus.
    (3) The pericryptal fibroblasts replicate just under the stem cell zone in the base of the crypt. The fibroblasts migrate and differentiate in synchrony with the epithelial cells they subtend, and maintain contact with the epithelial basal lamina as they migrate.

C. **Intestinal epithelial cells.** Mature intestinal epithelial cells are located on the surface of the villi and in the crypts. Immature and replicating cells are limited to the crypts. Mature cells include absorptive cells (enterocytes), goblet cells, enteroendocrine cells, Paneth cells, and microfold (M) cells.

    1. **Absorptive cells.** Absorptive cells are specialized for the **terminal digestion** of nutrients to molecules that can be absorbed, and for the **absorption** of those nutrient molecules, electrolytes, and water.
        a. **Cell junctions.** Mature absorptive cells are **tall columnar cells** that are bound to one another and to interspersed goblet and enteroendocrine cells by **junctional complexes** located at the apical end of the intercellular space (see Figure 5-2).
            (1) The junctional complex consists of a tight junction, a zonula adherens, and one or more desmosomes.
            (2) The junction establishes a **barrier** between the intestinal lumen and intercellu-

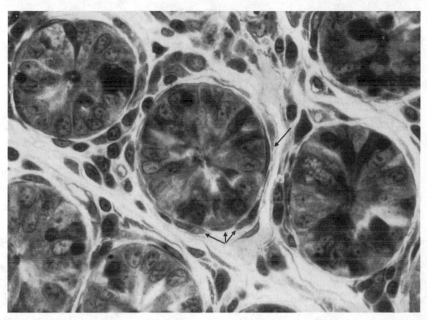

FIGURE 25-4. Jejunal crypts, cross-section, light micrograph. Pericryptal fibroblasts (*arrows*) are visible immediately deep to the epithelial basement membrane. Numerous mature goblet cells are visible interspersed among differentiating intermediate and absorptive cells. Note that in histologic sections of the crypt portion of the intestinal mucosa, the lamina propria surrounds the epithelial layer, rather than the epithelial layer surrounding the lamina propria, as in the villi (see Figure 25-2).

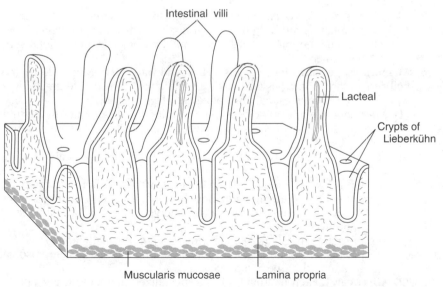

FIGURE 25-5. Crypts (mucosal glands) and villi of the mucosa of the small intestine. The epithelium forms a continuous sheet covering the villi and the crypts. Villi extend into the lumen from the surface, and crypts invaginate into the lamina propria. The muscularis mucosae is the deepest part of the mucosa and forms the boundary between the mucosa and the submucosa.

lar compartment of the epithelium. It also establishes two domains in the absorptive cell membrane, an **apical domain** and a **basolateral domain.**

   b. Absorption pathway. Substrates that enter across the apical cell surface must travel intracellularly to the lateral plasma membrane, where various transport mechanisms transfer the substrates across the lateral membrane into the intercellular space (see Figure 26-8).

     (1) Substances from the intercellular space diffuse across the basal lamina and enter the fenestrated capillaries immediately beneath.

     (2) Substances too large to enter the blood capillaries (e.g., lipoprotein particles, large proteins) diffuse to and enter the lymphatic lacteal.

     (3) Although most of the materials absorbed by the intestinal epithelial cells are for use by the rest of the body, the intestinal epithelial cells derive most of their own nutrition from the material that passes through them.

   c. Absorption mechanism. Transepithelial transport in the intestine is driven by **transport enzymes** called **pumps,** which are located in the lateral plasma membrane.

     (1) The principal membrane pump is **Na$^+$,K$^+$-ATPase,** the sodium pump enzyme.

       (a) This pump actively transports Na$^+$ ions from the cytoplasm to the lateral intercellular space, transiently lowering the cytoplasmic concentration of this ion.

         (i) Water follows the actively transported ions from the cell into the intercellular space so that a nearly isotonic solution eventually diffuses across the basal lamina to the fenestrated capillaries.

         (ii) Sodium and water cross the apical plasma membrane from the intestinal lumen, diffusing down their concentration gradients through membrane channels to replenish the sodium and water removed from the cytoplasm by the action of the pump.

       (b) The action of this pump drives absorption of many other molecules.

     (2) The **zonulae occludentes** of the junctional complexes participate in the absorption mechanism in two ways:

       (a) They seal the lateral intercellular space from the lumen of the intestine, ensuring that materials absorbed from the lumen pass through the cell, and preventing back-diffusion of transported materials from the intercellular space.

       (b) The zonulae occludentes restrict transport enzymes to the lateral plasma membrane, allowing the establishment of osmotic gradients between the cell and the intercellular space, and between the intercellular space and the lumen.

   d. Membrane specializations for absorption and transport. Microvilli on the apical cell surface and plications (i.e., folds) of the lateral cell surface greatly increase the surface area of the intestinal absorptive cell (Figure 25-6).

     (1) Microvilli. Up to 3000 closely packed microvilli are found on the luminal surface of each absorptive cell, **increasing the apical surface area** as much as 600 times.

       (a) Each microvillus on a typical jejunal absorptive cell is about 1.4 μm tall and 0.08 μm in diameter .

       (b) It has a vertical core of **actin microfilaments** anchored to the plasma membrane both at the tip and along the shaft. The actin filaments extend into the apical cytoplasm, where they merge with the actin filaments of the **terminal web.**

       (c) In routine histologic sections, microvilli collectively appear as a layer projecting from the apical surface forming a **brush border,** also called a striate border (see Figure 25-2).

     (2) Glycocalyx. Each microvillus has a specialized filamentous glycoprotein coat called a glycocalyx, which increases the surface available for **adsorption, binding,** and **digestion.**

       (a) The glycocalyx may measure as much as 0.5 μm thick at the tip of the microvillus (see Figures 21-2, 25-6).

       (b) The filamentous extensions of the glycocalyx from the plasma membrane contain several important digestive enzymes.

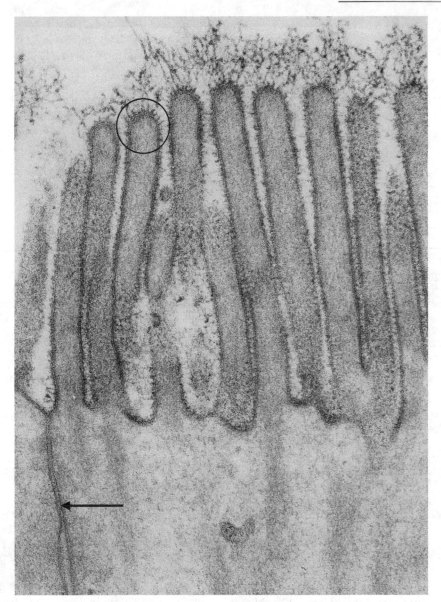

FIGURE 25-6. Microvilli of an intestinal absorptive cell, electron micrograph. At this level of resolution, the actin microfilament core of the microvilli, the trilaminar structure of the cell membrane, and the close relationship of the glycocalyx to the outer leaflet of the cell membrane (*circle*) are well shown, as is the occlusion of the intercellular space by a tight junction (*arrow*).

    (i) Disaccharidases and dipeptidases produce monosaccharides and amino acids that can then be absorbed by the cell. For example, lack of the disaccharidase lactase prevents breakdown of lactose to galactose and glucose, producing the clinical condition of lactose intolerance.

    (ii) Enterokinase is essential for the conversion of the inactive forms of pancreatic enzymes trypsinogen and chymotrypsinogen to trypsin and chymotrypsin.

(3) Lateral plications. The lateral surface of an intestinal absorptive cell shows extensive development of flattened processes, or plications, that interleave with processes of adjacent cells (Figure 25-7).

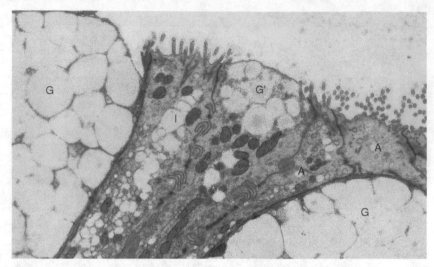

FIGURE 25-7. Human intestinal epithelium, middle portion of crypt. The large mucinogen droplets of two goblet cells (*G*) surround the apical portions of a developing goblet cell (*G*^{1}), *an intermediate cell (I)*, and two developing absorptive cells (*A*). Note the complex plications developing at the lateral margins between these cells, as well as the long actin microfilaments of the cores of the developing microvilli. Numerous desmosomes are visible between the differentiating cells.

        (a) This greatly increases the amount of lateral plasma membrane that contains transport enzymes.

        (b) The plications separate during active transport—especially transport of electrolytes, water, and lipids—allowing the development of an enlarged intercellular compartment that is often visible in living tissue examined by phase-contrast microscopy.

        (c) The hydrostatic pressure that develops as electrolytes and water accumulate in the intercellular space helps create a directional flow of fluid through the basal lamina toward the subepithelial capillaries.

  e. Cytoplasmic specializations for absorption and transport

    (1) Longitudinally oriented mitochondria are concentrated between the terminal web and the centrally located nucleus to provide energy for the membrane pumps in the apical portion of the lateral plasma membrane.

      (a) Vertically aligned stacks of Golgi cisternae are located in the central portion of the supranuclear cytoplasm.

      (b) Small apical secretory vesicles derived from the Golgi contain the glycoprotein enzymes destined for the plasma membrane of the microvilli.

    (2) Tubules and cisternae of smooth endoplasmic reticulum associated with the absorption of fatty acids and glycerol and the resynthesis of neutral fat are concentrated just beneath the terminal web.

    (3) Rough endoplasmic reticulum and free ribosomes are also concentrated in the supranuclear cytoplasm, lateral to the centrally located Golgi apparatus.

  f. Secretory functions of absorptive cells. Intestinal absorptive cells have significant secretory functions, evidenced by the synthesis of the digestive enzymes of the glycocalyx and the transport enzymes of the lateral plasma membrane.

2. Goblet cells. These are unicellular glands that secrete mucin (see Figure 25-4). They are present at all levels of the crypt and villus above the level of the replicative zone.

  a. Goblet cells increase in frequency from the proximal to the distal small intestine, and are most numerous in the terminal ileum.

  b. Goblet cells are characterized by the presence of a **large accumulation of mucinogen secretory droplets** in the apical cytoplasm.

    (1) The mucinogen droplets **distend the apex of the cell** and distort neighboring cells.

    (2) The nucleus and other cytoplasmic organelles are compressed into the narrower basal cytoplasm.

    (3) A large, cup-shaped array of flattened Golgi saccules surrounds the base of the accumulation of mucinogen droplets, immediately beneath the newly formed ones.

    (4) The basal cytoplasm is filled with rough endoplasmic reticulum and free ribosomes. This, along with the basally compressed heterochromatic nucleus, gives this region of the cell its characteristic intense basophilia.

  c. Microvilli are restricted to the apical membrane of the **thin rim of cytoplasm,** the **theca,** that surrounds the accumulated mucinogen droplets.

3. Enteroendocrine cells. The enteroendocrine cells are part of the **gastroenteropancreatic (GEP) system** (see Chapter 24 III A 4 e) and secrete hormones and regulatory peptides into the lamina propria between the base of the epithelium and the subepithelial absorptive capillaries.

  a. Although they are concentrated in the lower portion of the crypt, they migrate to all levels of the villus and, ultimately, are shed into the lumen (Figure 25-8).

  b. They secrete nearly all of the same peptide hormones as do enteroendocrine cells in the stomach.

    (1) Cholecystokinin (CCK), **secretin,** and **gastric inhibitory peptide** (GIP) are the most active regulators of gastrointestinal physiology and digestive function that are secreted by the enteroendocrine cells of the small intestine.

      (a) CCK stimulates both growth and secretory activity of the exocrine pancreas and contraction of the gallbladder, but inhibits gastric emptying.

      (b) Secretin stimulates pancreatic growth and secretion.

      (c) GIP inhibits gastric acid secretion but stimulates insulin release by the endocrine pancreas.

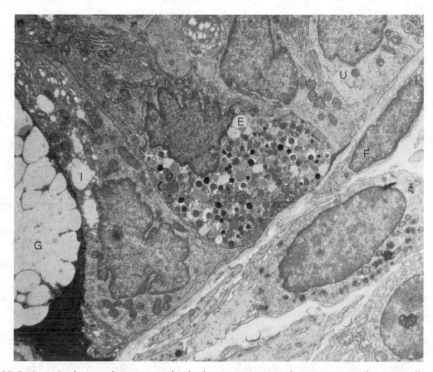

FIGURE 25-8. Intestinal crypt, lowest one-third, electron micrograph. An enteroendocrine cell (*E*) is visible in the middle of the field. Its dense secretory vesicles are concentrated in the basal portion of the cell. The variation in size and density of the vesicles suggests that this enteroendocrine cell is secreting several products. A pericryptal fibroblast (*F*) is visible immediately beneath the epithelial basal lamina. *G* = goblet cell, *I* = intermediate cell, *U* = undifferentiated cell.

(2) **Vasoactive inhibitory peptide** (VIP), **pancreatic polypeptide, motilin, entero-glucagon,** and **somatostatin** are among other peptides secreted by intestinal enteroendocrine cells that regulate digestive functions and other metabolic activities.

4. **Paneth cells.** Paneth cells are found in the bases of the crypts in the small intestine and, rarely, in the normal colon. Their number may increase in both sites under certain pathologic conditions.
   a. Paneth cells appear as typical serous cells, with a basophilic basal cytoplasm and intensely acidophilic zymogen granules.
      (1) The granules contain the **bactericidal enzyme lysozyme,** an **arginine-rich protein,** and **zinc.**
      (2) The cationic nature of the lysozyme and the arginine-rich protein are probably responsible for the intense acidophilia.
   b. Because secreted lysozyme digests the cell walls of certain bacteria in the lumen, and because Paneth cells are reported to phagocytize other bacteria and protozoa, it is believed that they play a role in regulating the normal bacterial flora of the small intestine.

5. **Microfold cells (M cells).** M cells are the epithelial antigen-transporting cells that cover accumulations of large lymphatic nodules, such as the Peyer patches of the ileum, that fill and distort the lamina propria.
   a. They are nearly squamous and have **microfolds** on their luminal surface, rather than microvilli.
   b. They take up macromolecules from the lumen in endocytic vesicles. The vesicles are transported across the cell, where they fuse and empty into the intercellular space.
      (1) The macromolecules are discharged in the vicinity of intercellular lymphocytes. These lymphocytes are the first line of cellular defense for the immune system.
      (2) Antigens that reach lymphocytes in this manner stimulate a response in the GALT (see I E).

6. **Intermediate cells.** Intermediate cells are immature cells, still capable of dividing. They have morphologic characteristics intermediate between those of developing goblet cells and developing absorptive cells (see Figure 25-7).
   a. Intermediate cells constitute the majority of cells in the lower one-half of the crypt.
      (1) They have short, irregular microvilli with long core filaments that extend deep into the cytoplasm.
      (2) They exhibit numerous desmosomal junctions with adjacent cells.
      (3) Small, mucin-like droplets form a vertical column in the center of the apical cytoplasm.
   b. Intermediate cells that are **committed to becoming goblet cells** develop a small, rounded aggregation of secretory droplets just under the apical plasma membrane.
   c. Intermediate cells that are **committed to becoming absorptive cells** lose the secretory droplets and develop concentrations of mitochondria, rough endoplasmic reticulum, and ribosomes in the apical cytoplasm.
   d. Intestinal tumors have many cells with the characteristics of intermediate cells. This can be an aid in identifying the origin of a metastatic lesion.

7. **Stem cells.** The stem cell population of the small intestine and colon is located in the bottom of the crypts. As in the stomach (see Chapter 24 II C 2 b), all the cells of the intestinal epithelium are derived from a **single stem cell population.**
   a. Stem cells are the most difficult of intestinal epithelial cells to recognize solely on the basis of morphologic characteristics. They have few organelles, little development of microvilli, and numerous desmosomes, but these characteristics do not distinguish them from most intermediate cells.
   b. The most reliable way to identify stem cells is to expose the intestine, in vivo or in vitro, to a pulse of tritiated thymidine.
      (1) This will label both stem cells and intermediate cells.

(2) Those cells that remain heavily labeled in the deepest part of the crypt 3 weeks after labeling are the stem cells.

D. **Epethelial cell renewal.** Cell replication is restricted to the lower one-half of the crypt.

1. **Initial division.** Stem cells divide to give rise to one daughter cell that will differentiate, and one that will remain in the stem cell pool.

2. **Additional divisions.** A cell that will differentiate into a goblet or absorptive cell undergoes two additional divisions as an intermediate cell after it originates as the daughter cell of a dividing stem cell.

3. **Epithelial cell migration.** Nearly all of the epithelial cells migrate from the crypt onto the villus and are shed from the tip of the villus.
   a. The turnover time for **absorptive cells** and **goblet cells** in the human small intestine is **5–6 days.** Virtually the entire epithelial lining of the small intestine is renewed in less than a week.
   b. **Enteroendocrine cells** also migrate, but appear to **turn over more slowly.** They normally undergo only one additional division after leaving the stem cell pool.
   c. **Paneth cells do not migrate,** nor do they divide again after arising from a stem cell.
      (1) Paneth cells have a turnover time of about 4 weeks.
      (2) When they die, they are replaced by differentiation of a nearby committed cell.

E. **Gut-associated lymphatic tissue (GALT).** The lamina propria throughout the length of the digestive tract is heavily populated with cells of the immune system.

1. **Cells and organization.** About one-fourth of the mucosa consists of lymphatic tissue, loosely organized as a zone of lymphocytes, lymphatic nodules, plasma cells, macrophages, and eosinophils in the lamina propria.
   a. Lymphocytes are also commonly insinuated in the intercellular space of the epithelium at all levels of the digestive tract.
   b. Mast cells are present in the lamina propria and interact with the immune cells.

2. **Functions.** In cooperation with the epithelial cells, the cells of the GALT sample the antigens in the intercellular space, process antigens, and synthesize several classes of antibodies. They also participate in **immune exclusion.**
   a. **Intraepithelial barrier.** Intraepithelial lymphocytes are the front-line elements of the immunologic barrier to antigens crossing the mucosa. Lymphocytes recognize antigens and process them, then migrate to lymph nodules in the lamina propria to **stimulate blastic transformation** and **antibody production** (see Chapter 15).
   b. **Immunoglobulin production.** Most of the plasma cells of the lamina propria synthesize dimeric immunoglobulin A (IgA), and others synthesize IgM and IgE.
      (1) Absorptive cells take up IgA from the lamina propria and re-secrete it by exocytosis as secretory IgA (sIgA). In the lumen of the intestine, sIgA binds to antigens, microorganisms, and toxins in the process of **immune exclusion** (see Chapter 21 III A 2 d).
      (2) IgM is also found in the intestinal lumen, and is believed to be secreted by the intestinal epithelial cells by a process similar to that for IgA.
      (3) Some of the IgE binds to the plasma membrane of mast cells in the lamina propria, sensitizing them to antigens that may reach them by absorption from the lumen.

F. **Submucosa, muscularis externa, and serosa**

1. **Submucosa** (see Chapter 21 II B). This dense connective tissue layer is distinguished in the **duodenum** by the presence of **Brunner glands,** which are branched tubuloalveolar submucosal glands (see I A 1 b). The duodenum is the only portion of the small intestine or colon in which submucosal glands are found.
   a. The secretory cells of these glands have characteristics of both mucus-secreting cells and zymogen-secreting cells.

    b. The secretion has a pH of 8.1 to 9.3 and contains neutral and alkaline glycoproteins and bicarbonate ions.

2. Muscularis externa (see Chapter 21 II C). The muscularis externa consists of two distinct, well-developed smooth muscle layers, an **inner circular layer** and an **outer longitudinal layer.**

    a. Local **contractions of the circular layer,** called **segmentation,** displace the intestinal contents both distally and proximally.

        (1) This action circulates the chyme locally and mixes it with the digestive enzymes.

        (2) It also moves the chyme into contact with the luminal surface of the epithelial cells for terminal digestion and absorption.

    b. Slower **contractions of the longitudinal layer,** called **peristalsis,** move the intestinal contents distally.

3. Serosa (see Chapter 21 II D). The serosa covers those parts of the small intestine that are free in the abdominal cavity. **Adventitia** covers those parts that are fixed to the abdominal wall (i.e., retroperitoneal).

II. **COLON.** The principal functions of the colon are the **reabsorption** of salt and water and the **elimination** of undigested foodstuffs and other wastes. The four layers characteristic of the alimentary canal (see Chapter 21 II, Figure 21-1) are present from the ileocecal junction to the rectoanal margin, although some unique features typify the colon (Figure 25-9).

A. **Anatomic segments.** The colon (large intestine) consists, in order along its length, of the cecum and appendix, ascending colon, transverse colon, descending colon, sigmoid colon, rectum, and anal canal. The segments at both ends of the colon differ somewhat from the rest of the colon.

1. Cecum and appendix. The cecum is a blind pouch just distal to the ileocecal valve. The appendix is a thin, finger-like extension from the cecum.

    a. Cecum. The cecum is the first portion of the large intestine and its structure closely resembles that of the rest of the colon.

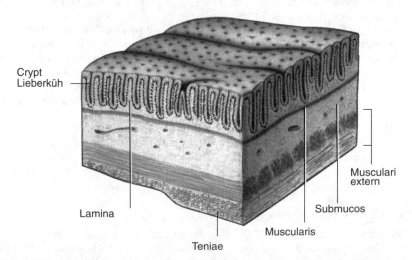

FIGURE 25-9. Colon, schematic representation. The smooth luminal surface appears as it would in a scanning electron micrograph. Simple, finger-like mucosal glands (crypts of Lieberkühn) invaginate from the free surface. The outer (longitudinal) layer of the muscularis externa is condensed into three broad bands of muscle, the teniae coli; part of one is illustrated here.

b. Appendix (see Chapter 16 IV). The appendix is characterized by a profusion of lymphatic nodules that often fuse and obscure the lamina propria and extend into the submucosa.

    (1) In many adults, the normal structure of the appendix is lost and the appendage is filled with scar tissue.

    (2) The appendix differs from the rest of the colon in having a uniform layer of longitudinal muscle in the muscularis externa. The teniae coli of the cecum converge at the base of the appendix.

2. Rectum and anal canal. The rectum is the dilated distal portion of the colon and is approximately 12 cm in length. The anal canal is the most distal portion of the alimentary canal and extends approximately 4 cm from the rectoanal junction to the anus.

    a. Rectum. The **upper rectum** is distinguished from the rest of the colon by the presence of semilunar folds called **transverse rectal folds.** The **lower rectum,** which is part of the anal canal, has longitudinal folds called **anal columns** that alternate with depressions called **anal sinuses.**

        (1) The mucosa of the rectum has straight tubular crypts with many goblet cells.

        (2) The longitudinal muscle layer forms a uniform sheet in the rectum. There are no teniae coli.

    b. Anal canal. The anal canal is usually defined as the distal rectum and the short, terminal, nonglandular segment of the alimentary tract that leads to the **anal orifice,** or **anus.**

        (1) In the upper portion of the anal canal, straight tubular **rectal glands** (colonic glands) secrete mucus onto the anal surface.

        (2) The lower portion of the anal canal is characerized by large, apocrine **circumanal glands.**

            (a) In many animals, the secretion of these glands acts as a sex attractant (pheromone).

            (b) At about 2 cm above the anus the epithelial lining abruptly changes from a simple columnar epithelium to a nonkeratinized stratified squamous epithelium that is continuous with that of the skin of the perineum.

            (c) Hair follicles and sebaceous glands underlie the lower portion of the anal canal.

        (3) The muscularis mucosae disappears at about the level of the rectoanal margin.

            (a) The circular layer of the muscularis externa thickens to form the internal anal sphincter.

            (b) Striated muscles of the perineum form the external anal sphincter.

B. Mucosa. The mucosa of the colon consists of a simple columnar epithelium organized into straight tubular glands that extend through the full thickness of the mucosa (Figure 25-10). The mucosal surface is flat throughout; **plicae and villi are absent.** It has a highly cellular lamina propria with a well-developed GALT.

1. Columnar epithelium. The epithelium of the large intestine contains the same cell types as that of the small intestine, although Paneth cells are not usually present.

    a. Absorptive cells predominate over goblet cells at a 4:1 ratio in most of the colon.

        (1) This distribution is not always apparent in routine histologic sections in which the margins of the more numerous but narrower absorptive cells may not be clearly visible.

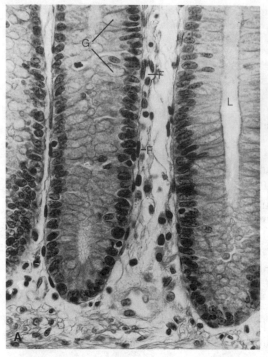
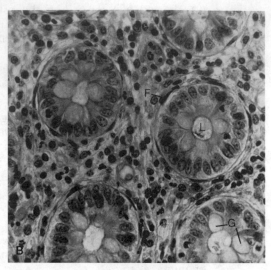

FIGURE 25-10. Colonic glands. (*A*) sagittal section; (*B*) cross-section. The tightly appliqued fibroblasts (*F*) of the pericryptal sheath are distinct from the other loosely arrayed elements of the lamina propria. The pericryptal fibroblast is a flattened cell, with the shape of a fried egg, that conforms to the contours of the intestinal crypt. *L* = lumen; *G* = goblet cells.

    (2) The ratio decreases, approaching 1:1, as goblet cells become more numerous near the rectum.

    (3) The absorptive cells are morphologically identical with those of the small intestine, having well-developed microvilli and lateral plications.

      (a) Na^+,K^+-**ATPase** is abundant in the lateral plasma membrane.

      (b) The **intercellular space** is usually dilated, indicative of active transport of fluids.

      (c) The **glycocalyx** of the microvilli is morphologically prominent. It has a rapid turnover, with membrane glycoproteins being shed and replaced every 16 to 24 hours. However, it lacks the digestive enzymes that characterize the glycocalyx in the small intestine.

  b. **Goblet cells** in the colon may differentiate deep in the crypts, even as deep as the replicative zone (Figure 25-11).

    (1) They secrete mucus continuously to lubricate the passage of waste materials along the colon.

    (2) At the luminal surface, the secretion rate of mucin often exceeds the synthetic rate, and cells with the appearance of exhausted goblet cells are frequently seen.

    (3) The infrequently observed **caveolated cell** (tuft cell) may be a form of exhausted goblet cell in which the microvilli are prominent.

  c. **Enteroendocrine cells** are present at all levels of the crypt and at the free surface.

 2. **Epithelial cell renewal.** The cell renewal pattern in the colon closely resembles that of the small intestine (see I D).

  a. All of the epithelial cells arise from a **single stem cell population** in the bottom of the crypts.

  b. The **zone of replication** is restricted to the **lowest one-third of the crypt,** with some goblet cells reaching full maturation there.

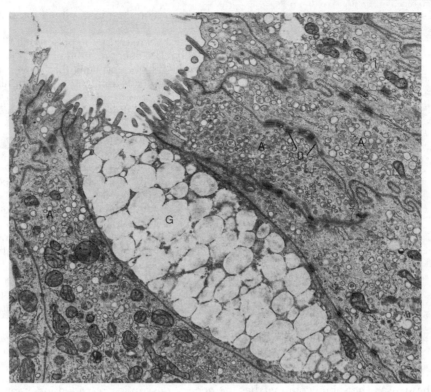

FIGURE 25-11. Colon, lowest one-third of crypt. A mature goblet cell (*G*) is surrounded by intermediate cells (*I*) and immature absorptive cells (*A*) with developing microvilli and numerous prominent desmosomes (*D*). Microvilli are also visible on the apical surface of the goblet cell.

    (1) Newly generated cells destined to become absorptive cells and goblet cells undergo 2 to 3 more divisions as they pass through the replicative zone on their migration to the luminal surface.

    (2) Absorptive and goblet cells have a turnover time of 5 to 6 days and are shed into the lumen at the midpoint between two adjacent crypts.

    (3) Enteroendocrine cells probably divide only once after arising from a stem cell. They turn over in 3 to 4 weeks.

3. Lamina propria. The lamina propria is a loose, highly cellular connective tissue layer similar to that of the rest of the digestive tract; there are, however, some significant differences.

    a. GALT. Lymphatic tissue is a prominent feature of the lamina propria throughout the length of the colon.

        (1) Large lymphatic nodules often distort the regular spacing of the crypts and cross the muscularis mucosae into the submucosa.

        (2) The extent of the immune barrier in the colon probably reflects the large numbers and variety of microorganisms present, as well as the noxious end-products of metabolism and cell breakdown normally found in the lumen.

    b. Absence of lymphatic vessels. Despite the extensive development of the GALT, there are no lymphatic vessels in the lamina propria of the colon.

        (1) Lymphatic vessels form a network around the muscularis mucosae, but no vessels extend toward the free surface in the lamina propria.

        (2) Thus, cancers that develop in the epithelium of large colonic polyps may grow quite large before they reach the level of the muscularis mucosae, where metastases may enter the lymphatic circulation.

    c. Pericryptal fibroblast sheath. The pericryptal fibroblast sheath is more easily recognized and more highly developed in the colon than in the small intestine (see Figure 25-10).

(1) The fine collagen fibers (reticular fibers) secreted by the pericryptal fibroblasts form the reticular layer of the epithelial basement membrane.

(2) The reticular fibers are arranged in a tightly wound helix that reflects the helical migration pattern of both the epithelial cells and the pericryptal fibroblasts.

(3) Under the free surface, these reticular fibers form a layer up to 5 μm thick between the basal lamina of the epithelium and the basal lamina of underlying fenestrated capillaries.

   (a) This thick layer is called the **collagen table.** It is secreted and maintained by the mature fibroblasts that have migrated to this level.

   (b) Variations in the degree of macromolecular organization of the proteoglycans in this layer may help to regulate the flow of transported electrolytes and water from the intercellular space to the blood capillaries.

(4) The pericryptal fibroblasts at all levels of the crypt and free surface retain some degree of morphologic apposition to the epithelial basal lamina.

   (a) Near the base of the crypt there is little secreted collagen and most of the superficial (adepithelial) surface of the fibroblast is in contact with the basal lamina.

   (b) As collagen is secreted, the body of the cell is pushed further from the basal lamina, but large processes retain extensive areas of contact with it.

   (c) Even under the free surface, the fibroblasts extend processes through the thick collagen table to make contact with the basal lamina.

(5) The fate of pericryptal fibroblasts is still unclear, although most of the cells associated with the collagen table take on the morphologic and histochemical characteristics of tissue macrophages (i.e., histiocytes).

C. **Submucosa.** The submucosa matches the general description provided in Chapter 21 II B.

D. **Muscularis externa.** The outer longitudinal layer of the muscularis externa is mostly compressed into three thick bands, the **teniae coli,** that are equally spaced around the circumference and are visible grossly. Between the teniae coli, the outer layer of longitudinal muscle is thin but continuous.

1. **Segmentation and haustra.** Bundles of muscle from the teniae coli penetrate the inner circular layer at intervals along the length and circumference of the colon.
   a. Contraction of these bundles leads to the formation of **sacculations,** called **haustra,** in the colon wall.
   b. These partial discontinuities along the length of the teniae coli allow segments of the colon to contract independently. This may expose more of the contents to the epithelial surface for absorption of water and electrolytes.

2. Contraction of long segments of the teniae coli produces massive peristaltic movements that move the colonic contents distally. Such mass peristaltic movements in the distal colon occur only once or twice a day in a healthy human in order to empty the sigmoid colon.

E. **Serosa.** The portions of the large intestine that are free in the abdominal cavity have a typical **serosa** as the outermost layer (see Chapter 21 II D 1). Where the large intestine is in direct contact with other structures, such as the posterior wall of the abdominal cavity, its outermost layer is **adventitia.**

Chapter 26

Liver and Gallbladder

I. **INTRODUCTION.** The hepatocystic system consists of the liver and the gallbladder.

    A. **Liver.** The liver is the largest internal organ in the body and the largest mass of gland tissue.

        1. It is both an **endocrine** and an **exocrine** organ. It is essential to the processes of **digestion** and **metabolism, detoxification** and **recycling,** and **homeostasis.**

        2. It is unique among the organs in that its **major blood supply is venous blood** from the intestine, pancreas, and spleen.

    B. **Gallbladder.** The gallbladder stores and concentrates the bile secretions of the liver.

II. **GENERAL STRUCTURE OF THE LIVER**

    A. **Parenchyma.** Liver parenchyma consists of anastomosing plates of epithelial cells called **hepatocytes.**

    B. **Stroma.** The liver is covered with a thin connective tissue capsule called the Glisson capsule. Blood vessels, nerves, lymphatic vessels, and bile ducts travel within loose connective tissue that is continuous with the capsule.

    C. **Sinusoids.** The plates of hepatocytes are separated by a system of sinusoidal capillaries.

    D. **Perisinusoidal space.** The perisinusoidal space (space of Disse) lies between the sinusoidal endothelium and the hepatocytes.

        1. It is the site at which nutrients and wastes are exchanged between the blood and the cells.

        2. The perisinusoidal space is also the site at which the endocrine secretions of the liver cells are delivered to the blood.

III. **HEPATIC CIRCULATION**

    A. **Blood supply.** The liver has a dual blood supply consisting of a venous (portal) supply and an arterial supply (Figure 26-1).

        1. **Hepatic portal vein.** The portal vein carries about 75% of the blood supply of the liver. In addition to normal blood cells, the following substances are carried to the liver in the portal blood:
            a. Nutrients and noxious substances absorbed across the intestinal epithelium
            b. Breakdown products of blood cells from the spleen
            c. Endocrine secretions of the pancreatic islets

        2. **Hepatic artery.** The hepatic artery is a branch of the celiac trunk.
            a. The hepatic artery carries oxygenated blood and supplies about 25% of the blood supply to the liver.
            b. Blood from the hepatic artery and the portal vein mixes in the sinusoids that

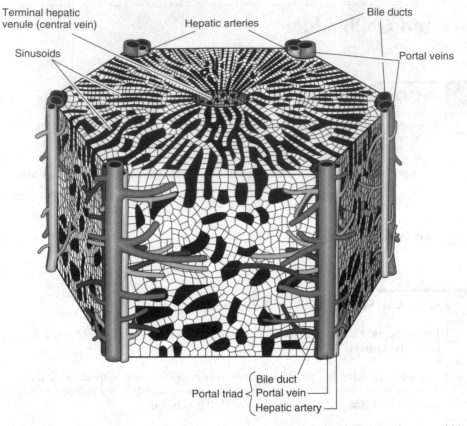

Terminal hepatic venule (central vein)   Hepatic arteries   Bile ducts

Sinusoids   Portal veins

Bile duct
Portal triad { Portal vein
Hepatic artery

FIGURE 26-1. Three-dimensional representation of the classic liver lobule, shown as a hexagonal block of tissue with the terminal hepatic venule (central vein) as its axis and the portal triads at each of the six corners. The hepatocytes are shown as radiating plates of cells separated by radiating venous sinusoids. Distributing branches of the portal vein and hepatic artery that extend along the sides of the tissue block between the portal areas empty into the sinusoids that perfuse the hepatocytes. (Adapted from Ross MH, Romrell LJ, Kaye GI: *Histology: A Text and Atlas,* 3rd ed. Baltimore, Williams & Wilkins, 1995, p 498.)

perfuse the liver parenchyma. Hepatocytes are, therefore, never exposed to fully oxygenated blood.

3. Distribution of vessels. Both the portal vein and the hepatic artery enter the liver at a hilum called the **porta hepatis.** The common hepatic duct (see VII C 1), which carries the exocrine secretions of the liver, leaves the gland at the same site.

  a. Distributing vessels. The distributing branches of the portal vein and hepatic artery travel together in the liver stroma, along with the draining branches of the bile duct system that lead to the common hepatic duct.

  b. Portal triads. Portal triads are morphologic landmarks that consist of the preterminal branches of the portal vein and hepatic artery, the smallest collecting duct of the biliary duct system, and one or more lymphatic vessels, encased in a connective tissue sheath. The term *portal triad* is a misnomer because the lymphatic vessels constitute a fourth element.

  c. Sinusoids. The terminal branches of the portal vein and the hepatic artery both drain into the sinusoids.

B. **Sinusoidal circulation.** The finest branches of the portal vein and hepatic artery drain into the sinusoids, which are the extensive capillary bed of the organ.

  1. Inlet venules. Fine vessels branch from the terminal branches of the portal vein and penetrate the periphery of the classic lobule, to lead into the sinusoids.

  2. Arterioles. Fine arterioles derived from terminal branches of the hepatic artery empty directly into the inlet venules. Other fine arterioles give rise to capillaries that supply the structures in the connective tissue of the portal area before draining into the inlet venules.

3. **Sinusoidal endothelium.** Hepatic sinusoids are lined with a **thin discontinuous endothelium.** Only a few discontinuous elements of basal lamina material underlie the endothelial cells.

    a. **Fenestrae and gaps.** The discontinuity of the endothelial layer is due to large fenestrae, without diaphragms, in the endothelial cells and to the presence of large gaps between neighboring endothelial cells.

    b. **Kupffer cells.** A second cell type, the **stellate sinusoidal macrophage** or Kupffer cell, is also a regular part of the vessel lining and usually resides in the gaps between endothelial cells.

        (1) Kupffer cells are part of the mononuclear phagocytic system and, like most cells of this system, are derived from monocytes that originate in the bone marrow.

        (2) Kupffer cells do not form junctions with adjacent endothelial cells.

        (3) Processes of Kupffer cells may overlie portions of the endothelium or may even span the sinusoidal lumen and partially occlude it.

            (a) Kupffer cells probably phagocytize and break down damaged or senile red blood cells that have not been captured by the macrophages of the spleen.

            (b) After splenectomy, this function increases and becomes essential.

C. Venous drainage

1. **Drainage pathway**

    a. **Terminal hepatic venules.** The sinusoids drain to terminal hepatic venules, or central veins, in the parenchyma.

        (1) The terminal hepatic venules have numerous pores in their thin walls.

        (2) The sinusoids empty through these pores into the systemic circulation.

    b. **Sublobular veins.** The terminal hepatic venules connect to sublobular veins that run at right angles to the venules.

        (1) The sublobular veins have a well-developed tunica adventitia containing both collagen and elastic fibers.

        (2) Because there is no tunica media, this layer is just external to the endothelium.

    c. **Collecting veins.** Sublobular veins run in the connective tissue trabeculae (when they exist) and join to form collecting veins.

        (1) Collecting veins, in turn, join to form the larger **hepatic veins** that empty into the **inferior vena cava.**

        (2) The hepatic veins **lack valves** but do have a relatively well-developed tunica media.

2. **Unaccompanied vessels.** The sublobular veins, collecting veins, and hepatic veins travel alone. Thus, they can readily be distinguished from the hepatic portal veins that travel with the other elements of the portal triad.

D. Lymph circulation. Plasma that does not return to the sinusoid from the perisinusoidal space drains to the periportal connective tissue, thus becoming lymph.

1. The plasma that drains from the perisinusoidal space to the periportal area flows first into the **space of Mall,** a small space between the stroma of the portal canal and the outermost hepatocytes of the classic lobule.

2. The fluid then enters lymphatic capillaries that travel with the other elements of the portal triad.

3. The lymph flows into progressively larger vessels that eventually leave the liver at the porta hepatis and ultimately drain into the thoracic duct.

    a. About 80% of the lymph that originates in the liver follows this pathway, constituting the major portion of the thoracic duct lymph.

b. The remaining hepatic lymph drains into lymphatic networks that accompany the large hepatic veins.

IV. ORGANIZATION OF LIVER PARENCHYMA.

Three models of microscopic units of structure of the liver parenchyma have been devised in order to relate the major functional activities of the liver to its structure. These are the **classic lobule,** the **portal lobule,** and the **liver acinus** (Figure 26-2).

A. **Classic lobule.** The classic lobule is the traditional description of the organization of the parenchyma. It is defined by the peripheral distribution of the penultimate branches of the portal vein and hepatic artery, by the central location of a terminal hepatic venule, and by the radial distribution of sinusoids between the plates of cells.

1. **Lobule shape.** The classic lobule is a roughly **hexagonal block of tissue** (see Figure 26-1), measuring about 2.0 mm by 0.7 mm, that contains radially arranged **anastomosing plates of hepatocytes** separated by an **anastomosing system of sinusoids.**

2. **Lobule axis.** At the **center** of the lobule is a **terminal hepatic venule,** hence the common name, **central vein.**

3. **Lobule boundary.** The corners of the hexagon are the **portal areas** containing the **portal triads** (see III A 3 b).

4. **Blood and bile flow.** In the classic lobule, the **flow of blood is centripetal,** from the portal areas at the periphery of the lobule toward the central vein. The **flow of bile and lymph is centrifugal,** from the center of the classic lobule toward the portal areas.

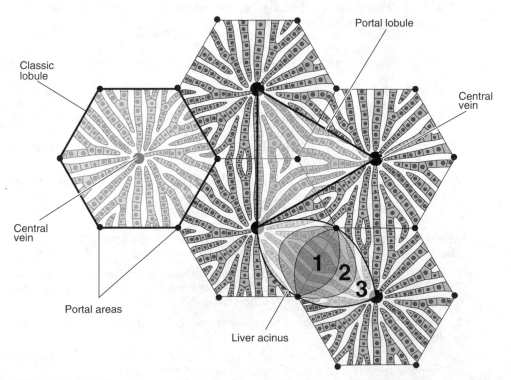

FIGURE 26-2. Schematic representations of the three models of the organization of hepatic tissue superimposed on the liver parenchyma. *Numerals* indicate acinar zones.

5. **Connective tissue.** In some species (e.g., the pig) the classic lobule is more readily seen because a relatively thick layer of connective tissue stretches between each portal area, surrounding the finest branches of the vessels and bile ducts. In humans, however, lobules are poorly defined because there is very little connective tissue between portal areas.

B. **Portal lobule.** This model emphasizes the exocrine functions of the liver. The axis of a portal lobule is the bile duct of the portal triad. This allows description of the hepatic parenchyma in terms comparable to those used to describe other exocrine glands, which are characterized by the presence of ducts.

1. **Lobule shape, axis, boundary.** The portal lobule is a roughly **triangular block of tissue** with a portal triad at its center. Its margins consist of imaginary lines drawn between the three terminal hepatic venules that are closest to that portal triad.

2. **Comparison with classic lobule.** A portal lobule includes those portions of three classic lobules that secrete the bile that drains to its axial bile duct.

C. **Liver acinus.** The concept of the liver acinus was introduced to correlate the blood perfusion of the parenchyma with metabolic activity of hepatocytes and hepatic pathology.

1. **Acinar shape.** The liver acinus is the smallest functional unit in the hepatic parenchyma. It is **diamond shaped** or lozenge shaped.

2. **Acinar axes.** The **short axis** of the acinus is defined by the terminal branches of two hepatic portal veins and two hepatic arteries that extend into the parenchyma from adjacent portal triads. The **long axis** is a line drawn between the two terminal hepatic venules closest to the short axis.

3. **Significance of liver acinus.** The acinar model allows correlation between blood perfusion and gradients of metabolic activity in the parenchyma.
   a. The liver acinus also allows interpretation of patterns of degeneration, regeneration, and specific toxic effects relative to the degree or quality of vascular perfusion of the hepatocytes.
   b. Because the smallest branches of the bile ducts are in the short axis, this concept also allows description of the exocrine functions of the liver in terms comparable to those used for other exocrine glands.

4. **Acinar zones.** The liver cells in each acinus are arranged in **three concentric elliptical zones around the short axis;** zone 1 is closest to the axis, zone 3 is closest to the terminal hepatic venule.
   a. **Zone 1.** The cells in zone 1 are the first to receive both nutrients and toxins in the blood.
      (1) They are generally the last to die if circulation is impaired, and are the first to regenerate.
      (2) They are the first to show changes following bile duct occlusion (bile stasis).
   b. **Zone 2.** Zone 2 has no sharp boundaries but is morphologically and functionally intermediate between zones 1 and 3.
   c. **Zone 3.** The cells in zone 3 are the first to show signs of ischemic necrosis (centrilobular necrosis).
      (1) They are the last to react to toxins or to bile duct occlusion.
      (2) They are the first to show fat accumulation in metabolic or drug-induced fatty livers.
      (3) Zones 1 and 3 also differ in enzyme activity, glycogen deposition and utilization, and cell organelle content and size.

V. **HEPATOCYTES** (Figure 26-3). Hepatocytes constitute the anastomosing plates of the liver parenchyma. These plates are 1 to 2 cells thick.

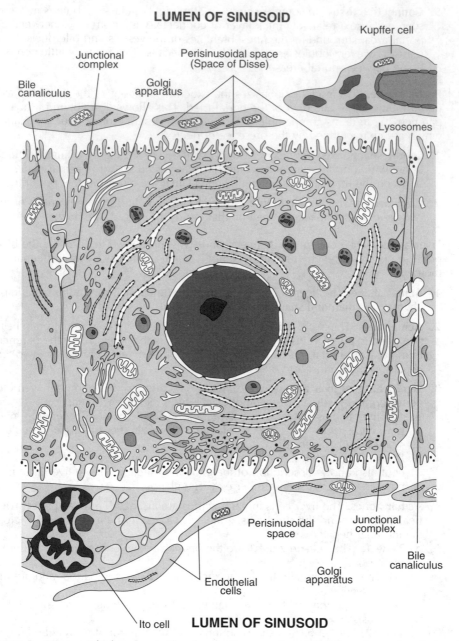

FIGURE 26-3. Diagram of a hepatocyte showing the large number and variety of cytoplasmic organelles present in this very active cell. The sinusoid is lined by fenestrated endothelial cells that are widely separated from each other and by perisinusoidal macrophages (Kupffer cells). Fat-storing cells (cells of Ito) are found in the perisinusoidal space. (Adapted from Ross MH, Romrell LJ, Kaye GI: *Histology: A Text and Atlas*, 3rd ed. Baltimore, Williams & Wilkins, 1995, p 503.)

A. **Morphologic characteristics**

1. **Size.** Hepatocytes are large polygonal cells that measure between 20 and 30 μm in each dimension.

2. **Surfaces.** The many surfaces of the hepatocyte can be classified into three categories.

a. **Basal surfaces** that form the border of the perisinusoidal space are equivalent to the basal surface of other epithelial cells.

    (1) Some hepatocytes also have surfaces that are in contact with the loose connective tissue of the portal area. These surfaces are also equivalent to the basal surface of other epithelial cells.

    (2) Unlike other epithelial cells, however, hepatocytes lack a basal lamina.

b. **Lateral surfaces** that are wholly in contact with similar surfaces of adjacent hepatocytes are equivalent to the lateral surfaces of other epithelial cells.

c. **Apical surfaces** that form one margin of a bile canaliculus are equivalent to the apical surface of other epithelial cells.

3. **Nuclei.** Hepatocyte nuclei are **large and round,** and usually occupy the center of the cell. Many hepatocytes are binucleate.

    a. Most hepatocytes in the adult liver are tetraploid (i.e., 4N amount of DNA). Some hepatocytes may have higher degrees of ploidy, with the size of the nucleus increasing with the degree of ploidy.

    b. Clumps of heterochromatin and two or more nucleoli are usually present in each nucleus.

4. **Cytoplasm.** The cytoplasm of hepatocytes is generally **acidophilic** but contains many organelles and inclusions described with routine light microscopy as granules. Special staining procedures allow the identification of some of these granules. The remainder can be identified by electron microscopy.

B. **Cytoplasmic organelles and inclusions** (Figure 26-4)

1. **Rough endoplasmic reticulum (rER) and free ribosomes.** Localized concentrations of rER and free ribosomes appear as basophilic granules using light microscopy.

    a. **rER.** The rER is responsible for the **synthesis** of various **plasma proteins** secreted by the hepatocyte into the perisinusoidal space. These proteins make up the endocrine secretion of the hepatocyte.

        (1) These include the major blood proteins albumin, fibrinogen, and nonimmune α- and β-globulins.

        (2) Also synthesized by the rER for secretion into the blood are the protein portions of the various lipoproteins, prothrombin, and soluble glycoproteins, including fibronectin.

    b. **Free ribosomes.** Numerous free ribosomes are also present in the cytoplasm of hepatocytes. They are usually arranged in spiral or rosette patterns as polyribosomes, indicating a high rate of synthesis of protein for internal use by the cell.

2. **Smooth endoplasmic reticulum** (sER). Hepatocytes contain a significant amount of sER. In some cells and under specific circumstances (see V B 2 b), this can be the predominant membranous compartment in the cell.

    a. **Function.** The sER has numerous synthetic functions related to both the exocrine and endocrine secretions of the hepatocyte, as well as important catabolic functions.

        (1) It is responsible for **glycogen metabolism** and for **cholesterol synthesis** and **bile salt formation.**

        (2) It is responsible for important **detoxification reactions** including conjugation of bilirubin, steroids, and other drugs with glucuronic acid to inactivate them and make them soluble.

        (3) The sER is the site of **deiodination of thyroxine (T_4),** yielding the much more active thyroid hormone **triiodothyronine (T_3).**

    b. **Hypertrophy of sER.** Certain drugs and hormones stimulate increased activity of the sER, as well as synthesis of new sER membranes and associated enzymes.

        (1) The sER hypertrophies after the hepatocyte is exposed to large amounts of phenobarbital, ethanol, anabolic steroids and progesterone, and certain cancer chemotherapeutic drugs.

        (2) Stimulation of the sER by one toxin (e.g., ethanol) enhances the ability of the hepatocyte to detoxify other agents, including certain carcinogens and pesticides. This cross stimulation can have important clinical implications.

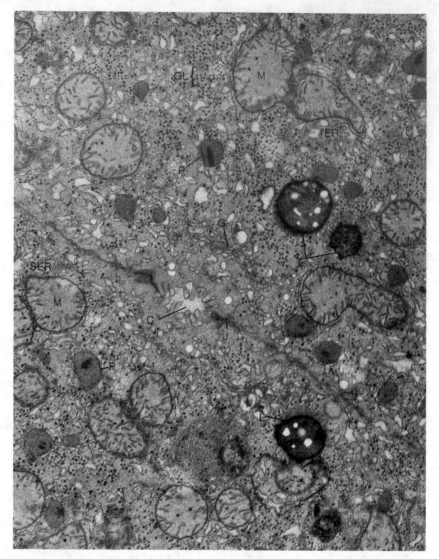

FIGURE 26-4. Electron micrograph of canine hepatocytes showing pericanalicular portions of two adjacent cells. The canaliculus (*C*) is separated from the rest of the intercellular space by two junctional complexes (*J*). Small microvillous processes extend into the bile canaliculus. The pericanalicular cytoplasm contains numerous mitochondria (*M*), several secondary and tertiary lysosomes (*L*), peroxisomes (*P*) that are recognized by the contained crystalloid of urate oxidase, elements of the Golgi apparatus (*G*), glycogen particles (*GL*), and cisternae of the smooth endoplasmic reticulum (*sER*) and rough endoplasmic reticulum (*rER*).

    (a) Inducing general anesthesia in chronic alcoholics can be difficult and potentially dangerous because greater amounts of anesthetic agents are needed due to the rate at which the liver can detoxify them.

    (b) Newborns, whose livers are primed by the high rate at which they are detoxifying the breakdown products of fetal hemoglobin, are also difficult to anesthetize.

  3. Golgi apparatus. Several small Golgi complexes are visible by light microscopy in each cell after appropriate staining. Electron microscopy reveals the Golgi apparatus in hepatocytes to be more elaborate than might be expected from examining light microscopic preparations.

a. Each Golgi complex consists of three to five closely stacked cisternae, numerous large and small vesicles, and associated primary lysosomes.

b. A Golgi complex may actually be branches of a single tortuous Golgi apparatus that can be appreciated only in heavy metal preparations of thick sections.

    (1) Elements of the Golgi apparatus concentrated near the **bile canaliculus** are associated with the **exocrine secretion of bile** (see VIII).

    (2) Elements of the Golgi apparatus concentrated near the **sinusoidal surfaces** are associated with the **endocrine secretion** of the hepatocytes.

        (a) These elements contain electron-dense granules 25 to 80 nm in diameter. The granules are **very low-density lipoproteins** (VLDLs) and other lipoprotein precursors that are released into the sinusoids as part of the endocrine secretion.

        (b) **Post-translational processing of plasma proteins** that are released into the sinusoids as part of the endocrine secretion also occurs in elements of the Golgi apparatus close to the sinusoidal surfaces.

4. Lysosomes. Numerous lysosomes can be identified by staining for **acid hydrolases.** Lysosomes of hepatocytes are extremely heterogeneous and may be identified positively only by histochemical means.

a. Secondary and tertiary lysosomes found near the bile canaliculus can be identified using electron microscopy. They correspond to the **peribiliary dense bodies** sometimes visible with light microscopy.

b. The contents of the secondary and tertiary lysosomes vary considerably. They include pigment granules (lipofuscin), partially digested cytoplasmic organelles, and myelin figures (i.e., membrane remnants made up of incompletely digested lipoproteins).

    (1) Lysosomes may be a normal site for **storage of iron** as a ferritin complex, and for accumulation of iron in certain hereditary iron-storage diseases (e.g., hemochromatosis).

    (2) Lysosomes increase in number under pathologic conditions ranging from simple obstructive jaundice (i.e., bile stasis) to anemia and viral hepatitis.

    (3) A surprising finding, however, has been that over a wide range of normal hepatocyte function, measured as the rate of bile secretion, there are no statistically significant variations in the size of the peribiliary Golgi apparatus or the number of associated lysosomes.

c. Lysosomal activity. Hepatic lysosomes function in the digestion of a broad range of endogenous and exogenous substrates.

    (1) They digest excess synthesized products of the hepatocyte, aged and exhausted organelles, and membranes of hypertrophied sER that are no longer needed.

    (2) They also digest partially broken down metabolites that are carried to the liver in the portal blood and taken into the hepatocyte from the sinusoid.

5. Peroxisomes. Staining for peroxidase activity can demonstrate the presence of numerous peroxisomes.

a. Electron microscopy resolves the peroxidase staining visible with light microscopy to demonstrate the presence of 200 to 300 peroxisomes per hepatocyte.

b. Hepatocyte peroxisomes have a role in numerous oxidative reactions, especially the β-oxidation of long-chain fatty acids and the oxidation of ethanol to acetaldehyde.

6. Mitochondria. As many as 800 to 1000 mitochondria per cell can be identified after vital staining or enzyme histochemical staining.

7. Glycogen. Large deposits of glycogen are identifiable after periodic acid–Schiff staining.

8. Lipid droplets of various sizes and frequency are also present in hepatocytes; their number and size vary with the health of the liver.

C. **Life span.** Hepatocytes are long lived when compared to other epithelial cells of the digestive system. Their average turnover time is about 5 months. However, they are capable of considerable, rapid regeneration when liver substance is lost through surgery, disease, or hepatotoxic processes.

VI. **PERISINUSOIDAL SPACE.** The perisinusoidal space, or **space of Disse,** lies between the hepatocyte and the sinusoidal endothelium and Kupffer cells (Figure 26-5).

A. **Exchange site.** It is the site of exchange of metabolic substrates and wastes as well as of secretory products, hormones, and recycled material between the blood and the hepatocytes.

1. **Enhanced hepatocyte basal surface.** Basal microvillous processes that extend into the perisinusoidal space from the hepatocytes increase the surface area available for exchange of materials as much as six times.

2. **Absence of cellular barrier.** Because of the gaps between endothelial cells, the numerous large fenestrae in the endothelial cells, and the absence of a basal lamina, there is no significant barrier between the blood plasma in the sinusoid and the plasma membrane of the hepatocyte.

3. **Site of endocrine secretion.** Proteins and lipoproteins synthesized by the hepatocytes are secreted into the perisinusoidal space. This constitutes the principal endocrine secretion of the liver. Glucose released from stored glycogen in the hepatocytes also enters the blood at this site.

B. **Adipose cell of Ito.** This is a type of lipocyte found in the perisinusoidal space (see Figure 26-3), often at sites where the sinusoid bends.

1. **Vitamin A.** These cells are the primary storage site for vitamin A, the essential precursor of the visual pigments of the retina.

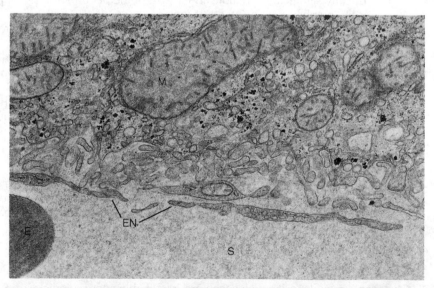

FIGURE 26-5. Electron micrograph showing a portion of the basal cytoplasm of a hepatocyte and a portion of the underlying sinusoid (*S*). The perisinusoidal space (space of Disse) lies between the widely separated sinusoidal endothelial cells (*EN*) and the basal plasma membrane of the hepatocyte. Short microvillous processes of the hepatocyte extend into the perisinusoidal space. Note that neither the endothelium nor the hepatocyte has a basal lamina. *E* = portion of erythrocyte in sinusoid, *M* = mitochondrion.

2. **Collagen secretion.** Ito cells are thought to secrete the fine **type III collagen fibers** (reticular fibers) that are present in the space of Disse. Lipid-depleted Ito cells are morphologically indistinguishable from fibroblasts.

   a. An increase in number and wider distribution of reticular fibers in the perisinusoidal space is an early sign of hepatic response to toxins.

   b. Continued insult to the liver can lead to the development of a continuous reticular stroma in the perisinusoidal space extending from the portal area to the terminal hepatic venule. This is the first indication of **bridging fibrosis,** an early morphologic indication of developing **cirrhosis.**

VII. **BILIARY SYSTEM.** The system of channels and conduits of increasing diameter that carries the bile from the hepatocytes to the small intestine via the gallbladder is called the **biliary tree.**

A. **Bile canaliculi.** The finest branches of the biliary tree are the bile canaliculi, which are **intercellular secretory channels** between apposed surfaces of two adjacent hepatocytes. Bile canaliculi form interconnecting rings around the hepatocytes (Figure 26-6; see also Figure 26-3).

1. **Apical secretory surface.** Because the surface of the hepatocyte that borders the bile canaliculus is equivalent to the apical surface of other exocrine glandular cells, the canaliculus is equivalent to the acinar or tubular lumen of the exocrine secretory unit.

   a. Canaliculi appear in both light microscopic and electron microscopic preparations as dilated portions of the intercellular space, ranging from 0.5 to 1.5 μm in diameter. Microvillous processes extend from the hepatocytes into the lumen of the canaliculus.

   b. Canaliculi may be demonstrated by retrograde infusion of a dye into the larger bile ducts, or by histochemical staining for ATPase and other alkaline phosphatases. The presence of ATPase at this site suggests that secretion of bile may be an active process.

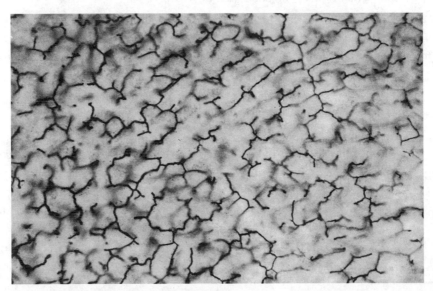

FIGURE 26-6. Light micrograph of a preparation of liver parenchyma back injected with India ink through a bile duct. The ink has filled the interconnecting network of bile canaliculi between the hepatocytes, demonstrating that these channels often form complete rings around hepatocytes.

2. Junctional complexes. The bile canaliculi are isolated from other portions of the intercellular space by tight junctions between the adjacent hepatocytes that form the canaliculus.
  a. Adhesion belts may also be found between adjacent hepatocytes at this site.
  b. Desmosomes and gap junctions provide intercellular adhesion and communication, respectively, between adjacent hepatocytes at other sites.

3. Centrifugal bile flow. Bile flow in the canaliculi is toward the portal space from the parenchyma (i.e., opposite to the direction of blood flow in the sinusoids).
  a. Near the portal space (but still within the lobule), canaliculi join to form small ductules, the **canals of Hering,** that are lined with cuboidal epithelial cells that are not hepatocytes.
  b. These small ductules, which carry the bile to the interlobular bile ducts in the portal triad, are subtended by a basal lamina, as is the rest of the distal biliary tree.

B. **Intrahepatic bile ducts.** The proximal bile ducts, the **interlobular bile ducts of the portal triad,** range in diameter from 15 to 40 μm. They are lined with a simple cuboidal epithelium that gradually becomes columnar as the ducts become larger and approach the porta hepatis.

  1. The cells of the intrahepatic bile ducts have well-developed microvilli as do those of the extrahepatic bile ducts and the gallbladder.
    a. Bile ducts gradually acquire a dense fibrous wall containing numerous elastic fibers.
    b. Smooth muscle cells appear in the duct walls as the ducts near the porta hepatis.

  2. Interlobular ducts form a network that gradually fuses into the left and right **lobar (hepatic) ducts** that join at the hilum to form the **common hepatic duct.**

C. **Extrahepatic bile ducts.** The extrahepatic bile ducts carry the bile from the liver to the gallbladder and then to the small intestine (see Figure 27-1).

  1. Common hepatic duct. The common hepatic duct is the proximal extrahepatic bile duct. It is about 3 cm long. It is lined by a tall columnar epithelium that closely resembles that of the gallbladder (see IX A 1 b).

  2. Cystic duct. The cystic duct branches from the common hepatic duct and leads to the gallbladder. It carries bile both into and out of the gallbladder.

  3. Common bile duct. Distal to the site at which the cystic duct originates from the common hepatic duct, the extrahepatic duct is called the common bile duct because it carries both unconcentrated bile from the liver and concentrated bile from the gallbladder.
    a. The common bile duct extends for about 7 cm to reach the wall of the duodenum at the **ampulla of Vater.**
    b. The **sphincter of Oddi,** a thickening of the muscle of the duodenal wall, surrounds the openings of both the common bile duct and the pancreatic duct at this site. It serves as a valve to regulate the entry of bile and pancreatic secretions into the duodenum.
    c. In animals that lack a gallbladder, such as the rat, or in humans after cholecystectomy, the common bile duct may exhibit some absorptive function to concentrate the bile.

VIII. **BILE.** Bile is the **major exocrine secretion of the liver.** The adult human liver secretes up to 1500 ml of bile per day. Bile is considered an exocrine secretion because it is secreted into a duct system. The bile canaliculus and the biliary tree are equivalent to

TABLE 26-1. Composition of Bile

Component	Principal Functions	Fate
Water	Solute for all other components	Recycled
Electrolytes: Na^+, Cl^-, HCO_3^-, K^+, Ca^{2+}, Mg^{2+}	Establish and maintain isotonicity of bile	Recycled
Bile acids: glycocholic and taurocholic acid	Emulsifying agents for lipids in the gut and for cholesterol and phospholipids in bile	Recycled
Bile pigments, principally bilirubin glucuronide	Detoxify bilirubin and carry it to the gut	Eliminated with feces
Cholesterol and phospholipids (e.g., lecithin)	Substrates for other cells; precursors of membrane components and steroids	Recycled

the acinar lumen and the duct system of other exocrine glands. The composition of bile is shown in Table 26-1.

A. **Bile acids** (bile salts). Bile acids act as emulsifying agents for lipids in the duodenum. They also serve to keep cholesterol and lecithin in solution in the bile.

   1. **Recycling from gut to liver.** About 90% of the bile acids are recycled by absorption in the gut and subsequent transport back to the liver in the portal blood.

   2. **Recycling by hepatocytes.** Bile acids are then absorbed from the portal blood and resecreted by the hepatocytes. The small amount lost in the gut is replaced by de novo synthesis by the hepatocytes.

   a. In addition to the bile acids, cholesterol and lecithin delivered to the gut in the bile are reabsorbed there and recycled via the portal blood.

   b. Also resorbed are most of the electrolytes and water that reach the gut in the bile, although the primary site of electrolyte and water absorption from the bile is the gallbladder.

B. **Hormones and immunoglobulins.** Insulin and immunoglobulin A appear in the bile but they are not synthesized or secreted by the hepatocytes. They are transported unchanged, in vesicles, across the hepatocyte from the sinusoidal blood into the bile for delivery to the gut.

C. **Bilirubin glucuronide.** Bilirubin, a primary breakdown product of hemoglobin, arrives in the portal blood from the spleen. It is conjugated with **glucuronic acid** in the hepatocyte sER and secreted as bilirubin glucuronide into the bile.

   1. Bilirubin glucuronide is not recycled. It is delivered to the duodenum and ultimately is excreted as a component of the feces to which it gives its color.

   2. Failure of the hepatocyte to absorb the bilirubin or failure to conjugate it and secrete the glucuronide can produce **jaundice.**

D. **Concentration of bile and control of bile secretion.** Bile is concentrated and stored in the gallbladder and delivered to the gut when needed for digestion.

   1. **Concentration.** The 1000 to 1500 ml of bile secreted by the liver each day is reduced to 100 ml or less by the concentrating activity of the gallbladder.

   2. **Hormonal regulation.** Bile flow from the liver, as well as emptying of the gallbladder into the common bile duct, is regulated by several of the hormones secreted by the enteroendocrine cells of the gastrointestinal tract.

   a. Secretin, cholecystokinin (CCK), and gastrin all increase the rate of bile flow from the liver. CCK stimulates emptying of the gallbladder by stimulating contraction of its smooth muscle.

  b. The rate of blood flow to the liver in the portal vein also exerts a regulatory effect of the rate of bile flow from the liver.

IX. GALLBLADDER. The gallbladder is responsible for the **storage and concentration of bile.** It is an elongate, distensible sac with a volume of about 50 ml in humans and is attached to the posteroinferior surface of the liver (see Figure 27-1). It concentrates the bile by **absorbing water and selected electrolytes** from the bile that reaches it from the liver.

A. Structure of the gallbladder wall

 1. **Mucosa.** The empty (or partially filled) gallbladder has numerous **deep mucosal folds,** many of which smooth out when the organ is distended (Figure 26-7).
    a. Stem cells. Other folds appear to be functionally significant. Stem cell populations for the columnar epithelium of the mucosa are located in the bottoms of these folds.
      (1) The stem cells are comparable to those located in the bases of the intestinal crypts (see Chapter 25 I C 7).
      (2) Cells that originate here migrate and differentiate along the folds and eventually are lost at the tips.
    b. Absorptive epithelium. The tall columnar epithelial cells that line the gallbladder have numerous microvilli, well-developed apical junctional complexes, apical and basal concentrations of mitochondria, and complex lateral plications.

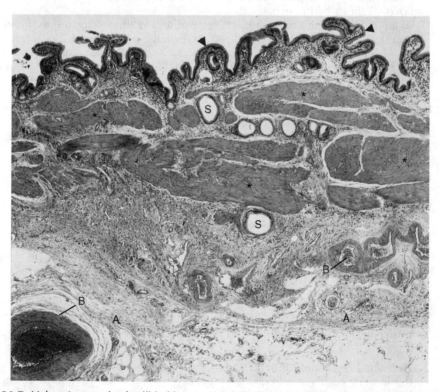

FIGURE 26-7. Light micrograph of gallbladder mucosa. This field shows the numerous mucosal folds (*arrowheads*) normally present in the undistended gallbladder. The muscularis externa is formed by irregularly arranged bundles of smooth muscle (*). A muscularis mucosae is absent. *A* = adventitia, *B* = blood vessels, *S* = Rokitansky-Aschoff sinuses. (Courtesy of Michael Ross.)

(1) These morphologic characteristics are similar to those of the absorptive columnar epithelial cells of the small intestine and colon.

(2) Na^+,K^+-ATPase is localized on the lateral plasma membrane of the epithelial cells.

(3) Secretory vesicles filled with glycoproteins destined for insertion in the glycocalyx are prominent in the apical cytoplasm.

c. Lamina propria. The lamina propria is particularly rich in blood vessels, especially fenestrated capillaries and small venules. It resembles the lamina propria of the colon, another organ specialized for the absorption of electrolytes and water.

(1) There are no lymphatic vessels in the lamina propria.

(2) Large numbers of lymphocytes and plasma cells are found in the lamina propria.

(3) Glands are sometimes present in the lamina propria close to the neck of the gallbladder and are more common in inflamed gallbladders. These glands contain mucin-secreting cells and some enteroendocrine cells.

d. The gallbladder has **no muscularis mucosae.** The outer limit of the lamina propria is the muscularis externa (muscularis propria).

2. Muscularis externa. The muscularis externa has numerous collagen and elastic fibers among the randomly oriented smooth muscle bundles.

a. Contraction of this layer reduces the volume of the gallbladder, forcing the concentrated bile back into the cystic duct.

b. Deep invaginations of the surface epithelium, called **Rokitansky-Aschoff sinuses,** sometimes penetrate through the muscularis externa (see Figure 26-7).

(1) They are most commonly found in and near the neck of the gallbladder, and are believed to be early indicators of pathologic changes in the gallbladder mucosa.

(2) Bacteria that lodge in these sinuses may cause chronic inflammation leading to obstruction.

3. Adventitia and serosa. A thick layer of dense connective tissue lies outside the muscularis externa. It is rich in adipose tissue and elastic fibers, and contains large blood vessels, an extensive lymphatic network, and autonomic nerves.

a. Where the gallbladder is attached to the liver this layer is an **adventitia.**

b. Where the gallbladder surface is exposed to the peritoneal cavity this layer is covered by a **serosa,** which is the **mesothelium** of the visceral peritoneum.

B. **Mechanism of bile concentration.** The concentration of bile is accomplished by the coupled transport of salt and water from the bile contained in the lumen of the gallbladder (Figure 26-8). Distension of the gallbladder with bile turns on an ion transport pump in the gallbladder epithelium.

1. Active salt transport. The absorptive epithelial cells of the gallbladder actively transport Na^+, Cl^-, and lesser amounts of HCO_3^- from the cytoplasm into the intercellular compartment of the epithelium. These ions are then replaced in the cytoplasm by diffusion across the apical plasma membrane from the bile in the lumen.

a. Ion pump enzyme. A transport ATPase that requires both Na^+ and an anion to function is located in the lateral plasma membrane.

b. Osmotic gradient. The active salt transport creates an osmotic gradient, making the intercellular space hypertonic to both the cytoplasm and the gallbladder lumen.

2. Passive water movement. Water moves from the cytoplasm and from the lumen of the gallbladder into the intercellular space because of the osmotic gradient.

3. Development of a hydrostatic pressure. Although the epithelial intercellular space can distend below the junctional complex by separation of the lateral plications, often to a degree visible with the light microscope, this distensibility is limited.

a. Thus, as water enters the intercellular space to equilibrate with the transported salt, a hydrostatic pressure develops in the space.

Lumen

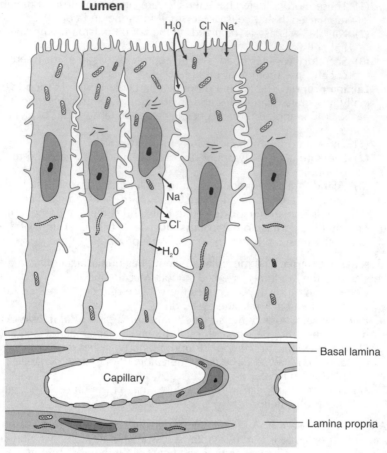

H₂0   Cl⁻   Na⁺

Na⁺
Cl⁻
H₂0

— Basal lamina

Capillary

— Lamina propria

FIGURE 26-8. Schematic representation of the gallbladder wall illustrating the mechanism and pathway of fluid transport responsible for the concentration of bile.

    b. This hydrostatic pressure forces a nearly isotonic fluid out of the intercellular space, across the basal lamina, and into the lamina propria.

    c. The tight junctions of the epithelium prevent backflow of the equilibrated fluid from the intercellular space to the lumen.

4. Role of underlying vessels. The entry of the salt solution into the lamina propria stimulates pinocytosis, resulting in rapid formation of new fenestrae in the fenestrated capillaries and small venules. The transported fluid is thereby quickly absorbed into the circulation.

5. Essential role of intercellular space. Studies of fluid transport in the gallbladder first demonstrated the essential role of the intercellular compartment of a transporting epithelium in allowing transport of an isotonic fluid across an epithelium.

6. Efficiency of bile concentration. The normal human gallbladder can transport from the lumen to the vascular compartment an amount of fluid nearly equal to its own volume in an hour (i.e., approximately 50 ml/hour).

    a. Thus, by removing salt and water, the gallbladder can concentrate bile acids and other components of bile up to 10 to 12 times.

    b. After cholecystectomy, a limited amount of bile concentration is achieved by the same mechanism operating in the epithelium of the common bile duct. However, a much more dilute bile is delivered at relatively steady rate to the duodenum.

Chapter 27

Exocrine Pancreas

I. **INTRODUCTION.** The pancreas is an abdominal organ that lies close to the stomach and the small intestine (Figure 27-1). The pancreas consists of two distinct components, the exocrine pancreas and the endocrine pancreas.

A. **Exocrine pancreas.** The exocrine component of the pancreas is a continuum throughout the organ. It is a **serous gland** (i.e., protein-secreting) [see Chapter 23 II A 1] that synthesizes and secretes enzymes essential for **digestion.** These enzymes are delivered to the duodenum via the pancreatic duct in an inactive form, as proenzymes.

B. **Endocrine pancreas.** The endocrine component (see Chapter 33) is dispersed throughout the organ as distinct cell masses called **islets of Langerhans.** The endocrine component synthesizes insulin, glucagon, and other peptide hormones that are released into the blood to regulate glucose, lipid, and protein **metabolism** throughout the body.

II. **HISTOLOGIC CHARACTERISTICS.** The **exocrine secretory units** of the pancreas are **serous acini** and **tubuloacini** that closely resemble those of the parotid gland (see Chapter 23 III).

A. **Simple epithelium.** The serous secretory units are formed by a simple epithelium of pyramidal epithelial cells that have a narrow luminal surface and a broad basal surface (Figure 27-2).

B. **Sparse connective tissue.** Periacinar connective tissue is sparse. Trabeculae that penetrate the gland from the capsule appear as rays or strands, seldom as partitions.

C. **Absence of lobules.** Because of the paucity of connective tissue, the human pancreas does not exhibit the distinct lobar/lobular structure that characterizes salivary glands (see Chapter 23 II).

D. **Duct system.** The exocrine pancreas contains a system of ducts, as do all exocrine glands. All the secretory units of the exocrine pancreas are drained by this duct system.

III. **SEROUS ACINAR CELLS.** The pancreatic acinar cells are typical of cells engaged in regulated protein secretion (Figure 27-3).

A. **Zymogen granules.** The acinar cells are characterized by the presence of **acidophilic** zymogen granules in the apical cytoplasm. The granules are more numerous in fasting individuals, often compressing the nucleus and rough endoplasmic reticulum (rER) into the basal cytoplasm.

1. Zymogen granules contain a variety of stored proenzymes that are synthesized and secreted by the acinar cells. These include inactive forms of peptidases, amylase, lipase, and nucleases.
   a. The **peptidase proenzymes** trypsinogen, chymotrypsinogen, and procarboxypeptidase are converted in the duodenum into the potent protein-digesting enzymes, trypsin, chymotrypsin, and carboxypeptidase [see Chapter 25 I C 1 d (2) (b)].
   b. **Amylase** digests carbohydrates, **lipase** digests lipids, and **deoxyribonuclease** and **ribonuclease** digest DNA and RNA, respectively.

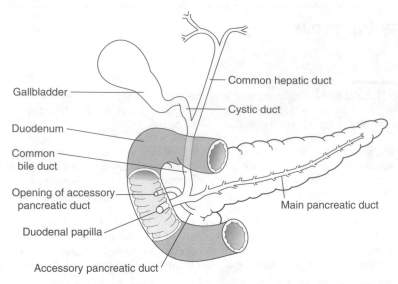

FIGURE 27-1. Diagram of the relationship between the pancreas and the duodenum. The main pancreatic duct receives the interlobular ducts along its length throughout the pancreas. The accessory duct arises in the head of the pancreas and enters the duodenum craniad to the conjoint main duct and common bile duct. The duodenal papilla marks the entry of the conjoint main pancreatic and common bile duct on the duodenal mucosa. (Adapted from Grant JCB: *A Method of Anatomy,* 10th ed. Baltimore, Williams & Wilkins, 1980, p 173.)

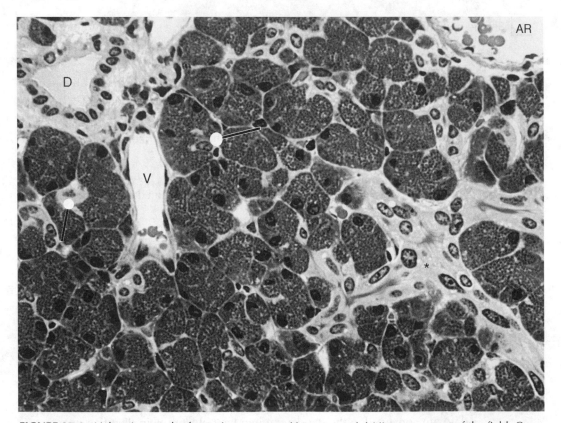

FIGURE 27-2. Light micrograph of exocrine pancreas. Numerous acini (*A*) occupy most of the field. Centroacinar cells (*arrows*) are evident in several of the acini. In one acinus, two centroacinar cells surround the lumen of the intercalated duct (*circle*). Several intercalated ducts merge in another area of the field (***). *D* = intralobular collecting duct, *AR* = arteriole, *V* = venule.

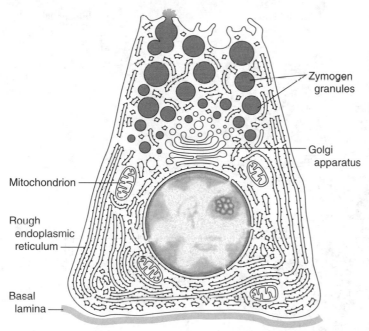

Zymogen granules

Golgi apparatus

Mitochondrion

Rough endoplasmic reticulum

Basal lamina

FIGURE 27-3. Diagram of a pancreatic acinar cell showing the abundant rough endoplasmic reticulum that imparts the basophilia to the subnuclear and perinuclear cytoplasm, the large supranuclear Golgi apparatus, and the numerous zymogen granules in the apical cytoplasm. (Adapted from Lentz T: *Cell Fine Structure.* Philadelphia, WB Saunders, 1971, p 195.)

2. Contents of zymogen granules are released from the acinar cells by **exocytosis** into the lumen of the acinus, from which they enter the duct system that eventually carries them to the duodenum.

B. **Basal cytoplasm.** The subnuclear portion of the acinar cells is characterized by a distinct **basophilia** due to an extensive **rER** and free ribosomes.

1. The extensive rER provides a structural basis for the **prodigious protein production** of the pancreatic acinar cells.

2. The basophilia visible with light microscopy may appear lamellar. Each lamella corresponds to a stack of rER cisternae.

3. This portion of the cell also stains metachromatically with thionin (basic) dyes, indicating a high concentration of anionic groups.

C. **Golgi apparatus.** A well-developed Golgi apparatus is located in the supranuclear cytoplasm.

1. This organelle receives the newly synthesized proenzymes from the rER.

2. The proenzymes undergo post-translational modification and packaging into the zymogen granules in the Golgi apparatus.

D. **Intercellular junctions. Junctional complexes** join the acinar cells at their apical poles, forming an isolated lumen into which the zymogen granules release their contents.

1. The membrane added to the apical surface by exocytosis is retrieved by endocytosis and reprocessed.

2. Small microvillous processes extend into the lumen from the apical cell surface.

IV. **DUCT SYSTEM.** The pancreas is unique among exocrine glands in having a duct system that begins in the lumen of the acinus.

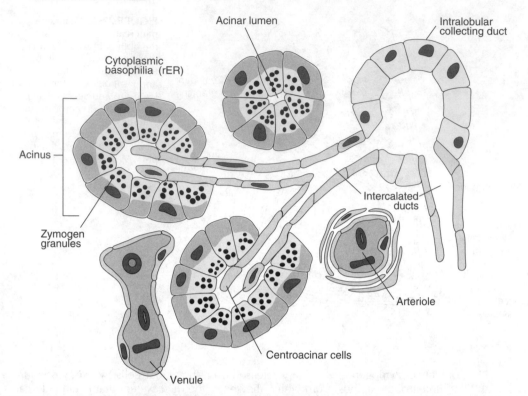

FIGURE 27-4. Diagrammatic representation of three acini of the exocrine pancreas. The location of centroacinar cells, the relationship of centroacinar cells to intercalated ducts, and the convergence of intercalated ducts into an intralobular collecting duct are illustrated.

A. **Centroacinar cells and intercalated ducts.** Centroacinar cells are intercalated duct cells (see Chapter 23 II C 2 a) that are displaced into the lumen of the acinus (Figure 27-4). The centroacinar cells are relatively pale squamous cells and, thus, are easily distinguished from the adjacent secretory cells.

1. Centroacinar cells are continuous with the cells of the intercalated ducts, which are short ducts that carry the secretion from the acinus to larger diameter intralobular ducts.

2. The relationship between the intercalated duct and the acinus resembles that between a small balloon (the acinus) and a drinking straw (the intercalated duct) that has been pushed through the neck of the balloon into its lumen.

3. An ideal plane of section in a light or electron microscopic preparation would show centroacinar cells inside an acinus that are continuous with the extra-acinar intercalated duct.

B. **Intralobular collecting ducts.** The intercalated ducts drain to a network of intralobular collecting ducts that are formed by a simple cuboidal epithelium.

1. The intercalated and intralobular ducts **secrete a large volume of fluid rich in Na$^+$ and HCO$_3$$^-$** that is added to the small volume of slightly viscous, protein-rich acinar secretion.
   a. The secretion of the intralobular ducts dilutes the acinar secretion so that it can flow more easily through the duct system.
   b. The bicarbonate ion in the secretion helps to neutralize the acidity of the chyme

that enters the duodenum, and to establish the optimum pH for the pancreatic enzymes.

2. The secretory activity of these ducts produces a final pancreatic secretion volume of about 1 liter per day.
   a. This is comparable to the initial volume of bile secreted by the liver.
   b. Whereas the bile is concentrated in the gallbladder, the entire volume of the pancreatic secretion is delivered to the duodenum.

3. Because the intralobular ducts are primarily secretory rather than absorptive, there are **no striated ducts** in the pancreas.

C. **Interlobular ducts.** The interlobular ducts are large, conspicuous structures in the connective tissue trabeculae of the pancreas.

1. They are lined by a simple low columnar epithelium.

2. Occasional goblet cells and enteroendocrine cells are found in the epithelium of the interlobular ducts, emphasizing the embryonic origin of the pancreas from the foregut.

D. **Main pancreatic duct and accessory duct.** All interlobular ducts drain into either the main duct, the **duct of Wirsung,** or into the accessory duct, the **duct of Santorini** (see Figure 27-1).

1. The **main pancreatic duct** runs through the length of the gland, parallel to its long axis. The entry of interlobular ducts into the main duct imparts a herringbone pattern to this portion of the duct system.

2. The **accessory pancreatic duct** is located in the head of the gland and drains those interlobular ducts not drained by the main pancreatic duct.
   a. This duplicate duct system also reflects the embryology of the pancreas, which arises as two separate evaginations of the foregut that later fuse into a single gland.
   b. Both the main duct and the accessory duct are lined with a simple tall columnar epithelium that contains occasional goblet cells and enteroendocrine cells.

3. The **main pancreatic duct** and the **common bile duct** unite to form a dilated segment (hepatopancreatic ampulla, ampulla of Vater) before opening through a short common duct into the duodenum. Occasionally the main pancreatic duct and the common bile duct enter the duodenum separately.
   a. The **accessory pancreatic duct** enters the duodenum a short distance craniad to the main duct.
   b. The **sphincter of Oddi** (see Chapter 26 VII C 3 b) regulates the flow of pancreatic juice (through the main pancreatic duct) and bile (through the common bile duct) into the duodenum.

V. **CONTROL OF PANCREATIC EXOCRINE SECRETION.** Hormones secreted by the enteroendocrine cells of the duodenum are the principal regulators of pancreatic exocrine secretion.

A. **Secretin and cholecystokinin.** The coordinated activity of these two peptide hormones leads to the delivery to the duodenum of a large volume of enzyme-rich, alkaline fluid.

1. **Secretin.** Secretin stimulates the intralobular duct cells to secrete large amounts of **fluid** and HCO_3^-. It has only a minor effect on enzyme secretion.

2. **Cholecystokinin (CCK).** This hormone, also called **pancreozymin,** stimulates the acinar cells to release their stored proenzymes. It has only a minor effect on duct secretory activity.

3. Both of these hormones, along with **gastrin,** also **stimulate pancreatic growth,** thus indirectly stimulating exocrine secretion.

B. **Other hormones.** Other peptide hormones secreted by both enteroendocrine cells and endocrine cells of the pancreatic islets also exert regulatory effects on pancreatic exocrine secretion.

1. **Vasoactive intestinal peptide** (VIP) stimulates pancreatic exocrine secretion, probably by increasing HCO_3^- secretion by duct cells.

2. **Pancreatic polypeptide** (PP) inhibits both proenzyme secretion by the acinar cells and HCO_3^- secretion by the duct cells.

C. **Neural influences.** The pancreas also receives autonomic innervation.

1. **Parasympathetic fibers** stimulate proenzyme secretion by the acinar cells, resembling the action of cholecystokinin.

2. **Sympathetic fibers** are principally involved in regulation of pancreatic blood flow and are only indirectly involved in regulation of secretion.

Chapter 28

Respiratory System

I. **INTRODUCTION.** The respiratory system consists of the nasal cavity, pharynx, larynx, trachea, bronchi, bronchioles, and lungs (Figure 28-1). The system performs several functions: air conduction, gas exchange, olfaction (reception of odor), and phonation (production of sound).

II. **NASAL CAVITY.** The nasal cavity is the site of **filtration, hydration,** and **temperature regulation** of inspired air.

A. **Anatomy of the nasal cavity.** The nasal cavity is formed by **paired chambers** separated from each other by the **nasal septum.**

1. Each chamber communicates anteriorly with the environment through the **nares** (nostrils) and posteriorly with the nasopharynx through the **choana.**

2. The lateral wall of each chamber is remarkably irregular because of the presence of the superior, middle, and inferior **chonchae** (turbinate bones).

3. The nasal cavity is lined by a **ciliated pseudostratified columnar epithelium.** This type of epithelium is commonly found throughout the larger diameter regions of the respiratory system and, because of this, is occasionally called **respiratory epithelium.**

B. **Functions of the nasal mucosa**

1. **Air hydration.** The secretions of serous and mucous exocrine glands coat and moisten the surface of the nasal cavity.
   a. The secretions add water vapor to the inspired air.
   b. Goblet cells in the epithelial lining, and their secretions, also contribute to the fluid layer.

2. **Air filtration.** Turbulent airflow is created in the nasal cavities by interruption of the airstream by the conchae.
   a. **Turbulent precipitation** is a mechanism for cleaning inspired air. Particulate matter contained in the inspired air is thrown out of the airstream by centrifugal force and adheres to the nearby moist mucosal surface.
   b. Cilia beat synchronously to move mucus and trapped particulate debris to the pharynx, where it is either swallowed or expectorated.

3. **Temperature regulation.** The nasal mucosa has an extensive superficial **vascular bed** that **warms or cools inspired air.**

C. **Olfactory mucosa.** The olfactory mucosa is a **localized sensory region** in the dome of each nasal cavity that is thicker than the surrounding, nonsensory mucosa of the nasal cavity.

1. **Olfactory epithelium** is a specialized pseudostratified columnar epithelium that is part of the olfactory mucosa and contains four types of cells (Figure 28-2).
   a. **Olfactory cells.** These **bipolar sensory neurons** span the thickness of the epithelium.
      (1) **Axon and dendrite.** The neuron has an apical (supranuclear) **dendritic process** and a basal (infranuclear) **axonal process.**
         (a) The dendrite extends to the free surface of the epithelium, where it forms a bulbous dilatation (called a dendritic knob or olfactory vesicle) that projects slightly above the epithelial surface.

FIGURE 28-1. Overview of the respiratory system.

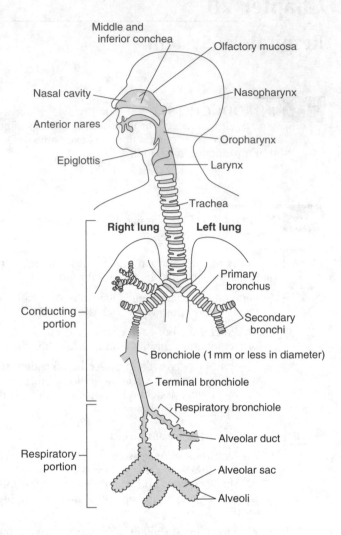

Middle and inferior conchea

Olfactory mucosa

Nasal cavity

Nasopharynx

Anterior nares

Oropharynx

Epiglottis

Larynx

Trachea

Right lung   **Left lung**

Primary bronchus

Conducting portion

Secondary bronchi

Bronchiole (1 mm or less in diameter)

Terminal bronchiole

Respiratory bronchiole

Alveolar duct

Respiratory portion

Alveolar sac

Alveoli

(b) The axon extends basally and leaves the epithelium to become part of the olfactory nerve (cranial nerve I).

(2) **Olfactory cilia.** Several **extremely long cilia** originate from the dilatation of each olfactory cell.

(a) The cilia are non-motile, bent over, and are immersed in the surface mucous layer. The typical $9+2$ array of microtubules (see Chapter 3 III) is present only in the proximal parts of these unusual cilia.

(b) **Chemoreceptors** are found in the large surface area of the long olfactory cilia. The receptors recognize the structural differences of odiferous substances.

(3) **Neuron turnover.** Olfactory cells are a **slowly renewing population of neurons** that are able to regenerate after injury.

(a) The **life-span of a mammalian olfactory neuron** is about 30 days. New neurons arise from the basal cells in the olfactory mucosa.

(b) Olfactory cells are one of a small population of neurons known to replicate throughout life. Other neurons that replicate are ganglion cells of the enteric nervous system and neuroepithelial cells of taste buds.

b. **Supporting (sustentacular) cells** are the columnar cells of the pseudostratified olfactory epithelium. Their free surface is characterized by the presence of **microvilli.**

c. **Basal cells** contact the basal lamina but do not extend to the free surface. They

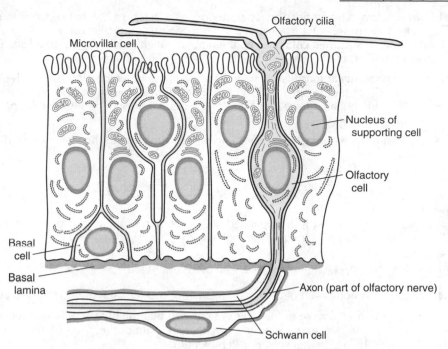

FIGURE 28-2. Drawing of olfactory epithelium based on electron micrographs. The height of the epithelium is reduced in this illustration.

are **stem cells** that differentiate into columnar supporting cells and into olfactory cells.

d. **Microvillar (brush) cells** are small, infrequently encountered, pear-shaped cells found in the superficial level of the olfactory epithelium.

   (1) A tuft of short microvilli projects from the cell into the nasal cavity.

   (2) A long, slender process arises from the basal part of the microvillar cell and extends toward the basal lamina. The process resembles an axon.

   (3) Microvillar cells are also found in other regions of the respiratory system (e.g., tracheal epithelium) and are thought to be a second type of chemoreceptor in the respiratory system.

e. Goblet cells are not present in the olfactory epithelium, but are found elsewhere in the lining of the nasal cavity.

2. **Serous exocrine glands (Bowman's glands)**

   a. These are found in the connective tissue deep to the olfactory epithelium.

   b. The secretions are released onto the surface of the olfactory region. Odiferous substances are suspended or dissolved in this fluid layer.

III. PARANASAL SINUSES AND NASOPHARYNX

A. **Paranasal sinuses.** The **frontal, maxillary, ethmoidal,** and **sphenoidal** sinuses are air-filled spaces in the bones that form the wall of the nasal cavity. The mucosal surface of the sinuses is a **thin ciliated pseudostratified columnar epithelium.**

   1. The sinuses communicate with the nasal cavity via narrow openings. Mucus produced in the sinuses drains into the nasal cavity through the openings.

   2. Inflammation that occludes the drainage openings of a sinus can result in sinusitis and recurrent sinus infections.

B. **Nasopharynx.** The air-filled space posterior to the nasal cavity and superior to the soft palate is the nasopharynx. Most of the nasopharyngeal mucosa is covered by a **ciliated pseudostratified columnar epithelium,** although patches of stratified squamous nonkeratinized epithelium may spill over from the oropharynx.

    1. The **pharyngeal tonsil** (see Chapter 16) is a mass of lymphatic tissue in the posterior wall of the nasopharynx. When enlarged, this tonsil is called the "adenoids." Diffuse lymphatic tissue and solitary nodules are present throughout the nasopharynx.

    2. The **auditory (eustachian) tubes** join the nasopharynx to the cavity of each middle ear.

V. **LARYNX.** The larynx is an expanded hollow portion of the respiratory system located between the nasopharynx and the trachea.

A. Air passing through the larynx produces speech and other vocalizations.

B. The larynx is composed of cartilages, ligaments, muscle, and a mucosal surface.

    1. The **mucosal surface** of the larynx is covered by a **highly variable epithelium.**
        a. Areas subject to abrasion (e.g., by the airstream during speech) are characterized by a stratified squamous epithelium.
        b. Parts of the epiglottis, which directs food into the esophagus and prevents food from entering the larynx, are also covered by a stratified squamous epithelium.
        c. Pseudostratified ciliated columnar epithelium covers most of the remaining laryngeal mucosa; stratified columnar epithelium may occur in transitional zones.

    2. **Laryngeal cartilages** are **hyaline** or **elastic,** or occasionally combinations of both cartilage types. Cartilages often show evidence of calcification.

    3. **Laryngeal muscles** are skeletal muscle.

V. **TRACHEA.** The trachea carries air between the larynx and the bronchi.

A. **Anatomy**

    1. The trachea is a tube about 10 cm long and about 2.5 cm in diameter that is supported by **C-shaped rings of hyaline cartilage.**

    2. The trachea bifurcates at the level of the sternal angle to form the **primary (extrapulmonary) bronchi.**

B. **Histologic characteristics.** The tracheal wall is formed by an inner mucosal epithelial layer, a submucosal connective tissue layer, numerous glands, cartilage rings, and an outer adventitial layer.

    1. **Tracheal epithelium.** The trachea is lined by a **ciliated pseudostratified columnar epithelium** in which the following cell types may be identified:
        a. **Ciliated columnar cells** have numerous cilia that project into the mucus and move the mucous layer toward the pharynx. The columnar cell spans the full thickness of the epithelium, and is the most prominent cell type in tracheal epithelium.
        b. **Basal cells** rest on the basal lamina but do not reach the luminal surface. Basal cells are stem cells capable of differentiating into the other cell types in the epithelium.
        c. **Goblet cells** synthesize and secrete mucus. The cell is dilated apically by muci-

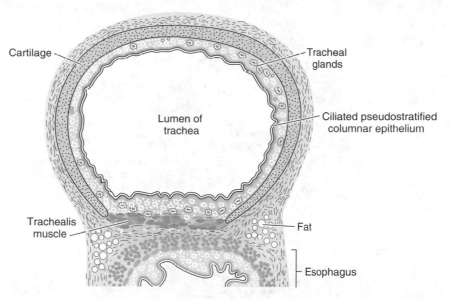

FIGURE 28-3. Trachea, transverse section through a cartilage ring. Cartilage rings assure the patency of the tracheal lumen. The trachealis muscle is visible in the cartilage-free segment of the tracheal wall, adjacent to the esophagus. (Adapted with permission from Kelly DE, Wood RL, Enders AC: *Bailey's Textbook of Microscopic Anatomy,* 18th ed. Baltimore, Williams & Wilkins, 1984, p 625.)

gen droplets. It also contains a prominent Golgi apparatus and a large quantity of basally located rough endoplasmic reticulum.

    d. Microvillar (brush) cells are interspersed among the other epithelial cells and are similar to those found in the epithelium of the nasal cavity (see II C 1 d).

    e. Small granule cells are present in the basal level of the epithelium and are filled with granules 100–300 nm in diameter that contain catecholamine-like materials.

        (1) These cells are part of the amine precursor uptake and decarboxylation (APUD) cell classification, a subset of the diffuse neuroendocrine system (DNES). These cells were formerly referred to as argyrophilic and argentaffin cells because of their staining characteristics with silver salts.

        (2) The secretions of these cells may exert a paracrine effect on goblet cell secretion and on ciliary activity. Small granule cells are also found in bronchi and bronchioles.

2. Tracheal cartilages. The patency of the tracheal airway is maintained by C-shaped rings in the submucosal connective tissue (Figure 28-3). Approximately 15–20 cartilaginous rings support the trachea.

    a. The open portion of the ring is directed posteriorly, toward the esophagus, and is bridged by smooth muscle fibers of the trachealis muscle.

    b. The perichondrium of each tracheal cartilage merges with the fat-laden connective tissue of the adventitia, which also contains blood vessels, nerves, and lymphatic vessels.

3. Lymphatic tissues. Evidence of localized immune reactions to antigen contained in inspired air is present in the tracheal mucosa as diffuse lymphatic tissue and nodules with germinal centers.

VI.   **BRONCHI.** Bronchi are extrapulmonary and intrapulmonary cartilage-supported airways.

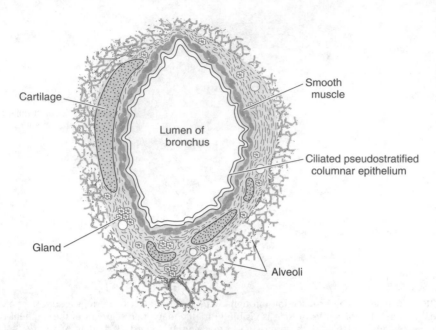

FIGURE 28-4. Bronchus, transverse section. This bronchus is approximately 2 mm in diameter. Its small size, intrapulmonary location, and sparsity of supporting cartilaginous plates suggest that this is a segmental (tertiary) bronchus. (Adapted with permission from Kelly DE, Wood RL, Enders AC: *Bailey's Textbook of Microscopic Anatomy*, 18th ed. Baltimore, Williams & Wilkins, 1984, p 630.)

A. **Extrapulmonary (primary) bronchi** are formed by the bifurcation of the trachea. Extrapulmonary bronchi resemble the trachea but are slightly smaller in diameter.

B. **Intrapulmonary bronchi** are surrounded by the parenchyma of the lung and divide repeatedly to form **lobar (secondary)** and **segmental (tertiary)** bronchi (Figure 28-4).

  1. Lobar bronchi
    a. The largest intrapulmonary bronchi are lobar bronchi.
    b. Five lobar bronchi can be identified, one to each of the five lobes of the lungs.

  2. Segmental bronchi
    a. Lobar bronchi divide to form segmental bronchi. A segmental bronchus is smaller in diameter than a lobar bronchus.
    b. Eighteen segmental bronchi can be identified, one to each bronchopulmonary segment of the lungs.

C. **Histologic characteristics of bronchi**

  1. Bronchi are lined by a **ciliated pseudostratified columnar epithelium,** similar to the trachea. Goblet cells occur in the epithelium and mucous and serous exocrine glands are present in the subepithelial connective tissue.

  2. All bronchi contain **cartilage.** Any intrapulmonary conducting part of the system that has cartilage in its wall is a bronchus.
    a. Extrapulmonary bronchi. The cartilage of a primary, extrapulmonary bronchus is in the form of C-shaped rings like those of the trachea.
    b. Intrapulmonary bronchi
      (1) The cartilage in the wall of lobar and segmental bronchi is in the form of **irregular cartilage plates** that form a complete but not continuous circumferential support.
      (2) The smallest bronchi have only widely scattered cartilaginous plates in their walls.

3. **Smooth muscle** in the wall of an intrapulmonary bronchus encircles the lumen. This is in contrast to the trachea and extrapulmonary bronchi, in which the smooth muscle is restricted to the cartilage-free area.

 BRONCHIOLES. The smallest bronchi lead into bronchioles. A large number of bronchioles exist in a lung. Bronchioles branch repeatedly until, finally, terminal bronchioles and respiratory bronchioles are formed (Figure 28-5).

A. **Histologic characteristics** that differentiate bronchioles from bronchi include:

1. **Size.** Bronchioles are always smaller than bronchi (less than 1 mm in diameter). Smaller bronchioles are of microscopic diameter.

2. **Epithelium.** Bronchioles are lined by a **ciliated columnar or cuboidal epithelium.** Occasionally, pseudostratified epithelium extends into a larger bronchiole from a bronchus.

3. **Lack of cartilage and exocrine glands.** Bronchioles lack both supporting cartilaginous plates and subepithelial glands.

4. **Smooth muscle.** Bronchioles have a relatively thick layer of circumferential smooth muscle.

5. **Goblet cells.** Mucus-secreting goblet cells are present in larger bronchioles but not in smaller ones.

6. **Bronchiolar (Clara) cells.** These secretory cells are present in the epithelium of bronchioles and are different from goblet cells.

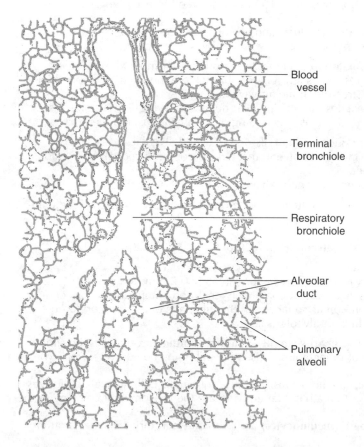

Blood vessel

Terminal bronchiole

Respiratory bronchiole

Alveolar duct

Pulmonary alveoli

FIGURE 28-5. Distal airways. The branching of a terminal bronchiole is depicted. (Adapted with permission from Kelly DE, Wood RL, Enders AC: *Bailey's Textbook of Microscopic Anatomy*, 18th ed. Baltimore, Williams & Wilkins, 1984, p 631.)

a. Bronchiolar cells have a characteristic **domed apex** that contains numerous secretory granules. The granules are not well characterized chemically but probably contain a **surfactant-like material** that is secreted onto the bronchiolar surface.

b. Bronchiolar cells are less numerous than columnar ciliated cells in larger bronchioles. In smaller bronchioles, however, the relative proportion of bronchiolar cells increases.

B. **Terminal bronchioles** are the smallest, most distal bronchioles that **function exclusively in air conduction;** they lead into respiratory bronchioles.

C. **Respiratory bronchioles.** Respiratory bronchioles are transitional structures, partly devoted to **air conduction** and partly devoted to **gas exchange.**

1. A respiratory bronchiole is a small (post-terminal) bronchiole with noncontiguous (i.e., scattered) alveoli punctuating its wall. These alveoli have the same microscopic structure as alveoli found more distally.

2. In a respiratory bronchiole, alveoli alternate with nonalveolar regions.
   a. **Air conduction** occurs in **nonalveolar regions,** which are lined by cuboidal or columnar epithelial cells.
   b. **Gas exchange** occurs in **alveolar regions,** which are lined by squamous epithelial cells.

VIII. **ALVEOLI.** Alveoli are blind, spheroidal compartments that are the terminal part of the respiratory system. The alveolus is the **functional unit of gas exchange** in the respiratory system. There are approximately 100 million alveoli in each lung.

A. **Structural organization.** Alveolar ducts and alveolar sacs are multi-alveolar units of structure that originate from the respiratory bronchioles (see Figure 28-5).

1. **Alveolar duct.** A respiratory bronchiole leads into one or more alveolar ducts.
   a. An alveolar duct resembles a respiratory bronchiole in which alveoli become the predominant structure in the airway wall.
   b. Smooth muscle extends into the alveolar duct and is visible in histologic sections as "knobs" of tissue at the opening of each alveolus into the duct.

2. **Alveolar sac.** Alveolar ducts end in culs-de-sac called alveolar sacs.
   a. Alveolar sacs are clusters of alveoli that have a common central space into which alveoli open.
   b. Smooth muscle is not present in alveolar sacs.

3. **Alveoli.** In a typical section of lung tissue, most of the tissue sample will be composed of alveoli.

B. **Histologic characteristics of alveoli** (Figure 28-6)

1. **General characteristics**
   a. Alveoli are thin-walled structures approximately 0.2 mm in diameter.
   b. The alveolar air space is not a completely enclosed compartment. It is confluent at some point on its surface with the air space of a respiratory bronchiole, alveolar duct, or alveolar sac.

2. **Alveolar cell types.** A **primarily simple squamous epithelium** replaces the simple cuboidal epithelium of bronchioles. This epithelial lining comprises several types of cells:
   a. **Type I cells (type I pneumocytes)** are thin, squamous cells specialized for **gas exchange.** They rest on a basal lamina and are the predominant cell type of the alveolar lining.
   b. **Type II cells (type II pneumocytes)** are cuboidal **secretory cells** that protrude

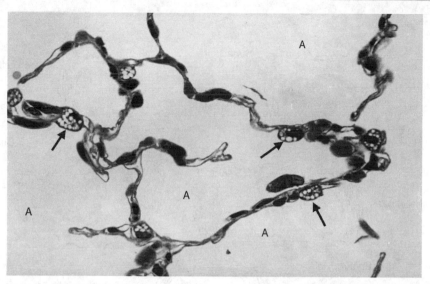

FIGURE 28-6. Lung alveoli, light micrograph. Several cuboidal type II cells with characteristically vacuolated cytoplasm are indicated (*arrows*). Most of the alveolar surface area is formed by squamous type I cells. *A* = alveolar air space.

into the alveolar space (see Figure 28-6). They are integral components of the alveolar lining, joined to type I cells by tight junctions.

    (1) Type II cells are widely scattered in the alveolar lining: 5–10 type II cells are found in each alveolus.

    (2) Type II cells have an extensive rough endoplasmic reticulum and a large Golgi apparatus, which are characteristics typical of secretory cells.

    (3) Type II cells secrete membrane-bounded **multilamellar bodies,** which accumulate in the apical cytoplasm and have been shown to contain phospholipid-rich **pulmonary sufactant** (see X).

  c. Alveolar macrophages (dust cells)

    (1) Alveoli are sites of phagocytic activity (Figure 28-7). Alveolar macrophages are part of the mononuclear phagocytic system and are derived from blood monocytes.

    (2) Alveolar macrophages are not permanent components of the alveolar surface and they do not form junctional complexes with pneumocytes.

      (a) Alveolar macrophages may traverse the intercellular space of the alveolar lining to protrude into the alveolar space.

      (b) Macrophages may also pass completely into the lumen of the alveolus to phagocytize foreign material that has penetrated the respiratory system to its distal extremity.

      (c) Macrophages are also present in the interalveolar connective tissue.

    (3) Alveolar macrophages are obvious in histologic sections of lung if they have removed large amounts of foreign material from the inspired air.

C. **Interalveolar septum.** An interalveolar septum is formed where two or more alveoli abut.

  1. The **components** of the septum are:

    a. Type I or type II cells of the two abutting alveoli, and their basal laminae

    b. Capillaries, connective tissue cells, collagen and elastic fibers, and ground substance, which fill the intervening space

  2. The abundant elastic fibers in the interalveolar septum are partially responsible for the **elastic recoil of the lung.**

  3. An **extensive capillary bed** permeates the interalveolar septum and the capillaries

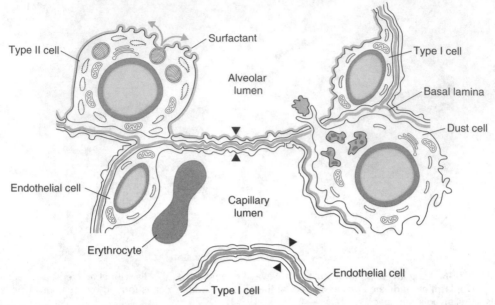

FIGURE 28-7. Lung alveoli and capillary, drawing based on electron micrographs. A squamous type I cell and a cuboidal type II cell form a portion of the wall of an alveolus. An alveolar macrophage (dust cell) with several lysosomes extends a process into the alveolar lumen. The minimal air–blood barrier is formed by part of a type I cell, part of an endothelial cell, and their fused basal laminae (*arrowheads*), and is shown in an electron micrograph in Figure 28-8.

closely invest each alveolus. Any one capillary may be shared by two or more alveoli.

D. **Collateral air circulation** occurs in the lung via openings in the interalveolar septum.

1. Adjacent alveoli are often connected by pores in the interalveolar septa that allow air circulation between the alveoli.

2. If a bronchiole is blocked, the alveoli distal to the blockage may continue to function if they are joined by pores to adjacent alveoli unaffected by the blockage.

3. Pores allowing collateral air circulation also occur between bronchioles and alveoli, and between adjacent bronchioles.

IX. **AIR–BLOOD BARRIER.** The richly vascularized, thin wall of the alveolus is specialized for the **exchange of gases** between **inspired air** in the lumen of the alveolar space and **blood-borne gases** in the perialveolar capillaries. The air–blood barrier is a thin, structurally heterogeneous layer of cells and cell products across which gases must move between the alveolar and vascular compartments (see Figure 28-7).

A. **Minimal air–blood barrier.** The components of the thinnest air–blood barrier are resolvable only with the electron microscope (Figure 28-8). The thinnest air–blood barrier is formed by:

1. A type I epithelial cell

2. A capillary endothelial cell

3. The fused basal laminae of the type I cell and the endothelial cell.

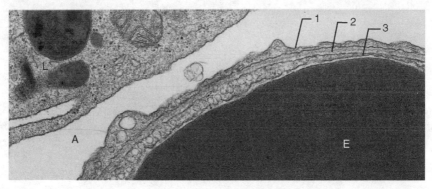

FIGURE 28-8. Lung alveolus, electron micrograph. The components of the minimal air–blood barrier are indicated: *1* = type I cell; *2* = fused basal laminae; *3* = endothelium of alveolar capillary. An erythrocyte (*E*) fills the lumen of the capillary. A portion of an intra-alveolar macrophage with lysosomes (*L*) is visible in the upper left. *A* = alveolar air space. (Courtesy of F. L. Minnear, Albany Medical College.)

B. **Thicker air–blood barrier.** More often, connective tissue cells, fibers, and ground substance are present between the two basal laminae, widening the air–blood barrier and increasing the distance across which gases must move.

X. **SURFACTANT.** Phospholipid surfactant is secreted by type II cells (see Figure 28-7).

A. Surfactant **reduces alveolar surface tension** by forming a **monomolecular layer** on the luminal surface of the alveolus.

1. An **air–phospholipid interface** is established. The air–phospholipid interface has a lower surface tension than an air–water interface.

2. An adequate supply of surfactant reduces the work involved in breathing.

B. In the absence of surfactant, a **high surface tension** develops at the air–water interface on the luminal surface of an alveolus.

1. A high surface tension can collapse the alveolus or prevent its inflation during inspiration.

2. **Hyaline membrane disease** (respiratory distress syndrome) occurs in newborns when surfactant synthesis by type II cells is inadequate.

Chapter 29

Urinary System

I. **INTRODUCTION.** The urinary system consists of the paired **kidneys,** the paired **ureters,** the **bladder,** and the **urethra** (Figure 29-1A).

II. **GENERAL CHARACTERISTICS OF THE KIDNEYS**

A. **Gross appearance.** The kidneys are paired, reddish, bean-shaped organs that lie on either side of the spinal column in the retroperitoneal space of the posterior abdominal wall. Their concave border is medial and their convex border is lateral. Each kidney is approximately 10 to 12 cm long, 6 to 7 cm wide (concave to convex margin), and 3 to 4 cm thick.

B. **Gross structure**

1. Each kidney is embedded in a thick layer of **perirenal adipose tissue** that cushions the organ. At the upper pole of each kidney, also embedded in the perirenal fat, is an **adrenal (suprarenal) gland** (see Chapter 32).

2. The **hilum** is a depression on the concave medial border of each kidney through which the renal blood vessels, lymphatic vessels, and nerves pass and through which the ureter leaves the kidney.

3. The **renal sinus** is the cavity within the hilum in which the vessels distribute to the kidney parenchyma and that contains the funnel-shaped origin of the ureter. The sinus is visible only in the sectioned kidney (Figure 29-1B).

4. A thin, tough **capsule** covers the kidney. It may be divided into an outer layer of dense irregular connective tissue and an inner layer characterized by numerous myofibroblasts. These aid in resisting the volume and pressure changes that accompany variations in kidney function.

C. **Functions**

1. **Recycling.** The kidneys retrieve essential materials, such as water, essential electrolytes, and small metabolites.

2. **Excretion.** The kidneys remove waste products of metabolism, particularly urea, from the body.

3. **Secretion.** The kidneys are endocrine organs that secrete or modify several hormones. **Renin** and **medullipin I** participate in the regulation of blood pressure. **Erythropoietin** is a growth factor that regulates red blood cell formation. Kidneys also hydroxylate **vitamin D,** a steroid prohormone, to produce its active form.

III. **ORGANIZATION OF THE KIDNEY PARENCHYMA**

A. **Cortex and medulla.** A fresh kidney, hemisected in a sagittal plane, shows a distinct outer cortex and an inner medulla (see Figure 29-1B).

1. **Cortex.** The cortex is a reddish-brown band, 1 to 2 cm thick, underlying the capsule. It consists of **renal corpuscles, convoluted portions of the proximal and distal tubules,** and only short lengths of the straight portions of the tubules. These components constitute the **cortical labyrinth.**

A

B

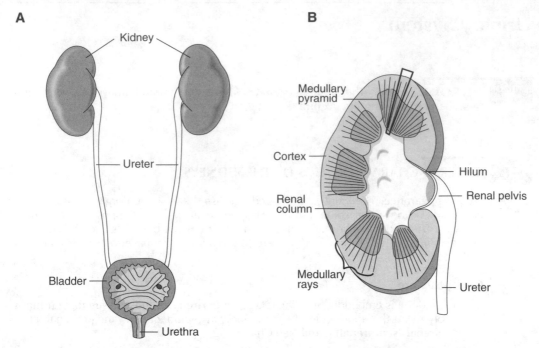

FIGURE 29-1. (*A*) Components of the urinary system. (*B*) Diagram of a hemisected kidney, indicating the principal cortical and medullary structures, and proximal components of the excretory passages. The region enclosed in a *rectangle* is enlarged in Figure 29-2. (Figure 29-1B adapted from Ross MH, Romrell LJ, Kaye GI: *Histology: A Text and Atlas,* 3rd ed. Baltimore, Williams & Wilkins, 1995, p 563.)

    a. The cortex is **highly vascularized.** Its red color is due to the fact that 90% to 95% of the blood that passes through the kidney is in the cortex.

    b. In fresh sections of kidney cortex, the **renal corpuscles** (see V A) are visible, with the unaided eye, as small red dots surrounded by tubular portions of the cortical labyrinth.

  2. Medulla. The medulla is the lighter, inner portion of the kidney parenchyma. It consists of varying lengths of the **straight portions of the proximal and distal tubules,** the **loops of Henle, collecting ducts,** as well as the **vasa recta,** which are unusually straight blood vessels.

    a. It is organized into 8 to 18 radially striated, conical structures called **medullary pyramids.**

    b. The base of each pyramid is adjacent to the cortex. The apex of each pyramid projects into the renal sinus.

B. **Renal columns and medullary rays.** Renal columns are cortical tissue that projects into the medullary domain; medullary rays are medullary tissue that projects into the cortical domain.

  1. Renal columns. The cortical tissue that caps each medullary pyramid also extends along the lateral margins of the pyramid toward the sinus, forming the renal columns (columns of Bertini or Bertin).

  2. Medullary rays. 400 to 500 parallel bundles of tubules project into the cortex from the base of each medullary pyramid. Each bundle is a medullary ray.

    a. Each medullary ray contains straight collecting tubules that connect to a collecting duct (see VI A) surrounded by many straight tubular portions of nephrons (see V C, E).

b. The nephron and the collecting tubule to which it is connected together form the **uriniferous tubule.**

C. **Lobes and lobules**

1. **Lobes.** Each lobe of the kidney consists of one medullary pyramid and the cortical tissue at its base and sides. Thus, there are normally 8 to 18 lobes in each human kidney. Some animals, notably rodents, have only one medullary pyramid and, thus, a unilobar kidney.

2. **Lobules.** A renal lobule is a narrow, cylindrical, multinephron unit of structure. Each lobule consists of a single medullary ray and the cortical tissue that drains to the collecting ducts of that medullary ray.

IV. **INTERSTITIUM OF THE KIDNEY.** The interstitial tissue is the **connective tissue** that surrounds the components of the nephrons, the ducts, and the blood and lymphatic vessels of the kidney.

A. **Cortical interstitium.** In the cortex, the principal interstitial cells are fibroblasts that are located between the tubules and the adjacent peritubular capillaries.

B. **Medullary interstitium.** In the medulla, the principal interstitial cells more closely resemble myofibroblasts and may have a role in compressing the tubular elements of the kidney.

1. Medullary interstitial cells also contain prominent lipid droplets that are associated with secretion of **medullipin I,** an antihypertensive prohormone.

2. Medullipin I is probably converted to the active hormone **medullipin II** as it circulates through the liver.

V. **NEPHRON.** The nephron is the **basic unit of structure and function** in the kidney. There are 1.5 to 2 million nephrons in each human kidney. A nephron consists of several sequential components that extend from the renal corpuscle to the collecting tubule. These are, in order, the **renal corpuscle,** the **proximal convoluted tubule,** the **straight portion of the proximal tubule,** the **thin limb of the loop of Henle,** the **straight portion of the distal tubule,** and the **distal convoluted tubule** (Figures 29-2, 29-3). The distal convoluted tubule drains through a curved **connecting tubule** to a **collecting tubule** in a medullary ray.

A. **Renal corpuscle.** The renal corpuscle (Malpighian corpuscle) is the beginning of the nephron. Renal corpuscles are found exclusively in the cortex. Those close to the medulla are corpuscles of **juxtamedullary nephrons;** the others are corpuscles of **cortical nephrons.** A corpuscle consists of a double-layered epithelial cup, the **renal capsule,** surrounding a tuft of anastomosing capillary loops, the **glomerulus** (Figures 29-4, 29-5).

1. **Renal capsule.** The renal capsule (Bowman capsule) is the portion of the nephron in which blood is **filtered** to produce **glomerular filtrate.**
   a. **Capsule structure.** The capsule consists of an inner visceral layer and an outer parietal layer. The space between the two layers of the renal capsule is the **urinary space.**
      (1) **Visceral layer.** The visceral layer is highly specialized and closely applied to the glomerular capillaries.

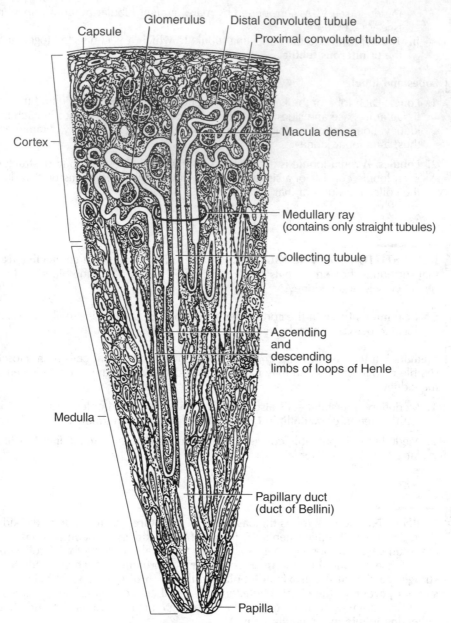

Capsule Glomerulus Distal convoluted tubule

Proximal convoluted tubule

Cortex

Macula densa

Medullary ray
(contains only straight tubules)

Collecting tubule

Ascending
and
descending
limbs of loops of Henle

Medulla

Papillary duct
(duct of Bellini)

Papilla

FIGURE 29-2. Enlarged drawing of the portion of the kidney outlined in Figure 29-1B. This drawing emphasizes the relationships of two nephrons and the collecting system to the structures of the cortex and medulla. The upper, midcortical nephron has a short loop of Henle that extends only a short distance into the medulla. The lower, juxtamedullary nephron extends a long loop of Henle deep into the medulla. Each drains through short connecting tubules into a collecting tubule and duct that are in the core of the medullary ray. (Adapted from Ross MH, Romrell LJ, Kaye GI: *Histology: A Text and Atlas*, 3rd ed. Baltimore, Williams & Wilkins, 1995, p 563.)

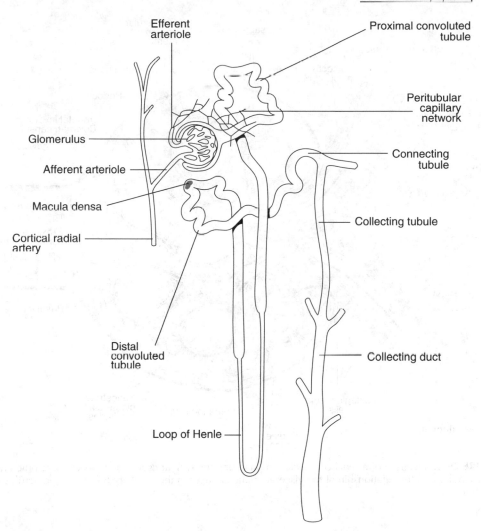

Efferent
arteriole

Proximal convoluted
tubule

Peritubular
capillary
network

Glomerulus

Connecting
tubule

Afferent arteriole

Collecting tubule

Macula densa

Cortical radial
artery

Distal
convoluted
tubule

Collecting duct

Loop of Henle

FIGURE 29-3. Drawing of a midcortical nephron, emphasizing blood supply and drainage of the glomerulus.

      (2) Parietal layer. The parietal layer is a simple squamous epithelium that is continuous with the cuboidal epithelium of the proximal convoluted tubule.

      (3) Vascular pole. The open end of the cup-shaped capsule is the vascular pole of the renal corpuscle, where an **afferent arteriole** enters the renal corpuscle and an **efferent arteriole** leaves it. The parietal layer is continuous with the visceral layer at the vascular pole.

      (4) Urinary pole. The opposite side of the renal capsule is the urinary pole of the renal corpuscle. Here, the urinary space is continuous with the lumen of the proximal convoluted tubule.

   b. Podocytes. Podocytes are the epithelial cells of the visceral layer of the renal capsule. They are specialized for filtration. The portion of the podocyte containing the nucleus sits in the urinary space. Each podocyte extends processes toward the glomerular basement membrane of several capillary loops of the glomerulus.

      (1) Pedicels. Podocyte processes ramify and form fine, finger-like cellular exten-

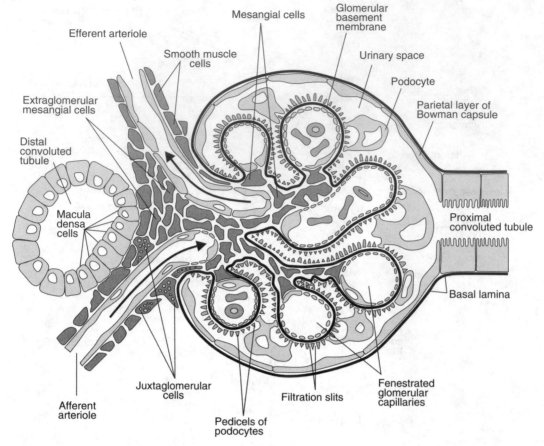

FIGURE 29-4. Diagram of a renal corpuscle, emphasizing the structures found at the vascular pole and urinary pole, and the relationship of the visceral epithelial layer to the capillary tuft of the glomerulus (not drawn to scale).

sions called pedicels, or foot processes, that wrap around the capillary loops.

(a) Pedicels are the only portions of the podocytes that are in intimate contact with the glomerular basement membrane.

(b) In addition to their role in filtration, pedicels probably help to maintain the integrity of the fine glomerular capillaries against the hydrostatic pressure exerted on them.

(2) **Filtration slits.** Pedicels of several podocytes interdigitate on each capillary loop, creating an elaborate pattern of narrow filtration slits adjacent to the glomerular basement membrane.

(a) Filtration slits are **narrow extracellular spaces,** about 25 nm wide, that allow the filtrate from the glomerular capillaries to enter the urinary space.

(b) The filtration slits are bridged by a **filtration slit membrane,** a 6-nm-thick layer that resembles the diaphragm of a capillary fenestra.

(3) The complex relationships between podocytes and their processes, and the anastomosing capillary loops of the glomerular tuft, are best appreciated in scanning electron microscope preparations.

2. **Glomerulus.** The glomerulus is formed by capillaries derived from several small ar-

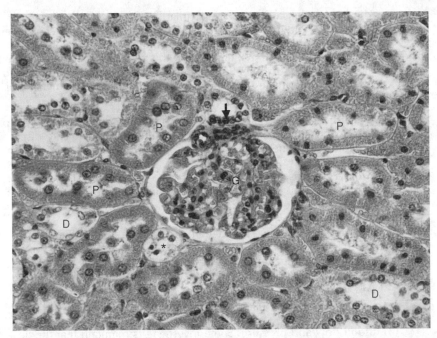

FIGURE 29-5. Light micrograph of the cortical labyrinth showing a renal corpuscle surrounded by sections through proximal (*P*) and distal (*D*) convoluted tubules. A macula densa (*arrow*) is visible in the distal tubule immediately above the afferent arteriole that supplies the glomerular capillary tuft (*G*) of this corpuscle. The cellular layer between the macula densa and the glomerulus is formed by juxtaglomerular cells. A small connecting tubule (*) is visible next to the renal corpuscle, and can be identified by the clarity of the lateral cell margins. The squamous epithelial cells of the parietal layer of the Bowman capsule are also visible.

terioles that branch from the afferent arteriole that supplies each renal corpuscle (see Figure 29-4).

a. **Glomerular lobule.** The portion of the capillary tuft derived from each small arteriole is a **lobule,** which has a connective tissue core called the **mesangial region.** The lobule is not apparent in routine histologic sections.

b. **Glomerular outflow.** The capillaries of the several lobules unite to form the efferent arteriole, which leaves the renal corpuscle and subsequently branches to form either **vasa recti** or a **peritubular capillary network** (see VII E). The glomerulus is thus the first capillary bed of an **arterial portal system.**

c. **Glomerular endothelium.** The glomerular capillary endothelium is highly fenestrated and rests on the glomerular basement membrane.

3. **Glomerular basement membrane.** The glomerular basement membrane is actually the **fused basal laminae** of the capillary endothelium and the visceral layer of the renal capsule. It is thick enough (300–350 nm) to be visible with light microscopy. The glomerular basement membrane is the principal component of the filtration barrier in the renal corpuscle, and acts both as a **physical barrier** and an **ion-selective filter.**

a. **Composition.** The glomerular basement membrane contains type IV collagen, sialoglycoproteins, and other non-collagenous glycoproteins (including laminin); as well as proteoglycans and glycosaminoglycans (particularly heparan sulfate proteoglycan).

b. **Substructure.** These components of the glomerular basement membrane are localized in three layers:

(1) The **lamina rara interna,** adjacent to the capillary endothelium, is rich in **heparan sulfate** and other polyanions and specifically impedes the passage of positively charged molecules.

      (2) The **lamina densa** is composed primarily of **type IV collagen** that is arranged in a feltwork that serves as a physical filter for molecules larger than approximately 70,000 daltons (e.g., albumin and hemoglobin).

      (3) The **lamina rara externa,** adjacent to the pedicels of the visceral epithelium, resembles the lamina rara interna in both composition and function. **Sialoglycoproteins** in both laminae rarae attach the endothelial cells and the podocytes to the glomerular basement membrane.

  4. Glomerular filtration. The filtration barrier of the renal corpuscle consists of both cellular and extracellular components. The cellular components are discontinuous; the extracellular component (the glomerular basement membrane) is continuous.

    a. Components of the filtration barrier

      (1) Glomerular basement membrane. This is the principal component of the filtration barrier. The appearance of significant amounts of protein in the urine, usually hemoglobin or albumin, indicates damage to the glomerular basement membrane.

      (2) Glomerular capillary endothelium. The fenestrated endothelium of the glomerular capillaries restricts the movement of blood cells and other formed elements from the capillaries.

      (3) Filtration slits and slit membranes. The filtration slits formed by the pedicels, and their slit membranes, act as physical barriers to bulk flow of fluid. In addition, the glycoproteins of the pedicel glycocalyx and the slit membrane may also specifically impede positively charged molecules.

      (4) Blood flow and pressure. Some investigators maintain that the flow rate and pressure in the glomerular capillaries actually serve as important regulators of the filtration process in the glomerulus.

    b. Glomerular filtrate. Nearly 180 liters of glomerular filtrate are produced in 24 hours in a normal adult human.

      (1) The initial filtrate is isosmotic with the blood and contains principally the nonprotein components of plasma (i.e., water, salts, amino acids, sugars, peptides) as well as metabolic substrates and urea.

      (2) Through the absorptive and secretory activities of the rest of the nephron and of the collecting tubules and ducts, a final volume of about 1500 ml of hypertonic urine is produced daily—less than 1% of the volume of primary filtrate.

  5. Mesangium. The mesangium is a complex of mesangial cells and extracellular matrix found in the interstitial spaces between glomerular capillary loops, and in association with the vessels of the vascular pole.

    a. Glomerular mesangial cells are located within the basal lamina of the glomerular capillaries. In this regard, they resemble the pericytes of postcapillary venules in other parts of the body.

      (1) Mesangial cells **phagocytize** trapped residues and protein aggregates from the glomerular basement membrane, clearing the glomerular basement membrane of debris.

      (2) They provide **structural support** for the capillary loops where the endothelial basal lamina may be absent or incomplete.

      (3) They may have a role in **regulating blood flow** through the glomerulus. They are derived from smooth muscle precursors and are **contractile.** They respond to angiotensin II, a vasoconstrictor, as well as to atriopeptides, which are vasodilators.

    b. Extraglomerular mesangial cells located outside the renal corpuscle at the vascular pole are also called **lacis cells** and form part of the **juxtaglomerular apparatus** (see V G).

B. **Proximal convoluted tubule.** The urinary space of the renal capsule drains to the proximal convoluted tubule. The proximal convoluted tubules are approximately 15 mm long and, collectively, constitute the largest part of the renal **cortical labyrinth.** The proximal convoluted tubule and the proximal straight tubule together constitute the

proximal thick segment of the nephron (see Figure 29-2). The complex processes of absorption and secretion that produce the final urine begin in the proximal tubule.

1. **Cytologic characteristics.** The proximal convoluted tubule is lined with cuboidal cells that have elaborate **surface amplifications** usually associated with **absorption** and **fluid transport.** In well-fixed preparations, these characteristics help to distinguish the cells of the proximal convoluted tubule from those of other parts of the nephron (Figure 29-6).

   a. **Apical brush border.** A well-developed microvillous border faces the lumen of

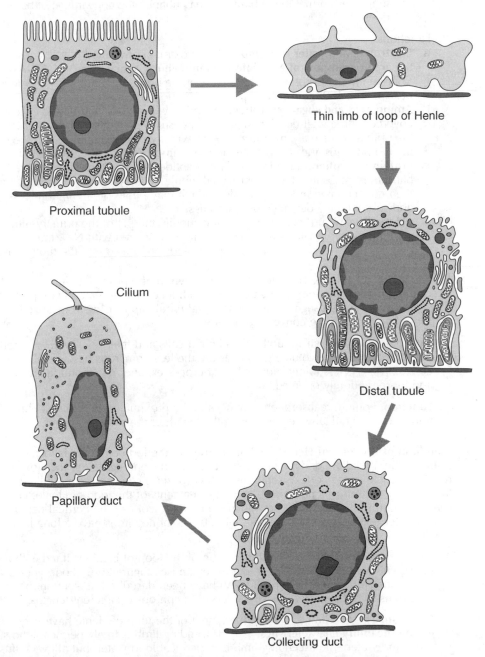

FIGURE 29-6. Drawings of cell types typical of various parts of the tubular portion of the nephron and the collecting system.

the tubule. A shallow junctional complex seals the apical end of the intercellular space and separates the apical plasma membrane domain from the lateral membrane domain.

    b. Lateral plications. Large, flattened processes on the lateral margins of the cells implicate with similar processes of adjacent cells.

    c. Basal interdigitations. There is extensive interdigitation of basal processes of adjacent cells.

        (1) This gives the base of the proximal tubule cell a **striated** appearance when viewed with the light microscope.

        (2) Mitochondria concentrated in the basal processes and oriented with their long axes normal to the basal lamina enhance the appearance of basal striations.

2. Functions

    a. Electrolyte and water resorption. The proximal convoluted tubule cells use the **active transport of Na^+ into the intercellular space by a Na^+,K^+-ATPase** to drive the reabsorption of about 80% of the primary filtrate, thus recycling approximately 150 liters of fluid per day.

    b. Amino acid and sugar resorption. The microvilli of proximal tubule cells are covered with a well-developed glycocalyx. Small peptides and disaccharides in the primary filtrate are hydrolyzed by enzymes in the glycocalyx, and the resulting amino acids and monosaccharides are absorbed by the tubule cells.

    c. Protein resorption. Proteins and large peptides that get through the filtration barrier are reabsorbed by the proximal tubule cells by endocytosis. They are then concentrated in large vacuoles, which may be visible by light microscopy, and subsequently degraded by lysosomes.

    d. pH modification. Proximal tubule cells modify the pH of the primary filtrate by resorbing bicarbonate as a secondary anion associated with Na^+ transport, and by secreting specific exogenous organic acids and bases into the tubular fluid.

C. **Proximal straight tubule.** The thick straight segment of the proximal tubule is the **thick descending limb of the loop of Henle.** It has both a cortical and medullary portion. The cells of the straight segment of the proximal tubule appear less specialized for absorption than those of the convoluted portion.

    1. Cytologic characteristics. Both the cuboidal cells and their microvilli are shorter than those of the convoluted tubule, as are the less numerous basolateral processes. There is less implication of lateral processes, and mitochondria are smaller and more randomly oriented.

    2. Function. Sodium reabsorption continues in the proximal straight tubule, but the transport rate gradually declines along the length of the straight segment.

D. **Thin limb of the loop of Henle.** The thin portion of the loop of Henle is located exclusively in the medullary domain and is short or long depending on the location of its renal corpuscle in the cortex. Nephrons with corpuscles close to the medulla (i.e., juxtamedullary nephrons) tend to have long thin segments of the loop of Henle. Nephrons with corpuscles located more superficially in the cortex (i.e., cortical nephrons) have shorter thin segments. In humans, about 15% of nephrons have a long loop of Henle.

    1. Cytologic characteristics. The thin portion of the loop of Henle is lined with a **simple squamous epithelium** throughout its length (see Figure 29-6). Four types of squamous epithelial cells (types I to IV) have been described in electron micrographs of different portions of the loop in nephrons of different lengths.

    2. Function. The two limbs of the thin segment of the loop of Henle have very different **permeability characteristics.** The descending limb is freely permeable to salt, urea, and water. The ascending limb is impermeable to water, but allows diffusion of salt and urea. This difference is essential for concentration of the urine (see VIII A).

E. **Distal straight tubule.** The thick straight segment of the distal tubule is the **thick ascending limb of the loop of Henle.** It has both medullary and cortical portions.

1. **Cytologic characteristics.** In routine histologic sections, the distal tubule epithelial cells stain lightly with eosin and the margins are indistinct (see Figure 29-6).
   a. The nucleus is more apically located than in cells of the proximal tubule, often causing the apical portion of the cell to bulge into the lumen.
   b. The epithelial cells have numerous large mitochondria associated with basal plications, but have considerably fewer apical microvilli than proximal tubule cells.

2. **Function.** This segment also allows movement of ions from the tubule lumen to the interstitium of the kidney.
   a. Cl^-, Na^+, and K^+ diffuse into the cell from the lumen. Cl^- and Na^+ then diffuse out of the cell across the basolateral plications; K^+ largely diffuses back into the lumen to be recycled.
   b. This spatial redistribution of ions gives the misleading impression of a Cl^- pump operating in this segment.

3. **Macula densa.** This specialized portion of the distal tubular epithelium is involved in blood pressure regulation (see V G). It is located approximately at the junction between the straight and convoluted portions of the distal tubule.

F. **Distal convoluted tubule.** The distal convoluted tubule is located in the cortical labyrinth. It is only about one-third as long as the proximal convoluted tubule.

1. **Cytologic characteristics.** The cells of the distal convoluted tubule are similar to those of the distal straight tubule.

2. **Function.** The distal convoluted tubule is the site of several absorptive and secretive activities.
   a. **Na^+ is reabsorbed** from the urine and K^+ is secreted into the urine. **Aldosterone** secreted by the adrenal gland under stimulation by angiotensin II (see V G 2) increases the reabsorption of Na^+ and secretion of K^+. This increases blood pressure and volume.
   b. **Reabsorption of bicarbonate** takes place, with concomitant secretion of hydrogen ions into the lumen to increase the acidity of the urine.
   c. **Ammonia is converted to ammonium ions,** which then enter the urea cycle, thereby avoiding the toxic effects of ammonia.

G. **Juxtaglomerular apparatus.** The juxtaglomerular apparatus is composed of the macula densa, juxtaglomerular cells, and extraglomerular mesangial cells. It **regulates systemic blood pressure** through a complex series of enzymatic and regulatory steps.

1. **Components**
   a. **Macula densa.** This is a portion of wall of the distal segment of the nephron close to the junction between the straight and convoluted portions. It lies directly adjacent to the vascular pole of its renal corpuscle (see Figures 29-4, 29-5). The distal tubule cells at this site are taller and more closely packed than other distal tubule cells and their nuclei often seem to overlap, hence the name.
   b. **Juxtaglomerular cells.** At this same site, smooth muscle cells in the wall of the afferent arteriole (and, sometimes, the efferent arteriole) are modified into secretory cells, called juxtaglomerular cells (JG cells). They contain stored secretory granules.
   c. **Extraglomerular mesangial cells.** The extraglomerular mesangium is in immediate proximity to these specialized structures at the vascular pole.

2. **Blood pressure regulation**
   a. The cells of the macula densa monitor blood sodium concentration and blood volume. Decreases in either of these cause release of a factor by the macula densa cells that stimulates JG cells to secrete an aspartyl peptidase called **renin.**

(1) In the blood, renin catalyzes the hydrolysis of circulating **angiotensinogen** to the **angiotensin I.** Angiotensin I is then hydrolyzed to the active octapeptide **angiotensin II** by an enzyme in lung tissue.

(2) Angiotensin II then stimulates the release of the hormone **aldosterone** from the zona glomerulosa of the adrenal gland (see Chapter 32 III B).

  b. Aldosterone increases resorption of sodium in the distal tubule, and consequent resorption of water, thus raising blood volume and blood pressure.

VI. DUCT SYSTEM OF THE KIDNEY. The duct system of the kidney begins at the end of the distal convoluted tubule in the cortical labyrinth, proceeds through the medullary rays into the medullary pyramids, and ends at the tip of the renal papilla (see Figure 29-2).

A. Organization of the duct system

1. Connecting tubules. The distal convoluted tubules empty into tubules in the cortical labyrinth that connect them to the small-diameter, straight collecting tubules in the medullary ray.

  a. Superficial cortical nephrons have relatively straight connecting tubules.

  b. Midcortical and juxtamedullary nephrons have arched connecting tubules.

2. Collecting ducts

  a. Cortical ducts. Small-diameter collecting tubules in the medullary rays merge to form the large-diameter cortical collecting ducts that define the core of the medullary ray.

  b. Medullary ducts. As the cortical collecting ducts enter the medulla to become the medullary collecting ducts, they continue to merge at acute angles, eventually forming the large papillary ducts (ducts of Bellini).

3. Papillary ducts. The papillary ducts measure 200 to 300 μm in diameter and drain into the **minor calyces** at the surface of the papillary apex. The **area cribrosa** is the portion of the papillary surface on which the ducts empty.

B. Epithelium of the duct system

1. Cell types. The lining epithelium of the connecting tubules and collecting ducts contains several types of cells. Lateral margins are usually obvious in histologic preparations because of the paucity of lateral implication of adjacent cells. This can help distinguish these cells from epithelial cells of tubules of the nephron.

  a. Distal convoluted tubule cells may extend for varying distances into the collecting system.

  b. Connecting tubule cells (CNT cells) are low cuboidal to squamous cells that have a small Golgi apparatus and numerous small mitochondria but few other organelles. The apical surface is relatively smooth, but there are numerous basal infoldings between which the mitochondria are concentrated.

  c. Collecting duct cells (CD cells, principal cells, light cells) are pale-staining cells with a round, centrally located nucleus and **numerous basal infoldings** (see Figure 29-6).

  (1) As in the CNT cells, these are true infoldings, not merely implicated processes of adjacent cells.

  (2) CD cells contain small spherical mitochondria in the apical cytoplasm above the infoldings, and have a few short microvilli and a single, centrally located cilium.

  d. Intercalated cells (IC cells, dark cells) are characterized by the presence of numerous microplicae on their apical surface and a dense cytoplasm with numerous mitochondria and vesicles. They do not have basal infoldings.

2. Distribution of cell types. The many cell types of the connecting tubules and collecting ducts gradually diminish in the cortical and medullary collecting ducts, leaving only CD cells and IC cells.

    a. CD cells gradually increase in height until they become columnar in the papillary ducts.

    b. The number of IC cells gradually decreases in the medullary collecting ducts, and they are not present in the papillary ducts.

    c. At the area cribrosa, the epithelium gradually changes from the columnar epithelium of the ducts to the transitional epithelium characteristic of the excretory passages of the urinary system.

C. **Hormonal regulation of collecting duct function.** The collecting ducts are not merely conduits; the final concentration of urine depends on regulation of the permeability of the collecting system by antidiuretic hormone (ADH) released from the neurohypophysis of the pituitary gland (see Chapter 30 IV A 1, Table 30-2).

1. **ADH increases the permeability of the epithelium** of the collecting tubules and collecting ducts, thereby promoting the movement of water from the lumen of the duct into the medullary interstitium, and movement of urea from the interstitium into the papillary ducts.

2. **When ADH secretion is increased,** an extremely hypertonic urine is produced, thereby conserving body water.

3. **When ADH secretion is diminished** or absent, a copious watery urine is produced. When this is a pathologic situation, it is called **diabetes insipidus.**

VII. RENAL CIRCULATION

A. **Renal arteries and interlobar arteries.** Paired **renal arteries** arise from the abdominal aorta and usually divide into two branches before entering each kidney. The renal arteries branch in the renal sinus into **interlobar arteries** that course toward the periphery in the renal columns, between the medullary pyramids.

B. **Arcuate arteries and interlobular arteries.** As an interlobar artery approaches the corticomedullary junction, it branches into several **arcuate arteries.**

1. **Arcuate arteries.** The arcuate arteries run along the bases of the medullary pyramids, parallel to the convex surface of the kidney.

2. **Interlobular arteries.** Interlobular arteries, also called **cortical radial arteries,** branch at right angles from the arcuate arteries and run radially toward the periphery of the cortex in the cortical labyrinth.

    a. The interlobular arteries are generally located at the midpoint between the medullary rays, indicating the lateral margins of the adjacent lobules.

    b. As they traverse the cortex , interlobular arteries give off numerous **afferent arterioles** (Figure 29-7).

C. **Arterioles**

1. **Afferent arterioles** enter the renal corpuscle at the vascular pole and branch into the anastomosing loops of fenestrated capillaries that constitute the glomerulus.

2. **Efferent arterioles** are formed by the convergence of the glomerular capillaries and leave the renal corpuscle at the vascular pole.

D. **Postglomerular secondary capillary networks** arise from the efferent arterioles.

1. **Cortex. Peritubular capillaries** of the labyrinth arise from efferent arterioles from cortical glomeruli. Evidence is accumulating that the endothelial cells of these capillaries are the source of **erythropoietin.**

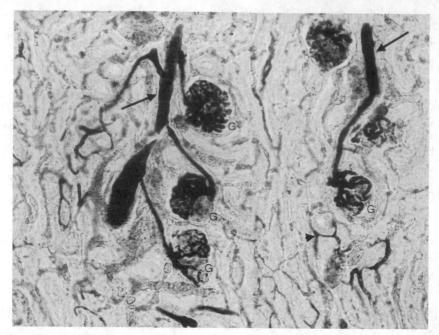

FIGURE 29-7. Light micrograph of kidney cortex from a specimen in which the vascular system has been injected with a contrast medium. Two interlobular arteries (cortical radial arteries, *arrows*) give rise to afferent arterioles that supply glomerular capillary tufts (*G*). Contrast medium that has left the glomerulus via the efferent arteriole is visible in several peritubular capillaries (*arrowhead*) in the cortical labyrinth.

2. **Medulla.** Efferent arterioles of juxtamedullary glomeruli form either **peritubular capillaries** in the medulla or **vasa recta.** These capillaries form networks at various levels in the medulla that perfuse the tubular structures of the pyramid and subserve the countercurrent exchange functions.

E. **Vasa recta.** The vasa recta form vascular loops parallel to the loops of Henle. They arise as unbranched **arteriolae rectae** from the efferent arterioles of the juxtamedullary renal corpuscles.

1. The arterioles descend into the medulla and make a hairpin turn deep in the medullary pyramid. The vessels then ascend as the **venulae rectae.**

2. Both the arterial and venous sides of the loop are thin-walled vessels. Plexuses of fenestrated capillaries connect them at various medullary levels.

F. **Venous drainage.** Venous flow in the kidney generally follows a reverse course to arterial flow, although there is considerable anastomosis in the venous drainage.

1. **Cortical capillaries** drain to **interlobular veins** that then drain to **arcuate veins, interlobar veins,** and the **renal vein.**

2. **Medullary capillaries** drain to venulae rectae that join the cortical outflow at the arcuate vein.

3. **Superficial cortical capillaries** and **capsular capillaries** drain to **stellate veins** in the peripheral cortex, that then drain to the interlobular veins. *Stellate* refers the appearance of the veins when viewed from the kidney surface.

G. **Renal lymphatic vessels.** The kidneys contain two networks of lymphatic vessels.

1. One network is located in the peripheral cortex and drains to large lymphatic vessels in the capsule.

2. The other network is more deeply located in the kidney parenchyma and drains to large lymphatic vessels in the renal sinus. There are numerous anastomoses between the two networks.

VIII. **HISTOPHYSIOLOGY OF THE KIDNEY.** The ability to produce a hypertonic urine derives from a combination of three morphologic specializations: the **loop of Henle,** the **vasa recta,** and the fact that the **collecting ducts pass through the medulla.**

A. **Countercurrent multiplier.** The loop of Henle creates and maintains a gradient of hypertonicity in the medullary interstitium from the corticomedullary junction to the renal papilla.

1. **The descending limb** of the loop of Henle is **freely permeable to Na^+, Cl^-, and water.**

2. **The ascending limb** of the loop of Henle is **impermeable to water,** but the thick limb allows movement of Na^+ and Cl^- from the lumen of the nephron to the surrounding interstitium.
   a. Because water cannot follow the ions out of the ascending limb, the **interstitium becomes hypertonic** relative to the luminal contents.
   b. Some of the Na^+ and Cl^- ions in the interstitium diffuse back into the nephron at the descending limb, only to be put back into the interstitium at the ascending limb.
   c. The opposite directions of flow in the descending and ascending limbs of the loop of Henle constitute a **countercurrent.** The cycling of Na^+ and Cl^- from ascending limb to interstitium to descending limb, and again into the flow to the ascending limb; added to the sodium chloride coming along the nephron with newly arriving preliminary urine; produces a **multiplier effect,** giving rise to the term **countercurrent multiplier system.**

3. **Medullary osmotic gradient.** In this manner, a standing gradient is produced, in which the concentration of sodium chloride in the interstitium gradually increases from the corticomedullary margin to the tip of the medullary papilla. Urea adds to the hypertonicity of the medullary interstitium by diffusing out of the medullary collecting ducts and papillary ducts.

B. **Countercurrent exchange.** The vasa recta and the medullary collecting ducts interact with the interstitium in a **countercurrent exchange system.**

1. The **arteriolae rectae** descend through the medulla, losing water to the interstitium and gaining salt from the interstitium. At the tip of the loop of the vasa recta, the blood is essentially equilibrated with the hypertonic deep medullary interstitium.

2. As the **venulae rectae** ascend through the medulla, the process is reversed; the blood loses salt to the interstitium and gains water from the interstitium.

3. This **exchange of salt and water** between the vasa recta and the interstitium, as the blood flows in opposite directions in the arterioles and venules, constitutes one aspect of the countercurrent exchange system.

4 As the collecting ducts and papillary ducts pass through the increasingly hypertonic interstitium on their way to the renal papilla, water passes from the urine to the interstitium and the urine becomes hypertonic.
   a. The **exchange of water** between the urine and the interstitium is regulated by ADH.
   b. When ADH levels in the blood are abnormally low, the walls of the collecting ducts and papillary ducts are relatively impermeable to water, and a hypotonic urine is produced.
   c. When ADH levels in the blood are abnormally high, the permeability of the col-

lecting system increases markedly, and an unusually hypertonic urine is produced.

IX.   RENAL NERVE SUPPLY.
The fibers that form the renal plexus are mostly derived from the sympathetic division of the autonomic nervous system. They cause the contraction of vascular smooth muscle to produce vasoconstriction.

A. Effects of sympathetic stimulation

1. **Constriction of the afferent arterioles** reduces the glomerular filtration rate and the production of urine.

2. **Constriction of the efferent arterioles** increases the glomerular filtration rate and increases the production of urine.

B. Nonessential role of nerve supply.
Despite these neural effects on glomerular filtration rate, the extrinsic nerve supply is not necessary for normal kidney function. Nerve fibers to the kidney are cut during renal transplantation and the transplanted kidney subsequently functions normally, implying that hormonal secretions are the more important factors in regulation of kidney function.

X.   EXCRETORY PASSAGES OF THE URINARY SYSTEM.
On leaving the papillary ducts at the area cribrosa, the urine enters a series of structures that do not modify it but that are specialized for its storage and conveyance to the exterior of the body. The urine passes sequentially to a **minor calyx,** a **major calyx,** the **renal pelvis,** and leaves each kidney through a **ureter.** The ureter carries it to the **urinary bladder,** where it is stored. The urine is finally voided through the **urethra** (see Figure 29-1).

A. Histologic characteristics

1. **Transitional epithelium.** Transitional epithelium (see Chapter 5 IV B 4) lines all of the excretory passages except for the final segments of the urethra. It is essentially impermeable to salts and water.

2. **Distensibility.** The ability of transitional epithelium to become thinner and flatter conveys distensibility to the lining of the excretory passages.
   a. In the **undistended state,** surface epithelial cells are rounded cells with occasional deep **clefts** invaginating their apical cytoplasm. These cells bulge into the lumen, giving the surface an irregularly scalloped appearance (Figure 29-8).
      (1) The apical cytoplasm of the epithelial cells contains numerous **fusiform vesicles** that are bounded by a membrane with the same characteristics as the plasma membrane.
      (2) Transmission electron microscopy resolves these vesicles as infolded **plaques of thickened plasma membrane.**
   b. In the **distended state,** the fusiform vesicles appear to be reinserted into the surface plasma membrane as the mucosa is stretched and the transitional epithelial cells change shape from cuboidal to squamous (see Figure 5-1).

3. **Connective tissue and muscle.** A dense collagenous **lamina propria** and **two layers of smooth muscle** underlie the transitional epithelium of the excretory passages. There is neither a muscularis mucosae nor a submucosal layer in the walls of the excretory passages.

B. Calyces.
The calyces are cup-like extensions of the renal pelvis that are the beginning of the excretory passages of the urinary system (see Figure 29-1).

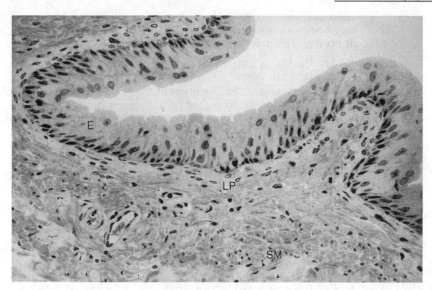

FIGURE 29-8. Light micrograph of urinary bladder mucosa. Transitional epithelium (*E*) is in its undistended state and shows its characteristically scalloped luminal surface. *LP* = lamina propria, *SM* = smooth muscle.

1. **Minor calyces** cap each medullary pyramid in the renal sinus and funnel into 3 or 4 major calyces.

2. **Major calyces,** in turn, fuse to form the funnel-shaped **renal pelvis,** which then narrows to form the proximal portion of the ureter.

C. **Ureters.** The ureters carry urine from the renal pelvis of each kidney to the urinary bladder (see Figure 29-1).

1. **Smooth muscle of the ureters.** The muscle layers are arrayed in two concentric helices. The inner layer is a **loose helix,** generally described as a **longitudinal layer.** The outer layer is a **tight helix,** generally described as a **circular layer.**
   a. This orientation is opposite to that of the smooth muscle of the muscularis externa of the intestinal tract.
   b. The smooth muscle is mixed with considerable connective tissue so that it forms parallel bundles rather than sheet-like layers (again, contrasting with the muscularis externa of the intestine).
   c. Near the entry of the ureter into the bladder, a third layer is found external to the outer layer, running parallel to the long axis.

2. **Ureter–bladder junction**
   a. The ureters follow an oblique path through the posterior wall of the bladder and the muscle of the ureters merges with that of the bladder.
   b. As the bladder distends with urine, the openings of the ureters into the bladder are compressed, reducing the possibility of reflux of urine from the bladder into the ureters and protecting the kidney from the potential spread of infection from the bladder.

D. **Urinary bladder.** The urinary bladder is a distensible reservoir for urine; its size and shape change as it fills.

1. **Smooth muscle and sphincter.** The smooth muscle of the bladder wall is even less regularly arranged than that of the tubular passages. Smooth muscle and collagen bundles are randomly mixed in the bladder wall.
   a. Contraction of the smooth muscle of the bladder compresses the entire hollow viscus, forcing the urine into the urethra.

b. In addition to compressing the ureteric orifices, the smooth muscle of the bladder forms a ring-like arrangement around the origin of the urethra, creating the **internal urethral sphincter.**

2. Innervation. The bladder is innervated by both the **sympathetic** and **parasympathetic** divisions of the autonomic nervous system.

  a. The parasympathetic fibers are the **efferent fibers** of the **micturition reflex.** Sympathetic fibers primarily innervate the blood vessels of the bladder.

  b. Sensory fibers from the bladder to the sacral spinal cord are the **afferent fibers** of the micturition reflex.

E. **Urethra.** The fibromuscular duct through which urine reaches the body surface is the urethra. The size, structure, and functions of the urethra are different in males and females.

1. Female urethra. The female urethra is 3 to 5 cm in length from the bladder to the vestibule of the vagina, where it normally terminates just below the clitoris.

  a. It has a crescent-shaped lumen and is lined through most of its length with a stratified squamous epithelium. Some mucin-secreting glands may be found in invaginations of the mucosal surface.

  b. The lamina propria is a highly vascularized connective tissue with abundant elastic fibers. It resembles the corpus spongiosum of the male.

  c. Striated muscle of the urogenital diaphragm forms the **external sphincter** of the female urethra.

2. Male urethra. The male urethra is about 20 cm long and serves as the terminal duct of both the urinary and reproductive systems. It can be divided into three segments: prostatic, membranous, and penile.

  a. The **prostatic urethra** begins at the neck of the bladder and extends for 3 to 4 cm through the prostate gland (see Chapter 36 VII B). It is lined with transitional epithelium continuous with that of the bladder.

  b. The **membranous urethra** extends about 1 cm from the apex of the prostate gland, through the urogenital and pelvic diaphragms, to the bulb of the corpus cavernosum of the penis.

    (1) Transitional epithelium ends in the membranous urethra and is replaced by stratified or pseudostratified columnar epithelium.

    (2) The skeletal muscles of the urogenital and pelvic diaphragms form what is called the **external (voluntary) urethral sphincter.**

  c. The **penile urethra** extends for about 15 cm through the length of the penis to the glans. It is lined with pseudostratified columnar epithelium except at the distal end, where it is lined with a stratified squamous epithelium continuous with that of the skin of the glans penis.

    (1) It is surrounded by the **corpus spongiosum,** a highly vascularized, loose, elastic connective tissue that is one of the three columns of erectile tissue of the penis (see Chapter 36 VIII A).

    (2) Ducts of the bulbourethral glands (Cowper glands), which secrete preseminal fluid, as well as ducts of the mucus-secreting glands of Littré, empty into the penile urethra.

Chapter 30

Pituitary Gland and Hypothalamus

I. **INTRODUCTION TO ENDOCRINE SYSTEM.** The pituitary gland, or hypophysis, and the hypothalamus are components of the two great coordinating systems of the body: the **nervous system** (Chapter 6) and the **endocrine system** (Chapters 30–34). Directly or indirectly, secretions by the cells of these two systems influence all the cells and tissues in the body.

A. **Endocrine glands.** Endocrine glands are **ductless glands** that release hormones into the bloodstream.

B. **Hormones.** Hormones are carried via the bloodstream to all parts of the body and exert their influence on **target** tissues and organs.

1. **Hormone receptors.** Target cells often lie a great distance away from the site of hormone release. These cells possess receptors specific for a particular hormone.

2. **Hormone effects.** Hormone effects are generally of **slower onset and longer duration** than those of the nervous system, which usually cease as soon as neurotransmitter release ceases. Hormonal responses are also more generalized because hormones reach target cells in widely dispersed sites in the body.

3. **Classes of hormones.** Cells of the endocrine system release more than 50 different hormones. They can be divided into three classes of compounds:
   a. **Steroids** are cholesterol-derived molecules that are synthesized and secreted by cells of the adrenal cortex, ovaries, and testes.
   b. **Peptides, proteins, and glycoproteins** are synthesized and secreted by cells of the hypothalamus, pituitary gland, adrenal gland, parathyroid gland, pancreas, pineal gland, and scattered endocrine cells of the gastrointestinal tract and respiratory system.
   c. **Amino acid analogs and derivatives** (e.g., catecholamines) are synthesized and secreted by cells in the adrenal medulla, as well as by many neurons. **Thyroxine,** an iodinated amino acid, is synthesized and secreted by cells in the thyroid gland.

C. **Blood supply of endocrine glands.** The endocrine glands are highly vascularized organs. This reflects their highly active metabolism, and the fact that the blood supply both brings to the glands the metabolites necessary for the synthesis of the hormones, and carries away the secreted hormones.

II. **PITUITARY GLAND** (Figure 30-1). The pituitary gland, or **hypophysis,** has been called the master gland because its secretions have general effects on cells of the entire body, including direct effects on the function of several other endocrine organs. The **hypothalamus,** the portion of the brain to which the pituitary gland is attached, and the pituitary gland together play central roles in a variety of regulatory feedback systems.

A. **Gross structure and development.** The pituitary gland is a small, compound endocrine gland located in the **sella turcica,** a saddle-shaped depression in the sphenoid bone. The pituitary is attached to the hypothalamus by a short stalk called the **infundibulum.** In humans, the pituitary gland weighs approximately 0.5 to 1.5 g. It contains both **glandular** and **neural** components, which derive from stomodeal ectoderm and brain ectoderm, respectively.

FIGURE 30-1. Diagram of a section through the human pituitary gland and regions of the hypothalamus.

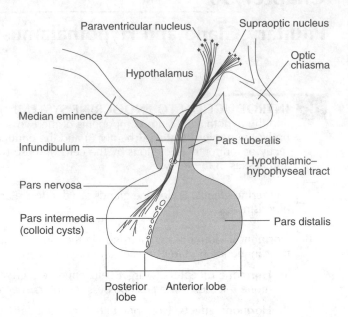

1. **Adenohypophysis**
   a. **Morphology.** The adenohypophysis consists of the **pars distalis** (anterior lobe), **pars tuberalis,** and **pars intermedia** (intermediate lobe).
   b. **Embryology.** The adenohypophysis is derived from a dorsal evagination of the roof of the pharynx known as the **Rathke pouch.** This evagination contacts and closely associates with a downward growth from the brain, the developing neurohypophysis. The Rathke pouch eventually loses its connection to the pharynx.
      (1) A hollow structure is thus formed. The posterior wall, attached to the neural evagination, becomes the pars intermedia of the pituitary. In humans, it is vestigial and remains as a collection of cysts.
      (2) The anterior wall proliferates and becomes the pars distalis. A dorsal extension partially wraps around the infundibular stalk and becomes the pars tuberalis.

2. **Neurohypophysis**
   a. **Morphology.** The neurohypophysis consists of the **pars nervosa** (posterior lobe), and the **infundibulum,** which is continuous with the **median eminence** of the hypothalamus.
   b. **Embryology.** The neurohypophysis is derived from a downward growth of the base of the midbrain toward the roof of the pharynx.

B. **Blood supply.** The vasculature of the pituitary is unique and plays an important role in the regulation of pituitary function. The pituitary receives blood from the **superior** and the **inferior hypophyseal arteries** (Figure 30-2). Both are branches of the internal carotid artery.

1. The **superior hypophyseal arteries** supply a capillary network in the median eminence, the infundibular stalk, and the pars tuberalis.

2. The **inferior hypophyseal arteries** supply a capillary network located primarily in the pars nervosa.

3. **Hypophyseal portal system** (Figure 30-3). The pars distalis receives no direct arterial supply. Instead, a venous portal system brings blood from the capillary bed in the median eminence (the **primary capillary bed**) to the capillary network of the anterior lobe (the **secondary capillary bed**).

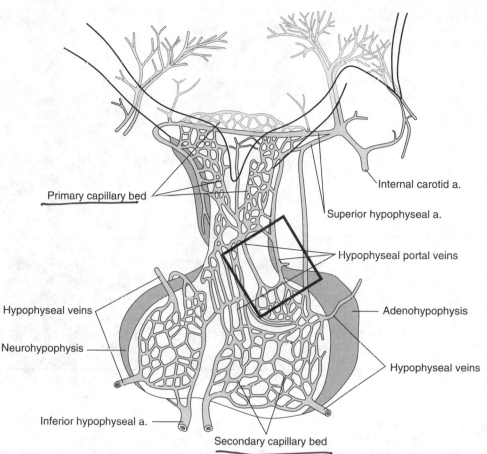

FIGURE 30-2. Diagram of the blood supply to the hypophysis. Branches of the carotid artery, the superior hypophyseal artery and the inferior hypophyseal artery, supply the adenohypophysis and the neurohypophysis. The blood supply to the adenohypophysis is indirect, first forming a capillary bed in the median eminence and infundibulum. This primary capillary bed is drained by the hypophyseal portal veins that empty into a secondary capillary bed in the adenohypophysis. The capillary bed in the neurohypophysis receives its blood supply directly from the arteries that supply it. Both capillary beds are drained by the hypophyseal veins. Histologic section of the region in the square is shown in Figure 30-3. (Adapted from Ross MH, Romrell LJ, Kaye GI: *Histology: A Text and Atlas,* 3rd ed. Baltimore, Williams & Wilkins, 1995, p 598.)

> **a.** These portal veins, the hypophyseal portal veins, carry neuroendocrine secretions of hypothalamic nerves that end in the median eminence directly to the cells in the pars distalis.
>
> **b.** These hypothalamic secretions help regulate the secretions of cells in the pars distalis.

4. Most of the blood from the pituitary gland drains into the cavernous sinus at the base of the diencephalon, and then into the systemic circulation.

> **a.** There is some evidence of the existence of short portal veins between the pars distalis and the pars nervosa. Thus blood could flow from the pars distalis to the pars nervosa, and from the pars nervosa toward the hypothalamus.
>
> **b.** These short pathways could provide a means for the hormones of the pars distalis to feedback directly to the brain without making a complete circuit of the circulatory system.

FIGURE 30-3. Section showing hypophyseal portal veins extending between the infundibulum and the pars distalis.

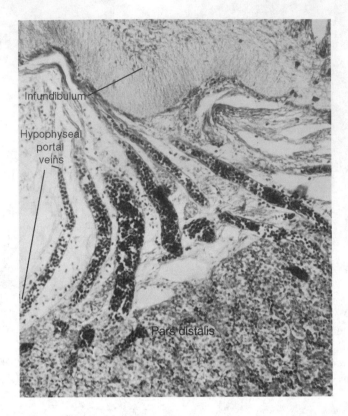

Infundibulum

Hypophyseal portal veins

Pars distalis

III. **ADENOHYPOPHYSIS.** The cells in the adenohypophysis are arranged in clumps and cords surrounded by large-diameter, fenestrated capillaries. These cells synthesize and secrete **tropic hormones,** which influence other endocrine glands and tissues throughout the body. The general nature and effects of these tropic hormones are summarized in Table 30-1.

A. **Morphologic classification**

1. **Staining characteristics.** The cells in the pars distalis were originally classified into groups based on the staining characteristics of the secretory granules within the cells. Using mixtures of acidic and basic dyes, three cell types were identified according to their staining reactions: **acidophils** (40% of cells), **basophils** (10%), and **chromophobes** (50%) (Figure 30-4).

2. **Immunohistochemistry.** More recently, the hormone contents of the cells in these groups have been identified positively by using hormone-specific antibodies and immunohistochemistry. The cells are now classified according to their hormone content.

3. **Cytoplasmic characteristics.** It is also possible to distinguish the cells in the adenohypophysis by electron microscopy. The secretory granules in each cell type have distinctive morphologic characteristics. In addition, the cells themselves can be distinguished by size, shape, and distribution of organelles.

B. **Pars distalis.** The cells of the anterior lobe of the pituitary gland synthesize and secrete several peptide and protein hormones.

1. **Acidophils.** The acidophils are subdivided into two cell types: **somatotropes** and **lactotropes** (mammotropes). These cells synthesize and secrete the simple polypeptides **growth hormone** (somatotropin) and **prolactin** (mammotropin), respectively.

TABLE 30-1. Tropic Hormones of the Adenohypophysis

Hormone	Structure	Molecular Weight	Functions
Somatotropin (growth hormone, GH)	Simple protein	21,700	Stimulates kidney and liver to synthesize and secrete somatomedin, which stimulates growth of long bones
Prolactin (PRL)	Simple protein	22,500	Promotes mammary gland development; initiates and maintains milk secretion
Adrenocorticotropic hormone (ACTH)	Small polypeptide	4500	Stimulates secretion of glucocorticoids by zona fasciculata of the adrenal cortex; maintains structure of zona fasciculata
Follicle-stimulating hormone (FSH, follitropin)	Two-chain glycoprotein	25,000	Stimulates follicular growth in ovaries and increases spermatogenic activity in testes
Leuteinizing hormone (LH, lutropin)	Two-chain glycoprotein	30,000	Stimulates corpora lutea formation and ovulation in female and stimulates testosterone secretion and maintenance of secondary sexual characteristics in male
Thyroid-stimulating hormone (TSH, thyrotropin)	Two-chain glycoprotein	26,600	Stimulates growth of thyroid epithelial cells and secretion of thyroid hormones to the blood
Lipotropin (LPH)	Small polypeptides	9900	No known function in humans; has lipotropic activity in other species

2. **Basophils.** The gonadotropes, thyrotropes, corticotropes, and lipotropes fall into this category. In addition to staining with basic dyes, basophils also stain with the periodic acid–Schiff (PAS) reaction for carbohydrates.
   a. **Gonadotropes** produce the glycoproteins **follicle-stimulating hormone** (FSH) and **leuteinizing hormone** (LH). Gonadotropes are the only secretory cell type of the adenohypophysis that secretes more than one hormone.
   b. **Thyrotropes** produce the glycoprotein **thyroid-stimulating hormone** (TSH).
   c. **Corticotropes** produce **adrenocorticotropic hormone** (ACTH) and **lipotropes** produce β-**lipotropin.** Both hormones are simple polypeptides that are derived from the same large precursor molecule, pro-opiomelanocortin (POMC), which is a glycoprotein (see III B 4).

3. **Chromophobes.** These cells were originally classified as chromophobes because they did not stain with any of the classic stains. The large percentage of cells identified as chromophobes was significantly reduced by the use of immunocytochemistry combined with electron microscopy. Most of the chromophobes were observed to have a small number of hormone-containing secretory granules. The small number of granules is below the limit of detection with routine staining procedures.

4. **Pro-opiomelanocortin.** POMC is a 31 kD glycoprotein that is synthesized by several

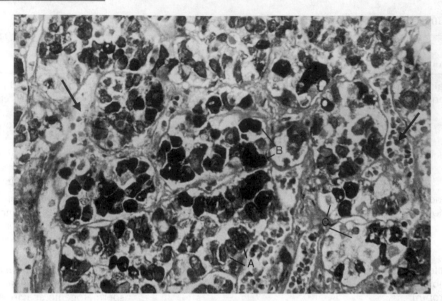

FIGURE 30-4. Light micrograph of a portion of the pars distalis. Acidophils (*A*), basophils (*B*), and chromophobes (*C*) are visible. The cells are arranged in cords and clumps, separated by a fine connective tissue stroma that contains blood vessels (*arrows*).

cell types in the pars distalis and the pars intermedia. It is a precursor for several peptide and polypeptide hormones.

a. The amino acid sequences for the hormones ACTH, melanocyte-stimulating hormone (α-MSH), β-lipotropin, endorphins, and enkephalins are all contained within the amino acid sequence of POMC. POMC is differentially cleaved into these hormones by proprotein convertases that are packaged with it in secretory granules.

b. Corticotropes, lipotropes, and melanotropes (see III C 1) can sometimes be stained with the same polyclonal antibody, an observation that suggests that they all produce the same hormones. However, the common staining pattern results because the antibody recognizes POMC, the precursor of the three hormones.

C. **Pars intermedia.** The intermediate lobe is a vestigial organ in the human. It consists of a series of small cysts that are remnants of the Rathke pouch (Figure 30-5). The cysts are filled with a colloid substance of unknown function.

1. In species other than man, the intermediate lobe is much more developed and contains **melanotropes,** cells that synthesize and secrete **melanotropins** (i.e., MSH). These cells are basophils that stain with the PAS reaction.

2. In the human adenohypophysis, melanotropes are scattered throughout the anterior lobe.

D. **Pars tuberalis.** The pars tuberalis is a highly vascularized upward extension of the anterior pituitary. The veins of the hypophyseal portal system run in this region. The endocrine cells, which are primarily gonadotropes, are arranged in cords in association with the vasculature.

IV. NEUROHYPOPHYSIS

A. **Pars nervosa** (see Figure 30-5). The posterior lobe of the pituitary gland contains the umyelinated axons and axonal endings of neuroendocrine cells, the cell bodies of

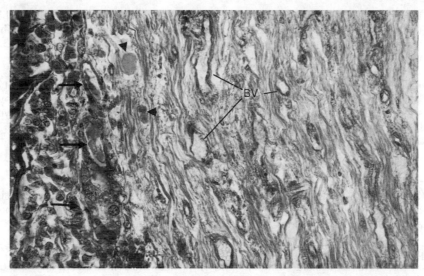

FIGURE 30-5. Light micrograph of a portion of the junction of the pars nervosa (*right*) and the pars distalis and pars intermedia (*left*). The pars nervosa is formed primarily by unmyelinated nerve processes. Stored neurosecretions (oxytocin and antidiuretic hormone) called Herring bodies are visible in the pars nervosa (*arrowheads*). Small cysts, adjacent to the pars nervosa, are evidence of the pars intermedia (*arrows*). *BV* = blood vessels.

which lie in the **paraventricular and supraoptic nuclei** of the hypothalamus. The axons terminate near the vessels of the capillary network in the pars nervosa.

1. **Site of hormone storage and release.** The pars nervosa is the site of storage and release of two hormones, **oxytocin** and **antidiuretic hormone** (ADH), also known as **vasopressin.** The general nature and effects of these hormones are summarized in Table 30-2.
   a. The hormones are **synthesized in the hypothalamus** in the cell bodies of neurosecretory cells.
   b. The secretory granules move by axonal transport (see Chapter 6 II C 3 e) in the infundibulum to the synaptic endings in the pars nervosa.
      (1) Oxytocin and ADH are synthesized in separate neurons and are thus released from separate axonal endings following the appropriate stimulation.
      (2) The axonal endings often aggregate to form **Herring bodies,** large fusiform swellings filled with secretory product, which are visible with the light microscope (see Figure 30-5).
         (a) Electron microscopy reveals that the axonal endings are filled with dense core vesicles, 50 to 80 nm in diameter, containing ADH or oxytocin.
         (b) Smaller (30 nm in diameter), clear vesicles containing acetylcholine are also found.

TABLE 30-2. Hormones of the Neurohypophysis

Hormone	Functions
Oxytocin	Stimulates contraction of uterine smooth muscle cells during parturition; stimulates contractile activity of myoepithelial cells of mammary ducts and ejection of milk (milk let-down factor).
Antidiuretic hormone (ADH, vasopressin)	Increases water permeability of luminal membrane of kidney collecting-duct epithelium, resulting in decreased urine output; increases blood pressure by stimulating smooth muscle cells in peripheral arterioles

2. Pituicytes. Surrounding the axons in the pars nervosa are specialized glial-like cells called pituicytes. Pituicytes contain the intermediate filament protein **glial fibrillary acidic protein,** a marker for central nervous system astrocytes (see Chapter 3 IV A 2 c). These cells are the only cell type that is specific to the neurohypophysis.

B. Infundibulum. The infundibulum connects the neurohypophysis to the brain. It contains the axons that carry the neurohormone containing secretory granules from the hypothalamus to the pars nervosa. The collection of axons is called the **hypothalamic–hypophyseal tract.**

V. HYPOTHALAMIC REGULATION OF HYPOPHYSIS.
In addition to oxytocin and ADH, cells in the hypothalamus secrete several neurohormones that regulate the synthesis and secretion of hormones by cells in the adenohypophysis.

A. Hypophyseal portal system and endocrine regulation. Axons of neurosecretory cells located in several hypothalamic nuclei end on or near the primary capillary bed of the hypophyseal portal system.

1. Following exocytosis, neurohormones secreted from these axons enter the primary capillary bed and are carried in portal veins to the secondary capillary bed, where they leave the circulation and bind to receptors on the plasma membrane of target cells.

2. These neurohormones are either stimulatory or inhibitory to the cells in the adenohypophysis with which they interact. The general nature and effects of these neurohormones are summarized in Table 30-3.

B. Feedback loops. Feedback loops regulate endocrine functions at two levels: tropic hormone production in the hypophysis and neurohormone production in the hypothalamus.

1. Hypophysis-initiated feedback loop. Hormones released by cells of the adenohypophysis stimulate distant target organs to secrete hormones. The hormones released by these organs, in turn, stimulate their own set of target cells. These distant organs

TABLE 30-3. Neurohormones of the Hypothalamus

Hormone	Structure	Functions
Thyrotropic-releasing hormone (TRH)	Tripeptide	Stimulates TSH and prolactin release
Gonadotropin-releasing hormone (GnRH)	Decapeptide	Stimulates FSH and LH release
Growth hormone–releasing hormone (GHRH)	Protein (40–44 amino acids)	Stimulates GH release
Corticotropin-releasing hormone (CRH)	Protein (41 amino acids)	Stimulates ACTH release
Somatostatin	Tetradecapeptide (14 amino acids)	Inhibits GH and TSH release (also inhibits insulin and glucagon release in pancreas)
Prolactin release–inhibiting factor (PIF; most likely dopamine)	Monoamine amino acid neurotransmitter	Inhibits prolactin release

TSH = thyroid stimulating hormone, FSH = follicle-stimulating hormone, LH = leuteinizing hormone, ACTH = adrenocorticotropic hormone, GH = growth hormone.

can also regulate their own secretions by feeding back on cells in the hypophysis and hypothalamus.

  a. **Feedback to the hypophysis—a one-step process** . Target tissue–released hormones can be carried back to the adenohypophysis, where they bind to tropic hormone producing cells to regulate tropic hormone release. For example, following stimulation of the adrenal cortex by ACTH, glucocorticoids bind to receptors in corticotropes in the hypophysis and reduce their secretion of ACTH.

  b. **Feedback to the hypothalamus—a two-step process.** Target tissue–released hormones can also interact with cells in the hypothalamus indirectly to regulate the activity of the target cells.

  (1) Target cell hormones modulate secretory activity of hypothalamic neuroendocrine cells.

  (2) Hypothalamic secretions, in turn, then regulate secretion of tropic hormones in the pars distalis.

  (3) For example, glucocorticoids can bind to corticotropin-releasing hormone (CRH)-producing cells in the hypothalamus, attenuating their secretions, which, in turn, results in reduced stimulation of corticotropes and reduced secretion of ACTH.

2. **Inputs from higher brain centers.** Information from physiologic and psychologic stimuli activates sensory pathways that can promote the release of stimulatory or inhibitory hormones by cells in the hypothalamus.

  a. Some of these hormones are released into the hypophyseal portal system and are transported to the adenohypophysis to regulate secretory activity there.

  b. Other hypothalamic neurons, whose axons travel to the neurohypophysis in the hypothalamic–hypophyseal tract, are stimulated to release oxytocin or ADH into the general circulation.

Chapter 31

Thyroid and Parathyroid Glands

I. **INTRODUCTION.** The thyroid and parathyroid glands are generally discussed together because they are close to each other anatomically, and because secretions of both play a major role in calcium homeostasis.

II. **THYROID GLAND.** The thyroid gland secretes **thyroxine (tetraiodothyronine, T_4)** and **triiodothyronine (T_3).** The thyroid hormones play a major role in regulation of the basal metabolic rate. **Calcitonin** is also secreted by the thyroid gland and is involved in calcium homeostasis.

A. **Structure and development.** The thyroid gland is a bilobed organ lying across the second and third cartilaginous rings of the trachea. The lobes are connected by a narrow isthmus. The thyroid weighs 15 to 20 grams, and is slightly heavier in the male than in the female.

1. The thyroid is derived from the **thyroid diverticulum,** an invagination of the endoderm that arises from the floor of the oropharynx near the root of the developing tongue.

2. The thyroid diverticulum grows and divides into two lateral lobes. The lateral lobes remain connected by the isthmus.

3. A rich network of fenestrated capillaries develops in the sparse connective tissue of the developing thyroid gland (Figure 31-1).

B. **Histologic characteristics.** The parenchyma of the thyroid gland is composed of groups of tightly packed **follicles,** spherical structures that range in diameter from 0.05 to 1.0 mm (Figure 31-2).

1. **Follicle epithelium.** The wall of the follicle is formed by a simple epithelium that synthesizes and secretes T_4 and T_3.
   a. Follicular cells have the ultrastructural morphology of a cell that is active in protein synthesis. The cytoplasm is filled with an extensive rough endoplasmic reticulum (rER) and prominent Golgi apparatus.
   b. The epithelial cells range in shape from low cuboidal to tall columnar, depending on the activity of a particular follicle. The apical surface of the cells faces the lumen of the follicle.
   c. The follicles are filled with thyroid **colloid,** a homogeneously staining, eosinophilic, proteinaceous material primarily consisting of **thyroglobulin,** which is secreted into the follicle by the epithelial cells.

2. **Parafollicular cells** (calcitonin cells, C cells). Parafollicular cells that synthesize and secrete calcitonin are the second type of endocrine cell found in the thyroid.
   a. Parafollicular cells have the ultrastructural characteristics of cells that are active in protein synthesis and in regulated secretion (i.e., abundant rER, prominent Golgi apparatus, numerous secretory granules).
   b. They occur as single cells or as clumps of cells associated with the thyroid epithelium or scattered in the interstitial connective tissue.
   c. Parafollicular cells are difficult to discern in routine histologic sections, but are readily identifiable with immunohistochemical procedures that employ antibodies to calcitonin.
   d. Parafollicular cells are derived from neural crest cells that migrate into the developing thyroid gland.

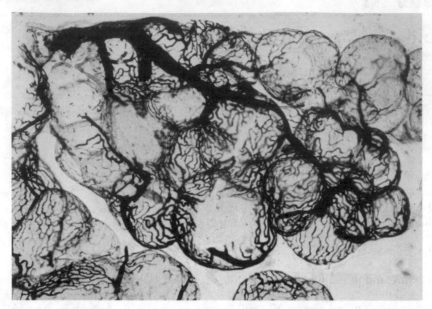

FIGURE 31-1. Injection of the vasculature of the thyroid gland showing the distribution of perifollicular blood vessels. Each follicle is surrounded by an intricate network of capillaries that carries secretions of the gland to the general circulation.

C. **Thyroid hormone** (Figure 31-3)

    1. Synthesis. The principal secretions of the thyroid gland are the thyroid hormones, T_4 and T_3. They are formed from iodinated tyrosine residues in thyroglobulin.

        a. Thyroglobulin. Thyroglobulin is a large (660 kD) glycoprotein that is synthesized on the rER, glycosylated in the rER and Golgi apparatus, and constitutively se-

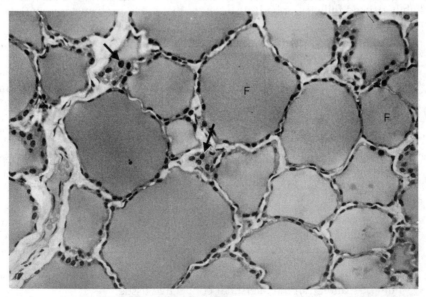

FIGURE 31-2. Thyroid gland, light micrograph. The wall of each thyroid follicle (*F*) is composed of a single layer of low cuboidal epithelial cells. The homogeneous mass in the center of the follicle is thyroglobulin (colloid), the glycoprotein precursor of thyroid hormone. Clumps of cells (*arrows*) are visible in the sparse interfollicular connective tissue and also in the follicle wall. These cells are most likely calcitonin-secreting parafollicular cells (C cells).

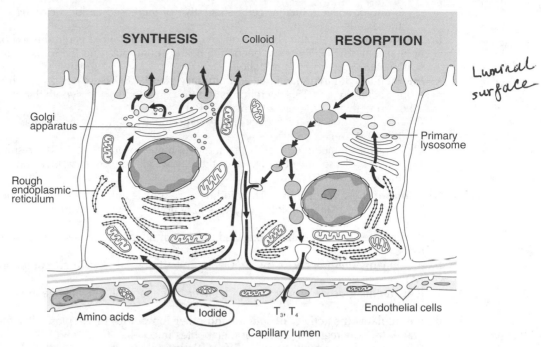

Luminal surface

FIGURE 31-3. Diagram illustrating structural–functional relationships in thyroid follicular cells. *Arrows* indicate the general metabolic pathways of thyroglobulin synthesis and iodination, and thyroglobulin resorption and processing, to form thyroxine (T_4) and triiodothyronine (T_3). The processes of synthesis and resorption are shown in the diagram as occurring in separate cells; however, both processes occur simultaneously in each follicular cell. (Adapted from Ross MH, Romrell LJ, Kaye GI: *Histology: A Text and Atlas,* 3rd ed. Baltimore, Williams & Wilkins, 1995, p 612.)

creted in small vesicles. Thyroglobulin is stored extracellularly in the lumen of the follicle as **colloid.**
  b. Iodination. Tyrosine residues are iodinated as thyroglobulin is secreted.
    (1) Follicle cells have an active iodide uptake mechanism in their basal membrane.
    (2) Iodide is transported to the luminal surface of the follicular cells, where it is oxidized to an activated form by a membrane peroxidase. Activated iodide is then coupled to tyrosyl residues in thyroglobulin, forming **monoiodotyrosine** (MIT) and **diiodotyrosine (DIT).**
  c. Formation of T_3 and T_4. In the colloid, iodinated tyrosines (MIT and DIT) undergo **oxidative coupling** that results in the formation of T_3 and T_4.
  d. Endocytosis and the release of thyroid hormone. Colloid is resorbed by the follicle cells by receptor-mediated endocytosis. These endocytic vesicles are larger than the secretory vesicles. Endocytic vesicles containing thyroglobulin then fuse with lysosomes.
    (1) Thyroglobulin is degraded by lysosomal proteases into constitutive amino acids, T_4, and T_3.
    (2) Thyroid hormones are released into the circulation as T_4 and T_3. The other amino acids are reutilized by the cells.

2. Regulation of synthesis. Thyroid hormone synthesis is regulated by **thyroid-stimulating hormone** (TSH), which is produced by the pituitary gland.
  a. Active follicles. Continued stimulation by TSH results in an increase in the amount and activity of the organelles of protein synthesis (i.e., rER, Golgi apparatus) in follicular cells.
    (1) The cells become columnar and the amount of colloid is greatly decreased.
    (2) Clear, nonstaining regions appear in the colloid near the apical plasma mem-

brane of active follicular cells, suggestive of increased endocytic activity by these cells.

   b. Inactive follicles. In the absence of TSH, synthesis of colloid is diminished or nonexistent. The cells flatten, becoming nearly squamous, and the follicle lumen remains enlarged and full of colloid.

   c. Interaction with hypothalamus and pituitary gland. TSH regulates thyroid hormone secretion, and TSH secretion is in turn regulated by the hypothalamic neurohormone thyroid-releasing hormone (TRH).

   (1) Thyroid hormone feeds back on the hypothalamus and on the pituitary to inhibit TSH secretion.

   (2) Exposure to acute cold activates the hypothalamus to release TRH, resulting in TSH release and stimulation of the thyroid gland to release thyroid hormone.

3. Functions of thyroid hormone. Thyroid hormone affects almost all organs in the body. Among the many physiologic roles and actions of thyroid hormone are the following:

   a. It **stimulates basal metabolic rate** and utilization of carbohydrates, lipids, and proteins.

   b. It **augments thermogenesis** by stimulating mitochondrial oxygen consumption and ATP production.

   c. It **augments glucose production** in the liver by enhancing gluconeogenesis and glycogenolysis.

   d. It **modulates the activity of sodium and other ion pumps** of the plasma membrane, thereby regulating entry of metabolites into cells.

   e. It is required for **nervous system differentiation** in early development.

4. Goiter. Goiter is an **enlarged thyroid gland** and is indicative of **abnormal thyroid function,** either **hypothyroidism** or **hyperthyroidism.** There are several etiologies; two examples follow.

   a. Iodine-deficiency (endemic) goiter. Endemic goiter and **hypothyroidism** can be caused by insufficient dietary iodine.

   (1) The hypothyroidism is characterized by deficient production of T_3 and T_4.

   (2) The low levels of thyroid hormone stimulate release of excessive amounts of TSH, causing enlargement of the thyroid through hypertrophy of the follicular cells and synthesis and increased storage of poorly iodinated thyroglobulin.

   b. Toxic goiter (Graves disease). In this form of **hyperthyroidism,** thyroid cells are continuously stimulated by autoantibodies that bind to follicular cells and stimulate them (Figure 31-4).

   (1) Continual stimulation produces an increase in the number and size of follicle cells, increasing follicular mass.

   (2) Because secretion is so rapid, there is little stored colloid. Toxic amounts of thyroid hormone are often produced.

   (3) Before it was discovered that the stimulating factor was an autoantibody, it was called long-acting thyroid stimulator (LATS).

D. Calcitonin. Parafollicular cells contain dense-core secretory granules that contain calcitonin.

1. Regulation of secretion. Calcitonin secretion appears to be controlled directly by blood calcium levels.

   a. Hypercalcemia, an increased blood level of calcium, is the stimulus for calcitonin secretion.

   b. Upon stimulation, calcitonin-containing secretory granules move to the plasma membrane and release their contents by exocytosis.

2. Function of calcitonin. Calcitonin lowers blood calcium levels and, together with secretions of the parathyroid gland, maintains blood calcium homeostasis.

III. PARATHYROID GLANDS. The parathyroid glands secrete **parathyroid hormone** (PTH), which is also involved in calcium homeostasis. The parathyroid glands are neces-

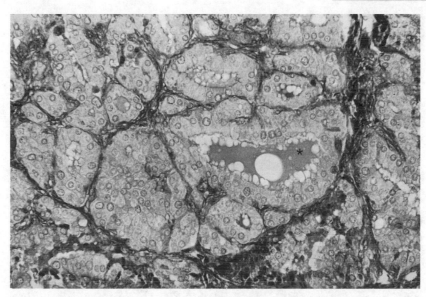

FIGURE 31-4. Light micrograph of thyroid gland from a patient with toxic goiter (Graves disease). The follicular epithelium is hyperplastic and is formed mainly by columnar cells. Most follicles do not contain colloid. Scalloping of the intrafollicular colloid is prominent in the follicle that contains colloid (*). Such scalloping also appears in very active, nonpathologic thyroid glands.

sary for life. Their removal results in a drop in blood calcium levels, resulting in tetanic convulsions and death.

A. **Structure and development.** In humans, four parathyroid glands are usually found embedded within the connective tissue capsule on the posterior surface of the thyroid gland: one each at the inferior and superior poles of the two lobes of the thyroid gland. Their precise location is variable, however.

1. Each gland is approximately 5 mm long, 3 mm wide, and 1 to 2 mm thick. Their size may vary depending on the age of the individual and state of calcium metabolism.

2. The glands are derived from the third and fourth branchial pouches.
   a. The glands that lie near the upper poles of the thyroid lobes derive from the fourth pouch.
   b. The glands at the lower poles of the thyroid lobes derive from the third branchial pouch. The locations of these glands vary the most, and they occasionally exist as ectopic glands in the mediastinum.

B. **Histologic characteristics.** The parathyroid glands consist of closely packed groups of cells that may occur as clumps, cords, or acini. Two cell types predominate: **chief cells** and **oxyphil cells** (Figure 31-5). Adipocytes may also be present. The glands are highly vascularized.

1. **Chief cells** synthesize and secrete parathyroid hormone. They are small (8–10 μm in diameter) and spherical in shape.
   a. Their ultrastructure is commensurate with cells that have an active regulated secretory pathway (i.e., abundant rER, prominent Golgi apparatus, numerous secretory granules).
   b. At certain stages of activity, chief cells contain abundant glycogen and lipid droplets. Because of this, in routine histologic preparations the cells may appear vacuolated, and are called **clear cells.**

2. **Oxyphil cells** are larger than chief cells and have a grainy eosinophilic cytoplasm. Their function is unknown.

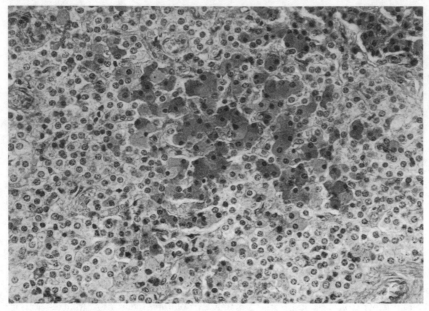

FIGURE 31-5. Light micrograph of portion of parathyroid gland. A clump of dark-staining oxyphil cells is surrounded by the smaller and more lightly stained chief cells.

     a. Their cytoplasm is filled with mitochondria, free ribosomes, and glycogen. Secretory granules, however, are absent.

     b. Oxyphil cells in humans appear around puberty and increase in number with age.

3. Adipocytes appear in the parathyroid glands at puberty and increase in number until approximately age 40, after which their proportional content in the gland remains relatively constant.

C. **Parathyroid hormone.** PTH is a polypeptide, 84 amino acids in length.

1. Synthesis. PTH is initially synthesized as a larger precursor protein, **preproparathyroid hormone.**

     a. This precursor protein undergoes two proteolytic cleavages to yield PTH.

     b. PTH is stored in secretory granules of chief cells and is released by exocytosis.

2. Regulation of secretion. Release of PTH is controlled by the level of calcium in the blood. Chief cells possess recognition sites for Ca^{2+} on their plasma membrane.

     a. Hypocalcemia. When serum Ca^{2+} concentration is low, PTH is released.

     b. Hypercalcemia. Serum Ca^{2+} levels also exert a negative feedback on chief cells, depressing PTH secretion when blood Ca^{2+} concentration rises above the normal range.

D. **Calcium homeostasis.** The reciprocal actions of PTH and calcitonin help to maintain blood Ca^{2+} at approximately 10 mg/100 ml.

1. Physiologic roles of PTH. PTH acts on a number of organs to raise plasma calcium concentration and to indirectly lower plasma phosphate concentration.

     a. Bone mineral metabolism. Osteoclasts are stimulated to mobilize calcium by secreting acid phosphatase that breaks down the hydroxyapatite, thus releasing Ca^{2+} and PO_4^{3-} into the blood. The initial effect of PTH stimulation is on osteoclasts, but prolonged stimulation will also mobilize osteocytes to participate in bone resorption (osteocytic osteolysis).

     b. Renal effects. PTH increases renal tubular absorption of Ca^{2+} and, at the same time, increases renal excretion of PO_4^{3-}.

    c. Intestinal effects. PTH directly enhances intestinal uptake of Ca^{2+}.

        (1) PTH also enhances intestinal uptake of Ca^{2+} indirectly, by stimulating biosynthesis of vitamin D by the kidney.

        (2) Vitamin D increases calcium uptake across the gut epithelium throughout the small and large intestines, particularly in the duodenum.

2. Physiologic roles of calcitonin. Calcitonin exerts its effects to lower serum Ca^{2+} by acting as an antagonist to PTH effects.

    a. Calcitonin inhibits the activity of PTH on osteoclasts by preferentially inhibiting osteoclastic bone-resorption activity without disturbing osteoblastic mineralization activity. In fact, calcitonin may enhance the movement of serum Ca^{2+} into the bone mineralization compartment.

    b. Calcitonin also enhances Ca^{2+} secretion by the kidney.

3. Rate of homeostatic activity. Several hours are required to reach the peak increase in serum Ca^{2+} levels due to PTH, a relatively **slow homeostatic action.** Calcitonin, on the other hand, lowers serum Ca^{2+} in less than an hour, a **rapid homeostatic action.**

Chapter 32

Adrenal Gland

I. **INTRODUCTION.** The adrenal gland is a **compound endocrine gland** composed of two tissues of different origin that produce two classes of hormones, which are structurally unrelated. The **adrenal cortex** is responsible for the synthesis and secretion of a number of **steroid hormones.** The **adrenal medulla** is responsible for the synthesis and secretion of **catecholamines** (epinephrine and norepinephrine).

II. **DEVELOPMENT AND STRUCTURE**

A. **Development of the adrenal gland.** The cortical and medullary tissues of the adrenal gland originate from separate primordia during embryonic development.

1. The **cortex** arises from coelomic mesoderm in the genital ridge of the embryo.

2. The **medulla** arises from presumptive sympathetic ganglion tissue, which is a neural crest derivative. The neural crest cells migrate into the developing gland.

3. The **fetal adrenal gland** is a temporary organ found only in the fetus. It arises from coelomic mesoderm and produces steroid hormones (see V).

B. **Gross structure.** The adrenal glands, which weigh 3.5 to 4.5 grams in humans, are flattened organs that are roughly pyramidal in shape. They lie at the superior pole of each kidney, hence the alternative term, **suprarenal glands.**

1. **Capsule.** The glands are encased in a thick connective tissue capsule.

2. **Vasculature**
   a. **Blood supply.** The glands are well vascularized and receive arterial branches from the phrenic arteries, renal arteries, and aorta. The vessels do not enter at a hilum, but penetrate the capsule over its surface.
      (1) **Cortical capillaries.** Capsular arteries form a plexus in the capsule and give off arterioles that supply the fenestrated capillaries surrounding the cortical cells. These capillaries eventually connect to the medullary capillaries.
      (2) **Cortical arterioles.** Other cortical arterioles pass through the cortex, terminating in the capillary network in the medulla.
   b. **Drainage.** The **medullary capillaries** perfuse the cords of medullary cells and then merge to form the single large **medullary vein** that drains the organ.
   c. **Implications of the dual blood supply.** The medullary tissues receive arterial blood directly, via the cortical arterioles, as well as blood that has passed through the cortex, via the cortical capillaries, after having bathed the cortical cells. This blood has given up some of its oxygen and contains cortical secretions, which influence the secretions of the cells of the medulla.

III. **ADRENAL CORTEX.** The cortex of the adrenal gland secretes three major classes of steroid hormones: **glucocorticoids, mineralocorticoids,** and **weak androgens.**

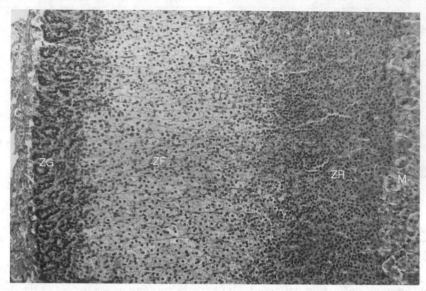

FIGURE 32-1. Adrenal cortex. Light micrograph of adrenal gland showing a section through the entire cortical region and part of the medulla (*M*). The cortex is divided into three zones: zona glomerulosa (*ZG*), zona fasciculata (*ZF*), and zona reticularis (*ZR*). A thick connective tissue capsule (*C*) surrounds the gland.

A. **Histologic organization of the cortex.** The adrenal cortex is divided into three morphologically and functionally discrete zones (Figure 32-1).

1. **Zona glomerulosa.** This is a thin **outer layer** that comprises 15% of the cortical volume. The cells of the zona glomerulosa are arranged in irregular clusters and curved columns that are surrounded by a rich network of fenestrated capillaries.
   a. The cells are small, columnar or pyramidal in shape, and stain darkly. They are continuous with the cords of cells in the zona fasciculata.
   b. The cells have morphologic characteristics typical of steroid-secreting cells: abundant smooth endoplasmic reticulum (sER), many Golgi elements, and numerous mitochondria. Lipid droplets are sparse. Free polysomes and some rough endoplasmic reticulum (rER) cisternae are also present.

2. **Zona fasciculata.** This is a thick **middle layer** that comprises 80% of the cortical volume. The cells of the zona fasciculata are arranged in long parallel cords, 1 to 2 cells thick, with the long axes of the cords perpendicular to the surface of the organ. The cords are separated by fenestrated sinusoidal capillaries.
   a. The cells are polyhedral or columnar, and stain lightly with eosin.
   b. The cytoplasm is filled with numerous, large lipid droplets. Because the lipid is extracted with organic solvents in routine histologic preparations, the cytoplasm appears highly vacuolated in section.
   c. These cells also contain abundant sER and mitochondria, a large Golgi apparatus, and many profiles of rER. The mitochondria contain tubular cristae, a characteristic of many steroid-secreting cells.

3. **Zona reticularis.** This is the **innermost layer** of the cortex, comprising 5% of cortical volume. The cells in the zona reticularis are arranged into a network of anastomosing cords, surrounded by fenestrated capillaries.
   a. The cells are smaller than those of the zona fasciculata. Both lightly and darkly stained cells appear in this layer.
   b. These cells resemble the steroidogenic cells of the other two layers of the cortex. Lipid droplets and rER are sparse. The darkly staining cells contain abundant lipofuscin granules.

B. **Mineralocorticoids.** The cells of the **zona glomerulosa** synthesize and secrete mineralocorticoids that regulate sodium and potassium homeostasis and water balance.

1. **Aldosterone.** The principal mineralocorticoid is aldosterone, which stimulates the resorption of Na^+ by distal and collecting tubules of the kidney, and by cells of salivary and sweat glands. Aldosterone also promotes excretion of K^+ by the kidney.

2. **Renin–angiotensin system.** Regulation of secretion by zona glomerulosa cells is under feedback control of the renin–angiotensin system.
   a. In response to lowered blood pressure or to a fall in serum sodium, juxtaglomerular cells in the kidney (see Chapter 29 V G 2) secrete the hormone **renin.**
   b. In the blood, renin catalyzes the cleavage of circulating **angiotensinogen** to **angiotensin I,** which is further cleaved to **angiotensin II** by **angiotensin-converting enzyme** (ACE) located in the plasma membrane of lung capillary endothelial cells.
   c. Angiotensin II then stimulates cells in the zona glomerulosa to secrete aldosterone.
      (1) Aldosterone stimulates the resorption of sodium by the kidney tubules, which increases the osmolarity of the blood. The juxtaglomerular cells respond to the resultant increase in blood pressure by attenuating renin secretion.
      (2) Drugs designed to interfere with the action of ACE in the lung (ACE inhibitors) are very effective in the treatment of essential hypertension.

C. **Glucocorticoids.** The cells of the **zona fasciculata** synthesize and secrete glucocorticoids, steroid hormones that have a general effect on virtually every tissue of the body through a wide range of effects on protein, fat, and carbohydrate metabolism.

1. **Hydrocortisone (cortisol).** Hydrocortisone, the principal secretion of the zona fasciculata, acts on many different cells and tissues to increase the availability of glucose and fatty acids. Glucocorticoids are anabolic in some cells (e.g., hepatocytes) but are catabolic in others (e.g., skeletal muscle, adipose tissue).
   a. **Anabolic effects.** Hydrocortisone stimulates **gluconeogenesis** (glucose synthesis) and **glycogenesis** (glycogen polymerization), and promotes the uptake of amino acids and fatty acids in the liver.
   b. **Catabolic effects.** In fat cells, glucocorticoids stimulate **lipolysis,** the breakdown of lipids to glycerol and fatty acids. In muscle cells, glucocorticoids stimulate **proteolysis.** The fatty acids and amino acids thus released become available as substrates for gluconeogenesis in hepatocytes.
   c. **Other effects.** Glucocorticoids have **anti-inflammatory** and **immunosuppressive** activities at higher than physiologic concentrations. Systemic levels of these steroids can be raised as the result of disease processes (e.g., Cushing disease) or by therapeutic administration.
      (1) Glucocorticoids inhibit the infiltration of macrophages and leukocytes into affected tissues during inflammation. They also reduce the inflammatory reaction by stabilizing lysosomal membranes, which prevents the secretion of enzymes that normally occurs during this process.
      (2) Glucocorticoids exert an immunosuppressive action through lympholytic actions that induce atrophy of the lymphatic system, thus lowering the circulating levels of lymphocytes.

2. **Hypothalamus–pituitary–adrenal interactions.** The regulation of synthesis and secretion of glucocorticoids is controlled by feedback interactions among the hypothalamus, the pituitary gland, and the zona fasciculata.
   a. **Stimulation. Corticotropin-releasing hormone** (CRH), secreted by hypothalamic neurosecretory cells, stimulates **corticotrophs** in the adenohypophysis to secrete **adrenocorticotropic hormone** (ACTH) [see Chapter 30 V B 1]. ACTH, in turn, stimulates cells in the zona fasciculata to synthesize and secrete glucocorticoids.
   b. **Inhibition.** The secreted glucocorticoids, in addition to their effects on other target cells, feed back onto CRH-producing cells in the hypothalamus and corticotrophs in the pituitary gland to inhibit production of these hormones. Blood glucocorticoid levels can thus be modulated.
   c. **Specificity of ACTH.** ACTH regulation primarily affects the zona fasciculata. In the presence of excessive ACTH, the zona fasciculata hypertrophies. Following hypophysectomy, the zona fasciculata atrophies.
      (1) ACTH has no effect on the structure or function of the zona glomerulosa.

(2) ACTH has a slight effect on cells in the zona reticularis, similar to its effect on the zona fasciculata.

D. **Adrenal androgens.** Cells in the **zona reticularis** primarily secrete the weak androgens **dehydroepiandrosterone** and **androstenedione.** Low levels of glucocorticoid secretion have also been noted.

1. **Secretion of androgens** by the adrenal gland is minimal compared to the secretion of these hormones by the gonads. Adrenal androgens may contribute to pubertal changes in the female by serving as substrates for extragonadal production of estrogens.

2. **Control of secretion** of adrenal androgens appears to be influenced by ACTH . Following hypophysectomy, the zona reticularis atrophies, and this atrophy can be reversed by exogenous ACTH administration.

E. **Mechanisms of steroid activity.** Adrenal steroids, like other steroids, freely enter cells because they are lipid soluble. They mediate their effects by initial interaction with receptors in the cytoplasm of target cells. The receptor–hormone complex then enters the nucleus, where it binds to specific nonhistone proteins of the chromatin.

1. This interaction results in the derepression of specific genes and the synthesis (transcription) of messenger RNA (mRNA) molecules. These mRNA molecules then move out of the nucleus into the cytoplasm, where they are translated into specific proteins.

2. The particular proteins translated vary with the target tissues, relating specifically to the characteristic functions of the tissue.
   a. For example, glucocorticoids released during intense exercise stimulate the transcription of genes in hepatocytes that encode enzymes involved in gluconeogenesis, such as tyrosine aminotransferase. This enzyme then functions in the conversion of tyrosine to glucose.
   b. In fat cells, however, glucocorticoids reduce the production of tyrosine aminotransferase.

IV. **ADRENAL MEDULLA.** The cells in the medulla, the central portion of the adrenal gland, synthesize and secrete the catecholaminergic neurohormones **epinephrine (adrenalin)** and **norepinephrine (noradrenalin).**

A. **Development.** The adrenal medulla is **comparable to a sympathetic ganglion** for several reasons:

1. The cells are derived from presumptive sympathetic ganglion tissue (i.e., neural crest).

2. The cells are innervated by cholinergic preganglionic sympathetic fibers.

3. The cells secrete catecholamines. Unlike sympathetic ganglion cells, however, adrenal medullary cells release their catecholamines to the blood instead of at synapses.

B. **Histologic characteristics.** The cells of the medulla are large, polyhedral, pale-staining epithelioid cells organized into clumps and anastomosing cords surrounded by a rich vasculature (Figure 32-2).

1. **Staining characteristic.** The cells are classified as **chromaffin cells** because they stain brown with chromium salts. This results from oxidation of catecholamines in the secretory granules.

2. **Ultrastructure.** The cells contain abundant profiles of rER, a well-developed Golgi apparatus, and numerous **chromaffin granules,** secretory granules with diameters of 100 to 300 nm.

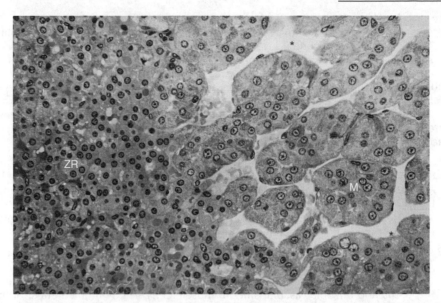

FIGURE 32-2. Adrenal medulla. Light micrograph showing the junction between the zona reticularis (*ZR*) and the medulla (*M*). The medullary cells are large, polyhedral cells arranged in clumps and surrounded by sinusoidal capillaries (*). The cells of the zona reticularis are smaller and are arranged into anastomosing cords.

3. **Cell types.** Epinephrine and norepinephrine are synthesized and secreted by two different cell types, which can be identified on the basis of secretory granule morphology, in conjunction with immunohistochemical specificity for each hormone.
   a. **Epinephrine-secreting cells** have small, lightly staining secretory granules, almost entirely filled with electron dense material.
   b. **Norepinephrine-secreting cells** have larger, dense-core granules. The core of the granules is irregularly shaped and often angulated.

C. Synthesis of adrenal catecholamines
   1. **Synthetic processes.** Epinephrine and norepinephrine are synthesized from tyrosine.
      a. **Initial cytoplasmic reaction.** Synthesis of the catecholamines begins in the cytoplasm.
         (1) Tyrosine is first converted into **dopa** (dihydroxyphenylalanine) by tyrosine hydroxylase.
         (2) Dopa is then converted into dopamine by dopa decarboxylase.
      b. **Initial intragranule reactions.** Dopamine is transported into chromaffin granules, where the enzyme **dopamine β-hydroxylase** (DβH) hydroxylates it, producing norepinephrine.
      c. **Second cytoplasmic reaction.** In epinephrine-secreting cells, norepinephrine is subsequently converted into epinephrine by the cytoplasmic enzyme **phenylethanolamine N-methyltransferase** (PNMT), and is then transported back into the chromaffin granules.
      d. **Storage of secretory products.** The catecholamines are stored in chromaffin granules, where they are complexed with Ca^{2+}, adenosine triphosphate (ATP), chromogranin (an acidic protein), and DβH. All of these products are released by exocytosis following stimulation of each medullary cell by cholinergic innervation.
   2. **Hormonal control of epinephrine synthesis.** In humans, epinephrine comprises 90% of the catecholamine secreted by the adrenal medulla.
      a. The predominance of epinephrine secretion appears to result from stimulation of medullary cells by glucocorticoids produced in the cortex.
      b. Glucocorticoids reach the adrenal medulla through capillaries that surround the cortical cells, and then drain into the medullary sinusoidal capillaries.

(1) These steroids regulate the synthesis of PNMT.
(2) In hypophysectomized animals, PNMT levels decline and norepinephrine predominates; normal levels of PNMT and epinephrine are restored by administration of ACTH or glucocorticoids.

D. **Effects of adrenal catecholamines.** Adrenal catecholamines play a significant regulatory role in metabolism because most cells in the body have adrenergic receptors. These adrenal medullary hormones have more generalized effects than do catecholamines that are released by neurons of the sympathetic nervous system because, as endocrine secretions, adrenal hormones are carried throughout the body by the blood supply.

1. **Metabolic effects.** Catecholamines increase oxygen consumption and heat production. They help regulate glucose and fat mobilization from storage sites.
   a. Catecholamines stimulate glycogenolysis in heart muscle and liver, leading to increased carbohydrate available for metabolism.
   b. They stimulate lipolysis in adipose tissue, releasing free fatty acids and glycerol into the circulation, making them available for metabolism.

2. **Physiologic effects.** Catecholamines have differing effects on similar tissues in different body sites.
   a. Catecholamines increase the rate and amplitude of contraction of myocardial cells and of some vascular smooth muscle cells. The combined effect of these two processes leads to **increased blood pressure.**
      (1) In other vessels, such as those supplying skeletal muscle and coronary arteries, catecholamines induce vasodilation.
      (2) Inhibitors of peripheral adrenergic receptors are thus used clinically to control blood pressure.
   b. Catecholamines also regulate the activity of extravascular smooth muscle. In some tissues, contraction is enhanced, whereas in others, relaxation is enhanced (e.g., relaxation and contraction of uterine myometrium, relaxation of intestinal and bladder smooth muscle, contraction of sphincters in the intestine and bladder).

3. **Fight-or-flight response.** The combination of the physiologic and metabolic effects of catecholamines are particularly important in the fight-or-flight response. Increased catecholamine secretion establishes conditions for maximum utilization of energy necessary for maximum physical effort.

V. FETAL ADRENAL GLAND. The adrenal gland develops and functions in the fetus. It consists of a thin, outer cortex, which is permanent, and a thick, inner fetal zone. During fetal life, the gland attains a size just slightly smaller than the adult kidney.

A. **Development.** The fetal adrenal gland arises from mesothelial cells that penetrate the underlying urogenital mesoderm and give rise to a large, eosinophilic tissue mass. Later, a secondary wave of mesothelial cells enters the mesenchyme and surrounds the primary cell mass. The permanent adrenal cortex develops from this secondary cell migration.

1. The fetal adrenal gland reaches its maximum size by the fourth fetal month. At birth, it is equivalent in size and weight to the adult gland, but secretes approximately twice the amount of steroids as the adult. The fetal adrenal gland rapidly regresses in the first month of postnatal life.

2. Neural crest cells migrate into and remain dispersed within this mass. A definitive medulla is not formed until after birth, when chromaffin cells aggregate.

B. **Histologic characteristics.** Histologically, the fetal adrenal gland resembles the adult adrenal cortex.

1. **Fetal zone.** The fetal adrenal gland consists of cords of large eosinophilic cells that make up approximately 80% of the mass and is referred to as the fetal zone.

2. **Permanent cortex.** The cells derived from the secondary mesothelial cell migration make up the remainder of the gland, and become the permanent adrenal cortex.
   a. These basophilic cells surround the larger fetal zone.
   b. The cells are arranged in small, irregular clusters and curved columns, thus resembling the zona glomerulosa of the adult gland.

3. **Ultrastructure**
   a. **Cells of the fetal zone** contain spherical mitochondria with tubular cristae, small lipid droplets, abundant rER, and multiple Golgi profiles.
   b. **Cells of the permanent cortex** have small mitochondria with shelf-like cristae, abundant free ribosomes, and small Golgi profiles.

C. **Function of the fetal adrenal gland.** The cells in the fetal zone interact with cells in the placenta. Together, they function as a steroid-secreting organ referred to as the **fetal–placental unit.**

1. Fetal adrenal cells lack certain enzymes for steroid synthesis that are present in placental cells; conversely, placental cells lack enzymes that the fetal adrenal cells possess.

2. Metabolic intermediates in steroid synthesis are therefore shuttled back and forth between the fetal adrenal gland and the placenta, enabling synthesis of glucocorticoids, aldosterone, androgens, and estrogens.

3. The fetal adrenal gland is under the control of the CRH–ACTH feedback system of the fetal pituitary gland.

Chapter 33

Islets of Langerhans

I. **INTRODUCTION.** The islets of Langerhans are an endocrine tissue compartment embedded within the exocrine compartment of the pancreas.

A. **Major secretions.** Islets are responsible for the secretion of two major hormones that play a role in serum glucose homeostasis: **insulin** and **glucagon.**

B. **Minor secretions.** In addition, islets secrete small amounts of other hormones that have more localized effects. These include **somatostatin, vasoactive intestinal polypeptide** (VIP), **pancreatic polypeptide** (PP), and **serotonin** (5-hydroxytryptamine, 5-HT).

II. **STRUCTURE AND DEVELOPMENT**

A. **Structure** (Figure 33-1). The islets are discrete, rounded clusters of cells dispersed among the larger mass of the exocrine pancreas (see Chapter 27).

  1. There are approximately 1 to 2 million islets in a normal human pancreas. This represents 10% to 15% of the pancreatic tissue.

  2. Islets are most numerous in the tail region of the pancreas. They vary widely in size and in the number of cells they contain.

B. **Development.** In humans, the pancreas arises during the fifth week of gestation from two diverticula of the duodenum, close to the hepatic diverticulum.

  1. Cells at this stage are undifferentiated low columnar epithelial cells similar to the primitive gut lining. They divide rapidly and produce lobulation of the developing gland.

  2. By the 14th week of gestation, the cells that will make up the islets bud off from acinar diverticula to form recognizable islets. The islets become vascularized by ingrowth of blood vessels that form the sinusoids of the mature endocrine gland.

C. **Histologic characteristics.** Three major cell types can be distinguished by histochemical and immunocytochemical methods (Figure 33-2). α **cells** (A cells) secrete **glucagon** and constitute 20% of islet cells. β **cells** (B cells) secrete **insulin** and constitute 70% to 75% of islet cells. δ **cells** (D cells) secrete **somatostatin** and constitute 5% to 10% of islet cells. Minor populations of cells can also be distinguished, including cells that secrete PP, cells that secrete VIP, and a population of enteroendocrine cells that secrete serotonin. The general nature and effects of these hormones are summarized in Table 33-1.

  1. **Ultrastructure.** These cells are typical of protein-secreting cells that possess a regulated secretory pathway.
    a. The cytoplasm contains abundant rough endoplasmic reticulum (rER), Golgi apparatus, and secretory granules.
    b. The three major cell types can be distinguished on the basis of secretory granule morphology.
      (1) α**-cell granules** have a dense core with an outer mantle that is less dense. They are relatively uniform in size, averaging 300 nm in diameter.
      (2) β**-cell granules** are also relatively uniform in size, averaging 200 nm in diameter. In man, they have a core of one or more polygonal crystals, embedded in a flocculent substance. The granules often appear to have halos.
      (3) δ **cell granules** are more varied in size than α or β cell granules. The

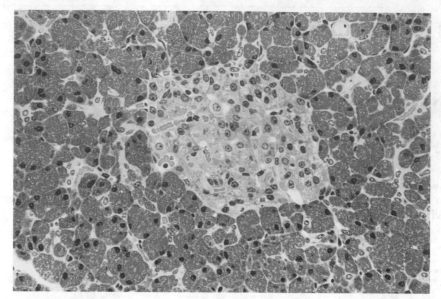

FIGURE 33-1. Light micrograph of an islet of Langerhans surrounded by acini of the exocrine pancreas. The cells in the islet are arranged in irregular cords and clumps. The islet is highly vascularized. α, β, and δ cells are not differentiated from one another in this preparation.

granules have a homogeneously staining character, some very dense and others less dense.

2. **Cellular distribution within an islet.** The α and δ cells are generally found at the periphery (mantle) of the islets, surrounding the more centrally located and more numerous β cells (see Figure 33-2). The minor cell types are scattered throughout the islets.

D. **Blood supply.** The endocrine cells are organized into cords, which are surrounded by an extensive network of sinusoidal capillaries lined by a fenestrated epithelium.

FIGURE 33-2. Diagram of an islet of Langerhans surrounded by acini of the exocrine pancreas, showing the relative number and distribution of the major cell types of the islets. Note the peripheral distribution of glucagon-secreting α cells, the central location of insulin-secreting β cells, and the intermediate location of somatostatin-secreting δ cells.

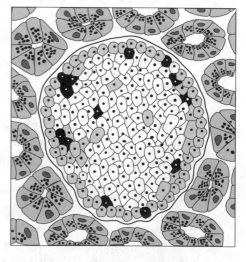

α cell
δ cell
β cell

TABLE 33-1. Hormones of the Islets of Langerhans

Hormone	Cell Type	Actions
Glucagon (29 amino acids)	α cell	Stimulates release of glucose into the blood, gluconeogenesis, and glycogenolysis
Insulin (51 amino acids)	β cell	Stimulates uptake of glucose from the blood, utilization of glucose, and storage of glucose as glycogen
Somatostatin (14 amino acids)	δ cell	Inhibits secretion of glucagon and insulin
Vasoactive intestinal peptide (VIP) (28 amino acids)	D_1 cell	Similar effects to glucagon; affects secretory activity and motility in the gut; stimulates pancreatic exocrine secretion
Pancreatic polypeptide (36 amino acids)	PP cell	Stimulates gastric chief cells, inhibits bile secretion and intestinal motility, inhibits pancreatic enzyme and HCO_3^- secretion

1. Celiac and mesenteric arteries give off arterioles that supply the capillaries of the mantle, and then continue into the central portion of the islet.
   a. α and δ cells are thus perfused before the more centrally located β cells.
   b. Because of this pattern of circulation, secretions from the α and δ cells can influence β cell function.

2. The capillaries then leave the islets and continue as a periacinar capillary network in the exocrine pancreas.
   a. A large fraction of the blood supplying the pancreas perfuses the islets first and then perfuses the exocrine cells.
   b. This places some of the target cells for islet secretions directly downstream from the site of release.

III. **CONTROL OF RELEASE OF INSULIN AND GLUCAGON.** Regulation of α- and β-cell secretion is complex and is influenced by metabolic, neural, and endocrine factors. The net effect of all of these stimulatory and inhibitory factors on any single cell determines if a hormone is secreted, and how much.

A. **Metabolic factors.** Insulin and glucagon function primarily in serum glucose homeostasis. By their actions on the liver, adipose tissue, and muscle, these two hormones help to maintain a balance between glucose production and utilization.

1. **Hyperglycemia.** If serum glucose levels go above 150 mg/100 ml, insulin release is stimulated. This, in turn, increases glucose utilization and storage as glycogen. Insulin directly lowers blood glucose levels.

2. **Hypoglycemia.** If serum glucose levels drop below 80 mg/100 ml, glucagon secretion is stimulated. Glucagon influences glucose production and utilization by stimulating gluconeogenesis and glycogenolysis.

3. **Other glycemic regulators.** Insulin and glucagon are not the only hormones that influence blood glucose; thyroid hormone, adrenal corticosteroids, and adrenal medullary catecholamines also have roles.

B. **Neural factors.** Pancreatic islets are innervated by the autonomic nervous system, with both sympathetic and parasympathetic inputs.

1. Approximately 10% of all the cells in the islet are innervated directly.
   a. Parasympathetic stimulation increases insulin and glucagon secretion.
   b. Sympathetic stimulation inhibits insulin release.

2. β cells are coupled to α cells and to other β cells by gap junctions that provide a mechanism by which neural stimuli are communicated to all cells. The depolarization of one islet cell thus leads to the depolarization of other islet cells.

C. **Endocrine factors.** Because of their anatomic location within the islet, hormonal secretions of islet cells can influence other cells in the islet. Such local hormonal effects are called **paracrine effects.**

1. Insulin release by β cells is directly stimulated by glucagon; conversely, glucagon secretion is directly inhibited by insulin.

2. Somatostatin is inhibitory to both insulin and glucagon release.

Chapter 34

Pineal Gland

I. **INTRODUCTION.** The pineal gland is considered a **neuroendocrine gland.** Its functions in humans are not yet fully understood.

A. **Development.** The pineal gland develops as an **evagination** of the posterior portion of the **roof of the diencephalon** and remains attached to the brain by a short stalk.

B. **Gross structure.** It is a flattened, cone-shaped structure that measures 3 to 5 mm at its base and 5 to 8 mm high. It weighs 100 to 200 mg. It is divided into lobules by connective tissue septa that extend into the gland from the overlying pia mater.

II. **PINEAL PARENCHYMAL CELLS.** The pineal contains two types of parenchymal cells: pinealocytes and interstitial cells.

A. **Pinealocytes.** Pinealocytes are the most common parenchymal cell, constituting nearly 95% of the cells. They are arranged in clumps and cords within the lobules.

1. **Histologic characteristics.** The pale-staining epithelioid cells have a large rounded or deeply indented nucleus with one or more prominent nucleoli.
   a. Lipid droplets are frequently found in the slightly basophilic cytoplasm.
   b. Silver-impregnation staining methods demonstrate long **cytoplasmic processes.** These processes end in club-like expansions that are associated with blood capillaries.

2. **Ultrastructure.** Transmission electron microscopy reveals both rough and smooth endoplasmic reticulum, a small Golgi apparatus, and annulate lamellae in the cytoplasm.
   a. Numerous dense-cored, membrane-bounded vesicles are present in the elongated cell processes, along with parallel bundles of microtubules.
   b. Pinealocytes contain numerous structures consisting of a dense rod or lamella, oriented perpendicular to the cell surface, surrounded by numerous small vesicles. These structures resemble **synaptic ribbons** of sensory cells of the retina and may be vestiges of the organ's evolution from a photoreceptor in lower vertebrates.

B. **Interstitial cells.** The insterstitial (glial) cells have features closely resembling those of astrocytes. They are similar to the pituicytes of the neurohypophysis.

C. **Corpora arenacea.** In addition to the two typical cell types, the pineal gland is characterized by the presence of **concretions** of calcium phosphates and carbonates in an organic matrix.

1. These concretions, also called **brain sand,** are probably derived from the carrier proteins, neuroepiphysins, that are released into the cytoplasm when pineal secretions are released by exocytosis.

2. The concretions are present in childhood, increase in number with age, and can serve as useful markers in radiographic and computerized tomographic examination of the brain.

III. **PINEAL FUNCTIONS.** The pineal gland mediates endocrine response to changes in light intensity.

A. **Seasonal breeders.** The pineal gland mediates the responses of the reproductive system of seasonally breeding animals to changes in day length.

1. **Light.** Information on day length and light intensity from photoreceptors in the retina is transmitted through the hypothalamus to the sympathetic nervous system, which then transmits the information to the pineal gland.

2. **Secretions.** The pineal gland is then stimulated to release its neurosecretions, which include **melatonin, arginine vasotocin, pineal antigonadotropin,** and a **gonadotropin-releasing factor** that is different from the gonadotropin-releasing hormone of the hypothlalamus.
   a. In periods of short day length, secretion of melatonin and other pineal hormones increases, and the gonads of seasonal breeders regress.
   b. As day length increases in the spring, pineal secretion decreases, and the gonadal atrophy is reversed.
   c. Arginine vasotocin appears to be even more effective than melatonin in gonadal suppression.

B. **Amphibians.** In amphibians, the responsiveness of the pineal gland to light is linked to regulation of skin color. Melatonin causes aggregation of melanosomes in amphibian melanophores.

1. **Photoreception.** In amphibians and other lower vertebrates, the pineal organs contain photoreceptor cells that resemble those of the mammalian retina (see Chapter 37 IX A 2). They have apical lamellar membrane stacks and a basal synapse.

2. **Parietal eye.** In some lizards, the photoreceptor is so well developed that it even contains a lens-like structure and is called a parietal eye.

C. **Humans**

1. **Reproductive system.** Although no direct evidence for pineal effects on reproductive activity in humans has yet been found, certain pathologic conditions and physiologic observations suggest that pineal secretions may affect gonadal development.
   a. Blood levels of melatonin in young boys are high and decline at puberty. Children with brain tumors that damage or destroy the pineal gland exhibit precocious puberty.
   b. Conversely, tumors of the pineal gland that secrete a greater than normal amount of pineal hormones may retard gonadal development and delay puberty.

2. **Responses to day length.** Recent studies suggest that the human pineal gland has a role in physiologic and emotional adjustment to changes in day length.
   a. Travelers suffering from jet lag, believed to be induced by sudden changes in day length and consequent disturbance of circadian rhythms, apparently respond positively to exposure for relatively short periods to intense light, which reduces the secretion of melatonin and other pineal hormones.
   b. Individuals who become clinically depressed by the short day lengths in winter in subarctic and temperate climates (seasonal affective disorder, SAD) report positive changes in mood when exposed to regular periods of intense artificial light during winter.

Chapter 35

Female Reproductive System

I. **INTRODUCTION.** The major components of the female reproductive system are the ovaries, fallopian tubes (oviducts), uterus, vagina, and mammary glands (Figure 35-1).

II. **OVARIES, OOCYTES, AND OVARIAN FOLLICLES**

A. **Gross aspects.** The ovaries are paired, palpable structures in the pelvic cavity that are ovoid in shape, 3 to 4 cm in length, and approximately 1 cm in thickness.

1. **Peritoneal covering.** The epithelial covering of the ovaries is the mesothelium of the **visceral peritoneum.** This epithelium was called the germinal epithelium in the older literature; however, it is not the source of germ cells (i.e., oogonia).

2. **Cortical compartment of the ovary**
   a. The cortex lies between the peritoneal epithelium and the medulla.
   b. The **most prominent cortical structures are oocyte-containing ovarian follicles.** Follicles in various stages of development are present in the cortex and are surrounded by the **ovarian stroma,** a cell-rich connective tissue.

3. **Medullary compartment of the ovary**
   a. The medulla lies deep to the cortex and contains large blood vessels.
   b. Ovarian follicles are absent from the medulla.

B. **Female germ cells: oogonia and oocytes**

1. **Embryonic source.** Oogonia differentiate from primordial germ cells that migrate from the yolk sac to the developing gonad.

2. **Mitotic expansion and arrested meiosis**
   a. **Mitosis.** The number of oogonia increases by **mitotic divisions** of the primordial germ cells and their progeny during gonad development in the embryo. Oogonia reach a maximum of **5 to 7 million** at approximately 5 months of fetal life.
      (1) In the second trimester of gestation, **oogonia stop dividing** and increase slightly in size.
      (2) The germ cells are now **primary oocytes.**
   b. **Meiosis.** The primary oocytes enter prophase of the first meiotic division at this time during fetal development (see Chapter 4 IX B 1) and the meiotic process is arrested.
      (1) The **first meiotic division** is not completed in any oocyte until its ovulation.
      (2) The **second meiotic division** is completed only after fertilization.

3. **Chromosome number and amount of DNA**
   a. **Primary oocytes are diploid cells.** Each cell contains 22 pairs of autosomes and two X chromosomes.
   b. Each primary oocyte, however, contains the 4N amount of DNA and never again passes through another S phase of the cell cycle.

C. **Ovarian follicles** are complexes formed by an oocyte and surrounding granulosa cells (Figure 35-2). Follicles vary considerably in appearance. Several distinct developmental stages can be recognized.

1. **Unilaminar follicles.** Primary oocytes have a sheath of cells that is one cell-layer thick. The ensheathing **granulosa cells** or **follicular epithelial cells** are derived from

FIGURE 35-1. (*A*) Sagittal section of the female pelvis showing the relationship of the uterus and vagina to the bladder and urethra and to the rectum. (*B*) Display of the dissected uterus and oviducts and their relationship to the ovaries.

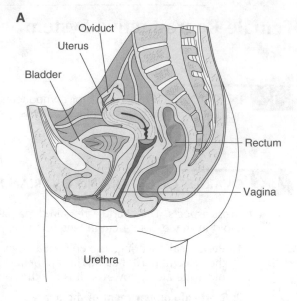

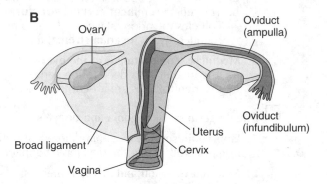

the **ovarian stroma.** The population of unilaminar follicles may be subdivided into primordial and primary follicles.

a. **Primordial follicles** are the least mature but most numerous ovarian follicles. A simple squamous epithelium of granulosa cells covers the primary oocyte.

b. **Primary follicles** are increased slightly in size. The granulosa cells have become cuboidal or columnar, but remain in a single layer.

2. **Multilaminar (secondary) follicles.** Granulosa cells divide and produce a stratified epithelium around the enlarging primary oocyte. Multilaminar refers to the stratified layer of granulosa cells.

a. A **zona pellucida** develops between the oocyte and granulosa cells.

(1) The zona pellucida is a glycoprotein layer of basal lamina-like material that is synthesized by the oocyte and first appears as a discontinuous layer. Later, the zona pellucida is seen as a thick, continuous layer surrounding the oocyte.

(2) Processes from the oocyte and granulosa cells enter the zona pellucida. Gap junctions connect the processes.

b. A **theca interna** develops from stromal cells (see Figure 35-2).

(1) Several layers of stromal cells become applied to the surface of the multilaminar follicle.

(2) These stromal cells acquire the fine structural characteristics of steroid secretory cells and, then, may be called the theca interna.

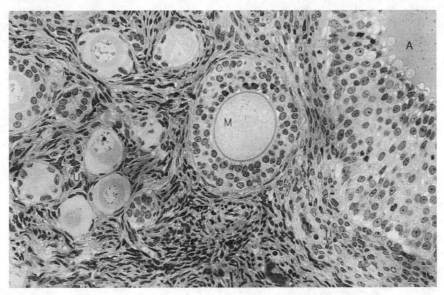

FIGURE 35-2. Several ovarian follicles. Unilaminar follicles (*U*), multilaminar follicle (*M*), and a portion of an antral follicle (*A*). A theca interna (*Ti*) surrounds the antral follicle.

      (3) The theca interna becomes richly vascularized and participates with the granulosa cells in the synthesis of estrogens.

    c. A **theca externa,** which is also formed by stromal cells, may be observed superficial to the theca interna. The theca externa is not a secretory structure.

3. Antral (tertiary) follicles. The antrum is a dilation of the intercellular space that develops within the layer of granulosa cells (Figure 35-3).

    a. An **antrum** is first visible as a small gap in the otherwise compact layer of granulosa cells. Later, the antrum increases tremendously in volume.

    b. A viscous, hyaluronic acid-rich **fluid accumulates in the antrum.**

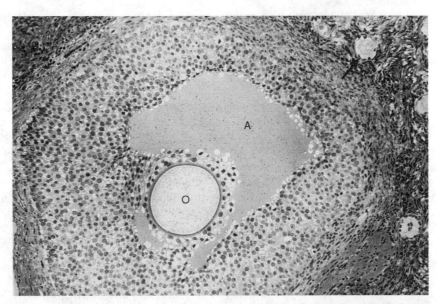

FIGURE 35-3. Antral follicle with an oocyte (*O*). The oocyte and its surrounding granulosa cells bulge into the antrum (*A*). Compare the large size of the antral follicle with a unilaminar follicle (*arrow*).

    c. The **oocyte reaches its maximum diameter** of 0.1 to 0.2 mm in the antral follicle.

  4. Graafian (mature) follicles. The Graafian follicle is the final stage in development of an ovarian follicle.

    a. The follicle reaches its **maximum diameter** of 0.5 to 1.0 cm and is visible macroscopically as a bulge on the surface of the ovary.

    b. The **antrum** is the single largest component of the mature follicle.

    c. **Granulosa cells** are seen as a stratified epithelium between the antrum and the theca interna. The antrum is enclosed completely by granulosa cells.

      (1) The **cumulus oophorus** is the mound of granulosa cells that encloses the oocyte.

      (2) The **corona radiata** is the layer of granulosa cells immediately adjacent to the zona pellucida to which it is anchored by cell processes.

D. **Ovarian follicles and age of the female.** The number of ovarian follicles and evidence of follicle development vary widely with the age of the individual.

  1. Ovaries of the fetus. After reaching the maximum number during fetal development (see II B 2), the number of germ cells gradually decreases by **atresia** (see II E).

  2. Ovaries of the child. At birth, each ovary contains approximately 1 million oocytes, most of which are unilaminar follicles (see II C 1).

  3. Ovaries of the sexually mature woman. At puberty, each ovary contains approximately 150,000 oocytes. A spectrum of developmental stages of follicles is seen at any one time in an ovary.

  4. Ovaries of the postmenopausal woman. At menopause, examination of the ovarian cortex reveals only a few scattered follicles widely separated by stromal connective tissue. Also noted in the cortical stroma are **corpora albicans** (see III B 3 c) and **atretic follicles** (see II E 3).

E. **Atresia of ovarian follicles.** Atresia is an example of **apoptosis** (i.e., programmed cell death) that occurs in the ovary (Figure 35-4).

  1. Reduction of number of oocytes. Atresia is the process by which the number of oocytes in the ovary is constantly decreased by the death and resorption of specific ovarian follicles.

    a. Atresia may be observed in the ovaries of the fetus, infant, child, adolescent, and sexually mature woman.

    b. Atresia may occur at any time during the maturation of an ovarian follicle. A small, unilaminar follicle may undergo atresia; a Graafian follicle may undergo atresia; and any follicle between these developmental extremes may undergo atresia.

  2. Evidence of a subtractive process is seen in the ovary. Although several million oocytes exist at one point during fetal development, only **about 400 oocytes mature** and are released by ovulation in the sexually mature woman. **Only a few follicles remain** in the ovaries of the postmenopausal woman. Most follicles will have undergone atresia.

  3. Histologic indications of atresia

    a. Atresia of unilaminar and small multilaminar follicles may be difficult to recognize because of dispersion of the follicular components into the stroma. The incidence of atresia is greatest in the least mature follicles.

    b. Large multilaminar, antral, and Graafian follicles undergoing atresia may show one or various combinations of the following characteristics.

      (1) The compact layer of granulosa cells in antral follicles becomes **loosened and frayed** as atresia commences (see Figure 35-4).

      (2) The oocyte shows evidence of **degeneration and disintegration.**

      (3) The **zona pellucida persists,** partially collapsed, long after disintegration of the oocyte.

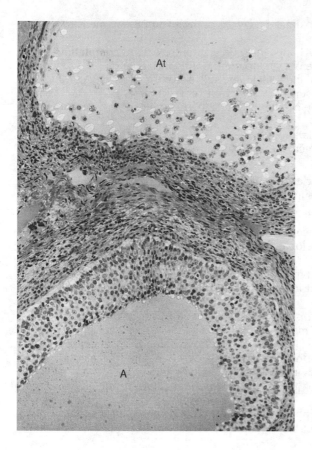

FIGURE 35-4. A developing antral follicle (*A*) and an atretic antral follicle (*At*). The granulosa epithelium of the atretic follicle is no longer a cohesive tissue, and its cells are free in the antrum.

(4) The basement membrane between the granulosa cells and the theca interna thickens and is called a **glassy membrane.**
(5) The **theca interna hypertrophies.**
(6) The follicle is **invaded by connective tissue.**
(7) Gap junctions between the oocyte and granulosa cells are lost. Close association between oocyte and granulosa cells appears to be essential for continued maturation of the oocyte.

4. Interstitial gland tissue and atretic follicles. Interstitial gland tissue, which appears as vascularized clumps of endocrine-like cells, is sometimes seen in the ovarian stroma. The interstitial gland tissue may derive from the theca interna of atretic follicles and is a possible source of estrogens.

III. OVULATION AND CORPUS LUTEUM FORMATION

A. **Ovulation.** The presence of a Graafian follicle is essential for ovulation to occur.

1. Follicle location. The Graafian follicle is **located in the superficial cortex** of the ovary and, because of its size and location, causes a **bulge** (called a **stigma**) on the surface of the ovary.

2. Oocyte detaches. The oocyte and attached granulosa cells may be **free in the antrum** for a short time before their expulsion from the follicle (and ovary).

3. Meiosis, ovulation, and the luteinizing hormone (LH) surge. A surge in the secretion of LH is detected at approximately day 14 of the ideal 28-day menstrual cycle (see VIII B 3 a).

    a. **Continuation of meiosis.** LH appears to be a stimulus for the **completion of the first meiotic division** of the oocyte around the time of ovulation.

    b. **Oocyte release.** Rupture of the follicle and release of the oocyte occur approximately 1 day after the LH surge.

        (1) The follicle releases the oocyte, with attached granulosa cells, and some follicular fluid.

        (2) At the moment of ovulation, the oocyte exists free in the peritoneal cavity but, normally, soon enters the infundibulum of the oviduct.

B. **Luteinization of the ovarian follicle.** Following ovulation, the partially collapsed wall of the Graafian follicle, under the influence of LH, develops into the corpus luteum (Figure 35-5).

  1. **Histologic appearance of the corpus luteum**

    a. **Size of structure.** The developing corpus luteum increases considerably in size and becomes much larger than the Graafian follicle from which it was derived.

        (1) The large size of the corpus luteum is due to the **hypertrophy** of its cells and not to a significant increase in cell number. The wall of the corpus luteum becomes folded.

        (2) The corpus luteum forms the largest single compartment of the ovary during the last half of the menstrual cycle.

    b. **Cells of the corpus luteum.** The wall of the corpus luteum is formed by **granulosa lutein cells** (originally the granulosa cells of the mature follicle) and by **theca lutein cells** (originally the cells of the theca interna).

        (1) The two populations of luteal cells may be difficult to distinguish from each other.

        (2) Usually, the more peripheral cells in the corpus luteum are the theca lutein cells, which are smaller than the more centrally located granulosa lutein cells.

    c. **Other landmarks of the corpus luteum**

        (1) The center of the corpus luteum, originally the antrum of the Graafian folli-

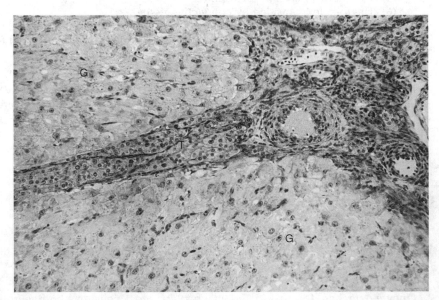

FIGURE 35-5. Edge of a fully developed corpus luteum. Granulosa lutein cells (*G*) are larger than the more peripherally located theca lutein cells (*T*). Note the blood vessels associated with this endocrine organ.

cle, becomes partially filled with loose connective tissue, clotted blood, and unexpelled follicular fluid.

(2) Blood vessels originally associated with the theca interna of the Graafian follicle invade the developing corpus luteum, which rapidly develops into a richly vascularized **endocrine organ.**

2. **Function of the corpus luteum**
   a. The corpus luteum primarily secretes **progesterone** and also secretes some **estrogens.**
   b. The progesterone secreted by the corpus luteum **prepares and maintains the endometrium** of the uterus (see VIII C) for implantation and subsequent development of a fertilized ovum.

3. **Regression of the corpus luteum**
   a. If the ovum is not fertilized, the corpus luteum degenerates 10 to 12 days after ovulation.
   b. Progesterone secretion ceases.
   c. The corpus luteum is rapidly reduced in size and forms a connective tissue scar, called a **corpus albicans.** The corpus albicans gradually reduces in size until, after several months, it merges with the ovarian stroma.

4. **Corpus luteum of pregnancy**
   a. If fertilization and implantation occur, the corpus luteum does not regress. It enlarges to 2 to 3 cm in diameter to form the **corpus luteum of pregnancy.**
   b. The corpus luteum of pregnancy continues as a **steroid-secreting organ** for approximately the first 8 weeks of pregnancy. The endocrine function of the corpus luteum of pregnancy is gradually taken over by the placenta.
      (1) Luteal progesterone is necessary to support the early stage of pregnancy.
      (2) Human chorionic gonadotropin (hCG) secreted by the placenta [see XI E 2 b (2)] has an LH-like effect and maintains the corpus luteum during the first 8 weeks of pregnancy.
   c. The corpus luteum of pregnancy then regresses to form a large corpus albicans, evidence of which may persist for years.

IV. MITOSIS AND MEIOSIS OF THE FEMALE GERM CELL. Both types of cell division occur at different times in the ovary.

A. Oogonia

1. Oogonia are **diploid cells.**
2. During the first trimester and early second trimester, the **number of oogonia in the fetal ovary rapidly and massively increases by mitotic division** (see II B 2).

B. Primary oocytes (see II B 2, 3)

C. Secondary oocytes

1. The LH surge at the time of ovulation provides the **stimulus for the completion of the first meiotic division.**
2. **Products of the first meiotic division** include a secondary oocyte, which has the **haploid number of chromosomes and 2N amount of DNA,** and a polar body of similar chromosomal content.
3. The secondary oocyte then enters the second meiotic division but is **arrested at metaphase.**

D. Ova

1. Attachment to and penetration of the secondary oocyte by the sperm at fertilization provide the **stimulus for completion of the second meiotic division.**

2. **Products of the second meiotic division** include an ovum and a second polar body. The ovum and the polar body each have the **haploid number of chromosomes** (each chromosome is formed by one chromatid) and **1N amount of DNA.**

V.   OVIDUCTS. The oviducts, or **fallopian tubes,** are tubular structures that provide a channel for the transport of the ovum from the ovary to the uterus and also provide an environment for fertilization.

A. Regions of the oviduct

1. The **infundibulum** is the flared opened end of the oviduct that is adjacent to the ovary. **Fimbriae** are the delicate, finger-like projections that extend from the infundibulum toward the ovary.

2. The **ampulla** is the longest segment of the oviduct and the segment of greatest diameter. It is the usual **site of fertilization.**

3. The **isthmus** is the narrow segment of the oviduct between the ampulla and the uterus.

4. The **intramural segment** is the portion of the oviduct that is contained within the wall of the uterus.

B. Histologic structure of the oviduct

1. **Mucosal epithelium.** The lumen of the oviduct is lined by a simple cuboidal/columnar epithelium. Some of the cells are ciliated; some are secretory.
    a. **Epithelial heterogeneity.** The relative numbers of ciliated and secretory cells vary from region to region along the length of the oviduct, as well as from phase to phase of the menstrual cycle.
        (1) **Ciliated cells** are usually more numerous at the infundibular end of the tube and during the proliferative phase of the cycle (see VIII B).
        (2) **Secretory cells** tend to predominate at the uterine end of the tube and predominate during the luteal phase of the cycle (see VIII C). Secretory cells, after release of their contents, become **peg cells.** Peg cells are narrow, nonciliated cells that are numerous during pregnancy.
    b. **Ciliary beat.** Most cilia appear to beat in the direction of the uterus. Ciliary motion is a mechanism that helps propel the ovum along the oviduct.
    c. **Cell secretions.** Secretions of epithelial cells provide a favorable environment for maintenance of the oocyte and for fertilization and cleavage.

2. **Subepithelial layers of the oviduct wall**
    a. The **lamina propria** is a layer of loose connective tissue that separates the epithelium from the smooth muscle of the wall.
    b. **Smooth muscle** that encircles the tube consists of an inner circular layer and an outer longitudinal layer.
        (1) Peristaltic waves of contraction move along the oviduct.
        (2) These contractions may also help propel the oocyte toward the uterus.
    c. The **serosa** is the outermost layer of the wall of the oviduct. It is formed by the visceral peritoneum and a thin connective tissue layer.

3. **Regional variation in mucosal folds**
    a. The mucosa of the oviduct is thrown into a complex arrangement of longitudinal folds.
    b. The folds reach their greatest height and complexity in the ampulla. Their height and complexity are greatly reduced in the isthmus.

VI. FERTILIZATION

A. Site of fertilization and germ cell viability

1. Some sperm may reach the site of fertilization (i.e., the ampulla of oviduct) as soon as 5 minutes postcoitus. However, most of the 300 to 500 sperm that ultimately reach the ampulla may take as long as 3 hours to traverse the cervical canal, uterus, and proximal fallopian tube.

2. **Time of germ cell viability is variable.**
   a. Sperm retain the ability to fertilize for a few days in the female reproductive tract.
   b. The oocyte must be fertilized within 12 to 24 hours of ovulation.

B. Sperm–oocyte juncture

1. **Sperm penetrate the corona radiata and zona pellucida.**
   a. Sperm cells cross the corona radiata. Acrosomal enzymes possibly aid in the dispersal of the granulosa (corona radiata) cells.
   b. Sperm penetrate the zona pellucida. This process is facilitated by acrosomal enzymes. More than one sperm may penetrate the zona pellucida, but usually only one sperm enters the secondary oocyte.

2. The **zona (cortical) reaction,** which occurs after entry of the first sperm into the oocyte, prevents additional sperm from entering the oocyte and participating in fertilization.
   a. The zona reaction may be produced by the release of cortical granules from the secondary oocyte.
   b. Substances released from the granules affect the zona pellucida to prevent entry of more sperm.

3. The plasma membranes of the sperm and oocyte fuse, and the **sperm head and tail enter the oocyte.**

4. The **second meiotic division is then completed,** producing the mature ovum and the second polar body.

C. Zygote formation

1. The nucleus contributed by the sperm cell (**male pronucleus**) and the nucleus of the ovum (**female pronucleus**) approach each other and fuse to form the nucleus of the **zygote.**

2. The chromosomes intermingle, and the first mitotic division of the zygote occurs shortly thereafter. This signals the beginning of embryonic development.

VII. THE UTERUS is a muscular organ that encloses a narrow lumen, receives the oviducts, and is continuous with the vagina. The uterus provides a hospitable environment for the development of the embryo and fetus (Figure 35-6).

A. Regions of the uterus. The body and fundus of the uterus have a similar histologic structure, which is different from that of the cervical region.

1. The **body** of the uterus is the expanded part of the organ, below the entrance of the oviducts.

2. The **fundus** of the uterus is the rounded superior portion of the organ, above the entrance of the oviducts.

3. The **cervix** is the most inferior part of the uterus, and it projects into the vagina.

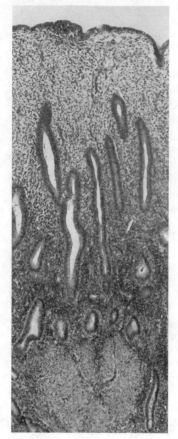 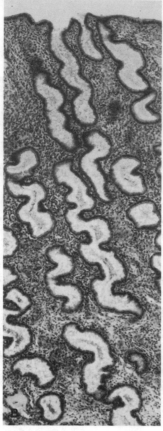 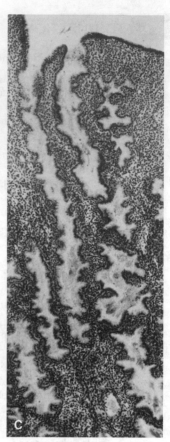

FIGURE 35-6. (*A*) Proliferating endometrium characterized by straight glands. (*B*) Early secretory endometrium characterized by coiled glands. (*C*) Late secretory endometrium characterized by sacculated glands.

B. **Perimetrium: outer covering of the uterus.** The perimetrium is formed by the peritoneum and a thin layer of connective tissue.

C. **Myometrium: muscular wall of the uterus**

1. The myometrium is the **thickest subcompartment of the wall** of the uterus.
   a. It is formed by **interlacing bundles of smooth muscle** (Figure 35-7).
   b. Small amounts of connective tissue separate adjacent muscle bundles and form the stroma of the myometrium.

2. During pregnancy, the uterine smooth muscle cells hypertrophy and also increase in number.

D. **Endometrium: mucosal lining of the uterus**

1. **Mucosa.** The fundus and body have structurally similar mucosal linings.
   a. A simple columnar epithelium forms the luminal surface.
   b. The endometrial stroma is connective tissue that underlies the endometrial epithelium and is continuous with the connective tissue stroma of the myometrium.

2. **Glands.** The epithelium forms simple tubular glands that invaginate the endometrial stroma (see Figure 35-6).
   a. The structure of the glands varies as the endometrium passes through the phases of the menstrual cycle.

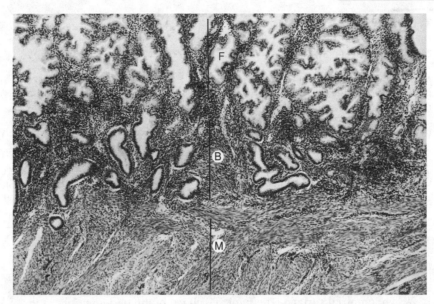

FIGURE 35-7. Junction of endometrium and myometrium, late secretory phase. Note the sacculated, sawtooth-like endometrial glands of the functional level of the endometrium (*F*), the relatively straight glands of the basal level of the endometrium (*B*), and the bundles of smooth muscle of the myometrium (*M*).

    b. The phase of the cycle may be recognized by the structure of the endometrial glands.

  3. Subdivisions of the endometrium. The endometrium may be divided into two layers parallel to the surface.
    a. The functional layer is the more superficial layer. It shows structural changes during the menstrual cycle and is lost during menstruation.
    b. The basal layer is a narrow layer deep to the functional layer and adjacent to the myometrium. It is relatively unaffected during the menstrual cycle and contains the deepest parts of the endometrial glands. The basal layer serves as a cell source for the cyclic regeneration of the endometrium.

  4. Endometrial blood vessels. The endometrium has a dual blood supply.
    a. Spiral arteries supply the functional layer.
    b. Straight arteries supply the basal layer.

E. **Cervix.** The wall of the cervix is mainly connective tissue; much less smooth muscle is found in the cervix than in the body or fundus of the uterus.

  1. The cervical canal is the narrow channel that joins the lumen of the uterus to the vagina.
    a. The canal is lined by a simple columnar epithelium from which several branched, tubular, mucus-secreting glands arise.
    b. The glands may become blocked and produce nabothian cysts.

  2. Cervical epithelium, together with the glands and surrounding connective tissue, is relatively unaffected during the menstrual cycle. However, the chemical and physical nature of the mucus produced by cervical glands does change during the cycle.
    a. During the proliferative phase, cervical mucus is watery.
    b. During the secretory phase, the mucus becomes more viscous.

  3. Cervical–vaginal junction. An **abrupt transition** is seen in the region of the vaginal cervix between the simple columnar epithelium of the cervical canal and the stratified squamous epithelium of the vagina.

VIII. **THE MENSTRUAL CYCLE** is a continuum of developmental stages that affects primarily the functional layer of the endometrium (see VII D 3 a). The cycle repeats approximately every 28 days.

A. **Menstrual phase** (days 1–4). The convention usually followed is that the first day of menstrual bleeding is day 1 of the cycle. This phase lasts approximately 4 days and is described in more detail in section VIII E.

B. **Proliferative phase** (days 4–15). This phase begins when menstrual bleeding stops, and ends the day after ovulation.

1. The term **proliferative** refers to the recovery of the endometrium from the degenerative events of menstruation. Both epithelial and connective tissue components of the basal layer of the endometrium proliferate. Other terms are also used to describe this phase.
   a. **Estrogenic phase.** Events occurring in the endometrium at this time are primarily influenced by estrogens.
   b. **Follicular phase.** The ovarian follicle is the major source of estrogens, which are of critical importance at this time.

2. **Histologic characteristics of proliferative phase**
   a. **Endometrial surface.** The luminal surface of the endometrium at the start of the proliferative phase (i.e., day 4 of the cycle) is formed only by the basal layer.
      (1) Stumps of glands project from the bare stroma into the uterine lumen.
      (2) Epithelial cells and stromal cells divide and proliferate. The functional layer is re-established.
   b. **Endometrial glands.** Glands develop and appear as widely spaced, simple, straight tubular glands (see Figure 35-6A).
      (1) The structure of the glands is an important characteristic of the proliferative stage.
      (2) Some watery mucus is secreted.

3. **The duration of the proliferative phase** is the **most variable portion of the cycle** because of variability in the day of ovulation.
   a. In the ideal menstrual cycle, ovulation occurs on day 14.
   b. Ovulation may occur normally between day 8 and day 20, however.

C. **Secretory phase** (days 15–27). This phase begins the day after ovulation and ends approximately 1 day before menstrual bleeding. It is less variable in duration than the proliferative phase.

1. The term **secretory** refers to the activity of the endometrial glands. Other terms are also used to describe this phase.
   a. **Progestational phase.** Progesterone produced by the corpus luteum has an important role in development of the secretory endometrium.
   b. **Luteal phase.** The corpus luteum develops in parallel with the secretory endometrium and is the prime source of progesterone.
   c. **Gravid phase.** During this phase, the uterus is prepared for implantation.

2. **Histologic characteristics of the secretory phase**
   a. **Endometrial thickness.** The endometrium becomes thicker than it is in the proliferative phase. Most of the increase in thickness is caused by edema of the endometrium.
   b. **Endometrial glands.** The previously straight glands now follow a spiral path through the stroma (see Figure 35-6B). Later in this phase, the glands have a sacculated appearance because of the accumulation of secretions (see Figure 35-6C).
      (1) Early in the secretory phase, glycogen may be demonstrated in the basal part of the glandular epithelial cells.
      (2) Later in the phase, the glycogen shifts to the apical cytoplasm in preparation for its release from the cell as a component of the glandular secretion.

(3) The deeper parts of the glands, which lie in the basal level of the endometrium, do not develop sacculations (see Figure 35-7).

3. **Significance of endometrial development.** The dramatic morphologic changes that occur in the endometrium, culminating in the late secretory endometrium, assure a receptive environment for implantation of the embryo.

D. **Premenstrual phase** (day 28). This is also referred to as the **ischemic phase** because it is characterized by reduced blood flow to the endometrium.

1. **Endometrial changes.** The endometrium regresses, or shrinks, during this phase.
   a. The maintenance of the endometrium depends on progesterone from the corpus luteum.
   b. Late in the cycle, the corpus luteum starts to involute, and its output of progesterone wanes.

2. **Endometrial blood vessels.** As the endometrium shrinks, the spiral arteries are compressed (i.e., the vessels buckle) to fit into the reduced endometrial compartment.
   a. **Blood flow is impaired,** and regions of the endometrium normally supplied by the spiral arteries become ischemic. Both blood vessels and endometrial tissues are affected by the ischemia.
   b. Vessels become temporarily patent, but the ischemia-damaged vessel walls do not effectively contain the blood, and **blood leaks into the stroma.** The pooling of blood in the endometrial stroma is a readily observed histologic characteristic of this stage.

E. **Menstrual phase** (days 1–4). This phase is characterized by loss of the functional layer of the endometrium.

1. **Endometrial blood vessels.** Further constrictions and openings occur in vessels of the endometrium, parts of the endometrium break off, and finally there is bleeding directly into the uterine lumen.
   a. Within a few days, the entire functional layer is sloughed.
   b. The basal layer of the endometrium remains relatively unaffected because of its different blood supply.

2. **Menstruation, blood vessels, and progesterone.** Disintegration of the endometrium appears to be the result of impairment of its blood supply that, in turn, is closely related to decreased progesterone secretion by the degenerating corpus luteum.

IX. **THE VAGINA** is a fibromuscular tube that joins the female reproductive system to the external body surface.

A. **Vaginal wall**

1. **Epithelium.** The vagina is lined by a stratified squamous, nonkeratinizing epithelium. The epithelial cells, under the influence of estrogens, accumulate large amounts of glycogen by midcycle.

2. **Muscle.** Both smooth muscle and skeletal muscle are found in the wall of the vagina. A **ring of skeletal muscle** circles the opening of the vagina. **Interlacing bundles of smooth muscle** form a major layer in the wall of the vagina.

3. **Connective tissue.** An irregular junction is noted between the vaginal epithelium and its subtending connective tissue. Considerable elastic tissue occurs in the wall of the vagina and this, in part, accounts for its remarkable distensibility.

B. **Vaginal secretions**

1. **Vaginal mucus** is produced by **cervical glands.** Glands are not found in the wall of the vagina.

2. Additional mucus is produced by the **greater vestibular glands** (glands of Bartholin) and by the numerous, small, **lesser vestibular glands.** Both the greater and lesser vestibular glands empty into the vaginal vestibule.

X.   THE MAMMARY GLAND is derived embryologically from epidermis. In the adult, the secretory compartment of the mammary gland retains connection with the epidermis by its duct system. The mammary gland shows some similarity to the cutaneous apocrine gland.

A. Basic gland structure

1. The mammary gland is a **compound, tubuloalveolar, exocrine gland** surrounded by variable amounts of dense irregular and adipose connective tissue.

2. There are approximately **20 lobes in each gland,** and each lobe opens onto the apex of the **nipple** via a duct.

3. Depending on functional state and hormonal stimulation, the glandular (secretory) compartment of the gland consists largely of either duct-like tubules (inactive gland) or tubuloalveolar secretory units (active gland).

B. Prepubertal mammary gland (e.g., 7-year-old girl)

1. Epithelial tubules originate at the nipple and radiate into the subcutaneous connective tissue.

2. Tubules are usually clustered into lobar and lobular arrangements.

3. There is little, if any, evidence of secretory activity.

C. Postpubertal mammary gland

1. **Inactive, nonsecreting gland** (e.g., 27-year-old, nonpregnant woman; Figure 35-8)

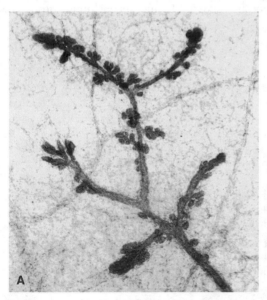
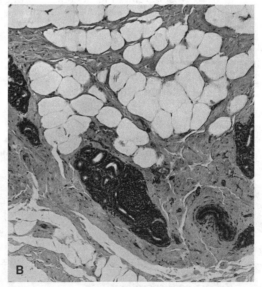

FIGURE 35-8. Mammary gland, inactive. (*A*) Demonstration of the branching duct system of the gland, which is capped by small tubuloalveolar secretory units. (*B*) Ductular and secretory epithelia are surrounded by a relatively large amount of fibrous and adipose connective tissue.

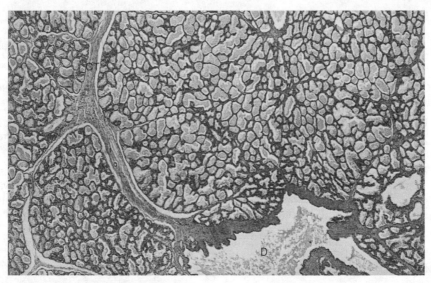

FIGURE 35-9. Mammary gland, active. Note the large number of tubuloalveolar secretory units and the compression of connective tissue (*CT*) into narrow interalveolar septa. Interlobular duct (*D*).

    a. Connective tissue has been synthesized in the pectoral region to produce the gross contour of the breast.

    b. Most of the gland tissue appears to be duct; little evidence of secretory activity exists. The lobar and lobular organization of the gland becomes more evident at this time.

    c. Some variation in gland structure is encountered during the menstrual cycle.

        (1) Estrogens, early in the cycle, promote development of ducts.

        (2) Progesterone, later in the cycle, promotes development of secretory alveoli.

2. Active, proliferating gland during pregnancy. The mammary gland at this time is being prepared for secretion but is not yet a secretory structure (Figure 35-9).

    a. Prolonged elevated levels of estrogens and progesterone of ovarian and placental origin stimulate full development of the gland.

    b. Growth hormone, prolactin, and other hormones of hypophyseal, adrenal, and placental origin are necessary for full development and function of the mammary gland.

    c. Connective tissue, the predominant tissue of the mammary gland in the nonpregnant woman, is reduced to narrow partitions between epithelial lobes and lobules during pregnancy.

3. Active, lactating gland following pregnancy. This is the fully developed, secreting mammary gland that provides nourishment for the infant. Lactation depends on prior preparation of the gland by estrogens, progesterone, and other hormones.

    a. The synthetic activity of the glandular epithelial cells is regulated by **prolactin,** which is secreted by the mammotropes of the pars distalis of the pituitary gland (see Table 30-1).

    b. The first secretion of the mammary gland, occurring in late pregnancy and for a few days after parturition, differs chemically from the milk secreted later.

        (1) Secretions of the mammary gland in the perinatal period are particularly rich in antibodies, which benefit the infant.

        (2) The secretion at this time is called **colostrum.**

    c. The milk ejection (or milk let-down) reflex is the release of milk from the mammary gland.

        (1) Mechanical stimulation of the nipple generates afferent impulses to the hypothalamus.

(2) **Oxytocin** is released from the neurohypophysis into the blood (see Table 30-2).

(3) Oxytocin causes release of milk from the gland, presumably by causing contraction of myoepithelial cells that surround the alveoli.

D. **Cellular aspects of mammary gland secretion.** The secretion of lipids and proteins from glandular cells involves different mechanisms.

1. **Apocrine secretion of lipids.** Lipid droplets are synthesized in the epithelial cells that form the tubuloalveolar secretory units of the gland. The droplets are released from the cells by an apocrine mechanism (see Chapter 23 II D 3).

2. **Exocytotic secretion of proteins.** Milk proteins are also synthesized in the secretory epithelial cells of the mammary gland by the same intracellular pathway used by other protein-synthesizing cells. The proteins are released from the luminal surface of the cell by exocytosis (see Chapter 23 II D 1). This is also referred to as **merocrine secretion.**

XI. **THE PLACENTA** is the point of exchange of metabolites, gases, and waste products between the fetus and mother.

A. **Cleavage, blastocyst formation, and implantation**

1. **Morula.** The **zygote undergoes cleavage** while still in the oviduct. A solid mass of approximately 16 cells, called a morula, arrives in the uterus approximately 4 days after fertilization.

2. **Blastocyst.** Continued divisions of cells of the morula and development of the early embryo produce a blastocyst. Three areas of the blastocyst may be recognized.
   a. The **trophoblast** is the epithelium that forms the wall of the blastocyst.
   b. The **inner cell mass** is a clump of cells, enclosed by the trophoblast, that forms the embryo.
   c. The **blastocoel** is the space enclosed by the trophoblast and not occupied by the inner cell mass.

3. **Implantation of the blastocyst in uterine wall.** Approximately 6 days after fertilization, the blastocyst erodes through the endometrial epithelium into the stroma.
   a. The endometrium is in the secretory phase of the menstrual cycle at the time of implantation.
   b. By 11 or 12 days postfertilization, the blastocyst is completely enclosed by the endometrial stroma.

B. **Development of syncytial trophoblast and cellular trophoblast.** At approximately the time of implantation, the trophoblast forms a double layer of cells.

1. **Syncytial trophoblast** (syncytiotrophoblast, syntrophoblast). This is the outer layer of the trophoblast, and it is a true syncytium. The syncytial trophoblast is a continuous, multinucleate, protoplasmic compartment that is not divided into cells.
   a. Later in development, this layer may be very thin.
   b. Exchanges between maternal and fetal blood must occur across the syncytial trophoblast.

2. **Cellular trophoblast** (cytotrophoblast, Langhans cells). The cytotrophoblast is a continuous simple cuboidal epithelium deep to the syncytial trophoblast.
   a. Later in development, the cytotrophoblast does not form a continuous epithelium but is seen as scattered cells deep to the syncytial trophoblast.
   b. Dividing cells of the cytotrophoblast contribute to the overlying syncytiotrophoblast.

C. **Formation of placental villi.** The surface of the syncytial trophoblast becomes irregular soon after implantation. The irregular spaces and cavities in the syncytial trophoblast are called **lacunae.** The lacunae become continuous with maternal blood vessels, and maternal blood circulates in the lacunar spaces.

1. The **trophoblastic processes** that border the lacunae **differentiate into villi.**
   a. **Primary villi.** Initially, the villi are formed just by the syncytial trophoblast and the cellular trophoblast.
   b. **Secondary villi.** Later, the villi acquire connective tissue cores.
   c. **Tertiary villi.** Finally, the villi become vascularized.

2. **Fetal villi–maternal blood interface.** Villi produce the **vast surface area** that is necessary for exchanges between the fetal and maternal circulation.
   a. Maternal blood flows through the intervillous spaces, and the blood is in contact with the surface of villi.
   b. The branching of placental villi is complex.

D. **Blood circulation through the placenta**

1. **Fetal side of the placenta**
   a. Blood that is poor in oxygen flows through the two umbilical arteries. These arteries supply capillaries in the placental villi.
   b. Oxygen-rich blood is drained from the placenta by the umbilical vein.
   c. The **chorion** is formed by the syncytial trophoblast, cellular trophoblast, and associated connective tissue. Placental villi arise from the **chorionic plate.**

2. **Maternal side of the placenta**
   a. Uterine arteries carry blood to the intervillous spaces.
   b. The villi (from the fetus) are bathed by oxygen-rich maternal blood.
   c. **Decidual cells** develop from endometrial stromal (connective tissue) cells and have the fine structural appearance of metabolically active cells. Decidual cells are a maternal response to implantation and are shed at parturition with the placenta.

3. **Placental barrier**
   a. Exchange of gases and metabolites occurs between fetal and maternal blood across the placental barrier.
   b. The cells and layers across which materials must be transported are the **syncytial trophoblast, cellular trophoblast** (discontinuous later in pregnancy), **basal lamina of the trophoblast, connective tissue of the villus,** and the **basal lamina and endothelium of the placental capillary.**

E. **Functions of the placenta**

1. **Nutrition and maintenance of the fetus**
   a. Nutrients, oxygen, some hormones, some immunoglobulins, and certain drugs and toxins cross the placental barrier from the maternal circulation to the fetal circulation.
   b. Wastes produced by the metabolism of the fetus leave the fetal circulation and enter the maternal circulation in the placenta.

2. **Synthesis and release of hormones**
   a. The placenta produces many hormones; it is an endocrine organ.
   b. The syncytial trophoblast appears to be the site of synthesis of most placental hormones.
      (1) Progesterone and estrogens are produced by the placenta.
      (2) The hormone hCG is produced early in pregnancy, and its presence forms the basis of pregnancy tests.
      (3) Other hormones [e.g., human chorionic somatomammotropin (hCS)] are also produced by the placenta. Hormone synthesis by the placenta is prodigious.

Chapter 36

Male Reproductive System

I.   **INTRODUCTION.** The male reproductive system (Figure 36-1) consists of the paired **testes,** the **genital ducts,** the **accessory glands,** the **urethra,** and the **penis.**

   A.   **Testes as secretory organs.** The testes are secretory organs that produce **sperm** (the male gamete) and **hormones.** The development of the male gamete (i.e., spermatogenesis) is described in section III.

     1. **Androgens,** especially **testosterone,** are steroid hormones secreted by the **interstitial cells** of the testes (i.e., Leydig cells)
       a. **Embryonic development.** Androgens are essential in embryonic development for the genotypic male embryo to develop as a phenotypic male fetus.
       b. **Puberty.** At puberty, testosterone is responsible for the initiation of sperm production (spermatogenesis) and secretion by the accessory sex glands. Testosterone is also responsible for the development of secondary sex characteristics.
       c. **Adult.** In the adult, testosterone is essential to maintain spermatogenesis and the normal secondary sex characteristics, as well as to maintain the structure and function of the genital ducts and accessory sex organs.

     2. **Other hormones and related substances.** The **Sertoli cells** (sustentacular, or supporting, cells) of the testicular epithelium secrete the hormone **inhibin, androgen-binding protein** and other binding proteins, and the fluid that aids passage of the maturing sperm into the genital duct system.

   B.   **Accessory sex glands** include the **seminal vesicles,** the **prostate gland,** and the **bulbourethral** (Cowper) glands.

     1. **Nutrients, hormones, and enzymes.** The genital ducts and the accessory sex glands secrete nutrients, enzymes, and hormones necessary for sperm survival and **semen** production.

     2. **Lubricants.** The bulbourethral glands, which secrete into the penile urethra, produce a mucus-like secretion that probably serves as a lubricant.

II.   **TESTES.** The human testes are ovoid organs, 4 to 5 cm in length, 2.5 cm in width, and 3 cm in thickness (Figure 36-2).

   A.   **Location and blood supply.** The testes are located outside the body cavity in the scrotum. They descend to this location through the inguinal canal shortly before birth. The anterolateral surface is covered with the **tunica vaginalis,** an **extension of the peritoneum** carried through the inguinal canal by the descending testis.

     1. Within the scrotum, the testes are maintained at **2° to 3°C below body temperature.** This lower temperature is essential for spermatogenesis. If testes are kept at body temperature, either artificially or because they fail to descend during development (**cryptorchidism**), they do not produce sperm.

     2. Each testis is supplied with blood by the **testicular artery,** which is highly convoluted near the organ.
       a. The artery is surrounded by the **venous pampiniform plexus,** forming a heat exchanger.
       b. The venous blood returning from the testes and scrotum cools the arterial blood entering the testes.

A

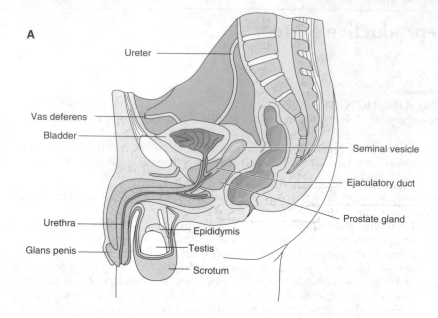

Ureter

Vas deferens

Bladder

Seminal vesicle

Ejaculatory duct

Prostate gland

Urethra

Epididymis

Glans penis

Testis

Scrotum

B

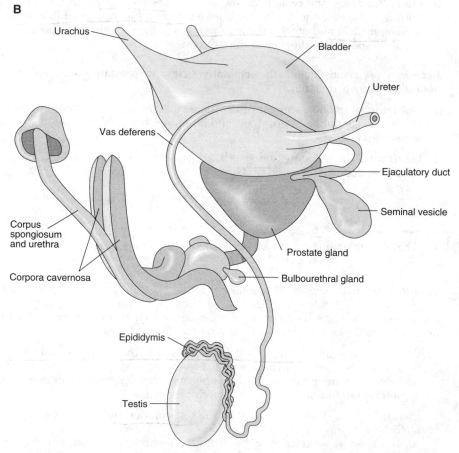

Urachus

Bladder

Ureter

Vas deferens

Ejaculatory duct

Seminal vesicle

Corpus
spongiosum
and urethra

Prostate gland

Corpora cavernosa

Bulbourethral gland

Epididymis

Testis

FIGURE 36-1. (*A*) Sagittal section of the male pelvis showing the location of the major urogenital organs. (*B*) Display of the corresponding dissected urogenital organs of the male.

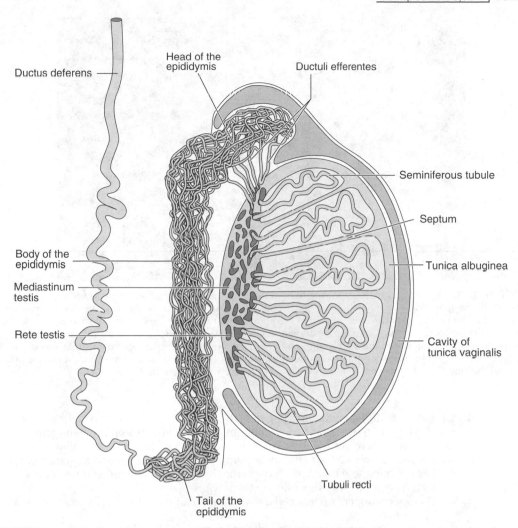

Ductus deferens

Head of the epididymis

Ductuli efferentes

Seminiferous tubule

Septum

Tunica albuginea

Body of the epididymis

Mediastinum testis

Rete testis

Cavity of tunica vaginalis

Tubuli recti

Tail of the epididymis

FIGURE 36-2. Diagram of a sagittal section through the testis and excurrent duct system, including the epididymis and ductus deferens. (Adapted from Weiss L (ed): *A Textbook of Histology,* 6th ed. Baltimore, Urban & Schwarzenberg, 1988, p 932.)

B. **Capsule and mediastinum.** Each testis is covered with a thick fibrous capsule, the **tunica albuginea.** Along the posterior surface, the tunica albuginea thickens to form the **mediastinum** of the testis.

1. The inner surface of the capsule is the **tunica vasculosa,** which is a thin, loose connective tissue layer that contains blood vessels. This layer is not always evident in routine histologic sections.

2 The mediastinum projects into the testis, containing blood and lymphatic vessels, the rete testis, and the proximal portions of the efferent ductules. Incomplete connective tissue septa that project from the mediastinum toward the capsule divide each testis into approximately 250 lobules.

C. **Seminiferous tubules.** Each lobule contains 1 to 4 highly coiled seminiferous tubules. Each tubule is 30 to 80 cm in length and 150 to 250 μm in diameter. Each seminiferous tubule forms a loop that ends in a short **straight tubule;** collectively, these are the **tubuli recti.**

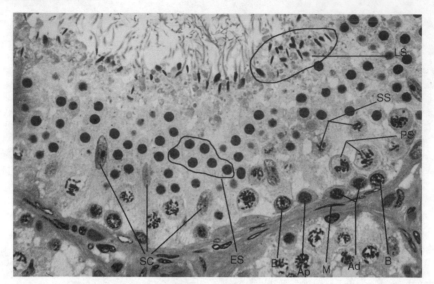

FIGURE 36-3. Light micrograph of monkey testis showing seminiferous epithelium. This fortuitous section shows all the major developmental stages of spermatogenesis in one location. Spermatogonia of types *Ap*, *Ad*, and *B* are visible just above the basement membrane and myoid (*M*) cells. Primary spermatocytes (*PS*) occupy the periphery of the luminal compartment and a few secondary spermatocytes (*SS*) are visible above them. The majority of the cells in the seminiferous epithelium are early spermatids (*ES*) and late spermatids (*LS*). All of these cells are embedded in invaginations of the surface of the Sertoli cells (*SC*) that extend through the full thickness of the epithelium. Compare with Figure 36-4.

1. **Complex stratified epithelium** (Figures 36-3, 36-4). The seminiferous tubules are lined with a complex stratified epithelium, the **seminiferous epithelium** (germinal epithelium). There are two basic and distinct cell populations in the epithelium.
   a. **Spermatogenic cells** are the **male germ cells** that replicate and migrate from the basal lamina to the lumen, through the thickness of the epithelium, as they mature. They consist of the following cell types.
      (1) **Spermatogonia (stem cells)** divide mitotically to give rise to other spermatogonia.
         (a) The spermatogonia reside adjacent to the basal lamina.
         (b) Some mitotically replicating spermatogonia remain as stem cells, whereas others differentiate into **primary spermatocytes.**
      (2) **Primary and secondary spermatocytes** undergo **meiotic division** to give rise to secondary spermatocytes and spermatids, respectively.
      (3) **Spermatids** reside in the apical portion of the epithelium. They differentiate into the **sperm** (spermatozoa).
   b. **Sertoli (sustentacular) cells** are the true epithelial cells of the seminiferous tubules. Each Sertoli cell extends through the full thickness of the seminiferous epithelium.
      (1) They are columnar cells with complex basal, lateral, and apical cell margins that surround the developing spermatogenic cells that are embedded in their surfaces.
      (2) Sertoli cells do not migrate nor do they replicate after puberty.
2. **Peritubular tissue.** A multilayered connective tissue closely surrounds each of the seminiferous tubules.
   a. The **tunica propria** consists of a typical basal lamina, a collagenous layer, three to five layers of **myoid cells** (peritubular contractile cells), blood vessels, and lymphatic vessels.
   b. The myoid cells have characteristics of both fibroblasts and smooth muscle cells. They secrete the external lamina and fibrillar collagen that surrounds them and separates them into layers.

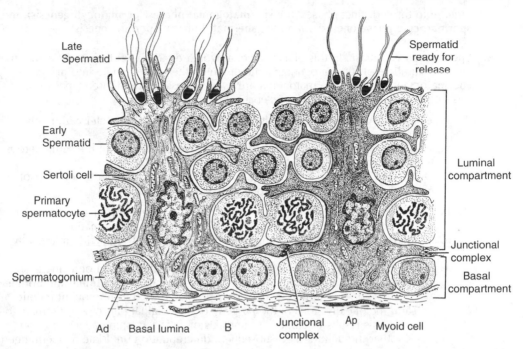

FIGURE 36-4. This drawing of human seminiferous epithelium illustrates the relationships of the Sertoli cells to the differentiating spermatogenic cells. The epithelium is subtended by a basal lamina and a layer of peritubular myoid cells. Type A pale (*Ap*), type A dark (*Ad*), and type B (*B*) spermatogonia are located in the basal compartment of the seminiferous epithelium, below the junctional complex between adjacent Sertoli cells. Primary spermatocytes, secondary spermatocytes (not shown in this diagram), early spermatids, and late spermatids reside in the compartment on the luminal side of the Sertoli–Sertoli junctional complex. (Reprinted with permission from Krause WJ and Cutts JH: *Concise Text of Histology,* 2nd ed. Baltimore, Williams & Wilkins, 1986, p 414.)

D. **Interstitial tissue.** The loose connective tissue between the seminiferous tubules contains **interstitial endocrine cells (Leydig cells),** blood and lymphatic vessels, nerves, fibroblasts, macrophages, and mast cells.

1. **Leydig cells secrete testosterone.** These cells are under the control of pituitary **luteinizing hormone** (LH), also called **interstitial cell–stimulating hormone** (ICSH).
   a. Active Leydig cells are large, irregularly polygonal, acidophilic cells that are often filled with lipid droplets. They have an elaborate smooth endoplasmic reticulum and mitochondria with tubulovesicular cristae. Inactive Leydig cells, however, are very difficult to distinguish from fibroblasts.
   b. Human Leydig cells often contain highly refractile, rod-shaped cytoplasmic crystals of unknown function known as the **crystals of Reinke,** which are seen easily with the light microscope.

2. **Role of Leydig cells in development.** Leydig cells differentiate early in fetal life and secrete the testosterone that is essential for development of the genotypic male embryo as a phenotypic male.
   a. The Leydig cells involute at approximately 5 months of fetal life and are then morphologically indistinguishable from fibroblasts.
   b. At puberty, Leydig cells are exposed to gonadotropic stimulation from the pituitary gland and again differentiate into androgen-secreting cells that produce the testosterone necessary for sexual maturation and continued sexual function in the male.

III. **SPERMATOGENESIS** is the process by which spermatogonia that reside in the basal portion of the germinal epithelium divide and differentiate into sperm. It can be di vided into three distinct phases: the **spermatogonial phase (spermatocytogenesis),** the **spermatocyte phase (meiosis),** and the **spermatid phase (spermiogenesis).**

A. **Spermatogonial phase.** In this phase, spermatogonia divide by **mitosis** to produce increased numbers of spermatogonia, some of which then differentiate into **primary spermatocytes.** In man, spermatogonia are usually classified into three types on the basis of their nuclear staining characteristics.

1. **Type A dark (Ad) spermatogonia** have darkly staining ovoid nuclei with finely granular chromatin.
   a. These spermatagonia are believed to be the true stem cells in the seminiferous tubules in man, and they **divide very infrequently.**
   b. Division of a type Ad spermatogonium may give rise to either a new pair of type Ad spermatogonia or to a pair of type Ap spermatogonia.

2. **Type A pale (Ap) spermatogonia** are the replicating population of spermatogonia. They have lightly staining ovoid nuclei with finely granular chromatin.
   a. The Ap spermatogonia are committed to differentiate. They divide mitotically and increase rapidly in number.
      (1) The pair of Ap spermatogonia produced from the division of a single Ad spermatogonium remain attached to one another by a **cytoplasmic bridge.** So, too, do the numerous daughters produced by the subsequent mitotic and meiotic divisions of the progeny of the original pair of Ap spermatogonia. This results in clones of hundreds of cells remaining attached to one another throughout their subsequent differentiation until late in spermiogenesis.
      (2) This is essential for the **synchronous development of each clone.**
   b. After several divisions, type Ap spermatogonia differentiate into type B spermatogonia.

3. **Type B spermatogonia** represent the last step in the spermatogonial phase. They have generally spherical nuclei with large clumps of chromatin along the nuclear envelope and around the nucleolus. Type B cells also divide mitotically to give rise to more type B spermatogonia, still connected by cytoplasmic bridges.
   a. At some point, all of the connected type B progeny of one pair of Ap spermatogonia differentiate into **primary spermatocytes.**
   b. The primary spermatocytes replicate their DNA shortly after they form from type B spermatogonia. Thus, a primary spermatocyte contains the **4N (tetraploid) amount of DNA.**

B. **Spermatocyte phase.** In this phase, **two meiotic divisions** reduce both the chromosome number and the amount of DNA to the **haploid** condition (22 autosomes + 1 sex chromosome; 1N amount of DNA). [Meiosis is described in detail in Chapter 4 IX; only a brief summary is presented here.

1. **Prophase of the first meiotic division,** the stage in which the chromatin condenses into visible chromosomes, is long (up to 22 days in humans). The stages of prophase are called **leptotene, zygotene, pachytene,** and **diplotene.**
   a. **Chromosomes.** The name of each stage describes a degree and complexity of coiling of the chromatin that ultimately results in the condensing of **44 autosomes** and the **X and Y chromosomes.**
      (1) Each chromosome has two chromatin strands called **chromatids.**
      (2) A unique feature of the first meiotic division is that **homologous chromosomes are paired** as they line up on the metaphase plate (**synapsis**).
   b. **Crossing over.** The paired homologous chromosomes, called **tetrads** because they consist of four chromatids, exchange genetic material in a process called **crossing over** (see Chapter 4 IX B 1 b). This ensures that the four sperm produced from each primary spermatocyte are different.

2. **Metaphase, anaphase, and telophase of the first meiotic division.** After crossing over is completed, the paired homologous chromosomes at the metaphase plate

move away from each other and toward opposite poles of the spindle. **Tetrads separate to form dyads.**

 a. The two chromatids of each chromosome remain together. This is the opposite of what happens in mitotic divisions, in which the chromatids normally separate.

 b. The movement of a particular chromosome of a homologous pair to either end of the spindle is random. Maternally derived and paternally derived chromosomes do not sort themselves as they leave the metaphase plate.

 c. The cells resulting from the first meiotic division are the **secondary spermatocytes,** which are still connected by cytoplasmic bridges.

3. **Prophase of the second meiotic division.** The secondary spermatocytes immediately enter the prophase of the second meiotic division **without passing through an S phase** (i.e., they do not synthesize DNA before dividing).

 a. Each secondary spermatocyte has **22 autosomes** and an **X or a Y chromosome,** each consisting of two chromatids.

 b. Each secondary spermatocyte has the **2N (diploid) amount of DNA.**

4. **Metaphase, anaphase, and telophase of the second meiotic division.** The mechanics of the second meiotic division resemble a mitotic division except that there has been **no DNA replication** immediately preceding it, and the **two chromatids of the dyad are not identical.**

 a. The chromosomes line up on the equatorial plate, and the **sister chromatids separate** and move to the opposite poles of the spindle.

 b. As the second meiotic division is completed, the nuclear envelope reforms, and two spermatids are formed from each secondary spermatocyte. These cells, too, are still connected by cytoplasmic bridges.

 c. The spermatids derived from each secondary spermatocyte have **22 autosomes** and an **X or a Y chromosome,** but each chromosome consists of **only a single chromatid.** Thus, the spermatid has only the **1N (haploid) amount of DNA.**

 d. The normal diploid condition is restored only if a sperm fertilizes an ovum, and the two haploid pronuclei of the gametes fuse.

C. **Spermatid phase.** Spermiogenesis is the process by which spermatids produced by meiosis differentiate into sperm. It is described as having four successive phases: **Golgi phase, cap phase, acrosome phase,** and **maturation phase.** All the phases involve major morphologic changes in the spermatids. They occur while the spermatids are embedded in invaginations of the luminal surface of the Sertoli cells.

1. **The Golgi phase** is characterized by the appearance of periodic acid–Schiff (PAS)-positive granules in the Golgi apparatus. These are **proacrosomal granules,** and they are rich in glycoproteins.

 a. The granules coalesce within a membrane-bounded vesicle called the **acrosomal vesicle,** which lies next to the nuclear envelope and **determines the anterior pole** of the developing sperm.

 b. Also characteristic of this phase is the **migration of the paired centrioles** from the juxtanuclear region to the newly established posterior pole of the spermatid, where the distal centriole aligns at a right angle to the plasma membrane and initiates synthesis of the **axonemal complex** of the developing sperm tail (flagellum).

2. **The cap phase** is characterized by the condensation, flattening, and spreading of the acrosomal vesicle over the entire anterior half of the nucleus, forming the **acrosomal cap.** The nuclear envelope beneath the acrosomal cap thickens and loses its pores, while the nuclear contents become further condensed and more intensely basophilic.

3. **Acrosome phase.** During this phase, the spermatid reorients itself so that the head points toward the basal lamina of the seminiferous tubule, and the developing sperm tail extends into the lumen.

 a. The **condensed nucleus elongates and flattens,** and the cytoplasm is displaced posteriorly.

b. Cytoplasmic microtubules organize into a cylindrical sheath called the **manchette,** which extends from the caudal rim of the acrosome toward the developing tail.

c. The centrioles return to the posterior surface of the nucleus, drawing the proximal portion of the tail into the cytoplasm. The proximal centriole becomes attached to a shallow groove in the nucleus.

  (1) The centrioles are then modified to form the **connecting piece** or **neck region** of the developing sperm.

  (2) Nine coarse fibers develop from the centriole attached to the nucleus and extend into the tail as the **outer dense fibers** peripheral to the microtubules of the axoneme. This unites the nucleus with the flagellum, hence the name connecting piece.

d. Mitochondria migrate from the rest of the cytoplasm to form a helically wrapped sheath around the coarse fibers in the neck region and its immediate posterior extension.

  (1) This forms the **middle piece** of the tail of the sperm.

  (2) Distal to the middle piece, a **fibrous sheath** consisting of two longitudinal elements and numerous connecting ribs replaces the mitochondria surrounding the nine longitudinal coarse fibers in the **principal piece** and extends nearly to the tip of the flagellum.

4. Maturation phase. This phase is characterized by the pinching off of the excess cytoplasm as **residual bodies** that are phagocytized by Sertoli cells.

a. The cytoplasmic bridges that have characterized the developing gametes since the Ap spermatogonial stage remain with the residual bodies.

b. The **mature spermatids (immature sperm)** are therefore no longer attached to each other. They are then released from the surface of the Sertoli cells into the lumen of the seminiferous tubule.

D. **Mature sperm** (Figure 36-5). Spermiogenesis produces a structurally unique cell that, after further maturation in the epididymis, is capable of carrying its **haploid amount of DNA** to the ovum in the female reproductive tract. Having lost nearly all of its cytoplasm, it carries with its nuclear material only an **acrosome,** which contains the enzymes necessary for penetration of the membranes covering the egg, and **mitochondria,** which provide the energy for flagellar movement.

1. Structure. The mature sperm is approximately 60 μm in length and has a distinct **head** and **tail.**

a. The **head** is flattened and pointed, measuring 4.5 μm in length, 3.0 μm in width, and 1 μm in thickness.

b. The **acrosome** covers the anterior two-thirds of the nucleus.

  (1) The acrosome is a highly specialized lysosome that contains **hyaluronidase** and other enzymes essential for the penetration by the sperm of the corona radiata and the zona pellucida of the ovum.

  (2) The release of acrosomal enzymes as the sperm touches the egg is the first step in the **acrosome reaction.** The acrosome reaction is a complex process that facilitates sperm penetration and subsequent fertilization and prevents the entry of additional sperm into the ovum.

c. The long **tail,** or **flagellum,** is subdivided into the following sections:

  (1) The **neck,** which contains the **centrioles** and the **connecting piece**

  (2) The **midpiece** (approximately 7 μm in length), which contains the **mitochondria,** external to the **coarse fibers**

  (3) The **principal piece** (approximately 40 μm in length), which contains the nine **coarse fibers** and the external **circumferential sheath fibers**

  (4) The **end piece** (approximately 5 μm in length), which contains only the **axonemal complex**

2. Transport. Newly released sperm are nonmotile. They are transported out of the seminiferous tubules, through the **straight tubules** to the **rete testis,** in a fluid secreted by the Sertoli cells.

a. From the rete testis, sperm are carried out of the testis through the **efferent duct-**

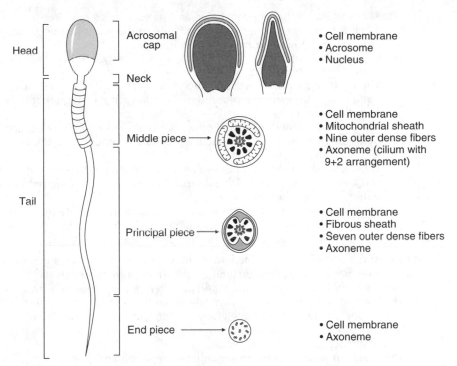

Head

Acrosomal cap

Neck

Tail

Middle piece →

Principal piece →

End piece →

• Cell membrane
• Acrosome
• Nucleus

• Cell membrane
• Mitochondrial sheath
• Nine outer dense fibers
• Axoneme (cilium with 9+2 arrangement)

• Cell membrane
• Fibrous sheath
• Seven outer dense fibers
• Axoneme

• Cell membrane
• Axoneme

FIGURE 36-5. Diagram of a human sperm. Regions of the mature sperm are shown on the *left*. Diagrams of sections through the head, and the major segments of the tail, are shown on the *right*.

ules into the proximal portion of the **ductus epididymis,** the first of the major extratesticular genital ducts.

(1) Most of the fluid secreted in the seminiferous tubules is reabsorbed in the efferent ductules. More of the fluid is absorbed by the proximal portion of the epididymis.

(2) Sperm develop motility as they pass through the 4 to 5 meters of the highly coiled ductus epididymis.

b. **Peristaltic contractions** of the smooth muscle that surrounds the efferent ductules and the epididymis propel the sperm to the distal portion of the ductus epididymis, where they are stored before ejaculation.

c. Mature sperm can live for several weeks in the male genital duct system but survive only 2 to 3 days in the female reproductive tract.

3. **Capacitation.** Sperm acquire the ability to fertilize an ovum only after existing for some time in the female tract. This process, called **capacitation,** remains incompletely understood but involves modification of glycocalyx components on the sperm plasma membrane.

E. Cycles of the seminiferous epithelium. Differentiating germ cells in the seminiferous epithelium are not arranged at random. There are regular **cell associations** that may be observed to **occur sequentially** at any given site in the tubule.

1. **Synchronized development.** These associations occur because intercellular bridges allow a clone of cells to develop synchronously. Also, the synchronized cells spend a specific time in each stage of maturation, and each stage of maturation is a different length.

a. A **cell association** is a recognizable grouping of cells in different stages of maturation that occurs repeatedly. Each cell association is considered a **stage in a cyclic process.**

    b. The series of stages that appears between two successive occurrences of the same cell association pattern at any given site in the seminiferous tubule constitutes the **cycle of the seminiferous epithelium.**

        (1) In man, six successive stages or cell associations define the cycle of the seminiferous epithelium.

        (2) The cycle in man lasts approximately 16 days; 4.6 cycles, or 74 days, are required for a spermatogonium to differentiate into a sperm that is released from the Sertoli cell.

    c. The cycle of the seminiferous epithelium has been most carefully studied in rats, where 14 successive stages occur in **linear sequence** along the length of the seminiferous tubule.

        (1) The six stages in man are not as clearly delineated, however, because the cell associations occur in irregular patches forming a **mosaic pattern** in the seminiferous epithelium.

        (2) Thus, a cross-section through a human seminiferous tubule may show only a few, or as many as all six stages of the cycle arranged in a pie-wedge fashion around the circumference of the tubule.

2. Waves of the seminiferous epithelium. In most mammalian species in which spermatogenesis has been studied, including subhuman primates, each stage in a cycle occupies a significant length of the total circumference of the seminiferous tubule.

    a. The stages appear to occur sequentially along the length of the tubule. A longitudinal section along the tubule gives the appearance of a wave of differentiation along the tubule. In the rat, there are estimated to be approximately 12 waves in each tubule.

    b. There are no waves in human seminiferous epithelium.

IV. SERTOLI CELLS are the true epithelium of the seminiferous tubule (see Figure 36-4).

A. **Structure.** Sertoli cells are nonreplicating, tall columnar epithelial cells that line the lumen of the seminiferous tubule and rest on a thick, multilayered basal lamina.

    1. They have an extensive smooth endoplasmic reticulum (sER), a well-developed rough endoplasmic reticulum (rER), and paracrystalline stacks of ER cisternae called **annulate lamellae.**

    2. The nucleus is euchromatic and is usually ovoid or triangular, often with several deep infoldings. In most mammalian species, the nucleus contains a unique tripartite structure consisting of an RNA-containing nucleolus flanked by a pair of DNA-containing bodies called **karyosomes.**

    3. In man, bundles of poorly ordered 15-nm filaments form characteristic inclusion bodies (of Charcot-Böttcher) in the basal cytoplasm. These may be large enough to be visible with the light microscope.

B. **Unique junctions.** Sertoli cells are bound to each other and to spermatids by an unusual junctional complex.

    1. Sertoli–Sertoli junctions. Sertoli cells are bound to one another, usually near the basal surface, by a junction that contains a highly developed tight junction and gap junctions, associated with cytoplasmic specializations.

        a. A **flattened cisterna of sER** lies parallel to the plasma membrane adjacent to the junction in each cell.

        b. Actin filament bundles are hexagonally packed and interposed between the sER cisternae and the plasma membranes.

    2. Morphologic compartmentalization. The Sertoli–Sertoli junctional complex establishes a **basal** compartment and a **luminal** (adluminal) compartment in the seminiferous epithelium.

a. Spermatogonia and early primary spermatocytes are restricted to the basal compartment, between the junctional complexes and the basal lamina.

b. More mature primary spermatocytes, secondary spermatocytes, and spermatids are restricted to the luminal compartment. Thus, the processes of meiosis and spermiogenesis are restricted to the luminal compartment.

  (1) The primary spermatocytes that derive from mitotic division of type B spermatogonia must "pass through" the junctional complex to move from the basal compartment to the luminal compartment.

  (2) This is accomplished by the formation of a new junctional complex between processes from adjacent Sertoli cells that extend beneath the newly formed spermatocytes and the subsequent breakdown of the junction immediately above the spermatocytes.

3. Sertoli–spermatid junctions. A similar-appearing junctional complex is found at the site where spermatids attach to Sertoli cells. There is no tight junction component, however, in the Sertoli cell–spermatid junctional complex. Only the Sertoli-cell side of the junction shows the flattened sER cisterna and the actin filament bundles. These elements are lacking in the spermatid.

C. **Functions of Sertoli cells.** Sertoli cells serve as **supporting cells** for the developing gametes, as **exocrine** and **endocrine secretory cells,** as **phagocytic cells,** and as the morphologic substratum of the **blood–testis barrier.**

1. Supporting cells. In both the basal and luminal compartments, the developing spermatogenic cells are surrounded by complex processes of the Sertoli cells.

  a. It is believed that Sertoli cells function in the exchange of metabolic substrates and wastes between the developing gametes and the circulatory system.

  b. A number of specific binding proteins, including **testicular transferrin** (an iron-binding protein) and **androgen-binding protein,** are secreted by Sertoli cells. They are important for transporting materials from the blood to the developing germ cells and for maintaining a luminal environment conducive to sperm differentiation.

2. Secretory cells. In addition to the binding proteins described above, Sertoli cells secrete **inhibin.**

  a. Inhibin is a component in the feedback loop that regulates release of **follicle-stimulating hormone** (FSH) by the adenohypophysis.

  b. Sertoli cells also secrete the fluid in which sperm are bathed as they move into the intratesticular genital ducts from the seminiferous tubules.

3. Phagocytic cells. Sertoli cells phagocytize and digest the residual bodies released in the last stage of spermiogenesis. They also phagocytize and digest cells of the germ cell line that fail to complete spermatogenesis.

4. Blood–testis barrier. The Sertoli–Sertoli junctional complex is the site of the blood–testis barrier.

  a. The blood–testis barrier creates a **physiologic compartmentalization** in the seminiferous epithelium that parallels the morphologic compartmentalization.

    (1) The ionic, amino acid, carbohydrate, and protein composition of the fluid in the seminiferous tubules is significantly different from that of the blood plasma.

    (2) In addition, the barrier allows the androgen-binding protein—and, therefore, testosterone—to be highly concentrated in the luminal compartment, which is an important factor for gamete development.

  b. The blood–testis barrier also serves as an **immunologic barrier,** creating an immunologically privileged site in the lumen of the seminiferous tubule. The genetically and, therefore, antigenically different haploid germ cells (i.e., secondary spermatocytes, spermatids, and sperm) are isolated from the immune system of the adult male.

    (1) Plasma proteins, particularly circulating antibodies (including sperm-specific antibodies present in some adult males), are excluded from the lumen of the seminiferous tubule.

(2) Conversely, antigens produced by or specific to the developing sperm are prevented from reaching the systemic circulation.

V. INTRATESTICULAR GENITAL DUCTS include the **straight tubules**, the **rete testis**, and the **proximal** portions of the **efferent ductules**.

A. **Straight tubules.** At each end of the loop of each seminiferous tubule there is an abrupt transition to the straight tubules, or **tubuli recti.**

1. This is a short terminal section of the seminiferous tubule that is lined solely by Sertoli cells.

2. As the straight tubule narrows near its opening into the rete testis, the lining changes to a simple cuboidal epithelium.

B. **Rete testis.** The rete testis is a complex series of interconnecting channels in the highly vascular connective tissue of the mediastinum testis.

1. The rete testis is lined throughout its tortuous course by a low cuboidal epithelium.

2. Each cuboidal cell has a single cilium on its apical surface and a few apical microvilli.

C. **Efferent ductules** (Figure 36-6; see also Figure 36-2). In man, approximately 15 efferent ductules (ductuli efferentes) leave the testis by penetrating the tunica albuginea and connect the rete testis to the proximal portion of the **ductus epididymis.**

1. **Coni vasculosi.** As the efferent ductules leave the testis, the 15 to 20–cm-long ductules become highly coiled and tightly packed into 6 to 10 conical masses called coni vasculosi. At the base of the cone, each efferent ductule empties into the single channel of the ductus epididymis.

2. **Saw-toothed epithelium.** Efferent ductules are lined with alternating clumps of tall

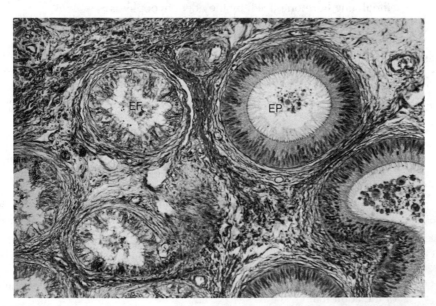

FIGURE 36-6. Photomicrograph of several cross-sections of efferent ductules (*EF*), and multiple cross-sections of the single, highly coiled ductus epididymis (*EP*). Note the saw-toothed luminal surface of the efferent ductules and the smooth luminal surface of the ductus epididymis.

and short columnar cells, thus giving rise to the saw-toothed appearance of the luminal surface.

  a. The **tall columnar cells** are generally ciliated and are believed to have a role in moving the sperm through the ductule.
  b. The **short nonciliated cells** have numerous microvilli and canalicular invaginations of the apical surface.
    (1) There are numerous pinocytotic vesicles, lysosomes, and other cytoplasmic components associated with intense endocytic activity.
    (2) Nearly 80% of the fluid secreted in the seminiferous tubules is reabsorbed in the efferent ductules.

3. **The muscular coat** that surrounds and, to some extent, characterizes the excurrent genital duct system is first seen at the level of the efferent ductules. The smooth muscle investment of the efferent ductules is several cell layers thick.
  a. The cells are arrayed as a circular sheath around the ductule, with elastic fibers interspersed between the layers.
  b. Contraction of this fibromuscular coat helps to move sperm from the efferent ductules to the epididymis.

VI. **EXTRATESTICULAR GENITAL DUCTS,** the **excurrent duct system,** include the **distal** portions of the **efferent ductules,** the **ductus epididymis,** the **ductus deferens,** the **ejaculatory duct,** and the **urethra.** The urethra is shared with the urinary system as a common duct for semen and urine.

A. **Ductus epididymis** (see Figure 36-2). This is a very long, highly coiled tube in which sperm undergo further maturation. The ductus epididymis is contained in the **epididymis,** which is a gross structure attached to the outside of the testis that measures approximately 7.5 cm in length.

1. The highly coiled **ductus epididymis** measures nearly **6 meters** in length. Because it is so compressed in the epididymis, a histologic section through this structure may show hundreds of sections of the continuous duct.

2. The ductus epididymis is described as having a **head (caput),** a **body (corpus),** and a **tail (cauda).** The efferent ductules empty into the head.

3. Sperm mature during their passage through the ductus epididymis.
  a. Essentially, mature sperm stored in the tail of the epididymis are capable of directional motion and are able to fertilize an ovum.
  b. This maturation, like their development, is androgen-dependent and involves addition to their glycocalyx of materials secreted by the epididymal epithelial cells.

4. **Pseudostratified epithelium** (see Figure 36-6). The ductus epididymis is lined with a pseudostratified epithelium consisting of tall columnar **principal cells** and short **basal cells.** The ductus epididymis differs from the efferent ductules in having a **smooth luminal surface.**
  a. **Structure and function of principal cells**
    (1) The principal cells vary from nearly 80 μm tall in the head to approximately 40 μm tall in the tail.
    (2) The principal cells of the head **reabsorb** most of the **fluid** that is not absorbed in the efferent ductules and **phagocytize** any residual bodies not removed by Sertoli cells. They also phagocytize any sperm that degenerate in the duct.
    (3) They are characterized by the presence on their apical surface of **long, modified microvilli** (erroneously named stereocilia) that extend in clumps into the lumen. These range from 25 μm in length (head) to approximately 10 μm in length (tail).
    (4) The apical cytoplasm of the principal cells exhibits numerous invaginations

at the bases of the stereocilia, as well as coated vesicles, multivesicular bodies, and numerous lysosomes.

(5) The principal cells are also **secretory.** They have a well-developed rER and an unusually large supranuclear Golgi apparatus. They are known to secrete glycerophosphocholine, sialic acid, and glycoproteins that are added to the glycocalyx of the sperm, and they may also secrete androgens that aid in sperm maturation.

b. The **basal cells** are believed to be the **stem cells** for the duct epithelium. Significant numbers of **lymphocytes,** called **halo cells,** are interspersed in the duct epithelium.

5. **Muscle coat.** The smooth muscle coat of the ductus epididymis also changes along its length.

a. In the head and most of the body, the smooth muscle consists of a thin layer of **circular muscle.** In the tail, both an **inner and outer longitudinal layer** are added. These three layers are then continuous with those of the ductus deferens.

b. **Peristaltic movements of the thin circular muscle layer** serve to move the sperm along in the head and body of the ductus epididymis.

c. **Intense contractions of the three muscle layers** in the tail of the ductus epididymis occur in response to appropriate neural stimulation during sexual excitation.

(1) This forces the sperm stored in the tail into the ductus deferens.

(2) This is the initial muscular component of the ejaculatory response.

B. **Ductus deferens.** The ductus deferens, or **vas deferens,** is a continuation of the tail of the ductus epididymis.

1. **Location and course.** The ductus deferens ascends along the posterior border of the testis along with the vessels and nerves that serve the testis.

a. It enters the abdomen in the spermatic cord, passing through the inguinal canal, and then descends into the pelvis to the level of the bladder, where it connects to the prostatic urethra (see Chapter 29 X E 2).

b. The distal end of the ductus deferens enlarges to form the **ampulla,** where it is joined by the duct of the **seminal vesicle** and continues as the **ejaculatory duct** through the parenchyma of the prostate gland to enter the prostatic urethra.

2. **Pseudostratified epithelium.** A pseudostratified columnar epithelium that closely resembles that of the epididymis lines the ductus deferens, although, unlike the epididymis, the lumen is thrown into deep longitudinal folds that are probably the result of contraction of the thick muscular coat of the ductus deferens.

a. The tall columnar cells also have long microvilli (stereocilia) that extend into the lumen.

b. The basal cells rest on the basal lamina and may also be stem cells.

C. **Ejaculatory duct.** This is a short (1 cm) duct formed by the union of the ductus deferens and the duct of the seminal vesicle. The ejaculatory duct enters the urethra at the **prostatic utricle.**

1. The duct is lined with a mixture of simple columnar and pseudostratified columnar epithelium.

2. The ejaculatory ducts have no muscle coat. The power for ejaculation comes primarily from the smooth muscle of the ductus deferens and caudal portion of the epididymis and, to a lesser extent, from the smooth muscle of the seminal vesicles and prostate gland.

VII. ACCESSORY SEX GLANDS include the **seminal vesicles,** the **prostate gland,** and the **bulbourethral (Cowper) glands.**

A. **The seminal vesicles** originate as evaginations from the ductus deferens distal to the ampulla. They are paired, elongated, folded tubular glands with a muscular and fibrous coat.

1. Although the **mucosa** is thrown into numerous primary, secondary, and tertiary folds that increase the surface area for secretion, all of the irregular chambers thus formed communicate with the lumen. Their development, normal adult morphology, and secretory function are under the control of testosterone.

2. The **pseudostratified columnar epithelium** contains tall nonciliated cells and short round cells that rest on the basal lamina.
   a. The columnar cells have the morphologic characteristics of **protein-secreting cells** (e.g., a well-developed rER, large secretory vacuoles in the apical cytoplasm).
   b. The secretion of the seminal vesicles is a whitish-yellow, viscous material that contains **fructose** (the principal metabolic substrate for sperm) along with other simple sugars, **amino acids, ascorbic acid,** and **prostaglandins.**

3. **Contractions** of the smooth muscle of the seminal vesicles during ejaculation discharge the secretion into the ejaculatory ducts and help to flush sperm out of the urethra.

B. **The prostate gland** (Figure 36-7) is the largest accessory sex gland. It secretes **acid phosphatase, fibrinolysin,** and **citric acid.**

1. **Multiple glands.** The prostate gland is a collection of 30 to 50 tubuloalveolar glands that surround the proximal urethra.

2. **Concentric layers.** The glands are arranged in three concentric layers: a mucosal layer of short glands that secrete directly into the urethra; a submucosal layer of glands; and the outer, or main, glands. Both the submucosal and main glands have ducts that carry their secretions to the prostatic urethra.

3. **Columnar epithelium.** The epithelium of the prostate gland is generally simple columnar, although patches of cuboidal, squamous, or pseudostratified epithelium may be found.
   a. The epithelium secretes **fibrinolysin,** which serves to liquefy the semen.
   b. In addition to acid phosphatase sequestered in lysosomes, the epithelium also

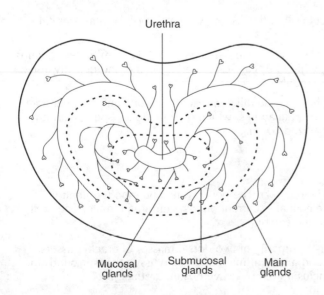

Urethra

Mucosal glands   Submucosal glands   Main glands

FIGURE 36-7. Diagram of a transverse section of the prostate gland, showing the relationship of the three concentric layers of prostatic glands to the prostatic urethra into which they secrete.

FIGURE 36-8. Cross-section of the penis of an adult male. The section is from the mid-portion of the shaft of the penis (skin removed).

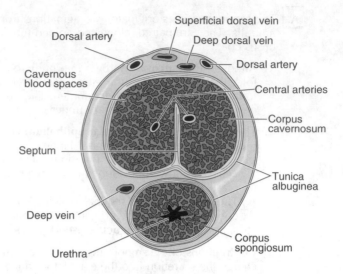

secretes large amounts of acid phosphatase, some of which enters the circulation.

4. **Concretions.** The prostatic alveoli, especially those of older males, usually contain concretions of variable form and size that may be as large as 2 mm in diameter.
    a. These are also called **corpora amylacea.**
    b. The concretions are believed to be formed by precipitation of secretory material around cell fragments. They may become calcified.

C. **Bulbourethral glands.** The paired bulbourethral glands (Cowper glands) are pea-sized structures located near the beginning of the membranous urethra. They are connected to the penile urethra by long ducts [see Chapter 29 X E 2 c].

1. The glands are compound tubuloalveolar glands that resemble mucus-secreting glands. Erotic stimulation causes release of the secretion, which constitutes the major portion of the preseminal fluid.

2. The clear, mucus-like secretion contains large amounts of galactose, galactosamine, galacturonic acid, sialic acid, and methylpentose, which probably serve to lubricate the penile urethra.

D. **Semen** is the combined product of all of the secretory elements of the male genital system—cells, solvent, and solutes.

1. The **volume** of the average ejaculate is approximately 3 ml. Each milliliter contains up to 100 million sperm, of which 20% are estimated to be morphologically abnormal, and nearly 25% are nonmotile.

2. Semen is alkaline and may help to neutralize the acid environment of the urethra and vagina. It also contains prostaglandins, which may influence sperm transit as well as implantation of a fertilized ovum.

VIII. **PENIS** (Figure 36-8; see also Figure 36-1). The penis is the common termination of both the urinary system and the genital excurrent duct system in the male. The urethra carries both semen and urine to the exterior.

A. **Erectile tissue.** The penis consists primarily of two dorsal masses of erectile tissue, called the **corpora cavernosa,** and a ventral mass of erectile tissue that surrounds the urethra, called the **corpus spongiosum** (corpus cavernosum urethrae).

1. A dense fibroelastic layer, the **tunica albuginea,** binds the three cavernosa together as well as forming a capsule around each one.

2. The corpora cavernosa are lined with vascular endothelium. They increase in size and rigidity by filling with blood.
   a. The **helicine arteries** that supply the corpora cavernosa dilate under sexual stimulation and increase the blood flow to the penis.
   b. An arteriovenous (AV) anastomosis between the deep artery of the penis and the peripheral venous system closes, also increasing blood flow to the penis.
   c. In addition, the peripheral veins that drain the penis are increasingly compressed as the erectile response develops, further amplifying the response.

B. **Skin of the penis.** The thin skin is loosely attached to the underlying connective tissue, which contains no adipose tissue. Only at the **glans** is the skin firmly attached.

1. There is a thin layer of smooth muscle in the skin that is continuous with the dartos layer of the scrotum.

2. In uncircumcised males, the glans is covered with a fold of skin, the **prepuce,** which has characteristics of a mucous membrane on its inner aspect.

C. **Innervation.** The penis is innervated by spinal, sympathetic, and parasympathetic nerves.

1. The skin of the penis is rich in sensory endings; sympathetic and parasympathetic visceral nerves innervate the smooth muscle of the tunica albuginea and the blood vessels.

2. Both the sensory and visceral motor fibers have essential roles in the erectile and ejaculatory reflexes.

Chapter 37

Eye

I. **INTRODUCTION.** The eye **receives images** of the environment and **processes and transmits** those images to integrative centers in the brain via the **optic nerve.**

A. **Location.** The paired human eyes are spherical organs (globes) located in bony orbital sockets.

B. **Size and suspension.** The eye measures approximately 25 mm in diameter. It is suspended in the socket by **six extrinsic muscles** that move it in horizontal and vertical planes around an anteroposterior axis.

C. **Function.** As the principal sensory organ, the eye is specialized to:

1. **Refract light through two dioptrics** (i.e., refractive elements), the **cornea** and the **lens**

2. **Focus** the image thus produced on a **photosensitive layer,** the **retina**

D. **Concentric layers** (Figure 37-1)

1. **Corneoscleral layer.** The **outermost layer** forms both a **tough fibrous protective coat** and the **cornea.** It completely encloses the other two layers, except where it is penetrated by the optic nerve.

2. **Uveal layer.** The **middle layer** includes the **choroid,** and the stroma of the **ciliary body** and **iris.**

3. **Retinal layer.** This is the **inner layer.**
   a. **Posteriorly,** it includes the **neural retina** and **pigment epithelium.**
   b. **Anteriorly,** it forms the **nonpigmented** and **pigmented epithelial layers of the ciliary body** and the double-layered **pigmented epithelium of the iris.**

II. **SPECIFIC FUNCTIONS OF OCULAR TISSUES** (Figure 37-2)

A. **Primary image formation.** The **cornea** and the **lens** transmit light.

1. **Aqueous and vitreous humors**
   a. The **aqueous humor** fills the internal space of the eye behind the cornea and in front of the lens (**anterior** and **posterior chambers;** see VI,VII).
   b. The **vitreous humor,** or **vitreous body,** fills the space behind the lens and in front of the retina (**vitreous space**) and helps to maintain the shape of the eye.
   c. The **refractive index** of the humors approximately matches that of the cornea and lens.

2. **Focusing role of lens.** Changing the shape of the deformable lens changes the focal distance of the eye. This is the process of **accommodation.** The lens becomes more rounded in order to bring objects that are close to the eye into focus.

B. **Photoreception. Rods** and **cones,** specialized cells in the neural retina, are the photoreceptors of the eye.

1. The **photoreceptors,** the **connecting neurons** in the retina, and the **ganglion cells** whose axons form the **optic nerve,** differentiate from neurectoderm (see Table 37-1).

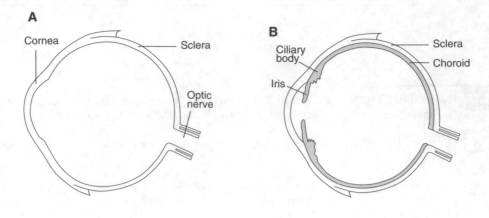

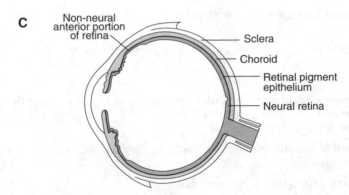

FIGURE 37-1. Concentric layers of the eye. (*A*) Outer supporting layer, the corneoscleral coat; (*B*) middle layer, the uveal layer, which includes the choroid and the stroma of the ciliary body and iris; (*C*) inner layer, the retinal layer, which includes the photosensitive layer and the anterior extensions that form the epithelium of the ciliary body and iris. (Adapted from Ross M, Romrell L, Kaye G: *Histology: A Text and Atlas,* 3rd ed. Baltimore, Williams & Wilkins, 1995, p 741.)

  2. Large **radial glia** of the retina called **Müller cells,** also derived from neurectoderm, extend through the thickness of the neural retina.

C. **Nutrition.** The **highly vascularized** tissues of the **uveal layer** provide nutritional support for most of the other ocular tissues.

  1. The ciliary body secretes the aqueous humor that provides nutritional support for the lens and the cornea, which are avascular.

  2. The retina has its own blood supply via the retinal artery. It also receives some nutritional support from the pigment epithelium.

D. **Pigmentation.** Pigment absorbs scattered and reflected light and minimizes glare within the eye.

  1. The structures of the uveal layer are heavily pigmented.

  2. Pigment is concentrated in the outer layer of epithelium of the retinal layer, which forms the retinal pigment epithelium, the nonsecretory layer of the ciliary epithelium, and the outer (anterior) layer of the iris epithelium.

  3. The inner (posterior) layer of the iris epithelium is also heavily pigmented, as is the stroma of the iris.

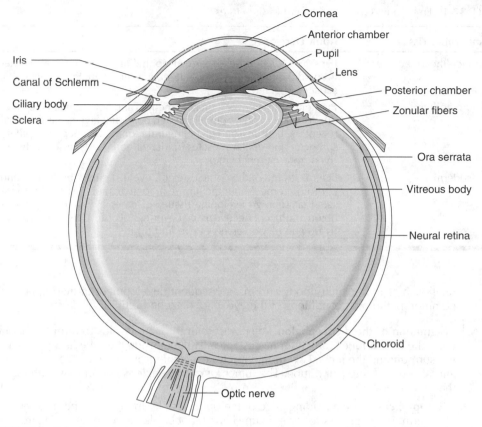

FIGURE 37-2. Principal structures of the anterior and posterior segments of the eye (meridional section).

E. Protection

1. **Lids** protect and help to lubricate the anterior surface of the eye.

2. The **corneosclera** is the tough outer coat of the eye. This dense fibrous connective tissue layer and its covering epithelium physically protect the inner structures of the eye.

   a. The **conjunctiva** is the stratified columnar epithelium that lines the inner surface of the lids (**palpebral conjunctiva**), covers the anterior portion of the sclera (**bulbar conjunctiva**), and is continuous with the corneal epithelium.

   b. The **corneal epithelium** is a nonkeratinized stratified squamous epithelium that renews regularly and heals rapidly if scratched or abraded.

3. **Lacrimal glands** secrete the **tears** that lubricate and clean the anterior surface of the eye.

4. **Pigment,** particularly in the retinal pigment epithelium, protects the retina from bright and ultraviolet light.

5. **Intraorbital fat** is a shock-absorbing cushion for the eye.

III. **EMBRYONIC DEVELOPMENT.** Knowledge of the embryonic origins of the structures of the eye (Table 37-1) is essential to understanding functional and morphologic

TABLE 37-1. Embryonic Origins of Adult Eye Structures

Embryonic Tissue	Adult Derivative
Surface (head) ectoderm	Lens and lens capsule; corneal epithelium; conjunctival epithelium; lacrimal gland, lacrimal duct, and lid epithelium; eyelashes; sebaceous glands
Neurectoderm	Pigment epithelium of retina; pigmented and nonpigmented epithelium of ciliary body; both pigmented epithelial layers of iris; photoreceptors, neurons, and glia of neural retina; optic nerve; pupillary sphincter and dilator muscles in iris; vitreous body (also partly derived from mesenchyme)
Mesoderm	Sclera; stroma of the cornea, sclera, eyelids, ciliary body, iris, and choroid; corneal endothelium; extraocular muscles; hyaloid vessels that supply developing tissues of inner eye (and degenerate before birth); connective tissue coverings of optic nerve; connective tissue and blood vessels of eye and orbit

relationships in the ciliary body and iris, subsequent development of the retina, and common pathologic conditions of the eye (e.g., detached retina).

 A. **Evagination of the diencephalon.** After closure of the neural folds to form the neural tube, the neural tube epithelium has its apical surface inside the tube and its basal lamina surrounding the tube. Two **optic vesicles** evaginate from the diencephalon shortly after closure of the neural tube. The lumen of each vesicle is continuous with that of the neural tube.

1. **Optic cup.** As the leading edge of the optic vesicle approaches the head ectoderm, it invaginates to form a cup-shaped, double-layered structure (Figure 37-3). Thus, cells of both layers of the cup lie with their apical surfaces abutting (head-to-head) and their basal surfaces facing away from one another.

2. **Derivatives of optic cup layers**
   a. The **inner layer** of the cup forms the **neural retina,** the **nonpigmented** (secretory) layer of the **ciliary epithelium,** and the **posterior iris epithelium.**
   b. The **outer layer** forms the **retinal pigment epithelium** (RPE), the **pigmented** (non-secretory) layer of the **ciliary epithelium,** and the **anterior iris epithelium.**
   c. A **potential space** in the retina, between the pigmented layer and the neural layer, is a vestige of the space between the two layers of the optic cup.

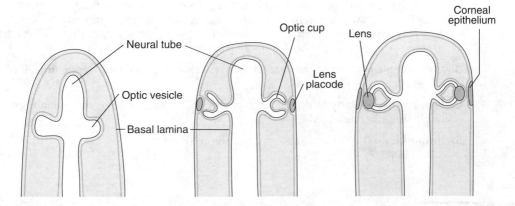

FIGURE 37-3. Formation of the optic cup from an evagination of the diencephalon of the developing neural tube and induction of the surface epithelium to form the lens and then the cornea.

B. **Induction of lens and cornea.** As the optic cup forms, its connection to the diencephalon constricts into an **optic stalk,** and the **surface ectoderm** external to the optic cup thickens to become a **lens placode.**

1. **Lens placode and vesicle.** The lens placode invaginates and pinches off to become the **lens vesicle.**
   a. **Lens.** The basal lamina surrounding the lens vesicle thickens to become the **lens capsule;** the lens vesicle differentiates into the **lens.**
   b. **Pupil.** The developing lens migrates to the mouth of the optic cup. The leading edge of the cup develops into the iris, which forms the pupil of the eye, in front of the lens.

2. **Cornea.** The **surface ectoderm** from which the lens vesicle has pinched off undergoes a **second induction** and becomes the **corneal epithelium.**
   a. **Stroma.** The space between the corneal epithelium and the lens is invaded by **mesenchymal cells** that give rise to the **definitive stroma.**
   b. These mesenchymal cells also give rise to the simple squamous epithelium at the back of the cornea, the **corneal endothelium.**

IV. CORNEA. The **transparent** cornea is the primary dioptric of the eye (see I C).

A. **Characteristics**

1. **Location.** The most anterior portion of the eye, it forms about one-sixth of the corneoscleral (fibrous) coat (see I D 1).

2. **Size.** In humans, the cornea is approximately 11 mm in diameter and 0.55 mm thick at its center.

3. **Vascularity.** The cornea is **avascular.** It conducts most of its metabolic exchanges with the aqueous humor. Blood vessels of the sclera end at the **corneoscleral margin,** the **limbus.**

4. **Innervation.** The cornea has an unusually rich sensory nerve supply. It is exquisitely sensitive to touch because free nerve endings penetrate nearly to the surface layers of the epithelium.

B. **Layers** (Figure 37-4)

1. **Corneal epithelium.** This **nonkeratinized stratified squamous** epithelium is about 50 μm thick and usually comprises 5 to 7 cell layers.
   a. Normal **turnover time is about 7 days.**
   b. Epithelial injuries heal more rapidly, however, by immediate migration of adjacent cells and more rapid turnover of nearby epithelial cells.

2. **Bowman membrane.** This acellular fibrous layer immediately beneath the epithelial basal lamina does not regenerate after injury.
   a. It is about 8 μm thick and has a hyaline appearance in routine histologic sections.
   b. It contains thin (~18 nm), randomly oriented type II collagen fibrils.
   c. It is not considered a specialized basement membrane because it does not stain for glycosaminoglycans.

3. **Corneal stroma.** The stroma constitutes 90% of the corneal thickness. It consists of about 60 thin lamellae between which are flattened fibroblasts that synthesize the stromal components. Corneal fibroblasts are called keratocytes.
   a. **Collagen fibrils**
      (1) Each lamella contains type III collagen fibrils, oriented at approximately right angles to those of the two adjacent lamellae. All fibrils run parallel to the free surface of the cornea.

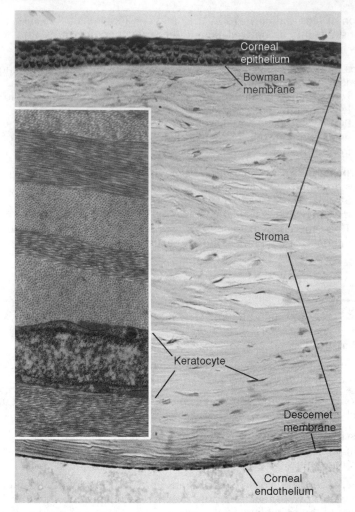

FIGURE 37-4. Principal layers of the human cornea, light micrograph. (*Inset*) Electron micrograph of the stroma shows regularity of size and spacing of the collagen fibrils in several lamellae as well as right-angle orientation of fibrils in adjacent lamellae. A portion of a keratocyte is visible between two of the lamellae.

(2) This arrangement, and the very regular size and spacing of the fibrils, underlie the transparency of the cornea.

    b. Proteoglycans. Along with collagen type V, sulfated proteoglycans regulate the diameter and spacing of the fibrils and underlie the intense metachromasia of the stroma.

    c. Injury. Disruption in the precise array of collagen fibrils can lead to temporary or permanent corneal translucency or opacity.

4. Descemet membrane. This membrane separates the endothelium from the posterior stroma.

    a. It is a thick (5–10 μm) basal lamina secreted by the corneal endothelium.

    b. It is readily regenerated after injury if the endothelium is intact.

5. Corneal endothelium. This sheet of squamous or low cuboidal mesenchymal epithelial cells covers the posterior surface of the cornea.

    a. It is responsible for metabolic exchanges between the cornea and the aqueous humor.

    b. Cells are joined by well-developed zonulae adherentes and desmosomes, but they have relatively leaky tight junctions.

c. Endothelial morphologic integrity and normal metabolic function are essential for corneal transparency.

V. **SCLERA.** This **opaque** layer of **dense connective tissue** constitutes the posterior five-sixths of the corneoscleral coat.

A. **Opacity** of the sclera, like that of other dense connective tissues, results from the irregularity of size and direction of the flat collagen bundles that constitute its structure.

B. **Layers** of sclera are the **episclera,** the **sclera proper** (also called the **Tenon capsule**), and the **lamina fusca.**

1. An **episcleral space** between the episclera and the Tenon capsule allows free rotation of the eye in the orbit.

2. The tendons of the extraocular muscles attach to the sclera proper.

VI. **ANTERIOR CHAMBER AND ASSOCIATED STRUCTURES**

A. **Characteristics**

1. **Location.** This compartment lies between the cornea and the iris (and the portion of the anterior surface of the lens exposed in the pupillary space).

2. **Size.** It is approximately 3 mm deep at the midpoint and has a volume of approximately 0.2 ml.

3. **Contents.** The anterior chamber is filled with aqueous humor under normal pressure of 20 mm Hg. Chamber pressure helps to maintain the shape of the cornea.

B. **Aqueous humor.** This clear fluid is secreted by the ciliary epithelium (see VII C 3). Aqueous humor approximates an ultrafiltrate of blood, but it has an extremely low protein content and a high concentration of ascorbic acid.

1. **Flow.** Aqueous humor has a flow rate through the posterior and anterior chambers of approximately 2 μl per minute.

2. **Drainage.** Aqueous humor leaves the anterior chamber by draining to the **chamber angle,** where it flows into the **trabelular meshwork** and the **canal of Schlemm.**

3. **Functions**
   a. The lens conducts all of its metabolic exchanges with the aqueous humor.
   b. The cornea conducts most of its metabolic exchanges with the aqueous humor across the **corneal endothelium.**
   c. Some oxygen and carbon dioxide are exchanged across the **corneal epithelium** as well.

C. **Chamber angle.** This acute angle is formed by the lateral margin of the cornea and the iris. It is immediately beneath the corneoscleral junction at the limbus (Figure 37-5).

1. Scleral structures at the chamber angle (see VI D) are essential for drainage of aqueous humor.

2. Scleral connective tissue fibers are continuous with those of the corneal stroma. Fluid-filled spaces in scleral tissue are continuous with the anterior chamber.

D. **Trabecular meshwork and canal of Schlemm.** The trabecular meshwork is continuous with the Descemet membrane. The endothelium that incompletely covers the strands of the trabecular meshwork is continuous with that of the cornea.

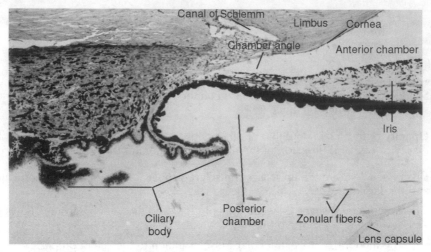

FIGURE 37-5. Angle of the anterior chamber of the eye (chamber angle).

1. **Spaces of Fontana.** These irregular spaces are created by the endothelium-covered strands of the trabecular meshwork.

2. **Canal of Schlemm.** Endothelium-lined channels anterior and lateral to the meshwork that run circumferentially around the cornea are collectively called the canal of Schlemm.
   a. They receive drainage from the spaces of Fontana.
   b. From the canal of Schlemm, aqueous humor passes through **aqueous veins** in the stroma to the **episcleral blood veins,** thereby leaving the interior of the eye.
   c. Obstruction or **restriction of drainage** at the chamber angle raises the intraocular pressure, causing one form of **glaucoma.**

VII. POSTERIOR CHAMBER AND ASSOCIATED STRUCTURES

A. Characteristics

1. **Contents.** The posterior chamber is the compartment into which **aqueous humor** is secreted.

2. **Margins.** This compartment is bounded:
   a. **Anteriorly** by the posterior surface of the iris
   b. **Posteriorly** by the lateral portion of the anterior surface of the lens and the zonular fibers, which lie just in front of the anterior surface of the vitreous body
   c. **Laterally** by the **ciliary body,** which secretes the aqueous humor

B. Iris

1. **Location.** This flattened, ring-like structure extends from the chamber angle, attaching to the sclera about 2 mm posterior to the limbus.

2. **Function**
   a. It separates the posterior chamber from the anterior chamber.
   b. It forms a contractile diaphragm anterior to the lens surface.

3. **Pupil.** The pupil is formed by the interior edge of the iridial ring. Its diameter varies inversely with the amount of light impinging on the eye.

4. Iridial epithelium. A double layer of epithelium covers the posterior surface of the iris.

    a. The **anterior iridial epithelium** is the layer whose basal lamina rests on the stroma.

    b. The **posterior iridial epithelium** is the layer whose basal lamina faces the posterior chamber.

5. Stroma and pupillary muscles. The bulk of the iris is connective tissue containing blood vessels, pigment cells, and both **sphincter** and **dilator muscles.**

    a. The **sphincter pupillae** is a compact bundle of smooth muscle cells that circles the pupillary margin. It is derived from the lip of the embryonic optic cup.

        (1) It is innervated by parasympathetic nerve fibers in the oculomotor nerve (cranial nerve III).

        (2) Its contraction reduces the pupillary opening in response to bright light.

    b. The **dilator pupillae** is a very thin layer that is actually composed of the basal portions of the anterior epithelial cells. The apical portion of each cell retains all its epithelial characteristics.

        (1) The dilator muscle fibers run radially from the pupillary region to the posterolateral edge of the iris.

        (2) Their contraction is stimulated by sympathetic nerve fibers.

6. Iridial pigment. Pigment-containing cells in the stroma of the iris absorb light that does not enter the pupil.

    a. The number of pigment cells in the iridial stroma determines the color of the iris.

    b. The more melanocytes present, the darker the color of the eye.

C. **Ciliary body.** The ciliary body lies between the iris and the neural retina, extending posterolaterally from the root of the iris to the ora serrata.

    1. Structure. The ciliary body is divided into **anterior** and **posterior portions.**

        a. The **pars plicata** (anterior portion) consists of about 75 folds (plicae) that radiate posteriorly.

            (1) These folds are the **ciliary processes** that secrete aqueous humor.

            (2) **Zonular fibers** extend from the grooves between the processes to the lens capsule, forming the **suspensory ligament of the lens.**

        b. The **pars plana** (posterior portion) is flat. It joins the neural retina at the **ora serrata,** a scalloped structure that is the margin between the **posterior** (neural) and **anterior segments** of the eye.

        c. As in the iris, a double-layered stroma is covered by a double layer of epithelium.

            (1) The outer layer of the stroma is the smooth ciliary muscle; the inner layer is vascular connective tissue that extends into the ciliary processes.

            (2) The epithelial layers covering the inner surface of the ciliary body are continuous with the two original layers of the retinal epithelium derived from the optic cup (see III A 2).

    2. Ciliary muscle. This muscle is divided into small compartments, each contained within a thick external lamina.

        a. Contraction of the circular and radial muscles relaxes tension on the zonular fibers, changing the shape and refractive power of the lens (see II A 2).

        b. Contraction of a meridional smooth muscle component stretches the choroid and tends to open the chamber angle to facilitate aqueous drainage.

    3. Ciliary epithelium. This double layer of epithelium **secretes aqueous humor** and **zonular fibers.**

        a. The **nonpigmented layer** is primarily a fluid-transporting epithelium.

            (1) Its cells also have a well-developed rough endoplasmic reticulum and Golgi apparatus, consistent with their role in secreting zonular fibers.

            (2) **Tight junctions** between nonpigmented epithelial cells are the major component of the **blood–aqueous barrier,** which is itself a component of the **blood–ocular barrier.**

    b. The **pigmented layer** is continuous with retinal pigment epithelium.
       (1) It has less well-developed apical junctions than the nonpigmented layer, and large intercellular spaces may develop.
       (2) The apical surfaces of the two layers face each other and are joined by desmosomes and gap junctions. Discontinuous luminal spaces thus formed are called **aqueous channels.**
    c. Secretory function
       (1) An ultrafiltrate of blood from the vessels in stroma of the ciliary body enters the intercellular spaces of the pigmented layer. It then percolates into the aqueous channels.
       (2) Solutes and solvents are transported into the intercellular compartment surrounding the nonpigmented epithelial cells by the action of Na^+, K^+-ATPase on their lateral plasma membranes.
       (3) Other components may be secreted by the nonpigmented cells directly into the intercellular space.

D. Lens. This **transparent, biconvex, avascular, wholly epithelial** structure is the **second dioptric** of the eye.
    1. Structure. The lens is approximately 10 mm in diameter and 5 mm thick at its center.
      a. The radius of curvature of the anterior surface is spherical; that of the posterior surface is paraboloid. The margin between these two surfaces is the **equator.**
      b. The lens is suspended between the pupil of the iris and the vitreous body by **zonular fibers** that stretch from the **ciliary body** to the **lens capsule.**

    2. Components
      a. Lens capsule completely surrounds the lens.
       (1) It is an unusually thick basal lamina, up to 10 μm on the anterior surface and about 5 μm on the posterior surface.
       (2) It is thickest at the equator, where the zonular fibers attach to it.
      b. Subcapsular epithelium is a layer of cuboidal cells present only on the anterior surface of the lens, beneath the capsule.
       (1) Organization. Apices of the epithelial cells are attached to the lens fibers by junctional complexes. Bases of the cells rest on the lens capsule, which is their basal lamina.
       (2) Replication. New epithelial cells arise in the anterocentral portion and migrate toward the equator, where they turn back on themselves and insinuate anteriorly between the lens fibers and the epithelium, and posteriorly between the lens fibers and the capsule.
        (a) Elongation. The insinuated cells elongate and lose their nuclei and their attachment to the capsule, thus becoming mature lens fibers.
        (b) Growth. The lens continues to add new fibers and to grow throughout life.
      c. Lens fibers are long, prismatic remnants of elongated epithelial cells that retain their plasma membranes and their complex intercellular relationships.
       (1) Mature peripheral lens fibers measure 8 to 10 mm by 8 to 10 μm by 2 μm. They are filled with densely packed proteins called **crystallins.**
       (2) At the **nucleus,** or center of the lens, lens fibers are compressed to the degree that individual fibers are difficult to recognize.
       (3) Despite the protein content and density of the fibers, the lens is transparent. Aging, disease, and environmental factors may cause loss of transparency (i.e., cataract).
    3. Zonule. The zonule (suspensory ligament of the lens) consists of **zonular fibers** that hold the lens capsule under tension [see VII C 1 a (2), 2 a]. The collagen fibrils of the zonular fibers resemble those of the vitreous body (see VIII A 1) and react strongly to periodic acid–Schiff staining.

VIII. VITREOUS BODY. The vitreous body is the transparent jelly-like substance that fills the space between the lens and the neural retina.

A. **Characteristics.** The vitreous body is a highly hydrated (more than 99% water) connective tissue gel. It consists of a dilute solution of glycosaminoglycans (principally hyaluronic acid) and collagen.

    1. Thin **collagen fibrils** that exhibit a 12 nm periodicity (similar to zonular fibers) are somewhat condensed at the periphery of the gel.

    2. **Hyalocytes** are also at the periphery. These rare, fibroblast-like cells likely secrete the components of the vitreous body.

B. **Functions**

    1. The vitreous body helps to maintain the shape of the eye.

    2. It holds the neural retina against the pigment epithelial layer. Shrinkage of the vitreous body expands the potential space between these two layers (see III A 2 c) and can lead to separation of these structures and retinal detachment.

IX. **RETINA.** The retina includes the **neural retina** and the **optic nerve** derived from it, and the **pigment epithelium** that physically and metabolically supports the neural retina. The neural retina contains **photoreceptors** (rods and cones). The pigment epithelium is attached to the choriocapillary layer of the choroid (see XI A).

A. **Neural retina.** This structure is usually described as having at least **6 major neuron types,** many different **synapse types,** and **10 layers** (Figure 37-6).

    1. **Retinal pigment epithelium** (RPE) is intimately associated with the neural retina and interacts with the photoreceptor layer metabolically, physically, and functionally.

        a. This single layer of cuboidal cells rests on the **Bruch membrane** (see XI B). Elaborate tight junctions and zonulae adherentes between the cells are the site of the **blood–retinal barrier.**

        b. RPE cells contain **elongated melanin granules** in processes that extend between the rods and cones of the photoreceptor cells.

        c. RPE cells contain the metabolic apparatus for the **restoration of photosensitivity to visual pigments** bleached by light.

        d. RPE cells phagocytize and recycle components of the membrane disks that break off rods and cones. **Retinal** of the visual pigment **rhodopsin** is the primary component for recycling.

    2. **A Layer of rods and cones** forms the outermost layer of the neural retina and the outer segment of the photoreceptor cells. Light that reaches the rods and cones must first pass through all of the other layers of the neural retina.

        a. **Rods** (about 120 million) are most numerous in the **periphery of the retina.** They are sensitive to **low levels of light.**

            (1) The **outer segment** of the rod cell contains 600 to 1000 transversely oriented **membrane disks,** stacked on one another like coins, surrounded by the plasma membrane.

            (2) The disk membranes contain the visual pigment **rhodopsin,** an aldehyde of vitamin A (retinal) bound to a protein (opsin).

        b. **Cones** (about 7 million) are more **centrally located,** respond to **intense levels of light,** and are responsible for **color vision.**

            (1) The **outer segment** of the cone cell is conical and also has a disk-like arrangement of membranes. In this receptor, however, the **membranes of the disk are continuous with the plasma membrane** (i.e., they are actually infoldings of the membrane).

            (2) Cones contain three different but similar pigments called **iodopsins.**

        c. **Photoreceptor cell function.** Photons striking the rod disks reduce retinal to retinol, triggering a cascade that promotes diffusion of Ca^{2+} from the disks into

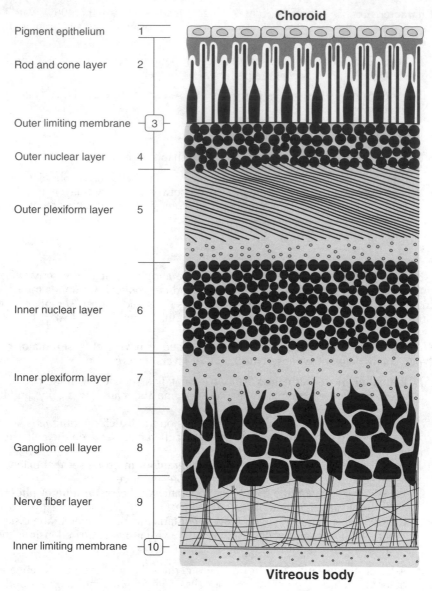

Choroid

Pigment epithelium	1
Rod and cone layer	2
Outer limiting membrane	3
Outer nuclear layer	4
Outer plexiform layer	5
Inner nuclear layer	6
Inner plexiform layer	7
Ganglion cell layer	8
Nerve fiber layer	9
Inner limiting membrane	10

Vitreous body

FIGURE 37-6. The 10 layers of the retina, based on information derived from study of specimens prepared by the Golgi method to impregnate the neuronal elements. (Adapted from Geneser F: *Textbook of Histology*, Philadelphia, Lea & Febiger, 1986, p 697.)

the cytoplasm, **hyperpolarization** of the receptor cell membrane, and generation of an electrical signal that passes to neighboring receptor cells through gap junctions and then through **synapses to bipolar neurons.**

   d. **Recycling of visual pigments.** Normal photoreceptor function and renewal lead to shedding of disks from both rods and cones. The superfluous disks are phagocytized by the RPE cells, each of which is estimated to dispose of about 7500 disks/day (see IX A 1 c, d).

3. **Outer limiting membrane** is not a biologic membrane, but a plane of demarcation formed by the **zonulae adherentes** between the apical ends of the Müller glial cells with each other and with the perikarya of the rods and cones (see II B 2).

4. **Outer nuclear layer,** immediately internal to the outer limiting membrane, contains the nuclei of rod and cone cells.

5. **Outer plexiform layer** contains the axons of rods and cones, dendrites of bipolar cells, and processes of amacrine and horizontal cells. Synapses occur between the receptor cells and the other three types. Blood vessels are first seen in this layer.

6. **Inner nuclear layer** contains the nuclei of bipolar cells, horizontal cells, amacrine cells, and Müller glial cells.

7. **Inner plexiform layer** subtends the inner nuclear layer. It contains axons of bipolar cells, dendrites of ganglion cells, and processes of amacrine cells. Retinal blood vessels are clearly visible.

8. **Ganglion cell layer** is the innermost cell layer of the neural retina.
   a. It is 8 to 10 cells thick at the **macula lutea** (the posterior pole of the eye), 1 cell-layer thick over most of the retina, and thin and sparsely populated at the periphery of the retina.
   b. Ganglion cells are absent over the **fovea.**

9. **Nerve fiber layer** is formed by the axons of the ganglion cells.
   a. Axons converge at the **optic head,** where the optic nerve leaves the globe. They vary from 0.2 to 3.0 μm in diameter and form bundles that often are surrounded by glial and Müller cells.
   b. Large blood vessels are found in this layer.

10. **Inner limiting membrane** is the basal lamina of the Müller cells. It is adjacent to the posterior surface of the vitreous body.

B. **Optic nerve.** The optic nerve is the link between the retina and the rest of the brain. Axons of the nerve fiber layer leave the globe through the posterior scleral coat (the **area cribrosa**) to form the optic nerve. The axons of the optic nerve are myelinated by glial cells after they leave the globe.

1. Absence of photoreceptors at the head of the nerve creates a **blind spot** in this portion of the retina.

2. The **central retinal artery** and **vein** that feed and drain the inner layers of the neural retina travel in the center of the nerve. Occlusion of the retinal artery is not unusual in aged individuals and leads to virtually instantaneous blindness in the affected eye.

C. **Fovea.** This shallow depression in the retina at the posterior pole of the optical axis is located about 3 mm lateral to the head of the optic nerve. It consists of the **macula lutea** and the **fovea centralis.**

1. **Macula lutea** surrounds the fovea centralis.
   a. Retinal vessels are absent from this region.
   b. Concentration of retinal cells and their processes on the sides of the macula allow light to reach the receptors in this sensitive zone of the retina unimpeded.

2. **Fovea centralis,** at the center of the fovea, is the zone of greatest visual acuity in the retina.
   a. It measures about 200 μm in diameter.
   b. It contains **only cone receptors** that are larger and longer than those in other parts of the retina.
   c. Cones in the fovea may connect through a single bipolar cell to only a single ganglion cell, thus accounting for the great acuity in this region.

X. **BLOOD–OCULAR BARRIER.** Like other blood–tissue barriers, the complex blood–ocular barrier resides in tight junctions in different cell layers in several parts of the eye.

A. Component barriers

   1. **Blood–aqueous barrier** consists of the tight junctions of the nonpigmented epithelial cells of the ciliary body.

   2. **Blood–iridial barrier** consists of elaborate tight junctions in the endothelium of the iridial blood vessels.

   3. **Blood–retinal barrier** has several components:
      a. Tight junctions in the blood vessels of the neural retina (as in the brain)
      b. Tight junctions between the cells of the retinal pigment epithelium
      c. Tight junctions that Müller cells form with each other and with receptor cells to form the outer limiting membrane (see IX A 3)

B. **Immunologically privileged site.** The interior of the globe, like the brain and the seminiferous tubule, is immunologically privileged. Although antigens may leave the eye, particularly through the outflow of aqueous humor, antibodies will not enter the eye if the blood–ocular barrier is intact.

XI. **CHOROID.** The choroid lies between the retina and the sclera and extends posteriorly from the ora serrata to surround the optic disk. **Pigment cells** are found in its connective tissue.

A. Posterior uveal layer

   1. The outer portion of this layer contains large venous vessels. The inner portion contains a complex network of small capillary sinuses, the **choriocapillaris.**

   2. Endothelium on the retinal side of each capillary sinus is thin and fenestrated. This facilitates metabolic exchanges between these vessels and the RPE.

B. **Bruch membrane.** This hyaline structure is a specialized basement membrane that separates the RPE from the choriocapillaris throughout the choroid. It has five layers: the basal lamina of the choriocapillaris; a thin collagen layer; a thin layer of elastic tissue; a thin subepithelial layer of collagen; and the basal lamina of the RPE cells.

XII. **EYELIDS.** The eyelids provide a protective cover for the anterior (corneal) surface of the eye.

A. **Structure.** The lids contain the **tarsal plate,** a dense elastic fibrous tissue.

   1. The inner surface of the tarsal plate is covered by the **palpebral conjunctiva** (see II E 2 a).

   2. The outer surface of the lids is covered by a loose, elastic layer of skin that can accommodate extreme swelling.

   3. The **orbicularis oculi** muscle closes the lids and the **levator palpebrae** muscle raises the **upper lid.**

B. Glands

   1. **Meibomian glands** (tarsal glands) are **elongate sebaceous glands** embedded in the tarsal plates.
      a. Their secretion produces the oily layer on the anterior surface of the tear film that retards evaporation.
      b. Although they are true sebaceous glands, they do not communicate with the hair follicles of the lid.

2. **Glands of Zeis** are **smaller sebaceous glands** that do empty their secretions into the hair follicles of the lids.

3. **Glands of Moll** are **sweat glands** with simple, unbranched, sinuous tubules.

C. **Eyelashes.** These short, stiff, curved hairs emerge from the most anterior edge of the lid margin, in front of the openings of the Meibomian glands. They have varying lengths and diameters, and may occur in double or triple rows.

XIII. **LACRIMAL APPARATUS. Lacrimal glands** secrete the **tears** that moisten and flush the conjunctival and corneal surfaces. **Lacrimal ducts** carry tear fluid from the glands to the conjunctival surface.

A. **Glands**

1. **Location**
   a. The main **lacrimal glands** lie beneath the conjunctiva in the **superolateral part of each orbital cavity.**
   b. **Accessory lacrimal glands** (tarsal lacrimal glands) are on the **inner surface of the upper and lower eyelids.**

2. **Structure**
   a. Lacrimal glands are tubuloacinar serous glands in which the acini have large lumina.
   b. Myoepithelial cells subtend the columnar acinar epithelial cells within the basal lamina.

B. **Ducts.** Approximately 12 ducts drain from each lacrimal gland to the superior fornix of the conjunctiva (i.e., under the upper lid, laterally).

C. **Tears**

1. **Composition.** Tears are sterile and contain the bactericidal enzyme **lysozyme.**

2. **Flow.** Tears flow across the corneal surface toward the medial angle, where the openings of the superior and inferior lacrimal canaliculi are located, just within the margin of the upper and lower lids.

3. **Drainage**
   a. The **common canaliculus,** the fusion of the superior and inferior canaliculi, drains medially to the **lacrimal sac.**
   b. In turn, the lacrimal sac drains through the **nasolacrimal duct,** which opens into the nasal cavity.

XIV. **EXTRAOCULAR MUSCLES.** Muscular attachments to each eye effect **vertical, lateral,** and **rotational movement** of the eye.

A. **Muscles.** The **six extraocular muscles** are the **medial, lateral, superior,** and **inferior rectus** muscles; and the **superior** and **inferior oblique** muscles.

B. **Coordinated action** of the muscles of both eyes moves the eyes in parallel (i.e., conjugate gaze).

Chapter 38

Ear

I. **INTRODUCTION.** The ear is a three-chambered sensory structure that functions in the sensation of movement, maintenance of balance, and perception of sound.

II. **EXTERNAL EAR**

A. **Auricle**

1. **Location.** The auricle, or pinna, is the oval appendage, known as the "ear," that projects from the lateral surface of the head.

2. **Shape.** Its characteristic shape is due to an internal supporting layer of elastic cartilage.

B. **External auditory canal.** The canal (meatus) is an air-filled tubular space. The **tympanic membrane** (ear drum) defines its inner limit.

1. **Wall of the canal**
   a. The **lateral segment** is cartilaginous and is continuous with the elastic cartilage of the auricle.
   b. The **medial segment** is contained within the temporal bone.

2. **Lining of the canal**
   a. The **lateral segment,** supported by cartilage, is lined by skin that contains hair follicles, sebaceous glands, and **ceruminous glands.** Ceruminous glands, thought to be apocrine glands, produce cerumen (ear wax).
   b. The **medial segment,** supported by bone, is lined by thinner skin, with fewer hairs and glands.

III. **MIDDLE EAR.** The middle ear is an air-filled space in the temporal bone.

A. **Tympanic membrane.** This membrane separates the lumen of the external auditory canal from the lumen of the middle ear.

1. The tympanic membrane is attached to the **auditory ossicles.**

2. It is the major functional landmark of the lateral wall of the middle ear.

B. **Auditory ossicles**

1. **Location.** These three small bones cross, in series, the space of the middle ear (Figure 38-1). They connect the tympanic membrane to the oval window, an opening in the bony wall between the middle and inner ear.

2. **Bones.** Auditory ossicles are named according to their approximate shape:
   a. **Malleus** (hammer), which is attached to the tympanic membrane
   b. **Incus** (anvil), or middle bone
   c. **Stapes** (stirrup), the footplate of which fits into the oval window

C. **Auditory (eustachian) tube.** This is a narrow channel that joins the cavity of the middle ear to the pharynx.

1. The auditory tube **vents the middle ear,** allowing air pressure in the middle ear to equalize with atmospheric pressure.

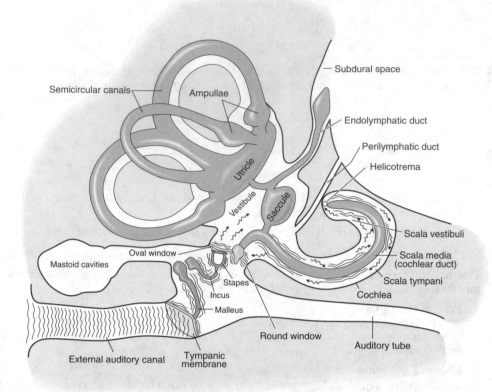

FIGURE 38-1. Pathway of sound energy through the external, middle, and inner ear. For clarity, the $2^3/_4$ turns of the cochlea are reduced to $^3/_4$ of a turn.

2. **Infections** may spread from the pharynx to the middle ear via the auditory tube, causing **otitis media.** The **tubal tonsil,** a small mass of protective lymphatic tissue, surrounds the pharyngeal orifice of the auditory tube.

D. **Muscles of the middle ear and the attenuation reflex**

1. **Tensor tympani muscle**
   a. This striated muscle lies in a bony canal above the auditory tube.
   b. Its tendon inserts on the malleus.
   c. Contraction increases tension on the tympanic membrane.

2. **Stapedius muscle**
   a. This is the smallest skeletal muscle in the body. It lies on the posterior wall of the middle ear.
   b. Its tendon inserts on the stapes.
   c. Contraction dampens movement of the stapes in the oval window.

3. **Attenuation reflex.** This protective neural mechanism is mediated by the tensor tympani and stapedius muscles.
   a. Contraction of these muscles produces a rigid chain of ossicles that reduces transmission of vibrations to the inner ear.
   b. The reflex protects the inner ear from the damaging effects of very loud sound.

IV. **INNER EAR.** The inner ear is formed by a **bony labyrinth** and a **membranous labyrinth.** Within the inner ear are **fluid-filled spaces** and several **sensory structures** (Figure 38-2; see also Figure 38-1).

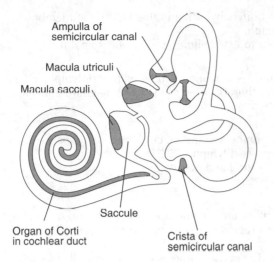

Ampulla of
semicircular canal

Macula utriculi

Macula sacculi

Organ of Corti
in cochlear duct

Saccule

Crista of
semicircular canal

FIGURE 38-2. Membranous labyrinth of the inner ear. *Shaded* areas indicate sensory regions.

A. **Bony labyrinth.** This is a complex system of connected cavities and canals contained within the temporal bone of the skull. It consists of the semicircular canals, the vestibule, and the cochlea.

1. **Semicircular canals.** These three narrow, bony-walled tubes lie at approximately right angles to each other.
   a. Each canal forms about three quarters of a circle (rather than a semicircle).
      (1) Bony walls of the canals are continuous with the bony wall of the vestibule.
      (2) The space enclosed by the semicircular canals is continuous with the lumen of the vestibule.
   b. One end of each canal, close to the vestibule, is dilated into an **ampulla.**

2. **Vestibule.** This region is the central chamber of the bony labyrinth.

3. **Cochlea.** This cone-shaped, bony helix arises from the vestibule on the side opposite the semicircular canals.
   a. The bony **cochlear canal** makes about $2^3/_4$ **helical turns** between its base and apex. It contains the membranous cochlear duct (see IV F 1).
   b. The **lumen of the cochlea,** like that of the semicircular canals, is **continuous with the lumen of the vestibule.**
   c. The **modiolus** is the central bony core around which the cochlea spirals. The spiral ganglion lies in the modiolus.

B. **Membranous labyrinth.** This compartment is **enclosed by the bony labyrinth.** It consists of small sacs and tubules joined to form a continuous, complex space (see Figure 38-1). Major regions of the membranous labyrinth are the membranous semicircular canals, the utricle and saccule, and the membranous cochlea (cochlear duct).

1. **Membranous semicircular canals** lie within the bony semicircular canals and are continuous with the utricle.

2. The **utricle** and **saccule** are dilations of the membranous labyrinth within the bony vestibule.

3. The **membranous cochlea,** or **cochlear duct,** is contained within the bony cochlea and is continuous with the saccule.

C. **Fluids and spaces.** The inner ear is a fluid-filled compartment, whereas the middle ear is an air-filled compartment.

1. **Perilymphatic space**

a. The space between the wall of the bony labyrinth and the wall of the membranous labyrinth is filled with **perilymph.**
   b. Perilymph is similar in ionic content to extracellular and cerebrospinal fluid.

2. **Endolymphatic space**
   a. The space enclosed by the membranous labyrinth is filled with **endolymph.**
   b. Endolymph is similar to intracellular fluid because of its high potassium concentration and low sodium concentration.

3. **Cortilymphatic space**
   a. The space between the basilar membrane and the reticular membrane of the organ of Corti (see V C) is filled with **cortilymph.**
   b. Cortilymph is similar to extracellular fluid and perilymph.

D. Sensory areas

1. **Sensory structures** project from the wall of the membranous labyrinth into the endolymphatic space (see Figure 38-2). Each region of the membranous labyrinth has a characteristic sensory structure.
   a. **Cristae of the semicircular canals.** One crista projects into the ampulla of each of the three semicircular canals (see V A 1 a).
   b. **Maculae of the vestibule.** One macula is found in the saccule and one in the utricle (see V B 1 a).
   c. **Organ of Corti.** This elongate, spiraling structure is found in the cochlear duct (see V C).

2. **Innervation**
   a. The membranous semicircular canals, utricle, and saccule are components of the vestibular system and are innervated by the vestibular division of the vestibulocochlear nerve (cranial nerve VIII).
   b. The membranous cochlea is part of the auditory system and is innervated by the auditory division of cranial nerve VIII.

E. **Hair cells** are the common receptor cell found in the sensory areas of the membranous labyrinth. They are transducers that perform the multiple sensory functions of the inner ear.

1. **Shared structural characteristics.** Hair cells from the various sensory areas share certain characteristics.
   a. They are **epithelial cells.**
   b. Each possesses **50 to 100 stereocilia** (elongate microvilli, also called sensory "hairs").
   c. Each hair cell in the vestibular system has a **single cilium** (kinocilium). Hair cells in the auditory system lack a cilium but have a basal body.
   d. The cells are associated with **afferent and efferent nerve endings.**

2. **Common basis of receptor cell function**
   a. All hair cells of the inner ear appear to function by the **bending of their stereocilia.**
   b. The **means by which the stereocilia are bent varies** from receptor to receptor.
   c. Stretching of the plasma membrane by bending of stereocilia **generates potentials** in the receptor cell. This information is conveyed to the afferent nerve ending associated with the hair cell.

F. **Cochlear canal.** The cochlear duct, which is a tubular part of the membranous labyrinth, divides the bony-walled cochlear canal, which is a tubular part of the bony labyrinth, into **three parallel compartments** called **scalae** (Figure 38-3).

1. The **scala media,** or **cochlear duct,** is the middle compartment. This endolymph-containing space is continuous with the lumen of the saccule. In transverse section, the scala media appears as an approximately triangular space.
   a. The **upper wall,** or roof, is the **vestibular (Reissner) membrane.** This separates the scala vestibuli from the scala media.

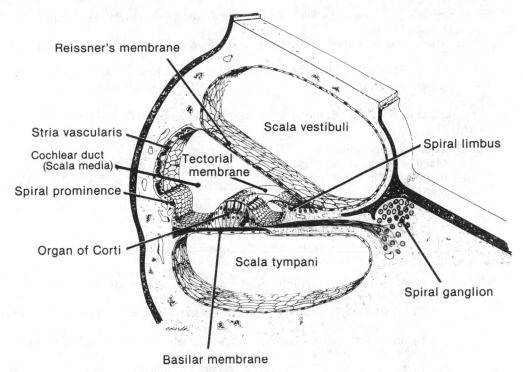

FIGURE 38-3. Schematic drawing of the cochlea shows the organ of Corti and surrounding structures. (Reproduced from Bloom W, Fawcett DW: *A Textbook of Histology,* 12th ed. New York, Chapman and Hall, 1994, p 929.)

    b. The **lateral (outer) wall** is formed by the **stria vascularis.** This thick pseudostratified epithelium appears to be the site of **synthesis of endolymph.**
    c. The **lower wall,** or floor, is the **basilar membrane.** The **organ of Corti** rests on the basilar membrane (see V C).

  2. The **scala vestibuli** and **scala tympani** are above and below, respectively, the scala media.
    a. These **perilymph-containing spaces** communicate with each other at the apex of the cochlea through a small channel called the **helicotrema.**
    b. The scala vestibuli begins at the **oval window** and the scala tympani ends at the **round window.**

V. FUNCTIONS OF THE INNER EAR

A. **Semicircular canals.** The semicircular canals are **sensors of angular movement.**

  1. Functional components
    a. A **crista** is a thickened epithelial ridge that lies in the ampulla of each semicircular canal, perpendicular to its long axis. It is formed by hair cells and supporting epithelial cells.
    b. A **cupula** is a gelatinous structure attached to the stereocilia of the hair cells. It projects into the lumen of the ampulla and is **surrounded by endolymph.**
    c. A **flexible attachment** formed by stereocilia functions as a **hinge** between cupula and hair cells.

  2. Effects of rotational movement
    a. During rotational movement of the head, the wall of the semicircular canal

moves, but the endolymph contained within the canal tends to lag behind because of inertia.
   b. The **cupula is swayed** by the movement differential between the crista and endolymph.
   c. **Stereocilia** in the narrow, hinge-like space between hair cell and cupula **bend,** generating nerve impulses in the associated afferent nerve endings.

B. **Saccule and utricle.** The saccule and utricle are **sensors of gravity and linear movement.**

   1. **Functional components**
      a. **Maculae** are localized thickened areas of the membranous labyrinth, facing the endolymph, in the saccule and utricle. A macula is formed by hair cells and supporting cells.
      b. The **otolithic membrane** is gelatinous material that lies on each macula. It contains particles of calcium carbonate called **otoliths.**
      c. **Stereocilia of macular hair cells** are embedded in the otolithic membrane. A hinge-like space spanned by stereocilia exists between the apical surface of the hair cells and the otolithic membrane.

   2. **Effects of movement.** The **otolithic membrane moves on the macula.**
      a. Stereocilia of hair cells are bent:
         (1) **By gravity,** in the stationary individual when the otolithic membrane pulls on the stereocilia
         (2) **By linear movement,** when the individual is moving in a straight line and the otolithic membrane drags on the macula because of inertia
      b. Bending of stereocilia by either means **generates impulses** in the associated afferent nerve endings.

C. **Organ of Corti.** The organ of Corti is a **sensor of sound vibrations** (see Figure 38-3).

   1. **Location.** The organ of Corti rests on the basilar membrane of the scala media [see IV F 1]. It spirals, following the $2\frac{3}{4}$ turns of the cochlea.

   2. **Structure.** The organ of Corti is a complex epithelial layer formed by hair cells and supporting cells.
      a. **Inner hair cells**
         (1) They form a single row of cells throughout the entire length of the cochlear duct.
         (2) The inner hair cells are closer to the modiolus [see IV A 3 c] than are the outer hair cells.
      b. **Outer hair cells**
         (1) The number of hair cells forming the width of the row is variable.
         (2) Three rows are found in the basal part of the coil. The width of the row increases to five cells at the apex of the cochlea.
      c. **Phalangeal cells**
         (1) Each hair cell is associated with a supporting phalangeal cell.
         (2) These cells have a slender process that passes to the surface of the organ of Corti, where it flares out to form part of the **reticular membrane.**
      d. **Reticular membrane**
         (1) The reticular membrane is a mosaic-like layer formed by the expanded processes of phalangeal cells and the apices of hair cells.
         (2) It adds rigidity to the apical surface of the organ of Corti.
      e. **Tectorial membrane**
         (1) The tectorial membrane attaches medially to the modiolus.
         (2) Its lateral free edge projects over and attaches to the organ of Corti by the stereocilia of the hair cells.

   3. **Sound perception** (see Figure 38-1)
      a. **Role of external and middle ear.** Sound energy is translated mechanically from the environment to the inner ear.

   (1) Sound waves **impinge on the tympanic membrane** and cause the **membrane to vibrate.**
   (2) Vibrations are **transmitted to the auditory ossicles,** which span the middle ear cavity.
   (3) The stapes **moves in and out** of the oval window, piston like, in response to the vibrations initiated by sound.
b. Inner ear and its fluid compartments. Sound energy is then transmitted to the perilymph–endolymph compartments of the inner ear.
   (1) Movement of the stapes in the oval window sets up vibrations in the peri-lymph of the scala vestibuli.
   (2) Vibrations are transmitted through the vestibular membrane to the scala media, which contains endolymph.
      (a) Vibrations are also propagated to the perilymph of the scala tympani.
      (b) Pressure changes in this closed perilymph–endolymph system are re-flected in movements of the membrane covering the round window (sec-ondary tympanic membrane).
c. Inner ear and the basilar membrane. Vibrations initiated by sound affect the basi-lar membrane of the scala media.
   (1) A **traveling wave** is set up in this membrane.
      (a) Sound of a specific frequency causes displacement of a relatively long segment of the basilar membrane.
      (b) Vibration of the basilar membrane is not uniform over this long segment, however. The region of maximum displacement is a relatively narrow band.
   (2) **High frequency sounds** cause maximum displacement of the basilar mem-brane near the base of the cochlea.
   (3) **Low frequency sounds** cause displacement closer to the apex.
   (4) The point of maximum displacement of the basilar membrane is specific for a given frequency. Different frequencies are discriminated on this basis.
d. Energy transduction. Distortion of stereocilia of hair cells changes the energy of sound vibrations to electric potentials.
   (1) **Hair cells** are attached, via the phalangeal cells, to the **basilar membrane,** which vibrates during sound reception.
   (2) **Stereocilia** of hair cells are attached to the **tectorial membrane.** This mem-brane also vibrates, but it is **hinged at a different point** than the basilar mem-brane.
   (3) Thus, a **shearing effect** occurs between the basilar membrane (and the cells attached to it) and the tectorial membrane when sound vibrations impinge on the inner ear.
      (a) Stereocilia are the only structures that connect the basilar membrane and its complex epithelial layer to the tectorial membrane.
      (b) The shearing effect between the basilar membrane and the tectorial mem-brane distorts these stereocilia.
   (4) **Stresses applied to the stereocilia,** or to the apical part of the hair cell, **gener-ate the potentials** that are conveyed to the central nervous system by the cochlear nerve.

Comprehensive Exam

CHAPTER KEY

This key lists the study questions that pertain to each chapter.

Chapter 1: 17, 26, 38, 143, 209–211
Chapter 2: 2, 18, 65, 172, 177, 180, 199, 225–229
Chapter 3: 68, 72, 80, 106, 171, 186, 194
Chapter 4: 31, 52, 60, 83, 115, 129, 163, 183, 192, 199
Chapter 5: 32, 39, 50, 81, 123, 132, 141, 252–256
Chapter 6: 12, 25, 40, 89, 102, 122, 131, 146, 225–229, 252–256
Chapter 7: 155, 208, 212–218, 225–229, 252–256
Chapter 8: 7, 19, 76, 85, 99, 178, 188, 194, 200, 212–218, 225–229, 252–256, 305–312
Chapter 9: 103, 173, 197, 203, 206
Chapter 10: 305–312
Chapter 11: 1, 35, 41, 51, 95, 109, 139, 161, 219–224, 305–312
Chapter 12: 9, 73, 118, 129, 130, 145, 148, 153, 158, 165
Chapter 13: 20, 56, 61, 90, 127, 164, 165, 166, 169
Chapter 14: 8, 10, 11, 13, 53, 101, 113, 125, 162, 168, 196, 208
Chapter 15: 34, 48, 57, 152, 174, 230–236
Chapter 16: 14, 70, 136, 174, 245–251, 277–280
Chapter 17: 27, 28, 29, 43, 156, 170, 230–236, 245–251
Chapter 18: 78, 91, 245–251
Chapter 19: 64, 66, 86, 107, 181, 245–251
Chapter 20: 126, 132, 134, 150, 262–266, 287–292
Chapter 21: 93, 122, 131, 187, 293–298
Chapter 22: 96, 181, 202, 277–280
Chapter 23: 49, 92, 94, 100, 137, 138, 191, 212–218, 277–280
Chapter 24: 3, 108, 112, 114, 117, 119, 237–241, 293–298
Chapter 25: 30, 42, 119, 120, 121, 122, 128, 147, 175, 179, 184, 204, 205
Chapter 26: 21, 44, 59, 62, 74, 144, 182, 190, 193
Chapter 27: 77, 82, 87, 159, 180, 195, 204
Chapter 28: 97, 104, 110, 116, 133, 140, 160, 167, 176, 198
Chapter 29: 15, 22, 23, 33, 36, 45, 55, 58, 79, 135, 189, 242–244
Chapter 30: 281–286
Chapter 31: 4, 84, 88, 281–286
Chapter 32: 257–261, 281–286
Chapter 33: 46, 138
Chapter 34: 67, 281–286
Chapter 35: 5, 6, 37, 71, 94, 105, 111, 124, 149, 151, 281–286
Chapter 36: 16, 47, 63, 75, 98, 154, 157, 185, 189, 201
Chapter 37: 24, 186, 207, 267–276
Chapter 38: 54, 69, 142, 299–304

DIRECTIONS: Each of the numbered items or incomplete statements in this section is followed by answers or by completions of the statement. Select the ONE lettered answer or completion that is BEST in each case.

1. Osteoid is most closely associated with the biochemical activity of

(A) osteoclasts
(B) chondrocytes
(C) osteoblasts
(D) chondroblasts
(E) osteocytes

2. Sulfation of sugars in proteoglycans occurs in which of the following cell structures?

(A) *Cis* Golgi
(B) *Trans* Golgi
(C) Late endosomes
(D) Rough endoplasmic reticulum (rER)

3. A histologic section of a portion of the alimentary canal shows the junction of a stratified squamous epithelium and a simple columnar epithelium. Submucosal mucus-secreting glands are visible under the stratified squamous epithelium. The columnar epithelium is a sheet of mucus-secreting cells. This section shows which of the following junctions?

(A) Gastroduodenal
(B) Rectoanal
(C) Ileocolic
(D) Esophagogastric
(E) Colorectal

4. Hypercalcemia stimulates secretion of

(A) aldosterone
(B) calcitonin
(C) epinephrine
(D) parathyroid hormone (PTH)

5. The antrum of a maturing ovarian follicle is denoted by which one of the following characteristics?

(A) Thickening of the zona pellucida
(B) Hypertrophy of the theca interna
(C) Dilatation of an intercellular space
(D) Vacuolization of the theca externa

6. Tissue from which one of the following organs is depicted in the accompanying micrograph?

(A) Prostate gland
(B) Mammary gland
(C) Parotid gland
(D) Thyroid gland
(E) Duodenal gland

7. A histologic section of connective tissue shows numerous cells containing large numbers of uniformly sized basophilic granules. The cells are ovoid, with a centrally located nucleus, and are aligned along blood vessels. The cells are most likely

(A) fibroblasts
(B) macrophages
(C) eosinophils
(D) mast cells
(E) plasma cells

Questions 8–11

The following questions are based on the accompanying transmission electron micrograph.

8. The micrograph depicts which of the following types of blood vessels?

(A) Elastic artery
(B) Muscular artery
(C) Arteriole
(D) Capillary
(E) Medium-sized vein

9. The structure indicated by the *asterisk* is which one of the following?

(A) Endothelial cell
(B) Erythrocyte
(C) Platelet
(D) Neutrophil
(E) Pericyte

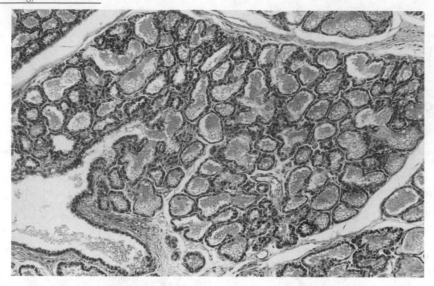

Question 6

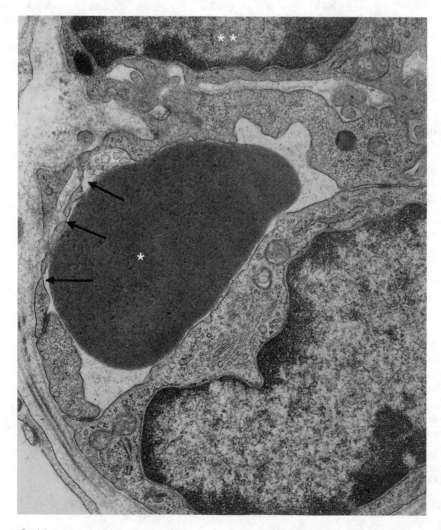

Questions 8–11

10. The cell indicated by the *double asterisk* is which one of the following?

(A) Erythrocyte
(B) Fibroblast
(C) Mast cell
(D) Pericyte
(E) Smooth muscle cell

11. The structures indicated by the *arrows* are which of the following?

(A) Basal laminae
(B) Endothelial fenestrations
(C) Pinocytotic vesicles
(D) Tight junctions

12. Release of a neurotransmitter into the synaptic cleft occurs by which one of the following processes?

(A) Endocytosis
(B) Exocytosis
(C) Diffusion
(D) Phagocytosis
(E) Pinocytosis

13. The bicuspid valve is found between which of the following cardiovascular system components?

(A) Venae cavae and right atrium
(B) Right atrium and right ventricle
(C) Right ventricle and pulmonary trunk
(D) Left atrium and left ventricle
(E) Left ventricle and aorta

14. An important histologic characteristic of the distal small intestine (ileum) is the

(A) absence of villi from the luminal surface
(B) concentration of outer smooth muscle layer into bands
(C) aggregation of lymphatic nodules in the mucosa and submucosa
(D) presence of submucosal glands that drain into the crypts of Lieberkühn

15. Which of the following renal vessels is found between an arcuate artery and an afferent arteriole?

(A) Interlobar artery
(B) Efferent arteriole
(C) Glomerular capillary
(D) Interlobular artery
(E) Arteriola recta

16. Which one of the following pituitary hormones is the principal controlling factor in regulating the interstitial endocrine cell (Leydig cell) of the testis?

(A) Growth hormone (GH)
(B) Thyroid-stimulating hormone (TSH)
(C) Luteinizing hormone (LH)
(D) Melanocyte-stimulating hormone (MSH)
(E) Follicle-stimulating hormone (FSH)

17. The structure of biologic membranes can best be described as

(A) a phospholipid bilayer interspersed with membrane proteins held together by covalent bonds
(B) a fluid-mosaic of proteins interspersed in a phospholipid bilayer
(C) a phospholipid bilayer with the hydrocarbon tails of the phospholipids oriented toward the cytoplasm
(D) an internal layer of protein covered on either side by a layer of phospholipid

18. Which of the following statements regarding primary lysosomes is correct?

(A) They reproduce by division
(B) They contain lysosomal DNA
(C) They are identifiable only after specific histochemical staining
(D) They contain enzymes synthesized on free ribosomes
(E) They are the site of β-oxidation of fatty acids

19. Which of the following statements accurately describes tropocollagen?

(A) It is an aggregate of collagen fibrils forming large banded fibers
(B) It is the basic molecule from which collagen fibrils self-assemble
(C) It is the precursor polypeptide of procollagen
(D) It can be recognized in electron micrographs by its 64–68 nm axial periodicity
(E) It is polymerized into collagen fibrils in the Golgi apparatus

20. An immature neutrophil may first be recognized in a stained smear of red bone marrow at which stage of granulopoiesis?

(A) Myeloblast
(B) Promyelocyte
(C) Myelocyte
(D) Metamyelocyte
(E) Band cell

21. Which of the following statements concerning bile canaliculi is correct?

(A) They are the site at which lipoproteins are secreted by hepatocytes
(B) They form between adjacent hepatocytes and are bounded by junctional complexes
(C) They are the space between the hepatic cell and the sinusoidal endothelium
(D) They drain into the terminal hepatic venule
(E) They are lined by simple squamous epithelium

22. A small protein (approximately 30,000 daltons) passes through the glomerular basement membrane into the glomerular filtrate. Cells of which of the following tissues would remove the protein from the filtrate?

(A) Visceral epithelium of the renal corpuscle
(B) Distal convoluted tubule
(C) Glomerular mesangium
(D) Proximal convoluted tubule
(E) Parietal layer of the renal corpuscle

23. Identification of a macula densa in a section of kidney also identifies an example of a

(A) proximal tubule
(B) loop of Henle
(C) distal tubule
(D) collecting duct
(E) papillary duct

24. An understanding of how the eye forms from the two layers of the optic cup is essential to explaining the morphologic basis of

(A) corneal swelling
(B) glaucoma
(C) retinal detachment
(D) cataract
(E) dry-eye syndrome

25. Collagen fibrils with 64–68 nm banding are visible adjacent to Schwann cells in an electron micrograph of peripheral nerve tissue. The collagen is evidence of

(A) external lamina
(B) endoneurium
(C) perineurium
(D) epineurium
(E) deep fascia

26. Freeze-fracture of membranes has provided information on the intramembranous distribution of

(A) phospholipids
(B) glycogen
(C) carbohydrates
(D) proteins
(E) ribosomes

Questions 27–29

The accompanying light micrograph shows a portion of the hilum of a lymph node.

27. The vessel enclosed by *arrowheads* in the micrograph is carrying

(A) blood to the lymph node
(B) blood away from the lymph node
(C) lymph to the lymph node
(D) lymph away from the lymph node

28. Based on the morphologic evidence in the micrograph, which of the following statements regarding the flow of lymph in the vessel indicated by the *asterisk* is correct?

(A) Flow is from left to right
(B) Flow is from right to left
(C) Flow is unrestricted in either direction
(D) Flow direction cannot be determined from the micrograph

29. What subcompartment of the lymph node is indicated by the *double asterisk*?

(A) Cortical sinus
(B) Germinal center
(C) Medullary sinus
(D) Medullary cord

30. The accompanying micrograph depicts tissue of which of the following organs?

(A) Colon
(B) Esophagus
(C) Gallbladder
(D) Small intestine
(E) Stomach

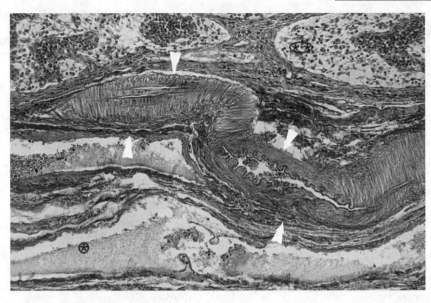

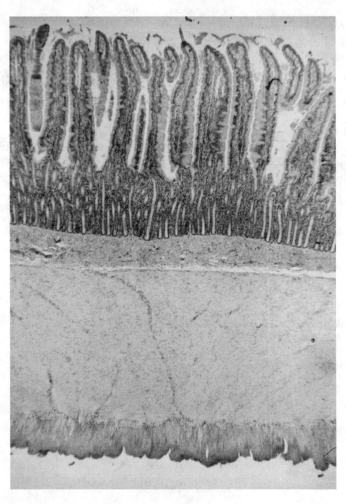

31. Which of the following statements correctly describes the nucleolus?

(A) It is a membrane-bounded intranuclear organelle
(B) It is the site of transcription of all genes that code for RNA in ribosomes
(C) It is not visible in the interphase nucleus
(D) It is the site of assembly of ribosomal subunits
(E) It is the site of synthesis of ribosomal proteins

32. Which one of the following cellular junctions prevents free diffusion of solutes and water through the transepithelial paracellular space?

(A) Gap junction
(B) Hemidesmosome
(C) Adhesion belt
(D) Tight junction
(E) Macula adherens

33. The greatest reduction in volume of initial glomerular filtrate occurs in which of the following structures?

(A) Urinary space of the renal capsule
(B) Proximal convoluted tubule
(C) Distal convoluted tubule
(D) Collecting duct
(E) Loop of Henle

34. An immunoglobulin-secreting plasma cell is developmentally most closely related to a

(A) B lymphocyte
(B) fibroblast
(C) mast cell
(D) colony-forming cell
(E) T lymphocyte

35. Which of the following processes has an osteoclast undergone?

(A) Neither karyokinesis nor cytokinesis
(B) Karyokinesis, but not cytokinesis
(C) Cytokinesis, but not karyokinesis
(D) Both karyokinesis and cytokinesis

36. Antidiuretic hormone (ADH) released from the posterior lobe of the pituitary gland acts primarily by modifying the permeability characteristics of which of the following renal structures?

(A) Thin ascending limb of the loop of Henle
(B) Foot processes of podocytes
(C) Thin descending limb of the loop of Henle
(D) Medullary collecting ducts
(E) Proximal convoluted tubule

37. Which one of the following steps is critical for ovulation?

(A) Prior completion of the second meiotic division
(B) Elevated levels of progesterone and estrogens
(C) Loss of oocyte–granulosa cell gap junctions
(D) Surge in the secretion of luteinizing hormone (LH)

38. Glycoproteins are asymmetrically distributed in the plasma membrane with their carbohydrate moiety oriented toward the extracellular environment. In what organelle is this asymmetry established?

(A) Plasma membrane
(B) Trans-Golgi network
(C) Rough endoplasmic reticulum (rER)
(D) Smooth endoplasmic reticulum (sER)

39. A cell junction that joins one epithelial cell to all of its immediately neighboring cells is a

(A) desmosome
(B) gap junction
(C) hemidesmosome
(D) tight junction

40. In a histologic section of spinal cord, rows of nuclei are seen aligned between myelinated axons in the white matter. The observed nuclei are evidence of which cell type?

(A) Astrocytes
(B) Satellite cells
(C) Oligodendrocytes
(D) Schwann cells
(E) Microglia

41. The layered appearance of lamellar bone results from the regular arrangement of

(A) canaliculi
(B) collagen
(C) cement lines
(D) hydroxyapatite
(E) lacunae

42. A histologic section of the intestine shows branched tubular glands in the compartment bounded by the muscularis mucosae and the muscularis externa. The glands drain into the crypts of Lieberkühn. This is a section of

(A) pylorus
(B) cecum
(C) ileum
(D) jejunum
(E) duodenum

43. At which point in the vasculature of a lymph node would a B lymphocyte leave the blood stream to enter the lymphatic tissue of the node?

(A) Capillaries of the superficial (nodular) cortex
(B) Venules of the deep (non-nodular) cortex
(C) Capillaries of the superficial medulla
(D) Venules of the deep medulla

44. The central, or axial, structure of the classic liver lobule is a

(A) portal triad
(B) sinusoid
(C) central vein
(D) space of Disse
(E) bile canaliculus

45. Which of the following is the central structure of a renal lobule?

(A) Cortical column
(B) Interlobular artery
(C) Renal hilum
(D) Arcuate artery
(E) Medullary ray

46. Insulin is synthesized and secreted by which pancreatic cell?

(A) Islet α cell
(B) Exocrine acinar cell
(C) Islet β cell
(D) Intercalated duct cell
(F) Islet δ cell

47. Which one of the following statements regarding cells of the seminiferous epithelium is correct?

(A) Spermatogonia are confined to the compartment on the basal side of the blood–testis barrier
(B) Sustentacular (Sertoli) cells divide during each cycle of the seminiferous epithelium
(C) Type A dark cells give rise to large numbers of primary spermatocytes by repeated meiotic divisions
(D) Interstitial endocrine (Leydig) cells clump together on the luminal side of the blood–testis barrier
(E) Spermatids and nearly mature sperm are separated from spermatocytes by the blood–testis barrier

48. Germinal centers in lymphatic nodules in the mucosa of the jejunum indicate

(A) formation of new epithelial cells and fibroblasts by a germinative pool of cells
(B) penetration of the epithelial barrier by intestinal microorganisms
(C) initiation of contraction in the smooth muscle layers of the jejunal wall
(D) absorption of fatty acids and their reassembly into triglycerides in the lamina propria

49. The defining characteristic of exocrine glands is the presence of

(A) both serous and mucous acini in the secretory portion of the gland
(B) myoepithelial cells between the secretory cells and the basal lamina
(C) stored zymogen droplets in the apical portion of the secretory cell
(D) ducts that convey the secretory product from the secretory cells to a body surface
(E) columnar cells in the duct system that transport sodium and water to concentrate the secretion

50. Fluorescently labeled molecules are microinjected into an epithelial cell. Ten minutes later, the presence of the probe molecules is detected in adjacent, uninjected cells. This is evidence that the cells are joined by

(A) desmosomes
(B) adhesion belts
(C) gap junctions
(D) tight junctions
(E) junctional complexes

51. Which of the following cell types is associated with the resorption of bone during the rapid growth of the fetal parietal bone of the skull?

(A) Osteoclast
(B) Osteocyte
(C) Osteoblast
(D) Osteoprogenitor cell

52. A nucleosome is a unit of structure of which of the following nuclear components?

(A) Nuclear matrix
(B) Nuclear lamina
(C) Nuclear pore
(D) Nuclear chromatin
(E) Nuclear envelope

53. The accompanying micrograph depicts which of the following pairs of vessels?

(A) Elastic artery and large vein
(B) Muscular artery and small vein
(C) Arteriole and venule
(D) Capillary and lymphatic vessel
(E) Vasa vasorum and medium vein

54. The part of a hair cell of the organ of Corti that is most distorted when sound vibrations impinge on the ear is the

(A) junctional complex
(B) stereocilia
(C) basolateral plications
(D) mitochondria
(E) basal lamina

55. The formation of a hypertonic urine is most closely related to which of the following factors?

(A) Filtering by the glomerular basement membrane
(B) Removal of small proteins from the filtrate by proximal tubule cells
(C) Reduction of filtrate volume in the proximal convoluted tubule
(D) Location of a macula densa in the wall of the distal tubule
(E) Establishment of a high salt concentration in the medullary interstitium

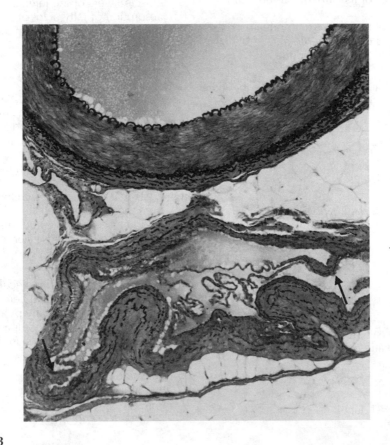

Question 53

56. In a smear of normal red bone marrow, a cell is observed to be obviously larger than an erythrocyte; to have a relatively large, unindented, euchromatic nucleus; and to have a scattering of purple-staining granules in the cytoplasm. The cell is a

(A) basophilic erythroblast
(B) promyelocyte
(C) neutrophilic metamyelocyte
(D) normoblast
(E) eosinophilic myelocyte

57. The predominant cell type found in a germinal center is a

(A) macrophage
(B) T lymphocyte
(C) reticular cell
(D) B lymphocyte
(E) plasma cell

58. The portion of the nephron that is least permeable to water is the

(A) proximal convoluted tubule
(B) thin descending limb of the loop of Henle
(C) straight portion of the proximal tubule
(D) thick ascending portion of the loop of Henle
(E) visceral layer of the renal corpuscle

59. The endocrine function of the liver is generally defined as secretion of

(A) gastrin into the perisinusoidal space
(B) cholesterol and lecithin into the bile canaliculus
(C) plasma proteins into the perisinusoidal space
(D) taurocholic and glycocholic acids into the perisinusoidal space
(E) insulin and immunoglobulin A into the bile canaliculus

60. An epidermal germinative cell has recently replicated its DNA in anticipation of mitosis but a mitotic spindle has not yet formed. In which of the following phases of the cell cycle is this cell?

(A) G_0 phase
(B) G_1 phase
(C) S phase
(D) G_2 phase
(E) M phase

61. Which one of the following hematopoietic cells of red bone marrow is postmitotic?

(A) Myelocyte
(B) Basophilic erythroblast
(C) Band cell
(D) Promyelocyte
(E) Polychromatophilic erythroblast

62. The liver derives approximately 75% of its blood supply from the

(A) hepatic portal vein
(B) celiac artery
(C) superior mesenteric vein
(D) hepatic artery
(E) terminal hepatic vein

63. Sperm cells in the human male begin to differentiate at which one of the following points in development?

(A) At 5 months of fetal life
(B) As soon as the embryonic Leydig cells secrete androgens
(C) At puberty
(D) As soon as primordial germ cells enter the genital ridge
(E) At birth

64. Surgical removal of the thymus from a neonate would result in drastically depleted numbers of which of the following cell types?

(A) B cells
(B) Mast cells
(C) T cells
(D) Plasma cells

65. Which of the following events is required to stimulate secretion of stored proteins?

(A) Influx of Na^+ into the cytoplasm
(B) Increase in cytoplasmic Ca^{2+} concentration
(C) Release of stored ATP from mitochondria
(D) Cleavage of a signal peptide from the stored protein
(E) Release of elementary particles stored in mitochondria

66. Hassall corpuscles are characteristic of which of the following?

(A) Blood
(B) Keratinizing cells
(C) Spleen
(D) Red bone marrow
(E) Thymus

67. In general, the role of the pineal gland may be described as

(A) controlling the functions of all the systemic endocrine glands
(B) regulating adenohypophyseal functions by release of several tropic hormones
(C) relating day length and light intensity to the function of other endocrine glands
(D) regulating thyroid function by secretion of arginine vasotocin
(E) releasing neuroendocrine factors that regulate renal electrolyte resorption

68. Colchicine inhibits cell division by which of the following processes?

(A) Inhibiting DNA synthesis in mitochondria
(B) Preventing assembly of the mitotic apparatus
(C) Stabilizing microtubules into a rigid structure
(D) Preventing cytokinesis by inhibiting membrane flow
(E) Inhibiting the ATPase activity of G-actin

69. The function of hair cells in an ampulla of a semicircular canal depends on attachment of their stereocilia to the

(A) cupula
(B) otolithic membrane
(C) modiolus
(D) tectorial membrane
(E) stapes

70. A histologic section shows an organ with a large amount of lymphatic tissue, including nodules with germinal centers and a deeply invaginated mucosal surface formed by a stratified but poorly defined epithelium. The section is an example of

(A) lymph node
(B) spleen
(C) palatine tonsil
(D) thymus gland
(E) Peyer patch

71. Fertilization usually occurs in which of the following locations?

(A) Lumen of the Graafian follicle
(B) Ampulla of the oviduct
(C) Lumen of the uterus
(D) Isthmus of the oviduct
(E) Lumen of the cervical canal

72. Tubulin polymerizes into microtubules that constitute which of the following cellular elements?

(A) Cores of microvilli
(B) Spectrin filaments in erythrocytes
(C) Mitotic spindles of dividing cells
(D) Glial filaments in astrocytes
(E) Neurofilaments of axons and dendrites

73. Which of the following is most frequently noted in a sample of peripheral blood?

(A) Eosinophils
(B) Lymphocytes
(C) Monocytes
(D) Neutrophils
(E) Platelets

74. A portion of what organ is shown in this electron micrograph?

(A) Gallbladder
(B) Kidney
(C) Liver
(D) Parotid gland
(E) Spleen

75. Secretion of testosterone, the primary androgen, is best described by which one of the following statements?

(A) It is secreted by the Sertoli cells of the seminiferous tubules
(B) It is secreted in response to cyclical variations in levels of follicle-stimulating hormone (FSH)
(C) It is secreted by the interstitial cells of the testis (Leydig cells)
(D) It is secreted only after stimulation by hypophyseal adrenocorticotropic hormone (ACTH)
(E) It is secreted by the gonadotropes of the anterior hypophysis

76. Which of the following statements best characterizes macrophages?

(A) They are easily distinguished from fibroblasts in routine histologic slides
(B) They contain phosphatases, esterases, and proteases that digest phagocytized material
(C) They can readily digest carbon, cellulose, asbestos, and tubercle bacilli
(D) They originate from granulocytes that leave the circulation to divide and differentiate
(E) They are essential in wound healing because they secrete newly formed collagen

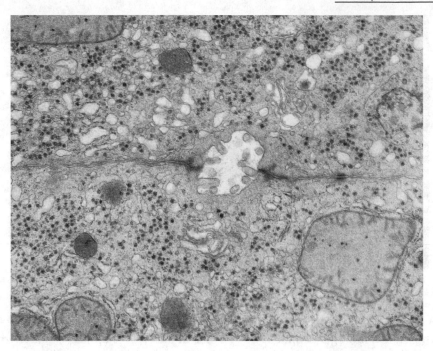

Question 74

77. Release of proenzymes from the pancreatic acinar cell is accomplished by which of the following processes?

(A) Exocytosis
(B) Transcytosis
(C) Apoptosis
(D) Endocytosis
(E) Phagocytosis

78. The development of nodules with germinal centers in the white pulp of the spleen is stimulated by

(A) accumulation of worn-out erythrocytes
(B) foreign antigens carried in the blood
(C) accumulation of breakdown products of erythrocytes
(D) foreign antigens carried in the lymph

79. Renin is secreted by

(A) proximal tubule cells
(B) visceral epithelial cells
(C) modified distal tubule cells
(D) gastric mucosal cells
(E) modified vascular smooth muscle cells

80. The beating of cilia and flagella is dependent upon which of the following processes?

(A) Polymerization and depolymerization of microtubules at the tip of the cilium
(B) Attachment of actin microfilaments to the membrane of the cilium
(C) Attachment and release of dynein side arms between adjacent microtubules of each doublets
(D) Attachment and release of doublet microtubules from the central pair of singlet microtubules
(E) Attachment and release of microtubule-associated proteins (MAPs) by doublet microtubules

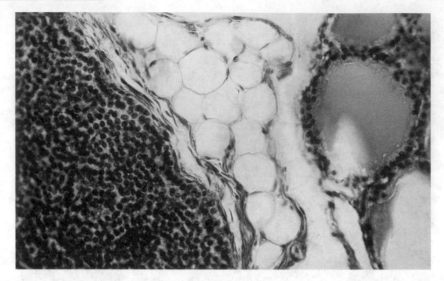

Question 84

81. Which of the following descriptions best characterizes the connective tissue–epithelium interface?

(A) A basal lamina, formed in part by a nonfibrillar collagen, separates the two basic tissue types
(B) Hemidesmosomes may be observed between the epithelial cells and the underlying fibroblasts
(C) A basement membrane consisting of fibroblasts surrounded by a basal lamina forms a continuous sheet between the two tissues
(D) Tight junctions join the basal epithelial cells to collagen fibers in the underlying connective tissue
(E) A basal lamina establishes an impermeable barrier to movement of materials between the two tissues

82. Stimulation of pancreatic exocrine secretion is accomplished primarily by

(A) sympathetic neurons of the autonomic nervous system
(B) secretin and cholecystokinin secreted by duodenal enteroendocrine cells
(C) insulin and glucagon secreted by the cells of the pancreatic islets
(D) stimulation of the olfactory mucosa by foodstuffs in the mouth
(E) pancreatic polypeptide (PP) secreted by F cells of the pancreatic islets

83. In meiosis, synapsis is characterized by which of the following activities?

(A) Exchange of neurotransmitters between daughter cells
(B) Pairing of homologous chromosomes during prophase I
(C) Formation of a narrow cleft between daughter cells
(D) Arrival of chromosomes at their respective poles

84. The accompanying light micrograph depicts the junction of the

(A) adrenal cortex and medulla
(B) ovary and fallopian tubes
(C) adenohypophysis and neurohypophysis
(D) pancreas and spleen
(E) thyroid and parathyroid glands

85. Which of the following statements regarding a cell synthesizing fibrillar collagen is most accurate?

(A) Its cytologic characteristics are those of a fibroblast
(B) It incorporates glycine and proline at a high rate from the extracellular space
(C) It stores collagen fibrils in secretory vacuoles in the cytoplasm
(D) It does not synthesize any other components of the extracellular matrix
(E) It is a terminally differentiated cell

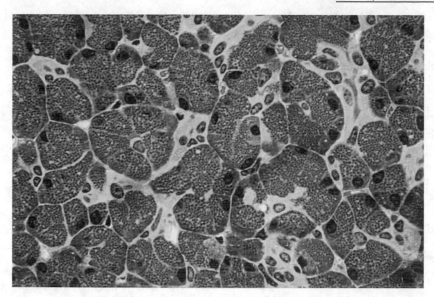

Question 87

86. T cells originate in which of the following structures?

(A) Thyroid
(B) Thymus
(C) Tonsils
(D) Testis
(E) Trachea

87. The accompanying light micrograph depicts which of the following glandular tissues?

(A) Parotid gland
(B) Adrenal cortex
(C) Submandibular gland
(D) Exocrine pancreas
(E) Thyroid gland

88. Decreased follicular storage of thyroglobulin results from

(A) toxic goiter
(B) dietary iodine deficiency
(C) decreased levels of thyroid-stimulating hormone (TSH) in the circulation
(D) increased protein synthesis by follicular cells

89. Positive identification of the central or peripheral nervous system source of a myelinated axon in an electron micrograph can be based on the presence or absence of

(A) external laminae
(B) major dense lines
(C) Nissl substance
(D) synaptic vesicles
(E) nodes of Ranvier

90. The greatest amount of nuclear DNA per cell in hematopoietic tissue is observed in

(A) promyelocytes
(B) metamyelocytes
(C) reticulocytes
(D) megakaryocytes
(E) proerythroblasts

91. In the red pulp of the spleen, the presence of large numbers of macrophages with secondary lysosomes indicates

(A) the breakdown of 120-day-old red blood cells (RBCs)
(B) the blastic transformation of B-lymphocytes
(C) the stimulation of the periarteriolar lymphatic sheath (PALS)
(D) the cytotoxicity of stimulated T-lymphocytes

92. A histologic section of an exocrine gland shows numerous serous secretory acini, some mucous acini, many prominent striated ducts, and distinct interlobular ducts. This section is a sample of which of the following types of glands?

(A) Sublingual gland
(B) Exocrine pancreas
(C) Eccrine sweat gland
(D) Parotid gland
(E) Submandibular gland

93. The human esophagus is lined with

(A) pseudostratified ciliated columnar epithelium
(B) simple columnar absorptive epithelium
(C) simple columnar mucus-secreting epithelium
(D) nonkeratinized stratified squamous epithelium
(E) stratified ciliated columnar epithelium

94. The mammary gland is classified as an exocrine gland because of which one of the following characteristics?

(A) Connective tissue capsule
(B) Extraepithelial location
(C) Association with myoepithelial cells
(D) System of drainage ducts
(E) Tubuloacinar secretory units

95. Examination of a hematoxylin–eosin (H& E)–stained section of decalcified bone reveals an irregular basophilic interface meandering through the bony matrix. This is an example of which one of the following structures?

(A) Canaliculus
(B) Sharpey fiber
(C) Lacuna
(D) Perforating canal
(E) Cement line

96. Which of the following statements best describes taste buds?

(A) They are small, keratinized, knob-like structures on the lingual mucosa
(B) They are present on fungiform, circumvallate, and foliate papillae of the tongue
(C) They form encapsulated nerve endings in the lamina propria of the oral mucosa
(D) They are secreted by the epithelial cells of the mucosa of the tongue
(E) They are capable of reacting to hundreds of different specific taste stimuli

97. Which of the following components of the respiratory system is lined by simple squamous epithelium?

(A) Alveolus
(B) Bronchus
(C) Nasal cavity
(D) Nasopharynx
(E) Trachea

98. Each secondary spermatocyte is best described by which one of the following characteristics?

(A) It has 22 autosomes and an X and Y chromosome
(B) It has 2N (diploid) amount of DNA
(C) It gives rise to four spermatids
(D) It is identical to its parent primary spermatocyte
(E) It replicates its DNA before dividing

99. Which of the following statements best describes proteoglycans (PGs) of the connective tissue extracellular matrix?

(A) They are large proteins with small polysaccharide side chains
(B) They are one of the fibrous components of the extracellular matrix
(C) They are identical to glycoproteins of the extracellular matrix
(D) They consist of multiple large polysaccharides attached to a protein core
(E) They are made up exclusively of repeating units of glucose and galactose

100. Purely serous salivary glands secrete which of the following substances?

(A) Mucinogen and other glycoproteins
(B) Enzymes and bicarbonate ions
(C) Fibrous proteins and proteoglycans
(D) Hormones and other regulatory agents
(E) Dead cells and pieces of cells

101. The tissue forming the impulse-generation and impulse-conduction system of the heart consists primarily of modified

(A) motor neurons
(B) collagen fibers
(C) myelinated axons
(D) smooth muscle
(E) myocardial fibers

102. Which of the following statements describes the fate of the membrane of a synaptic vesicle after release of neurotransmitter?

(A) It is incorporated into the postsynaptic plasma membrane
(B) It floats free in the extracellular space of the synaptic cleft
(C) It is incorporated into the presynaptic plasma membrane
(D) It is recycled into the microtubules of the presynaptic axon
(E) It is incorporated in the postsynaptic density

103. Under extreme conditions, fat, in addition to serving as a source of calories, can also be a source of

(A) amino acids
(B) glucose
(C) electrolytes
(D) hormones
(E) water

104. Turbulent precipitation occurs in what area of the respiratory system?

(A) Alveoli
(B) Bronchi
(C) Bronchioles
(D) Nasal cavity
(E) Trachea

105. The decreased number of oocytes in the ovaries of a 45-year-old woman is achieved primarily by which one of the following processes?

(A) Arrested mitosis
(B) Ovulation
(C) Crossing over
(D) Atresia
(E) Arrested meiosis

106. Nuclear lamins are intermediate filaments that

(A) bind to the nuclear envelope and prevent disassembly during mitosis
(B) form the channel of the nuclear pore complex
(C) form the membrane of the nucleolus
(D) line the inner aspect of the nuclear envelope

107. The production of new T lymphocytes in the thymus occurs in which of the following regions?

(A) Superficial cortex
(B) Corticomedullary junction
(C) Thymic nodules
(D) Deep medulla
(E) Thymic corpuscles

108. The replicative zone of the gastric epithelium is located in the

(A) base of the gastric gland, with all differentiating cells migrating toward the stomach lumen
(B) neck of the gastric gland, with all differentiating cells moving toward the base of the gland
(C) surface epithelium, with all differentiating cells moving toward the base of the gland
(D) neck of the gland, with some differentiating cells moving toward the surface of the gland, and some moving toward the base
(E) base of the submucosal glands, with all differentiating cells moving through the full thickness of the mucosa to the surface

109. Which structures listed below are found in a perforating (Volkmann) canal?

(A) Osteoclasts
(B) Blood vessels
(C) Osteocytic processes
(D) Sharpey fibers
(E) Osteoblasts

110. The epithelial lining of a lobar bronchus is which of the following tissue types?

(A) Simple columnar
(B) Ciliated pseudostratified
(C) Stratified squamous
(D) Transitional
(E) Simple squamous

111. An oocyte found in the ampulla of a fallopian tube of a celibate woman is referred to as

(A) an oogonium
(B) a primary oocyte
(C) a secondary oocyte
(D) an ovum
(E) a zygote

112. A cell in a gland of the stomach wall exhibits the following characteristics: it is large and ovoid, with granular-appearing, acidophilic cytoplasm and many mitochondria; electron microscopy reveals an elaborate intracellular canalicular system. This cell is

(A) a mucus-secreting cell of the mucous neck of a gastric gland
(B) a chief cell
(C) a stem cell from which the other cells of the gastric glands derive
(D) a parietal cell
(E) an enteroendocrine cell

113. The one tissue listed below that forms a continuum throughout the cardiovascular system is

(A) smooth muscle
(B) stratified cuboidal epithelium
(C) Purkinje fibers
(D) simple squamous epithelium
(E) cardiac muscle

114. Which of the following descriptions correctly characterizes the mucosal epithelium of the human esophagus?

(A) Pseudostratified columnar
(B) Nonkeratinized stratified squamous
(C) Simple columnar
(D) Keratinized stratified squamous
(E) Stratified cuboidal

115. Which of the following statements regarding the cell cycle is correct?

(A) It takes place once during the life of a cell (i.e., from origin to death)
(B) It is an ordered sequence of events during which the cell duplicates its chromosomes and divides into two cells
(C) It is divided into four phases: prophase, metaphase, anaphase, and telophase
(D) It is divided into karyokinesis and cytokinesis, which produce two identical cells from a single parent cell
(E) Its divisions represent diurnal variations in the protein synthetic activity of a cell

116. Pulmonary surfactant is secreted by which type of cells?

(A) Type I cells
(B) Type II cells
(C) Endothelial cells
(D) Dust cells
(E) Goblet cells

117. The muscularis externa of the human esophagus differs from that of the rest of the alimentary canal because it

(A) contains only a single thick layer of smooth muscle
(B) is continuous with the muscularis mucosae with no intervening submucosa
(C) contains exclusively striated muscle in the upper one-third of the esophagus
(D) forms three distinct longitudinal bands on the outside of the esophagus
(E) contains three distinct layers of smooth muscle in an orthogonal array

118. Which of the following lists of blood cell types is arranged in the sequence of most frequently to least frequently encountered cells in a smear of normal peripheral blood?

(A) Red blood cell (RBC), neutrophil, lymphocyte, basophil, monocyte, eosinophil
(B) Lymphocyte, neutrophil, RBC, monocyte, eosinophil, basophil
(C) RBC, neutrophil, lymphocyte, monocyte, eosinophil, basophil
(D) Neutrophil, RBC, lymphocyte, monocyte, eosinophil, basophil
(E) RBC, lymphocyte, neutrophil, monocyte, basophil, eosinophil

119. The surface epithelium that lines the stomach, small intestine, and colon is a regularly replicating cell layer. The turnover time for these epithelial cells in humans is

(A) 4 to 6 hours
(B) 4 to 6 days
(C) 4 to 6 weeks
(D) 4 to 6 months
(E) about once a year

Questions 120–122

The accompanying light micrograph of a portion of the small intestine shows the base of a crypt of Lieberkühn, the underlying muscularis mucosae, and part of the submucosa.

120. The cells indicated by *arrows* are

(A) absorptive cells
(B) chief cells
(C) enteroendocrine cells
(D) goblet cells
(E) Paneth cells

121. The two dark masses enclosed by the *circle* are evidence of which of the following processes?

(A) Bacterial phagocytosis
(B) Cell renewal
(C) Histamine secretion
(D) Lipid absorption

122. The cell indicated by an *arrowhead* is which of the following cell types?

(A) Neuron
(B) Fibroblast
(C) Goblet cell
(D) Epithelial cell
(E) Smooth muscle cell

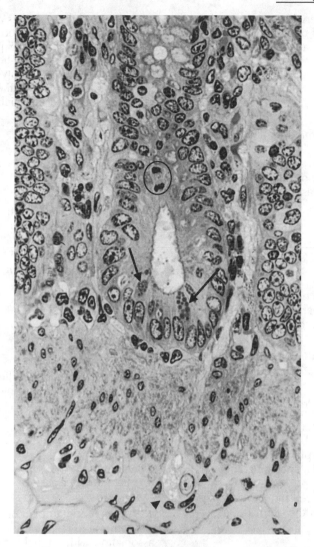

Questions 120–122

123. The terminal web of an epithelial cell is anchored peripherally to

(A) adhesion belts
(B) gap junctions
(C) desmosomes
(D) basal laminae
(E) tight junctions

124. The maximum number of oocytes that will ever occur in an ovary are found at what stage of development?

(A) 18-week-old fetus
(B) 1-week-old infant
(C) 7-year-old child
(D) 20-year-old woman
(E) 55-year-old woman

125. Purkinje fibers are most obvious in histologic sections of which of the following?

(A) Atrioventricular (AV) node
(B) Epicardium of the ventricles
(C) Interventricular septum
(D) Myocardium of the atria
(E) Sinoatrial (SA) node

126. In a routine histologic section of skin showing a full thickness of epidermis, mitotic cells are occasionally visible. These are characteristic of which level of the epidermis?

(A) Keratinized layer
(B) Granular layer
(C) Spinous layer
(D) Basal layer

127. A developing erythrocyte and a developing neutrophil in red bone marrow may be differentiated from one another by the presence of

(A) Golgi apparatus
(B) granules
(C) mitochondria
(D) peroxisomes
(E) rough endoplasmic reticulum (rER)

128. Villi are structural specializations of the mucosa that are found in which of the following portions of the gastrointestinal tract?

(A) Anal canal
(B) Colon
(C) Cardiac stomach
(D) Small intestine
(E) Appendix

129. A Barr body is noted in a neutrophil in a smear of normal peripheral blood. Which of the following most accurately describes this structure?

(A) A nuclear lobe that is formed primarily by heterochromatin and very little euchromatin
(B) A small appendage of a nuclear lobe that contains one X chromosome of a female
(C) A phagocytic vacuole containing a rod-shaped, bar-like bacterium
(D) A complex of a phagosome, an azurophilic granule, and a specific granule

130. The precursor cell of a macrophage in the papillary layer of the dermis is a

(A) lipocyte
(B) macrocyte
(C) neutrophil
(D) monocyte
(E) lymphocyte

131. A histologic slide of a transverse section through the duodenum shows large cells with large euchromatic nuclei and prominent nucleoli between two layers of smooth muscle that are oriented at right angles to one another. The large cells are

(A) enteroendocrine cells that secrete regulatory peptides
(B) Paneth cells that secrete bactericidal enzymes
(C) primordial cells that migrate into the epithelium to form stem cells
(D) neurons of the myenteric plexus that innervate the muscularis externa
(E) lymphocytes that have undergone blastic transformation

132. Tritiated thymidine is a radioactive nucleotide that is incorporated into newly synthesized DNA during the S phase of the cell cycle. Its intracellular location may be studied by autoradiography. Twenty minutes after its injection into a mouse, tritiated thymidine would be localized in which layer of the epidermis?

(A) Keratinized layer
(B) Granular layer
(C) Spinous layer
(D) Basal layer

133. In a section of lung tissue consisting predominantly of alveoli, a tubule about 2 mm in diameter is observed that contains smooth muscle and cartilage in its wall. The tubule is which one of the following?

(A) Alveolar duct
(B) Alveolar sac
(C) Bronchiole
(D) Bronchus
(E) Trachea

134. Which one of the following describes the secretory mechanism by which sebum is produced?

(A) Apocrine
(B) Cytocrine
(C) Eccrine
(D) Holocrine
(E) Paracrine

135. A cell containing numerous secondary lysosomes and residual bodies is seen in close association with a renal glomerular capillary. The cell is a

(A) visceral epithelial cell
(B) mast cell
(C) podocyte
(D) mesangial cell
(E) parietal epithelial cell

136. Lymphatic nodules with germinal centers are routinely noted in the

(A) deep cortex of a lymph node
(B) red pulp of the spleen
(C) medulla of the thymus gland
(D) palatine tonsil of the pharynx
(E) medulla of a lymph node

137. Which of the following statements about intercalated ducts of exocrine glands is correct?

(A) They constitute the named ducts of the major salivary glands
(B) They are composed of cuboidal and columnar epithelial cells that are often stratified
(C) They connect the secretory acini to the next larger portion of the duct system
(D) They contain basal membrane infoldings alternating with elongated mitochondria
(E) They are synonymous with the tubular secretory portions of tubuloacinar glands

138. Somatostatin secreted by δ cells of the islets of Langerhans affects the activity of the insulin and glucagon-secreting cells of the islets. This type of secretion is called

(A) apocrine
(B) endocrine
(C) holocrine
(D) merocrine
(E) paracrine

139. In a histologic section of bone examined at low magnification, a channel is visible that originates at the periosteal surface and penetrates the compact bone of the diaphysis. The width of the channel is several times the diameter of an erythrocyte. The channel is which one of the following structures?

(A) Perforating canal
(B) Osteocytic canaliculus
(C) Osteonal canal
(D) Howship lacuna

140. Most of the luminal surface area of a pulmonary alveolus is lined by which type of cells?

(A) Type II cells
(B) Endothelial cells
(C) Dust cells
(D) Clara cells
(E) Type I cells

141. A connexon is a structural component of the

(A) adhesion belt
(B) macula adherens
(C) gap junction
(D) tight junction
(E) desmosome

142. The auditory tube joins the pharynx to the

(A) scala tympani
(B) cochlear duct
(C) auditory meatus
(D) middle ear
(E) scala vestibuli

143. The molecules that form a continuum throughout a biologic membrane are made of

(A) cholesterol
(B) glycolipids
(C) glycoproteins
(D) phospholipids
(E) gangliosides

144. The gallbladder concentrates bile by which of the following mechanisms?

(A) Active transport of H^+ and Cl^- from the bile
(B) Active secretion of bile acids into the bile
(C) Active transport of Na^+ and Cl^- from the bile
(D) Active transport of water from the bile
(E) Active secretion of Na^+, Cl^-, and HCO_3^- into the bile

145. The presence or absence of which one of the following structures or secretions can be used to distinguish blood basophils and connective tissue mast cells?

(A) Histamine
(B) Basal lamina
(C) Heparin
(D) Cytoplasmic granules

146. The histologic basis of saltatory conduction of the nerve impulse is most closely associated with

(A) anterograde axonal transport
(B) distribution of Nissl substance
(C) spacing of nodes of Ranvier
(D) synaptic vesicle recycling
(E) presence of Schmidt-Lantermann clefts

147. Replicating populations of gastrointestinal epithelial cells are located

(A) in the crypt–villus junction in the jejunum
(B) in the basal one-third of the crypt in the colon
(C) at the free surface of the esophagus
(D) uniformly over the surface of the gastric pit
(E) in the base of the fundic gland of the stomach

148. The presence of a high concentration of neutrophils in the tracheal mucosa immediately deep to the epithelial lining is an indication of

(A) anaphylactic response
(B) blastic transformation
(C) acute inflammation
(D) immunoglobulin secretion
(E) parasitic infection

149. Placental villi are derived from which one of the following tissues?

(A) Epithelium of endometrial glands
(B) Inner cell mass of the blastocyst
(C) Spiral arteries of the endometrium
(D) Trophoblast of the blastocyst

150. The doughnut-shaped structures depicted in the light micrograph are

(A) Multilaminar ovarian follicles
(B) Hair follicles surrounded by dermis
(C) Blood vessels of the pampiniform plexus
(D) Osteons in spicules of spongy bone

151. A histologic section of endometrium containing examples of straight tubular glands is characteristic of which phase of the menstrual cycle?

(A) Luteal
(B) Menstrual
(C) Premenstrual
(D) Proliferative
(E) Secretory

152. The reticular cells of a lymph node most closely resemble

(A) macrophages
(B) squamous epithelial cells
(C) endothelial cells
(D) smooth muscle cells
(E) fibroblasts

153. The azurophilic granules of a neutrophil are which of the following cellular elements?

(A) Phagosomes
(B) Golgi apparatus
(C) Peroxisomes
(D) Residual bodies
(E) Lysosomes

154. The genetically and immunologically distinct secondary spermatocytes and spermatids are in a compartment that is isolated from the immune system by the blood–testis barrier. The barrier is formed by which one of the following?

(A) Basal laminae of seminiferous tubules
(B) Tight junctions between Sertoli cells
(C) Cytoplasmic bridges between spermatocytes
(D) Myoid cells subtending the seminiferous tubules
(E) Gap junctions between type B spermatogonia

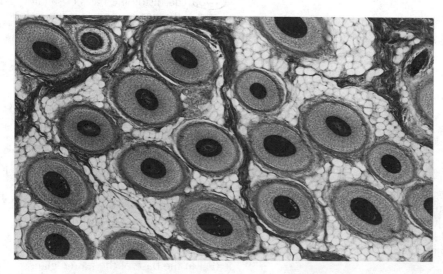

Question 150

155. In a sarcomere of skeletal muscle, which molecule or molecular aggregate connects Z disk to M line?

(A) Actin
(B) Myomesin
(C) Myosin
(D) Titin
(E) Tropomyosin

156. The convex, dome-shaped region of a lymph node is penetrated by numerous vessels of which of the following types?

(A) Arteriolar blood vessels
(B) Venular blood vessels
(C) Afferent lymphatic vessels
(D) Efferent lymphatic vessels

157. Capacitation of sperm is best described by which one of the following characteristics?

(A) It occurs entirely in the epididymis
(B) It is not necessary for fertilization to occur
(C) It includes removal of some sperm surface oligosaccharides while in the female reproductive tract
(D) It is completed in the vas deferens and seminal vesicle prior to ejaculation
(E) It includes removal of some sperm surface oligosaccharides by secretions of the prostate gland

158. A saline solution is added to a suspension of peripheral blood to produce a final sodium chloride concentration of 2.5% (isotonic saline = 0.9% NaCl). Microscopic examination of the red blood cells (RBCs) in the suspension would show

(A) microcytic RBCs
(B) crenated RBCs
(C) normal RBCs
(D) hemolyzed RBCs
(E) macrocytic RBCs

159. A section of gland tissue shows the following histologic characteristics: acini that are exclusively serous, intercalated ducts, non-serous cells in the lumen of the serous acini, and a herringbone pattern of smaller ducts leading to a large duct. This section is from which of the following glands?

(A) Parotid gland
(B) Sublingual gland
(C) Mammary gland
(D) Exocrine pancreas
(E) Submandibular gland

160. Which of the following pairs of cell types form the lining of a pulmonary alveolus and are joined by tight junctions?

(A) Surfactant-secreting cells and alveolar macrophages
(B) Alveolar macrophages and alveolar chondrocytes
(C) Squamous alveolar cells and surfactant-secreting cells
(D) Capillary endothelial cells and Type I cells

161. A mixed spicule that is formed during endochondral ossification is a combination of

(A) woven bone and lamellar bone
(B) hyaline cartilage and calcified cartilage
(C) compact bone and periosteal connective tissue
(D) calcified cartilage and new bone
(E) spongy bone and compact bone

162. Which one of the following characterizes a portal system of blood vessels?

(A) The absence of a capillary bed, thus shunting arterial blood directly to venules
(B) A capillary bed supplied and drained by a larger, noncapillary vessel
(C) Two capillary beds connected by a larger blood vessel
(D) A continuous capillary bed that extends from one organ to another

163. Crossing-over is the exchange of genetic material between

(A) sister chromatids in a tetrad
(B) non-sister chromatids during late anaphase
(C) regions on one chromatid during late prophase
(D) non-sister chromatids in a tetrad

Questions 164–166

The following questions are based on the accompanying light micrograph of stained bone marrow cells.

164. The cell labeled Y is committed to which line of myeloid differentiation?

(A) Erythropoiesis
(B) Megakaryocytopoiesis
(C) Granulopoiesis
(D) Monocytopoiesis

165. The cell labeled X is which of the following cell types?

(A) Band cell
(B) Neutrophilic myelocyte
(C) Reticulocyte
(D) Neutrophilic leukocyte
(E) Polychromatophilic erythroblast

166. The cell labeled Y is which of the following cell types?

(A) Erythroblast
(B) Myelocyte
(C) Normoblast
(D) Promyelocyte

167. Where in the body are intraepithelial bipolar neurons present?

(A) Nasal cavity
(B) Epidermis
(C) Gallbladder
(D) Urinary mucosa

168. A blood vessel 2 mm in diameter that, on histologic examination, is seen to have a distinct internal elastic lamina and a prominent tunica media is most likely which one of the following?

(A) Elastic artery
(B) Muscular artery
(C) Arteriole
(D) Pericytic venule
(E) Small vein

169. Loss of the nucleus from an erythroblast occurs between which two stages of erythropoiesis?

(A) Proerythroblast—basophilic erythroblast
(B) Basophilic erythroblast—polychromatophilic erythroblast
(C) Polychromatophilic erythroblast—normoblast
(D) Normoblast—reticulocyte
(E) Reticulocyte—erythrocyte

170. Which of the following regions of a lymph node is the thymus-dependent region?

(A) Nodular cortex
(B) Deep cortex
(C) Nodular medulla
(D) Medullary cords

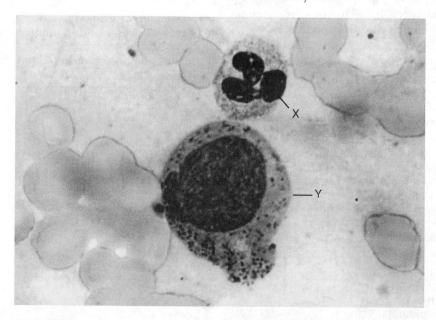

Questions 164–166

DIRECTIONS: Each of the numbered items or incomplete statements in this section is negatively phrased, as indicated by a capitalized word such as NOT, LEAST, or EXCEPT. Select the ONE lettered answer or completion that is BEST in each case.

171. Synthetic processes that occur in membrane-bounded cytoplasmic organelles include all of the following EXCEPT

(A) hydroxylation of proline and lysine in collagen synthesis
(B) glycosylation of proteins
(C) β-oxidation of fatty acids
(D) polymerization of G-actin to F-actin

172. Rough endoplasmic reticulum (rER) functions in the synthesis of all of the following molecules EXCEPT

(A) collagen triple helix
(B) lysosomal enzymes
(C) adenosine triphosphate (ATP)
(D) trypsinogen and pepsinogen
(E) N-linked glycoproteins

173. All of the following are functions of adult adipose tissue EXCEPT

(A) storage of energy in the form of neutral fats
(B) cushioning of sensitive organs and joints
(C) storage of energy in the form of glycogen
(D) thermal insulation in the skin
(E) cushioning of the soles of the feet and palms of the hand

174. A germinal center of a lymphatic nodule in a palatine tonsil would contain all of the following cells EXCEPT

(A) lymphoblasts
(B) killer cells
(C) T helper cells
(D) reticular cells
(E) B memory cells

175. All of the following cells are found in the epithelium of the small intestine EXCEPT

(A) absorptive cell
(B) Paneth cell
(C) pericryptal fibroblast
(D) enteroendocrine cell
(E) goblet cell

176. The alveolar air–blood barrier is formed by all of the following structures EXCEPT

(A) squamous alveolar cells
(B) basal laminae
(C) connective tissue
(D) endothelial cells
(E) smooth muscle cells

177. Post-translational modification of secretory proteins occurs in all of the following sites EXCEPT

(A) secretory granules
(B) Golgi apparatus
(C) rough endoplasmic reticulum (rER)
(D) plasma membrane
(E) smooth endoplasmic reticulum (sER)

178. All of the following statements concerning connective tissue are correct EXCEPT

(A) a general characteristic of connective tissue is an extensive extracellular space
(B) connective tissue may be classified as regular or irregular based on the arrangement of collagen fibers
(C) complex intercellular junctions between fibroblasts separate connective tissue from the other basic tissues
(D) one component of connective tissue is extracellular fibers that have cross-striations not visible with light microscopy
(E) macrophages, mast cells, fibroblasts, adipose cells, and undifferentiated mesenchymal cells constitute the resident cell population

179. Structural specializations that increase the absorptive surface of the small intestine include all of the following EXCEPT

(A) plicae circulares
(B) microvilli
(C) intracellular canaliculi
(D) villi
(E) glycocalyx

180. All of the following statements concerning protein secretion are correct EXCEPT

(A) zymogen granules contain stored proenzymes
(B) storage granules form at the *cis* face of the Golgi apparatus
(C) post-translational modification of proteins occurs in the rough endoplasmic reticulum (rER) and Golgi apparatus
(D) acid hydrolases are synthesized in the rER and targeted to lysosomes
(E) constitutive secretion is a continuous function of all cells

181. All of the following statements about the tongue are correct EXCEPT

(A) it is a muscular organ essential in speech and swallowing
(B) its dorsal surface is covered with numerous papillae of various shapes
(C) it uses both intrinsic and extrinsic muscles to perform its functions
(D) its lingual papillae and the taste buds associated with them constitute the specialized mucosa of the oral cavity
(E) it serves as the lymphatic organ that is the site of differentiation of certain lymphocytes, hence the name T lymphocytes

182. All of the following are normal functions of hepatocytes EXCEPT

(A) synthesis and breakdown of glycogen
(B) degradation and conjugation of drugs or toxins
(C) endocytosis of chylomicrons
(D) synthesis and secretion of immunoglobulins
(E) synthesis and secretion of bile acids

183. All of the following statements concerning meiosis are correct EXCEPT

(A) it results in the production of haploid gametes from diploid cells
(B) it is identical to mitosis but occurs only in germ cells in the postpubertal male and female
(C) it facilitates the exchange of genetic material between maternal and paternal chromosomes
(D) it produces cells that contain both the haploid number of chromosomes and the haploid amount of DNA
(E) it increases genetic diversity by the process of crossing over

184. All of the following are characteristics of intestinal absorptive cells EXCEPT

(A) an apical surface covered with as many as 3000 microvilli
(B) well-developed tight junctions with neighboring epithelial cells
(C) lateral plications with neighboring epithelial cells
(D) basal infoldings between which are vertically aligned mitochondria
(E) apical concentrations of mitochondria

185. All of the following are functions of the Sertoli cells EXCEPT

(A) secretion of transferrin
(B) phagocytosis of residual bodies
(C) secretion of a follicle-stimulating hormone (FSH) inhibitor
(D) creation of an immunologic barrier
(E) secretion of testosterone

186. All of the following are elements of the cytoskeleton EXCEPT

(A) keratin filaments
(B) vimentin
(C) actin filaments
(D) microtubules
(E) zonular fibers

187. All of the following cells or structures are components of the immunologic barrier present in the alimentary tract EXCEPT

(A) lymphocytes in the epithelial intercellular space
(B) plasma cells in the lamina propria
(C) junctional complexes in the epithelium
(D) macrophages and granulocytes in the lamina propria
(E) lymphatic nodules in the lamina propria

188. All of the following are connective tissues EXCEPT

(A) blood
(B) cartilage
(C) lamina propria
(D) capillary endothelium
(E) bone marrow

189. All of the following structures are part of the male genital system EXCEPT

(A) efferent ductules
(B) epididymis
(C) prostatic urethra
(D) ureters
(E) ductus deferens

190. The hepatic portal triad contains all of the following EXCEPT

(A) a branch of the portal vein
(B) one or more lymphatic vessels
(C) a hepatic arteriole
(D) a terminal hepatic venule
(E) one or more bile ducts

191. All of the following glands are salivary glands EXCEPT

(A) parotid
(B) sublingual
(C) buccal
(D) pancreas
(E) submandibular

192. All of the following statements concerning chromosomes are correct EXCEPT

(A) chromosomes are present only in actively dividing cells
(B) chromosomes contain all of the DNA in a eukaryotic cell except for the mitochondrial genome
(C) diploid human somatic cells contain 23 pairs of chromosomes
(D) chromosomes are composed of chromatin, which is a complex of DNA, histones, and nonhistone proteins
(E) chromosomes contain both transcriptionally active and transcriptionally inactive chromatin

193. All of the following statements about the sinusoids of the liver are correct EXCEPT

(A) sinusoids connect a vein to a vein
(B) perisinusoidal stellate macrophages form part of the cellular lining of the sinusoid
(C) a discontinuous fenestrated endothelium is characteristic of a hepatic sinusoid
(D) sinusoids carry a mixture of poorly oxygenated blood and oxygenated blood
(E) there is well-developed basal lamina between the sinusoidal endothelium and the hepatocyte

194. All of the following statements concerning collagen are correct EXCEPT

(A) it is a family of related glycoproteins
(B) it is a major component of the cytoskeleton
(C) it is not synthesized correctly in the absence of vitamin C
(D) it is synthesized by fibroblasts, epithelial cells, and muscle cells
(E) it has a tensile strength that approximates that of steel

195. All of the following are components of the duct system of the pancreas EXCEPT

(A) intercalated ducts
(B) striated ducts
(C) intralobular ducts
(D) interlobular ducts
(E) centroacinar cells

196. Each of the following items describes a passageway between two major cardiac structures. Which passageway is NOT guarded by a valve?

(A) Right ventricle–pulmonary trunk
(B) Left ventricle–aorta
(C) Right atrium–right ventricle
(D) Left atrium–pulmonary veins

197. All of the following statements correctly describe the cells from which adipocytes are derived EXCEPT

(A) undifferentiated mesenchymal cells
(B) monocytes that leave the circulation
(C) fibroblast-like cells with small lipid droplets and a thin external lamina
(D) lipoblasts
(E) cells that are morphologically indistinguishable from fibroblasts

198. Cartilage is found in all of the following parts of the respiratory system EXCEPT

(A) bronchi
(B) larynx
(C) trachea
(D) bronchioles

199. All of the following statements concerning the nuclear envelope are correct EXCEPT

(A) it is continuous with the membranes of the rough endoplasmic reticulum (rER)
(B) it serves as the boundary between the cytoplasmic and nuclear compartments
(C) it contains pores that regulate passage of materials in both directions between nucleus and cytoplasm
(D) it is the site of synthesis of proteins that will form elements of the nuclear matrix
(E) it is stabilized on its inner aspect by filaments of the nuclear lamina

200. All of the following statements about collagen are correct EXCEPT

(A) it is rich in hydroxyproline and hydroxylysine
(B) it is rich in glycine
(C) it has a triple-helical configuration
(D) it is rich in sulfur-containing amino acids
(E) it has an extremely high tensile strength in its fibrous form

201. Seminiferous tubules contain all of the following types of cells EXCEPT

(A) Sertoli cells in close association with spermatids
(B) Sertoli cells and spermatogonia only, prior to puberty
(C) Sertoli cells, primary spermatocytes, and late spermatids
(D) Sertoli cells in close association with Leydig cells
(E) Sertoli cells, spermatogonia, and secondary spermatocytes

202. All of the following statements about tooth enamel are correct EXCEPT

(A) it is the most heavily mineralized substance in the body
(B) it is secreted by ameloblasts
(C) it covers the exposed, visible portion (crown) of the tooth
(D) it is constantly renewed by secretion of new enamel
(E) it contains only enamelins and tuft protein when mature

203. Electron micrographs of white adipose tissue would show all of the following EXCEPT

(A) numerous mast cells
(B) numerous plasma cells
(C) numerous unmyelinated nerves
(D) a reticular fiber network
(E) a rich capillary network

204. All of the following enzymes are products of the exocrine pancreas EXCEPT

(A) trypsin
(B) ribonuclease
(C) amylase
(D) carboxypeptidase
(E) enterokinase

205. Pericryptal fibroblasts are a discrete population of cells that reside immediately under the basal lamina of the intestinal epithelium. They exhibit all of the following characteristics EXCEPT

(A) they secrete fibrous collagen
(B) they migrate in parallel with the epithelial cells
(C) they differentiate as they migrate up the side of the crypt
(D) their replicative zone is restricted to the crypt–villus junction
(E) they secrete glycosaminoglycans (GAGs) and proteoglycans (PGs)

206. Hormones involved in various aspects of adipose tissue regulation and function include all of the following EXCEPT

(A) thyroid hormone
(B) glucocorticoids
(C) insulin
(D) norepinephrine
(E) parathormone

207. All of the following statements describe aspects of the aqueous humor of the eye EXCEPT

(A) it circulates from the posterior chamber to the anterior chamber
(B) it provides for the metabolic support of the lens and cornea
(C) it is secreted by the epithelial cells of the ciliary body
(D) it is drained from the anterior chamber through the canal of Schlemm
(E) it is a highly hydrated connective tissue gel containing proteoglycans (PGs) and collagen

208. Which one of the following histologic characteristics does NOT apply to cardiac muscle?

(A) Central nuclei
(B) Large mitochondria
(C) Branching fibers
(D) Membranous triads
(E) Intercalated disks

DIRECTIONS: Each set of matching questions in this section consists of a list of four to twenty- six lettered options (some of which may be in figures) followed by several numbered items. For each numbered item, select the ONE lettered option that is most closely associated with it. To avoid spending too much time on matching sets with large numbers of options, it is generally advisable to begin each set by reading the list of options. Then, for each item in the set, try to generate the correct answer and locate it in the option list, rather than evaluating each option individually. Each lettered option may be selected once, more than once, or not at all.

Questions 209–211

(A) Na^+, K^+-ATPase
(B) Inositol trisphosphate
(C) Fluid-phase endocytosis
(D) Receptor-mediated endocytosis
(E) Phagocytosis

For each of the following cell functions, select the most appropriate molecule or process associated with it.

209. Uptake of large particles

210. Uptake of ligand in clathrin-coated vesicles

211. Increase of intracellular calcium concentration

Questions 212–218

(A) Cardiac muscle
(B) Myoepithelial cells
(C) Skeletal muscle
(D) Myofibroblastic cells
(E) Smooth muscle

For each histologic characteristic, select the most appropriate cell or tissue.

212. Transverse tubules are located at junctions between A bands and I bands

213. Cells are joined into fibers by adhesive and communicating junctions

214. Membranous complexes called triads are present

215. Responsible for the contraction of large skin wounds

216. Characterized by centrally located nuclei and branching fibers

217. Spindle-shaped cells surrounded by a network of reticular fibers

218. Associated with the secretory regions of exocrine glands

Questions 219–224

Match each description below with the appropriate lettered structure in the accompanying light micrograph.

219. Cell associated with bone resorption

220. Cells forming myeloid tissue

221. Cell that resides in a lacuna

222. Cells that synthesize osteoid

223. Junction between osteoid and calcified bone matrix

224. Cell that forms platelets

Questions 225–229

For each characteristic or function listed below, select the corresponding structure or area in the electron micrograph.

225. Site of unmyelinated axon–Schwann cell interaction

226. Site of glycosylation of extracellular matrix proteoglycans (PGs)

227. Site of actin and myosin overlap

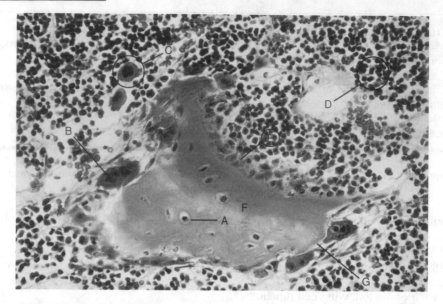

Questions 219–224

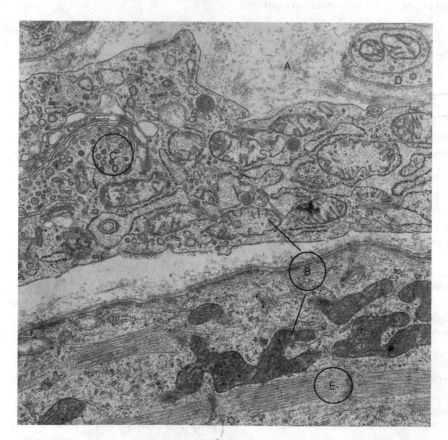

Questions 225–229

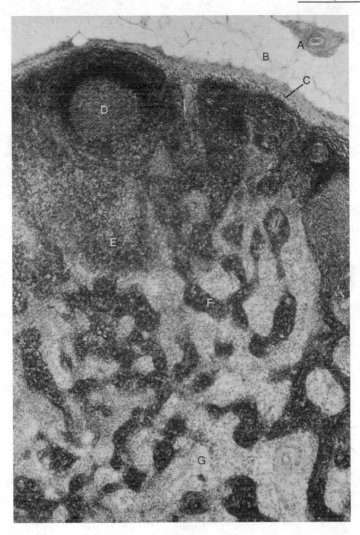

Questions 230–236

228. Site of oxidative phosphorylation and adenosine triphosphate (ATP) synthesis

229. Site of PG, collagen, and fibronectin accumulation

Questions 230–236

For each histophysiologic function or landmark of a lymph node, select the appropriate area in the light micrograph.

230. Region of B lymphocyte concentration

231. Location of mature, antibody-secreting cells

232. Zone dependent upon functional thymus for full development

233. Lumen of subcapsular (marginal) sinus

234. Site of blastic transformation of B lymphocytes

235. Space in direct continuity with the efferent lymphatic vessel

236. Area containing large numbers of lymphoblasts

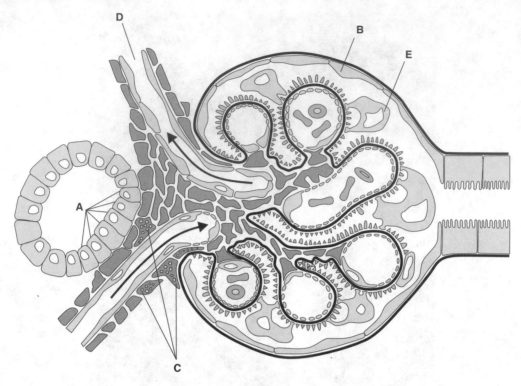

Questions 242–244

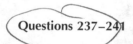

Questions 237–241

(A) Parietal cell
(B) Enteroendocrine cell
(C) Chief cell
(D) Surface mucous cell

Match the following cell products to the correct gastric epithelial cell type.

237. Visible mucus
238. Pepsinogen
239. Intrinsic factor
240. Hydrochloric acid
241. Gastrin

Questions 242–244

Match each of the following descriptions with the appropriate lettered structure in this diagram of components of the renal cortex.

242. Cell with processes that form part of the glomerular filtration barrier

243. Site of synthesis of a hormone that is important in regulation of blood pressure

244. Cells that monitor blood sodium concentration

Questions 245–251

(A) Lymph nodes
(B) Peyer patches
(C) Spleen
(D) Thymus gland
(E) Tonsils

For each histophysiologic characteristic, select the correct lymphatic structure.

245. Medulla characterized by large numbers of plasma cells

246. Presence of a subcapsular (marginal) sinus

247. Lymphatic nodules spanning gastrointestinal mucosal and submucosal layers

248. Numerous and distinct afferent lymphatic vessels

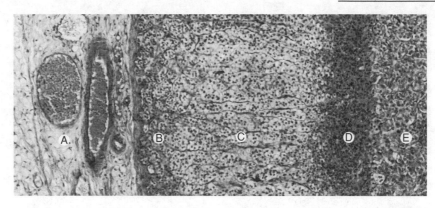

Questions 257–261

249. Lymphatic tissue encasing arteriolar blood vessels

250. Site of development of cells responsible for the cell-mediated immune response

251. Lymphatic nodules with germinal centers covered by a non-villous mucosal surface

Questions 252–256

(A) Simple columnar epithelium
(B) Striated skeletal muscle
(C) Myelinated peripheral nerve
(D) Dense irregular connective tissue

For each of the following histologic characteristics, select the appropriate tissue.

252. Cells are widely dispersed and noncontiguous

253. Plasma membrane and smooth endoplasmic reticulum (sER) are intimately associated

254. Constituent cells lack either a basal or external lamina

255. Tight junctions and desmosomes are typically present

256. Laminated plasma membrane forms a sheath

Questions 257–261

For each description, select the corresponding structure in the light micrograph.

257. It is derived from presumptive sympathetic ganglion tissue

258. It is regulated by renin–angiotensin system

259. Its secretions account for the predominance of adrenal epinephrine secretion in humans

260. It is the location of glucocorticoid synthesis

261. Its cells display the chromaffin reaction

Questions 262–266

Match the numbered cutaneous histophysiologic characteristics with the appropriate lettered structure in the accompanying light micrograph.

262. Site of organization of keratin filaments by filaggrin

263. Exocrine gland secreting by a holocrine mechanism

264. Smooth muscle bundle associated with a hair follicle

265. Portion of the duct of a thermoregulatory gland

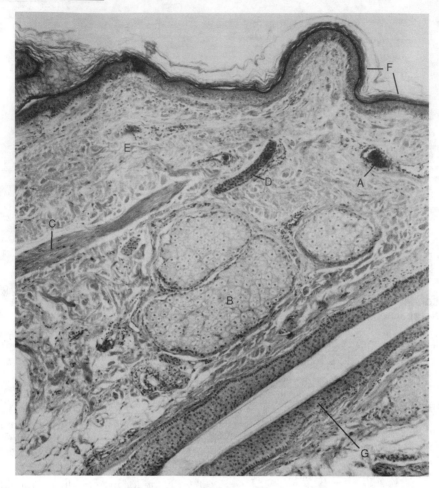

Questions 262–266

266. Epithelial structure producing a column of keratinized cells

Questions 267–276

The accompanying diagram shows a meridional section of a human eye. For each description, select the appropriate lettered structure.

267. Regulates the amount of light entering the eye

268. Changes shape in order to focus near objects on the retina

269. Is the primary dioptric of the eye

270. Carries visual information from the retina to the brain

271. Secretes *G*-labeled structures, as well as aqueous humor

272. Continues to grow throughout life but loses elasticity with age

273. Shrinkage of this hydrated connective tissue can lead to retinal detachment

274. Adult representation of the most anterior extension of the lip of the optic cup

275. Consists largely of regularly arrayed and precisely spaced fine collagen fibrils

276. Changes in tension on this structure lead to changes in the shape of the lens

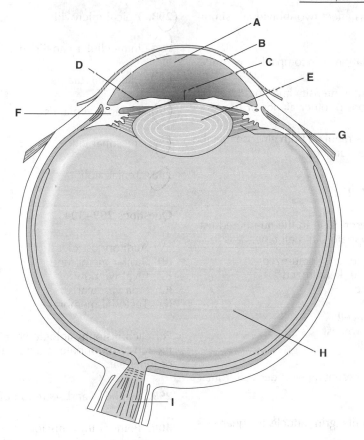

Questions 267–276

(A) Salivary gland
(B) Tooth
(C) Tongue
(D) Tonsil

Match the following descriptions with the most appropriate organ or structure.

277. Serves in grinding and macerating food

278. Secretes lubricants and enzymes

279. Forms an immunoprotective ring

280. Moves food during chewing and swallowing

Questions 281–286

(A) Adenohypophysis
(B) Adrenal cortex
(C) Adrenal medulla
(D) Neurohypophysis
(E) Pancreatic islet
(F) Parathyroid gland
(G) Pineal gland
(H) Placenta
(I) Thyroid gland

For each of the following items, select the endocrine gland or tissue that it most closely describes.

281. Specialized for the extracellular storage of a hormone precursor

282. Site of storage, but not of synthesis, of definitive peptide hormones

283. Secretions affect two individuals simultaneously

284. Total ablation is incompatible with life

285. Relates light intensity and duration to endocrine functions of other glands or tissues

286. Secretions regulate both glucose metabolism and kidney function

Questions 287–292

Match each description in the numbered list with the appropriate skin cell type.

(A) Keratinocyte, nonkeratinized
(B) Keratinocyte, keratinized
(C) Melanocyte
(D) Langerhans cell
(E) Sebaceous cell
(F) Dermal fibroblast
(G) Merkel cell

287. Antigen-presenting cell; derived from bone marrow

288. Contains filaggrin; anucleate squamous cell

289. Apoptotic; synthesizes lipid

290. Extraepithelial; protein-synthesizing cell

291. Exhibits keratin pattern; component of epidermal water diffusion barrier

292. Oxidizes tyrosine; neural crest derivative

Questions 293–298

(A) Absorption
(B) Propulsion
(C) Protection
(D) Secretion

Match each of the following morphologic specializations with the appropriate function associated with the alimentary canal.

293. Apical microvilli

294. Intracellular canaliculi

295. Plicae circulares

296. Extramural glands

297. Intestinal villi

298. Teniae coli

Questions 299–304

(A) Auditory ossicles
(B) Basilar membrane
(C) Oval window
(D) Stria vascularis
(E) Tectorial membrane

For each histophysiologic characteristic, select the most appropriate structure of the middle or inner ear.

299. Synthesis and secretion of endolymph

300. Point of transmission of sound energy into inner ear

301. Attached to stereocilia of hair cells of organ of Corti

302. Contains the traveling wave produced by sound vibrations

303. Junction of an air-filled space and a fluid-filled space

304. Connection between outer ear and inner ear

DIRECTIONS: Each set of matching questions in this section consists of a list of four to twenty- six lettered options followed by several numbered items. For each numbered item, select the appropriate lettered option(s). Each lettered option may be selected once, more than once, or not at all. EACH ITEM WILL STATE THE NUMBER OF OPTIONS TO SELECT. CHOOSE EXACTLY THIS NUMBER.

Questions 305–312

(A) Hyaline cartilage
(B) Loose irregular connective tissue
(C) Lamellar bone
(D) Dense irregular connective tissue
(E) Fibrocartilage
(F) Dense regular connective tissue
(G) Elastic cartilage

For each of the following histologic structures or processes, select the tissue or tissues that they characterize.

305. Canalicular channels (SELECT 1 TISSUE)

306. Lacunar compartments (SELECT 4 TIS-SUES)

307. Elastic fibers (SELECT 3 TISSUES)

308. Territorial matrix (SELECT 3 TISSUES)

309. Hydroxyapatite crystals (SELECT 2 TIS-SUES)

310. Appositional growth (SELECT 4 TISSUES)

311. Cement lines (SELECT 1 TISSUE)

312. Vascularized matrix (SELECT 4 TISSUES)

ANSWERS AND EXPLANATIONS

1. The answer is C [Chapter 11 III C]. Osteoid, which is synthesized by osteoblasts, is newly deposited bone matrix that is not yet calcified. It characteristically forms a narrow zone on the surface of the bone between a layer of osteoblasts and calcified matrix. New osteocytes, recently recruited from the nearby population of osteoblasts, may be contained within the layer of osteoid. Matrix vesicles, possibly with evidence of crystals of hydroxyapatite in them, may also be found in the osteoid layer.

2. The answer is B [Chapter 2 III B 4]. Sulfates are added to proteoglycans (PGs), and other molecules, in the *trans* Golgi by resident sulfotransferases, enzymes that catalyze this post-translational modification.

3. The answer is D [Chapter 24 I A 1 a, B 2; II C 1]. At the esophagogastric junction the lining of the alimentary canal changes from the protective stratified squamous epithelium of the esophagus to the secretory simple columnar epithelium of the surface mucous cells and gastric pits of the stomach. The other junctions listed are between portions of the gastrointestinal tract that are both lined with simple columnar epithelium. They can be distinguished, however, by the specific nature of the glands, or glands and villi, that constitute their lining mucosa.

4. The answer is B [Chapter 31 II D 1 a]. Hypercalcemia, an abnormally high concentration of calcium in the blood, is the stimulus for calcitonin secretion by parafollicular cells of the thyroid gland. Calcitonin reduces blood calcium levels. Parathyroid hormone (PTH) works in a manner reciprocal to calcitonin by stimulating an increase in blood calcium. Balance between the effects of calcitonin and PTH maintain calcium homeostasis.

5. The answer is C [Chapter 35 II C 3; Figure 35-3]. The antrum of an ovarian follicle is a dilatation of the intercellular space of the epithelial-like layer of granulosa cells that surrounds the oocyte. The presence of an antrum is an indication of a developing follicle. The antrum of a growing follicle can become the largest subcompartment of the ovary.

6. The answer is B [Chapter 35 X A]. A lobule of active mammary gland tissue is shown in the light micrograph accompanying this question. Note the irregularly shaped tubuloalveolar secretory units, which contrast with the regularly shaped follicles of the thyroid gland. Some secretory units are shown emptying into a large interlobular duct (*lower left*). Such a duct would not be found in the thyroid gland, which is an endocrine gland.

7. The answer is D [Chapter 8 IV A 3]. Mast cell granules contain several vasoactive and immunoreactive substances, most notably histamine and heparin. Histamine release initiates the vascular leakage that produces the edema typical of acute inflammation. Heparin is a highly sulfated glycosaminoglycan (GAG). It is an anticoagulant that increases vascular leakage in the acute inflammatory response. The anionic sulfate groups account for the intense basophilia of the granules. Mast cells are very long-lived, and they do not divide in the connective tissue. Degranulated mast cells synthesize and store new histamine and heparin in newly formed secretory granules.

8. The answer is D [Chapter 14 V C 1]. The wall of this vessel is formed by a single layer of endothelial cells. Even without knowing the absolute magnification of this micrograph, one can infer that this is an extremely small vessel based on its luminal contents and thin wall. All of the other blood vessels listed have much thicker walls in which the three tunics (intima, media, and adventitia) are identifiable.

9. The answer is B [Chapter 12 II A 1, B 1; Figure 14-7]. This is an erythrocyte, or red blood cell (RBC). Its biconcave discoidal structure is not apparent because of the plane of section. Note how the RBC fills nearly the entire lumen of the capillary, the wall of which is formed by endothelial cells. A neutrophil is a nucleated blood cell that also contains cytoplasmic granules. Platelets are membrane-bounded cell fragments that also contain granules and are smaller than an RBC. A pericyte is an extravascular cell.

10. The answer is D [Chapter 14 V C 2]. Pericytes are routinely observed to be associated with capillaries. The pericyte is enclosed by a basal (external) lamina and where the pericyte and capillary endothelial cell are apposed, their laminae are fused.

11. The answer is B [Chapter 14 V D 2]. Three fenestrae, or pores, are visible in the wall of this fenestrated capillary. The fenestrations are bridged by diaphragms. Note that in this plane of section of the vessel, one of the three endothelial cells forming the vessel wall shows a nucleus. In this same cell are a small system of Golgi membranes and a few cisterns of the rough endoplasmic reticulum (rER), which are morphologic evidence of the synthetic capability of these cells.

12. The answer is B [Chapter 6 III A 5 a (2)]. Synaptic vesicles release neurotransmitter into the synaptic cleft by exocytosis. Exocytosis occurs in many other cell types and is characterized by the fusion of vesicle (or vacuolar) membrane with the plasma membrane. The content of the vesicle is released into the intercellular space (i.e., into the synaptic cleft) and the membrane of the vesicle is added to the cell surface. Endocytosis, phagocytosis, and pinocytosis are all processes by which material is taken into, not released from, a cell.

13. The answer is D [Chapter 14 II A 2 a (1) (b)]. The bicuspid valve, or mitral valve, is found between the left atrium and left ventricle. It allows blood flow from the atrium to the ventricle and prevents flow in the reverse direction. The tricuspid valve is located between the right atrium and the right ventricle. The semilunar aortic valve allows blood to enter the aorta from the left ventricle. The pulmonary valve, also semilunar, allows blood to enter the pulmonary trunk from the right ventricle. A valve-like structure is located between the inferior vena cava and the right atrium, but it is physiologically incompetent.

14. The answer is C [Chapter 16 III A 1, 2]. The ileum is characterized by the presence of aggregations of lymphatic nodules. Each aggregate of nodules is a Peyer patch. The aggregations are restricted to the portion of the intestinal wall that is antimesenteric (120–180 degrees of the circumference). Other regions of the small intestine commonly include only scattered solitary nodules. The ileum does contain villi. The outer muscle layer of the muscularis externa is arranged into bands in the colon, not in the small intestine. Submucosal glands are found in the duodenum but not in other parts of the small intestine or colon.

15. The answer is D [Chapter 29 VII B 2]. Interlobular arteries (cortical radial arteries) branch at right angles from the arcuate artery and run radially in the cortical labyrinth. They give rise to numerous vessels, all of which end as afferent arterioles. Efferent arterioles carry blood away from the glomerular capillary loops and subsequently form either peritubular capillary networks or vasa recta. Efferent arterioles of juxtamedullary glomeruli give rise to arteriolae rectae. Glomerular capillaries form the glomerular tuft between the afferent and efferent arterioles. They are the site of filtration of the blood to form the primary urine. Interlobar arteries supply the arcuate arteries.

16. The answer is C [Chapter 36 II D 1]. The morphology and function of Leydig cells (interstitial cells of the testis) depend on pituitary luteinizing hormone (LH) to maintain their normal structure and function. Growth hormone (GH) has a more general role in growth of a whole individual. Thyroid-stimulating hormone (TSH) regulates the structure and function of the thyroid gland. Follicle-stimulating hormone (FSH) is essential for growth of the ovum and ovarian follicle in the female and for the function of the Sertoli cells in the male. Melanocyte-stimulating hormone (MSH) is not a functional hormone in humans, although MSH immunoreactivity to byproducts of post-translational processing of propiomelanocortin may be found in the pars intermedia of the pituitary gland.

17. The answer is B [Chapter 1 II A 3; Figure 1-1]. According to the current model, the biological membrane is a fluid-mosaic of proteins interspersed in a phospholipid bilayer. The phospholipids and proteins of biological membranes are held together primarily through noncovalent interactions, not by covalent bonds. The hydrocarbon tails of the phospholipids are hydrophobic and, thus, preferentially orient themselves away from the polar, aqueous compartment, associating with each other in the interior of the bilayer.

18. The answer is C [Chapter 2 VI A 1]. Primary lysosomes are 0.1 to 0.3 μm in diameter, a dimension that is just at the limit of resolution of the light microscope. Thus, they are not readily observable. By electron microscopy, primary lysosomes appear as membrane-bounded vesicles that lack a unique identifying structure. They can, however, be demonstrated readily using histochemical procedures based on the enzymatic activity of the acid hydrolases they contain.

19. The answer is B [Chapter 8 II A 2 c]. Tropocollagen is the molecule produced by the cleavage of the nonhelical ends of procollagen by the procollagen peptidase of the plasma membrane. Tropocollagen molecules are long thin molecules (1.5 x 280 nm) with a distinct "head" and "tail" that self-assemble head-to-tail and side-to-side, with a quarter-molecule stagger, to form collagen fibrils with a distinctive 64–68 nm axial periodicity. Tropocollagen molecules are composed of three intertwined polypeptide α chains arranged in a right-handed triple helix. This is characteristic of the fibrillar forms of collagen. The nonfibrillar collagens contain only short helical sections in the tropocollagen molecule.

20. The answer is C [Chapter 13 IV C 1 c (1)(a)]. Specific granules are first found in the developing granulocyte at the myelocyte stage. Specific granules are necessary for the identification of a myelocyte as a cell in the neutrophilic, eosinophilic, or basophilic line. A promyelocyte contains azurophilic granules but no specific granules and, therefore, it cannot be identified as neutrophilic, eosinophilic, or basophilic.

21. The answer is B [Chapter 26 VII A 2]. Bile canaliculi are the finest branches of the biliary tree, which carries the exocrine secretions of the hepatocytes from the liver to the duodenum. They are dilations of the intercellular space between adjacent hepatocytes and are isolated from the rest of the intercellular space by junctional complexes between the adjacent cells. The small portion of the hepatocyte surface that faces the bile canaliculus is equivalent to the apical plasma membrane of other exocrine gland cells and the canaliculus, itself, is equivalent to the intercalated duct of other exocrine glands. Lipoproteins of all sizes are secreted across the hepatocyte surface that faces the perisinusoidal space, or space of Disse, between the cell and the sinusoidal endothelium.

22. The answer is D [Chapter 29 V B 2]. Small proteins and peptides that pass the glomerular filtration barrier are reabsorbed by the proximal convoluted tubule cells by endo-cytosis and degraded by lysosomal enzymes. The amino acids produced are then recycled to the circulation. The visceral epithelial cell of the renal corpuscle is the podocyte, whose processes form a component of the filtration barrier of the renal corpuscle. The distal convoluted tubule cells are responsible for reabsorbtion of Na^+ from the urine that has passed through the loop of Henle. Mesangial cells are phagocytic cells that clear the glomerular basement membrane of accumulated debris that would include much larger proteins than the one described here. The parietal epithelial cells of the renal corpuscle are not noted for any particular function other than lining the outer wall of the urinary space.

23. The answer is C [Chapter 29 V E 3]. The macula densa, which is a component of the juxtaglomerular apparatus, is located in the wall of the distal tubule. Therefore, identification of a macula densa also identifies the distal tubule. The macula densa is found close to the transition of the distal straight tubule to the distal convoluted tubule.

24. The answer is C [Chapter 37 III A 2 c; VIII B]. The space between the two layers of the optic cup remains in the adult eye as a potential space between the pigmented layer of the retina and the neural layer. Swelling in this space or shrinkage of the vitreous humor can lead to separation of the two layers, which is retinal detachment.

25. The answer is B [Chapter 6 IX A 2]. Collagen in this location, close to the Schwann cell, is part of the endoneurium. The inner limit of the endoneurium is the external lamina of the Schwann cell. Perineurium is an epithelioid layering of cells around a nerve bundle. Epineurium is a dense fibrous connective tissue layer superficial to the perineurium.

26. The answer is D [Chapter 1 II F 3 b]. The distribution of transmembrane proteins in the phospholipid bilayer is readily apparent by the technique of freeze-fracture electron microscopy: the intramembrane particles visualized by the technique are considered to represent membrane proteins. Phospholipids are not imaged with the freeze-fracture technique. Although carbohydrates can be linked covalently to transmembrane proteins and these membrane-spanning portions can be visualized by freeze-fracture, the technique yields little information about the carbohydrate part of the molecule. Freeze-fracture tells us little about the distribution of membrane-associated ribosomes and glycogen because these particles lie on the cytoplasmic side of the phospholipid bilayer, and the fracture cleavage plane passes through the interior of the bilayer.

27. The answer is A [Chapter 17 VI A 1]. The vessel indicated is a small muscular artery carrying blood to the lymph node. This undulating vessel appears in longitudinal and oblique section. Note the smooth muscle of the tunica media and the internal elastic lamina.

28. The answer is B [Chapter 17 V E 2]. The orientation of the cusps of the valve in this lymphatic vessel, the efferent vessel, allows flow of lymph from right to left. Flow from left to right would cause the free edges of the valve cusps to approximate one another, thus impeding flow in that direction.

29. The answer is C [Chapter 17 III B 2 b]. The indicated subcompartment is a medullary sinus. A cord of medullary tissue is surrounded by the sinus. Cortical sinuses are less well defined and, generally, are distant from the hilum. A germinal center is a structure found in the cortical region of a lymph node. It is formed by lymphoblasts and not by the reticular connective tissue seen here.

30. The answer is D [Chapter 25 I B 2, 4; F 2]. This section shows the full thickness of the wall of the small intestine. Villi are unusually distinct and the inner layer of the muscularis externa is very thick. The colon has a mucosal surface that is free of villi—quite unlike the villus-covered surface visible in this section. The esophagus is lined by a thick stratified squamous epithelium, and it does not have villi. The gallbladder is characterized by a complex mucosal surface that, in sections, may resemble the villous surface of the small intestine. However, the muscle layer of the gallbladder is less regularly arranged than the muscularis externa of the small intestine. A section of stomach would show gastric pits and tubular glands, rather than the villi and crypts seen here.

31. The answer is D [Chapter 4 III]. The nucleolus is the site of assembly of ribosomal subunits. Ribosomal RNA is transcribed in the nucleolus, except for the 5SRNA molecule, which is transcribed outside of the nucleolus. Ribosomal proteins are synthesized on free polysomes in the cytoplasm and transported back into the nucleus for assembly with ribosomal RNA in the nucleolus.

32. The answer is D [Chapter 5 V D 3 a]. A tight junction, also called a zonula occludens, blocks the intercellular space and prevents free diffusion of materials through the paracellular route from one side of the epithelium to the other side. A gap junction is a communicating junction that allows diffusion of materials through the aqueous channels of connexon pairs from the cytoplasm of one cell to the cytoplasm of an adjacent cell. A hemidesmosome, an adhesion belt, and a macula adherens (desmosome) are all adherens junctions and do not function as intercellular gaskets, as does the tight junction.

33. The answer is B [Chapter 29 V B 2]. The proximal convoluted tubule resorbs nearly 80% of the primary glomerular filtrate. It accomplishes this by an active transport process similar to that for fluid and electrolyte absorption in the gallbladder and intestine. The urinary space of the renal capsule is the space into which the large volume of glomerular filtrate is delivered, which then drains to the proximal tubule. The distal convoluted tubule receives the urine from the ascending portion of the loop of Henle. It conserves Na^+ by reabsorbing Na^+ and secreting K^+. Neither the distal convoluted tubule nor the collecting ducts affect the volume of the initial glomerular filtrate. The loop of Henle does not affect the volume of the material passing though it. Its primary function is to establish the hypertonic medullary interstitium that is necessary for removal of water from the urine in the medullary collecting ducts.

34. The answer is A [Chapter 15 III C 2, D]. Plasma cells are produced by the blastic transformation of B lymphocytes. A B lymphocyte is stimulated to undergo blastic transformation by recognizing the antigenic site to which it is genetically programmed to react. The B lymphocyte enlarges to become a lymphoblast. The lymphoblast divides and produces plasma cells and B memory cells.

35. The answer is B [Chapter 11 II D 1 a]. The osteoclast, which is found in areas of bone remodelling and bone removal, achieves its large size and multinuclear characteristic by undergoing repeated karyokinesis, but not cytokinesis. Karyokinesis is nuclear division, which occurs repeatedly in the osteoclast, and cytokinesis is cytoplasmic division, which does not occur in osteoclasts.

36. The answer is D [Chapter 29 VI C 1]. The primary site of action of antidiuretic hormone (ADH) is the epithelium of the medullary collecting ducts. ADH increases their permeability to water, thereby promoting the movement of water from the duct lumen to the hypertonic interstitium. The thin ascending limb of the loop of Henle is impermeable to water. This is essential to the establishment and maintenance of the hypertonic medullary interstitium. Foot processes of podocytes rest on the glomerular basement membrane and slits between them are components of the filtration barrier in the renal corpuscle. The thin descending limb of the loop of Henle is freely permeable to water and electrolytes. The proximal convoluted tubules are responsible for reabsorbing 70% to 80% of the initial glomerular filtrate. This is an active isotonic process driven by a Na^+,K^+-ATPase in the lateral margins of the epithelial cells.

37. The answer is D [Chapter 35 III A 3 b]. A sudden increase in the level of luteinizing hormone can be detected at midcycle (day 14 of the ideal 28-day cycle), and this hormonal surge appears to be essential for ovulation. Completion of the second meiotic division occurs only after fertilization, which occurs sometime after ovulation. The loss of gap junctions is associated with atresia, not with ovulation.

38. The answer is C [Chapter 1 II D 2]. Of the organelles or their components listed in the question, the only one in which glycosylation occurs is the rough endoplasmic reticulum (rER). Asparagine-linked sugars are assembled in the rER as a cotranslational modification of most membrane glycoproteins. The sugars are added to the protein on the cisternal side of the rER. They are transported through the Golgi stacks to the trans-Golgi network, where they are sorted to vesicles that carry them to the plasma membrane. The sugar moieties of the membrane glycoproteins are then exposed to the outside as a result of exocytosis during the eversion of the vesicles that carry the proteins to the cell surface. The smooth endoplasmic reticulum (sER) is the site of synthesis of membrane lipids.

39. The answer is D [Chapter 5 V D]. One tight junction completely encircles an epithelial cell and joins it to all its adjacent cells. Because of this belt-like characteristic, the tight junction is also referred to as a zonular-type junction. A desmosome, a gap junction, and a hemidesmosome are all punctate (macular-type) junctions.

40. The answer is C [Chapter 6 IV A 1]. Oligodendrocytes are numerous in the white matter of the spinal cord, where they elaborate the myelin that is characteristic of this compartment of the cord. The oligodendrocytes are restricted to the spaces between fibers and, depending on the plane of section, may be seen aligned in rows. Astrocytes and microglia may also be found in the white matter but would lack the regular spacing characteristic of oligodendrocytes. Satellite cells and Schwann cells are cells of the peripheral nervous system, not the central nervous system.

41. The answer is B [Chapter 11 IV B 2]. The plywood-like appearance of lamellar bone is due to the alternating arrangement of layers of collagen and their subsequent effect on the deposition of hydroxyapatite. The collagen fibrils in any one lamella are all oriented in the same direction. Collagen fibrils of adjacent lamellae run at approximate right angles to each other.

42. The answer is E [Chapter 25 I A 1 b; I F 1]. The glands described are the submucosal (Brunner) glands that are characteristic of, and restricted to, the duodenum, the first anatomic segment of the small intestine. These glands secrete an alkaline mucin that helps to neutralize the acidity of the chyme that enters the duodenum from the stomach. The secretion also helps to establish the slightly alkaline pH that is optimal for the function of the pancreatic enzymes that are delivered to the duodenum. The jejunum is the middle segment of the small intestine. It is the primary site of nutrient absorption and does not contain Brunner glands. The pylorus is the terminal portion of the stomach; it is not a part of the intestine but might appear in a longitudinal section through the gastroduodenal junction. The ileum may be identified by large lymphatic nodules that fill the lamina propria on the anti-mesenteric side of the tube. The cecum, part of the colon, is characterized by straight tubular glands restricted to the mucosa.

43. The answer is B [Chapter 17 VI B 1]. Both B lymphocytes and T lymphocytes leave the blood stream from the postcapillary venules in the deep (non-nodular) cortex. The venules in this location have a cuboidal or columnar endothelial lining that is very different from the squamous endothelial cells found at most other sites in the vascular system. It is likely that these high endothelial venules facilitate diapedesis of cells across the wall of the blood vessel.

44. The answer is C [Chapter 26 IV A 2]. The central landmark of the classic liver lobule is a central vein (central venule, terminal hepatic venule). The periphery of the classic lobule is marked by portal triads. Sinusoids are radially arranged, capillary-like vascular channels that converge on the central vein. The space of Disse is the perivascular space between the sinusoidal endothelium and the basal surface of the hepatocyte. A bile canaliculus is the finest, terminal part of the biliary system and is not a landmark in the definition of a classic liver lobule.

45. The answer is E [Chapter 29 III C 2]. The renal lobule consists of a medullary ray and the cortical tissue (i.e., the renal corpuscles and associated tubules) that drain to the collecting ducts of that medullary ray. A cortical column is cortical tissue that extends along the sides of a medullary pyramid, thus defining the borders of the renal lobes. Interlobular arteries are located in the cortical labyrinth, approximately midway between medullary rays. Interlobular arteries define the lateral borders of renal lobules. The renal hilum is a depression on the medial border of the kidney through which blood vessels enter and leave the kidney, and through which the ureter leaves the kidney. Arcuate arteries are located at the corticomedullary junction of each renal lobe and branch into the interlobular arteries.

46. The answer is C [Chapter 33 II C]. It is well established that insulin is produced by β cells in the islet of Langerhans. α cells produce glucagon; exocrine (acinar) cells produce digestive enzymes; δ cells produce somatostatin. Intercalated duct cells are partially responsible for secretion of the aqueous component of pancreatic juice.

47. The answer is A [Chapter 36 IV B 2 a]. Spermatogonia and the earliest primary spermatocytes are confined to a compartment between Sertoli–Sertoli cell junctions and the

basal lamina of the seminiferous tubule. This is the basal compartment created by the blood–testis barrier. Primary and secondary spermatocytes, spermatids, and maturing sperm are found together in the luminal compartment created by the blood–testis barrier. Sertoli cells do not divide after puberty. Type A dark spermatogonia give rise to type A pale spermatogonia by mitotic division. Leydig cells are found in the connective tissue surrounding the seminiferous tubules; they are not part of the seminiferous epithelium.

48. The answer is B [Chapter 15 VIII B 2]. Nodules with germinal centers (secondary nodules) indicate that a humoral immune response is occurring. The most likely source of the antigen that initiated the immune reaction is from the lumen of the intestine. The bacterial flora of the gut normally is restricted to the lumen by the intestinal epithelium. Rupture of the epithelial barrier would allow intestinal microorganisms and other antigens to contact the gut-associated lymphatic tissue (GALT), causing the formation of nodules with germinal centers.

49. The answer is D [Chapter 23 I A]. Exocrine glands are defined as glands that secrete through a duct onto an epithelial surface. This contrasts with endocrine glands, which do not secrete into a duct. Exocrine glands may be purely serous, purely mucous, or mixed. Only serous glands store zymogen granules in the apical cytoplasm. Not all exocrine glands have myoepithelial cells; they are present in salivary and eccrine sweat glands, but they are absent from the pancreas. Also, although some glands concentrate their secretion, not all glands do so, nor do those that concentrate the secretion transport exclusively sodium and water.

50. The answer is C [Chapter 5 V C 3 b (1)]. This type of experiment demonstrates the existence of cell–cell coupling by gap junctions. The narrow (2 nm) channel enclosed by a connexon pair, which is the functional unit of a gap junction, allows the flow of ions and small molecules from one cell to another. One gap junction may be formed by thousands of connexon pairs, and a cell may have hundreds of gap junctions over its surface. Cell–cell coupling can be extensive.

51. The answer is A [Chapter 11 II D]. Osteoclasts are multinucleate giant cells that are found in areas where the resorption of bone matrix is occurring. Osteoclasts are solitary cells, as opposed to the epithelioid arrangement of osteoblasts. Occasionally, osteoclasts are seen in depressions (Howship lacunae) on the surface of a bone that they themselves have made by their osteolytic function. The resorption of bone by osteocytes (osteocytic osteolysis) also occurs, but is not as extensive as bone resorption by osteoclasts.

52. The answer is D [Chapter 4 II C 3 a]. The nucleosome is a unit of structure of chromatin. A nucleosome is composed of a core of eight histone proteins with approximately 1.8 loops of DNA wrapped around the core. None of the other nuclear structures listed has a unit of structure per se. The matrix and lamina are filamentous subcompartments of the nucleus. The envelope forms the membranous interface between the cytoplasm and nucleoplasm and is pierced by many openings called pores.

53. The answer is B [Chapter 14 B 3]. A muscular artery is visible at the top of the field. The internal elastic lamina of the vessel is prominent, as is the demarcation between the tunica media and the tunica adventitia. The accompanying small vein is collapsed, which is typical, and the leaflets of a valve are included in the plane of section. The origins of leaflets from the tunica intima are indicated (*arrows*). The arterial vessel (*top*) has too many layers of smooth muscle in its wall to be an arteriole. The venous vessel (*bottom*), by itself, has some charactyeristics of a lymphatic vessel but the accompanying vessel is far too large to be considered a capillary.

54. The answer is B [Chapter 38 V C 3 d]. Stereocilia span the narrow extracellular space between the apical surface of the hair cells and the overlying tectorial membrane. Because of the different hinging points of the basilar membrane and the tectorial membrane, the stereocilia are distorted during propagation of the traveling wave that is produced by sound impinging on the ear.

55. The answer is E [Chapter 29 VIII A, B 4]. The establishment of a gradient of salt concentration in the medullary interstitium that increases from the corticomedullary border to the tip of the medullary papilla is essential for the production of a hypertonic urine. The presence and specific functional characteristics of long loops of Henle in the medulla are essen-

tial to the establishment of this gradient. The collecting ducts are permeable to water, which passes from the ducts to the interstitium as the ducts pass through the full thickness of the medulla. None of the other factors listed has a significant effect on the final tonicity of the urine.

56. The answer is B [Chapter 13 IV B 1]. Of the five myeloid cells listed, only the promyelocyte has the characteristics of the observed cell. The presence of granules eliminates cells of the erythropoietic line from consideration (i.e., the basophilic erythroblast and normoblast). The unindented euchromatic nucleus eliminates the metamyelocyte. The eosinophilic myelocyte is eliminated both because its nucleus is indented, and also because it contains reddish-orange specific granules in addition to the purple-staining azurophilic granules.

57. The answer is D [Chapter 15 VIII B 4 a]. Germinal centers are indicators of a humoral immune response, and B lymphocytes are closely associated with this type of immune reaction. Recognizable macrophages are usually not noted in germinal centers. Helper T cells would be found in the center but would be outnumbered by B lymphocytes and their derivatives. Some reticular cells would be present but they would be masked by the more concentrated lymphocytes. Mature, recognizable plasma cells are not found in a germinal center.

58. The answer is D [Chapter 29 VIII A 2]. The thick ascending limb of the loop of Henle is impermeable to water. This characteristic is essential to the role of the loop of Henle in establishing and maintaining the hypertonicity of the medullary interstitium. The proximal tubule actively removes water from the glomerular filtrate by transporting electrolytes from the lumen. The thin descending limb of the loop of Henle is freely permeable to water, as is the visceral layer of the renal corpuscle.

59. The answer is C [Chapter 26 V B 1 a]. Plasma proteins and lipoproteins are secreted across the basal surface of hepatocytes into the perisinusoidal space and thence to the blood. Secretion toward the subepithelial connective tissue is the typical pathway of an endocrine secretion. Hepatocytes do not secrete gastrin. Taurocholic and glycocholic acids are components of the bile, as are cholesterol and lecithin, and are secreted into the bile canaliculus as part of the exocrine secretions of the hepatocytes. Insulin and immunoglobulin A (IgA) are transported across the hepatocytes from the blood to the bile, apparently unchanged, for delivery to the duodenum.

60. The answer is D [Chapter 4 VIII A 3]. The G_2 phase follows the S phase, during which DNA synthesis occurs, and precedes the M phase (mitosis), during which the mitotic spindle begins to form.

61. The answer is C [Chapter 13 III F 1; IV F 1]. Once a developing neutrophil has reached the band cell stage, it is no longer capable of dividing. Promyelocytes and myelocytes, however, are both mitotic cells, as are basophilic and polychromatophilic erythroblasts.

62. The answer is A [Chapter 26 III A 1]. The hepatic portal vein carries the large venous blood flow from the intestine, pancreas, and spleen to the liver. Thus, the liver is interposed between these organs and the systemic circulation and is the first organ to receive nutrients from the gut, hormones from the pancreas, and breakdown products of erythrocytes from the spleen. The myriad functions of the hepatocytes reflect the variety of substrates, wastes, and regulatory molecules that are brought to the liver in the portal blood.

63. The answer is C [Chapter 36 I A 1 b]. Proliferation of spermatogonia and differentiation of sperm begin at puberty, when pituitary gonadotropins stimulate the involuted Leydig cells to differentiate into the testosterone-secreting cells essential for normal sexual development and function in the male. Testosterone secretion by embryonic Leydig cells is essential for the normal phenotypic development of the genetic male embryo. These cells involute at about 5 months of fetal life and remain involuted until puberty.

64. The answer is C [Chapter 19 VIII C 1]. The thymus provides the site for development of T cells (T lymphocytes). Large numbers of T lymphocytes are released from the thymus during the neonatal period. Removal of the thymus at this time reduces the number of T lymphocytes in the blood and lymph, and also in those areas of peripheral lymphatic organs that are normally rich in T-cells.

65. The answer is B [Chapter 2 III C 2 c]. A rise in intracellular Ca^{2+} concentration is es-

sential for exocytosis to occur. The Ca^{2+} could come from intracellular storage sites, such as the smooth endoplasmic reticulum (sER), or from the extracellular space via ligand-gated Ca^{2+} channels in the plasma membrane. No such signal is required for secretion in the constitutive pathway.

66. The answer is E [Chapter 19 V B]. Hassall corpuscles, also called thymic corpuscles, are found in the medulla of the thymus. A corpuscle is a spheroidal arrangement of epithelial reticular cells. The layering of cells forming the corpuscle is suggestive of keratinizing epidermal cells. Hassall corpuscles are unique identifiers of the thymus.

67. The answer is C [Chapter 34 III]. Throughout the vertebrate kingdom, the several functions of the pineal gland may be summarized as relating day length and light intensity to the function of various other endocrine organs. In lower vertebrates it has specific photoreceptor cells, in seasonal breeding mammals it helps regulate reproductive function, and in humans it may have a role in gonadal development and in regulating physiologic and emotional responses to changes in day length.

68. The answer is B [Chapter 3 III G 1]. The mitotic spindle does not assemble in the presence of colchicine. Colchicine inhibits microtubule assembly by binding to tubulin monomers and preventing polymerization and promoting disassembly of existing microtubules.

69. The answer is A [Chapter 38 V A]. The hair cells of a semicircular canal of the inner ear are contained in the crista of the canal. Their stereocilia are embedded in the cupula, a gelatinous structure in the lumen of the semicircular canal that is above and attached to the hair cells by the cells' stereocilia.

70. The answer is C [Chapter 16 II B 2 a]. Of the lymphatic organs listed, only the palatine tonsil and Peyer patches have mucosal surfaces. The mucosal surface of the tonsil is pharyngeal stratified squamous epithelium, whereas the mucosal surface of the Peyer patch is small intestinal simple columnar epithelium. Often, tonsillar epithelium is difficult to classify because of the large number of intraepithelial lymphatic cells. Its stratified construction can usually be discerned, however.

71. The answer is B [Chapter 35 VI A 1]. The ampulla of the oviduct is the usual site of fertilization. Cleavage begins in the oviduct and progresses to the morula stage by the time the embryo reaches the lumen of the uterus.

72. The answer is C [Chapter 3 III E 1]. Mitotic spindles are formed from microtubules that grow out from the centriole, a microtubule organizing center of a cell. Actin filaments form the core of microvilli. Glial filaments in astrocytes and neurofilaments in neurons are intermediate filaments. Spectrin is an actin-binding protein.

73. The answer is E [Table 12-1]. Of the structures listed, platelets are the most numerous (approximately 300,000/μl). Red blood cells (RBCs), which were not included in the list of possible answers, are about ten times more numerous than platelets. The quantification of platelets from a smear is difficult because of their tendency to form clumps.

74. The answer is C [Chapter 26 VII A]. The presence of a bile canaliculus (center) indicates that this is liver. The bile canaliculus is a dilatation of the intercellular space between hepatocytes, sealed on either side by tight junctions, and is the beginning of the biliary system. The bile canaliculus is a unique structure that allows identification of the organ from a minuscule tissue sample.

75. The answer is C [Chapter 36 I A 1]. Testosterone is secreted by the interstitial cells of the testis, the Leydig cells. It is essential for normal embryonic development, maturation at puberty, and adult function of the male reproductive system. Sertoli cells secrete an androgen-binding protein (ABP) that concentrates testosterone in the luminal compartment of the seminiferous tubules. The secretion of ABP, but not testosterone, is dependent on follicle-stimulating hormone (FSH). Adrenocorticotropic hormone (ACTH) affects the structure and function of the adrenal cortex but has no apparent effect on the testis.

76. The answer is B [Chapter 8 IV A 2]. Macrophages contain numerous primary lysosomes containing various acid hydrolases, including phosphatases, esterases, and proteases. These lysosomes fuse with vacuoles containing phagocytized materials (phagosomes) to form phagolysosomes. Digestion of the phagocytized material or organisms takes place in phagolysosomes. Enzymatically active phagolysosomes are also called secondary lysosomes. Vacuoles that contain only the indigestible remains of phagocytized organisms or materials are called tertiary lysosomes, or residual bodies. Residual bodies also accumulate in macrophages that have phagocytized material they cannot digest, such as carbon, cotton fibers, and asbestos.

77. The answer is A [Chapter 27 III A 2]. The membrane of the zymogen granule fuses with the apical cell membrane to release the proenzymes synthesized by the pancreatic acinar cells into the acinar lumen. This is exocytosis. Transcytosis describes the transit through the cytoplasm of certain materials, such as immunoglobulin A, from one surface of a cell to another. Such materials are taken up into vesicles by receptor-mediated endocytosis and are subsequently released by exocytosis. Endocytosis and phagocytosis are processes by which materials are taken into cells by invagination or other deformation of the plasma membrane. Apoptosis is programmed cell death, an important cellular process, but not related to secretion.

78. The answer is B [Chapter 18 III A 2 b, B]. The spleen is interposed in the flow of blood, not lymph. The presence of immunoreactive cells in the splenic white pulp enables the organ to react to blood-borne antigens. Splenic red pulp functions in the removal from circulation of aged red blood cells (RBCs).

79. The answer is E [Chapter 29 V G 2 a]. Modified smooth muscle cells in the wall of the afferent arteriole of the glomerulus synthesize and secrete renin, a hormonal enzyme that is essential in the regulation of blood pressure. Neither proximal tubule cells nor visceral epithelial cells secrete any hormones. Macula densa cells are modified distal tubule cells that are believed to monitor the concentration of sodium chloride in the blood and secrete a paracrine regulatory agent that stimulates renin secretion. Gastric mucosal cells of calves secrete rennin, a coagulating enzyme used to precipitate milk proteins in cheese making.

80. The answer is C [Chapter 3 III F]. In cilia and flagella, the doublet microtubules in the outer ring are associated with adjacent doublets by dynein side arms. The hydrolysis of adenosine triphosphate (ATP) by the dyneins produce a sliding force between the doublets, producing motility in the form of beating.

81. The answer is A [Chapter 5 II D 1 c; VII]. Basal laminae and external laminae separate connective tissue from the three other basic tissue types. Epithelia rest on a basal lamina; muscle and nerve tissue are surrounded by external laminae. Basal and external laminae consist primarily of type IV collagen, laminin, entactin, and related proteoglycans. Also present are fibronectin and type VII collagen, which fix the basal lamina to the cell membrane and to the underlying fibrous tissue, respectively. The basal lamina is one component of the basement membrane, a structure, visible at the light microscopic level, that also includes other proteoglycans and a thick layer of reticular fibers. The basal lamina is a permeable meshwork that may help to regulate the rate at which electrolytes and water move between the epithelial and connective tissue compartments.

82. The answer is B [Chapter 27 V A]. Secretin stimulates fluid and bicarbonate secretion by the intralobular duct cells, and cholecystokinin stimulates proenzyme secretion by the acinar cells. Pancreatic polypeptide (PP) inhibits both of these activities. Glucagon and insulin regulate glucose metabolism throughout the body and are not regulators of exocrine secretion. Sympathetic nerves to the pancreas affect only blood flow to the gland.

83. The answer is B [Chapter 4 IX B 1 a]. Synapsis is characterized by the association of homologous chromosomes to form a tetrad. Synapsis occurs in prophase of the first meiotic division; it does not occur in mitosis. Crossing over occurs during synapsis. Meiotic synapsis should not be confused with a neuronal synapse.

84. The answer is E [Chapter 31 II B; III A, B 3]. Chief cells of the parathyroid gland (*left*) and follicles of the thyroid gland (*right*) are separated by adipose tissue. Parathyroid glands are embedded in the thyroid gland; therefore, close proximity of these two endocrine glands is to be expected in some histologic sections. The appearance of the densely packed chief cells is typical, as is the appearance of the thyroglobulin-containing follicles.

85. The answer is B [Chapter 8 II A 3; IV A 1 c]. Every third amino acid residue in collagen

is a glycine molecule, and nearly 25% of the amino acids are proline or hydroxyproline. Cells that secrete fibrillar collagen actually secrete only the tropocollagen molecule (collagen monomer). Tropocollagen then self-aggregates in the extracellular space. Fibroblasts are the principal cell type that secretes fibrillar collagen, but Schwann cells, developing corneal epithelial cells, and smooth muscle cells do so as well. Fibroblasts simultaneously secrete all of the extracellular matrix components of connective tissue, including elastin, proteoglycans, and other glycoproteins. Fibroblasts are neither terminally differentiated nor postmitotic. They can modulate, structurally and functionally, into cells indistinguishable from fat cells, smooth muscle cells, and macrophages. They are able to divide in wound repair, and regularly replicating populations of fibroblasts exist at several sites in the body.

86. The answer is B [Chapter 19 VIII A]. It is in the protected environment of the cortex of the thymus that T cells arise mitotically, are processed, and finally are released into the circulation. T cells may increase in number, however, by blastic transformation in the lymphatic tissue found in the other four organs listed.

87. The answer is D [Chapter 27 II; IV A]. This is a section of the pancreas; only exocrine pancreas is included in the field. Several acini are shown and some contain centroacinar cells, which are unique to the pancreas. A particularly clear example of a centroacinar cell is visible in the acinus to the left of center. Note also the transverse section of an intercalated duct in the upper left of the field.

88. The answer is A [Chapter 31 II C 4 b]. In toxic goiter (Graves disease), follicle cells are continually stimulated to synthesize and secrete excessive amounts of thyroid hormones by autoantibodies that bind to thyroid-stimulating hormone (TSH) receptors on follicle cells. Because secretion is rapid, there is little stored thyroglobulin. In this disease, goiter results from cellular hypertrophy and hyperplasia, rather than from storage of large amounts of thyroglobulin.

89. The answer is A [Chapter 6 VII C]. A myelinated axon of the peripheral nervous system (PNS) has an external (i.e., basal) lamina surrounding it, whereas a myelinated axon of the central nervous system (CNS) lacks an external lamina. Both types of axons have major dense lines in their myelin sheaths. Neither type has Nissl substance and neither axon contains recognizable synaptic vesicles. Nodes of Ranvier are found in myelinated axons from both the CNS and the PNS.

90. The answer is D [Chapter 13 V B 1]. The megakaryocyte is a polyploid cell. The promyelocyte, metamyelocyte, and proerythroblast are diploid cells. The reticulocyte lacks a nucleus and, therefore, has no nuclear DNA. Because of repeated replications of its DNA and its lack of karyokinesis, the megakaryocyte increases the amount of DNA in its nucleus. Both the nucleus and the cell itself increase dramatically in size to become the largest hematopoietic cell in the red marrow compartment.

91. The answer is A [Chapter 18 V D 1]. Red blood cells (RBCs) have a life-span of about 120 days. Effete RBCs are removed from circulation as blood passes through the red pulp of the spleen. The red pulp is a macrophage-rich area of the spleen and old RBCs are recognized and phagocytized by the macrophages. The secondary lysosomes of red pulp macrophages contain fragments of RBCs.

92. The answer is E [Chapter 23 IV B]. This is a description of a mixed exocrine gland that is primarily serous and that has prominent striated ducts. Only the submandibular salivary gland fits this description. The sublingual gland is also a mixed gland but is primarily mucous, and striated ducts are not readily seen. The exocrine pancreas and the parotid gland are purely serous glands, and the eccrine sweat glands are compound tubular glands (i.e., they do not have secretory acini).

93. The answer is D [Chapter 21 II A 1 a (1); III A 1 a]. The primary function of the esophagus is to serve as a conduit for undigested foods from the oropharynx to the stomach. As such, it is constantly subject to frictional stress and possible abrasion. Of the epithelial types listed in the question, a stratified squamous epithelium provides the greatest protection from these insults. Carnivores, which do not chew their food, derive further protection from the keratinization of the esophageal stratified squamous epithelium.

94. The answer is D [Chapter 23 I A; Chapter 35 X A]. The histologic characteristic that is

common to all exocrine glands is the presence of a duct system to convey secretions from a point of origin to an epithelial surface. The mammary gland is a compound exocrine gland (i.e., it has more than one duct), and each duct drains a lobe of the gland. A coronal section through the nipple would reveal approximately 20 ducts converging on the nipple.

95. The answer is E [Chapter 11 VIII F]. The structure described is a cement line. A cement line is generally interpreted to be a junction between newer and older bone. It is an indication of bone remodelling where bone resorption, or osteoclasia, ceased, and was followed by a new phase of osteogenesis. Cement lines often have no apparent relationship to the lamellar or osteonal structure of the bone.

96. The answer is B [Chapter 22 III D]. Taste buds are oval, pale-staining bodies that extend through the full thickness of the nonkeratinized stratified squamous epithelium of the fungiform, circumvallate, and foliate papillae of the tongue. The taste buds contain neuroepithelial (sensory) cells, supporting cells, and basal cells. The sensory and supporting cells are renewed about every ten days by division and maturation of the basal cells. Taste buds respond only to four stimuli, sweet, salty, bitter, and acid; most sensory information that gives the perception of taste is actually the result of olfactory stimulation.

97. The answer is A [Chapter 28 VIII B 2]. In the respiratory system, a simple squamous epithelium is found only in alveoli. This type of epithelium is associated with sites of gas exchange. Of the regions of the respiratory system listed, significant gas exchange occurs only in alveoli. The nasal cavity, nasopharynx, trachea, and bronchi are lined primarily with a ciliated pseudostratified columnar epithelium. Patches of stratified squamous epithelium may be present in the nasopharynx, as well.

98. The answer is B [Chapter 36 III B 3]. Each secondary spermatocyte has 2N (diploid) amount of DNA contained in 22 autosomes and an X or a Y chromosome. Exchange of genetic material between homologous chromosomes during synapsis of the first meiotic division (crossing over) makes the secondary spermatocytes genetically different from their parent primary spermatocytes. Secondary spermatocytes do not replicate their DNA before entering the prophase of the second meiotic division that produces two spermatids from each secondary spermatocyte.

99. The answer is D [Chapter 8 III A 2]. Proteoglycans (PGs) are very large macromolecules with a core of protein to which many glycosaminoglycans (GAGs) are attached, similar to bristles attached to the core of a bottle brush. Because GAGs are highly sulfated, these compounds carry a significant net negative charge. This accounts for their intense basophilia (and often metachromasia) as well as for their ability to retard the movement of positively charged molecules through connective tissue.

100. The answer is B [Chapter 23 II A 1]. Serous cells and serous glands are protein secreting. The secretion granules (zymogen granules) that accumulate in the apical cytoplasm before release by exocytosis contain mixtures of digestive enzyme precursors and electrolytes. Mixed salivary glands have both serous and mucous secretory acini, or mucous acini with serous demilunes. Mixed glands secrete both enzyme precursors and mucinogens. The parotid gland is the stereotypic serous salivary gland. Fibrous proteins such as collagen are secreted primarily by the fibroblasts of the connective tissue. Hormones are secreted by endocrine glands and neurosecretory cells. Holocrine secretion of hair follicle–associated sebaceous glands is characterized by the secretion of dead cells and pieces of cells.

101. The answer is E [Chapter 14 II C]. The impulse-generation and impulse-conduction system of the heart consists primarily of modified myocardial fibers. These modified heart muscle cells retain some of the structural characteristics of the working myocardial cells, such as myofibrils with cross-striations. The components of this system are the sinoatrial (SA) node, the atrioventricular (AV) node, the AV bundle (bundle of His), and the Purkinje fibers. Motor neurons and myelinated neurons might be suspected of having an impulse-generation and impulse-conduction function, but studies relating cardiac physiology to cardiac histology reveal that the generation and conduction system forms from modified cardiac muscle cells only.

102. The answer is C [Chapter 6 III A 5 a (3)]. During nerve stimulation, membrane is added by synaptic vesicle exocytosis to the presynaptic surface, facing the synaptic cleft, and membrane located more laterally in the presynaptic ending is internalized and recycled. Synaptic vesicle membrane is never released into the synaptic cleft; only the chemical neurotransmitter is released.

103. The answer is E [Chapter 9 I A 2]. The complete metabolism of stored fatty acids produces carbon dioxide and water. The carbon dioxide is exchanged for oxygen in respiration, but the water can be recycled in the body. Thus, metabolism of fat stores can provide sufficient water for survival under extreme conditions of water deprivation.

104. The answer is D [Chapter 28 II B 2 a]. Turbulent precipitation occurs when inspired air meets the irregular contours of the lateral wall of the nasal cavity. Dust particles and other foreign materials are thrown out of the airstream by centrifugal force and adhere to the moist, mucus-coated wall of the nasal cavity.

105. The answer is D [Chapter 35 II E]. Atresia accounts for the loss of most of the oocytes from an ovary. Of the large number of oocytes that exist in the fetal ovary, only a tiny fraction mature to the point of ovulation. Atresia is a type of programmed cell death (apoptosis).

106. The answer is D [Chapter 3 IV A 4]. Nuclear lamins form a meshwork on the inner aspect of the nuclear envelope, stabilizing the nucleus during interphase. The lamins disassemble during mitosis and may play a role in the disassembly of the nuclear envelope.

107. The answer is A [Chapter 19 IV]. T lymphocytes are produced in the superficial cortex. It is in this location, close to the capsule of the thymus, that lymphoblasts may be visible. Lymphoblasts are large lymphocytes and are germinative cells. Nodules do not exist in the normal thymus. Thymic corpuscles, or Hassall corpuscles, are unique to the thymus but have nothing to do with lymphocyte production.

108. The answer is D [Chapter 24 II C 1 b]. The stem cells of the gastric epithelium are located in the mucous neck between the gastric pit and the main portion of the gastric gland. Cells that originate here migrate in two directions: some move toward the surface to become mucus-secreting cells of the gastric pit and the mucosal surface, and others move toward the base of the gland to become parietal cells, chief cells and enteroendocrine cells. There are no submucosal glands in the stomach.

109. The answer is B [Chapter 11 VIII E 1]. Perforating canals enter compact bone from either the periosteal or the endosteal surfaces and subsequently branch extensively in the bony matrix. Blood vessels enter the bone and are distributed to osteons via these channels. Sharpey fibers are collagen fibers that extend from the tendon into the bony matrix. Osteoblasts and osteoclasts are always found on the surface of a bone. Osteocytic processes are found in canaliculi, which are much smaller in diameter and far more numerous than perforating canals.

110. The answer is B [Chapter 28 VI C 1]. A lobar (secondary) bronchus is lined by ciliated pseudostratified epithelium, as are all the larger diameter parts of the respiratory system. The epithelium gradually changes to simple columnar or cuboidal in bronchioles and then to simple squamous in the alveoli.

111. The answer is C [Chapter 35 IV C, D]. A germ cell found in the ampulla must have been stimulated a short time earlier by the surge of luteinizing hormone to complete the first meiotic division. In a celibate woman, fertilization could not have occurred with the resulting stimulation to complete the second meiotic division. Therefore, an oocyte in the ampulla of a fallopian tube of this woman would remain, until its death, a secondary oocyte.

112. The answer is D [Chapter 24 III A 2]. This is a description of a parietal (oxyntic), acid-secreting cell of a gastric gland. These cells secrete 0.16N hydrochloric acid, which acidifies the gastric juice to provide the optimum pH for the action of the peptidases secreted by the chief cells. The stem cell population of the gastric epithelium is located among the mucous neck cells. Some newly derived daughter cells of the stem cells may differentiate into mucus-secreting cells that form the secretory sheets of the gastric pit and the mucosal surface. Other daughter cells differentiate into chief cells, parietal cells, and enteroendocrine cells of the gastric glands.

113. The answer is D [Chapter 14 II B 1 a (1)]. The one component of the cardiovascular system that is continuous throughout the entire system is endothelium. Smooth muscle is a major component of arterial and venous blood vessels, but is sparse in the endocardium and absent from capillary walls. Purkinje fibers are restricted to the subendocardium and are never found in an extracardiac location. Cardiac muscle is primarily restricted to the heart, but may extend into the tunica media of the venae cavae and pulmonary veins.

114. The answer is B [Chapter 24 I A 1 a]. In humans, the esophagus is lined throughout with a nonkeratinized stratified squamous epithelium. This provides protection against abrasion by the partially macerated food that passes through it from the oral cavity to the stomach. In animals that do not chew their food, such as carnivores, the epithelium of the esophagus is keratinized. Pseudostratified columnar epithelium is characteristic of portions of the respiratory system. Simple columnar epithelium is characteristic of the lining of the stomach and intestine. Stratified cuboidal epithelium is rare, but it can be found in ducts of exocrine glands, such as the salivary and eccrine sweat glands.

115. The answer is B [Chapter 4 VIII]. The cell cycle is an ordered sequence of events during which the cell grows, duplicates its chromosomes, and divides into two cells. Cells ordinarily undergo many cell cycles before cell death occurs. Prophase, metaphase, anaphase, and telophase are phases within mitosis, which is just one of the steps in the cell cycle. Likewise, karyokinesis and cytokinesis describe only portions of the cell cycle.

116. The answer is B [Chapter 28 VIII B 2 b]. Type II cells produce surfactant, a phospholipid secretion that coats the interior of the alveolus to reduce surface tension in the lung. Type I cells are the squamous epithelial cells that line most of the alveolus. Endothelial cells are squamous cells that line the entire cardiovascular system, including alveolar capillaries. Dust cells are macrophages, and goblet cells secrete mucus.

117. The answer is C [Chapter 24 I A 3]. The muscularis externa of the upper one-third of the esophagus is formed by striated muscle that is continuous with that of the laryngopharynx. This striated muscle is important in the initial, voluntary phase of swallowing. In the middle one-third of the esophagus, the striated muscle becomes mixed with smooth muscle, which gradually replaces the striated muscle distally. Longitudinal bands of the muscularis externa are characteristic of the wall of the colon, where they form the teniae coli.

118. The answer is C [Table 12-1]. In a smear of normal peripheral blood, cells would be encountered with the following frequencies: Red blood cells (RBCs) [about 1000 times more numerous than any other cell]; neutrophils (approximately 60% of leukocytes); lymphocytes (approximately 30% of leukocytes); monocytes (approximately 5% of leukocytes); eosinophils (approximately 3% of leukocytes); and, basophils (approximately 0.5% of leukocytes).

119. The answer is B [Chapter 24 II C 1 b; Chapter 25 I D 3; II B 2 b]. Although they have different stem cell locations, the surface epithelial cells of stomach, small intestine, and colon turn over very quickly, averaging 5 days. In the stomach, the gland cells are much longer-lived, turning over about once a year. The enteroendocrine cells in all three parts of the gastrointestinal tract migrate more slowly than the mucus-secreting cells and absorptive cells; their turnover time varies from 1 to 3 weeks. Paneth cells, found only in the small intestine, do not migrate from the stem cell zone at the base of the crypt and are replaced by differentiation of newly derived cells about every 4 weeks.

120. The answer is E [Chapter 25 I C 4]. The cells are Paneth cells, which are characteristic of the small intestine. They do not migrate from this deep level of the crypt, as do other cells of the epithelium, but remain in the deepest recesses of the crypt. Paneth cells secrete lysozyme and also contain relatively large amounts of zinc. Absorptive cells are present in the same epithelial layer but lack distinctive granules. Enteroendocrine cells contain smaller granules that are located in the basal, rather than the apical, cytoplasm. Goblet cells contain mucinogen droplets and are usually not found at this level of the crypt–villus complex. Chief cells are located in gastric glands, not in glands of the small intestine.

121. The answer is B [Chapter 25 I D]. The lower half of the crypt is the region of the in-

testinal epithelium where mitoses occur. A dividing cell in anaphase is enclosed by the *circle*. The two dark masses are the recently separated chromosomes that later will be located in the two daughter cells.

122. The answer is A [Chapter 6 II A; Chapter 21 II B 3]. The indicated cell, with a large euchromatic nucleus and a prominent nucleolus, is a nerve cell body of the submucosal (Meissner) plexus, which is part of the enteric nervous system. This neuron likely participates in the innervation of the adjacent muscularis mucosae. Note the nuclei of satellite cells. Submucosal fibroblasts have smaller, heterochromatic nuclei and delicate cytoplasmic processes. Epithelial cells of the cryptal epithelium and smooth muscle cells of the muscularis mucosae are also visible in the micrograph.

123. The answer is A [Chapter 5 V E 2 b]. The filamentous terminal web is attached to the adhesion belt. Any contractile event that occurs in the actin-rich terminal web would be transferred to the cell surface by its attachment to the adhesion belt. Gap junctions are not associated with any filaments. Desmosomes are associated with intermediate filaments. Tight junctions are not associated with any cytoplasmic filaments.

124. The answer is A [Chapter 35 II D 1]. The ovaries of a second-trimester fetus contain the maximum number of oocytes that will ever be found in that individual. This number was produced by mitotic divisions of oogonia. Mitotic expansion of the population of germ cells stops during the second trimester, and oocytic mitosis never resumes in that female.

125. The answer is C [Chapter 14 II C 4 b]. Purkinje fibers in the human heart are found in the subendocardium of the interventricular septum and possibly in other areas of the ventricle. The terminations of the Purkinje fibers can be identified in the myocardium. Species variation exists, however, and Purkinje fibers may be encountered closer to the atrioventricular (AV) node in non-human hearts, such as the dog heart.

126. The answer is D [Chapter 20 II B 1]. Epidermis is a renewing epithelium. Cells are lost at the free surface of the skin as desquamating keratinized cells, new cells are added to the epidermis by mitotic division of cells in the basal layer. In recognition of this important function, the basal layer is also called the stratum germinativum.

127. The answer is B [Chapter 13 I C 3 a]. The presence or absence of granules in the cytoplasm of a developing blood cell immediately allows the categorization of the cell as a granulopoietic or erythropoietic cell. Developing red blood cells (RBCs) do not have granules. Developing granulocytes, beginning with the promyelocyte stage, always have granules (either azurophilic exclusively, or a mixture of azurophilic and specific granules).

128. The answer is D [Chapter 25 I B 2]. Villi are characteristic of the small intestine, where they increase the surface area available for terminal digestion and absorption of metabolic substrates. They are not found in the other portions of the alimentary canal listed, all of which have a smooth mucosal surface with glands that descend into the lamina propria.

129. The answer is B [Chapter 12 III B 2 a; Chapter 4 II A 2 a, b]. A Barr body of a neutrophil from a human female appears as a small, drumstick-like appendage of a nuclear lobe. The Barr body is formed by one of the X chromosomes that remains in a condensed, heterochromatic state. Males do not have Barr bodies.

130. The answer is D [Chapter 12 VII C 1]. The monocytes of peripheral blood are the precursor cells of phagocytic cells in general. Lymphocytes and neutrophils are also blood cells but they do not give rise to macrophages. Macrocytes are abnormally large red blood cells (RBCs) and are not precursor cells of macrophages. A lipocyte is a fat cell.

131. The answer is D [Chapter 6 II A; Chapter 21 II C 3 a]. The muscularis externa throughout the gastrointestinal tract is innervated by neurons of the enteric division of the autonomic nervous system. The cell bodies of these neurons are located in the myenteric (Auerbach) plexus between the inner (circular) and outer (longitudinal) layers of the muscularis externa. Enteroendocrine cells and Paneth cells are cells of the epithelium of the mucosa. The stem cells of the epithelium are located in the epithelium and arise there. Lymphocytes that have undergone blastic transfor-

mation would be found in lymph nodules in the lamina propria. Although the transformed lymphocytes are larger than normal lymphocytes, they are much smaller than nerve cells and do not exhibit the nuclear and nucleolar characteristics described above.

132. The answer is D [Chapter 20 II B 1; Chapter 5 VI B 1]. The tritiated thymidine would be incorporated by cells that are preparing for mitosis and, therefore, would be localized in the cells of the basal layer of the epidermis. The basal layer is also called the stratum germinativum because of its mitotic potential. Under normal conditions, mitosis does not occur in the more superficial layers of the epidermis. Tritiated thymidine may be present in these layers for 3–4 weeks, however, as previously labeled epidermal cells differentiate and migrate through the tissue.

133. The answer is D [Chapter 28 VI C 2]. Any tubule with cartilage in its wall and contained in the parenchyma of the lung is a bronchus. Alveolar ducts, alveolar sacs, and bronchioles do not contain cartilage. The trachea does contain cartilage but the trachea lies outside of the lung.

134. The answer is D [Chapter 20 V C]. Sebaceous glands secrete sebum by a holocrine mechanism. The terminal stage of sebaceous transformation is characterized by the breakdown of the cell, coalescence of accumulated lipid droplets, and the flow of cell debris and lipid (i.e., sebum) into the sebaceous gland duct. Destruction of the synthesizing cell in the secretory process is the hallmark characteristic of holocrine secretion in the sebaceous gland.

135. The answer is D [Chapter 29 V A 5 a, c]. The mesangial cell is a phagocytic cell that is responsible for clearing accumulated filtered debris from the glomerular basement membrane. None of the other cells listed is phagocytic. Visceral epithelial cells are podocytes and their processes are a component of the filtration barrier. Mast cells are secretory cells that produce histamine and heparin. The parietal epithelial cells line the non-glomerular surface of the renal capsule.

136. The answer is D [Chapter 16 II B 3 a]. Palatine tonsils are lymphatic organs that regularly contain nodules with germinal centers. The presence of germinal centers indicates the occurrence of a humoral immune response. Nodules and germinal centers are not characteristically found in the other lymphatic sites listed.

137. The answer is C [Chapter 23 II C 2 a]. Intercalated ducts are the first element in the duct system of exocrine glands. They are not part of the secretory portion of the gland, although they are surrounded by secretory acini. They are usually formed by a simple squamous epithelium and lead from the lumen of the acinus to the next larger portion of the duct system, hence the name. They may modify the serous secretion by exchanging bicarbonate for chloride. In serous salivary glands, intercalated ducts lead to striated ducts, which are characterized by cuboidal cells that contain basal infoldings alternating with mitochondria. In other serous glands, such as the exocrine pancreas, intercalated ducts may lead directly to interlobular ducts, the first element of the excretory duct portion of the system. The larger excretory ducts may be lined with stratified cuboidal and stratified columnar epithelium, pseudostratified columnar epithelium, or stratified squamous epithelium.

138. The answer is E [Chapter 33 III C; Chapter 23 II D]. Somatostatin is released in the mantle region of the islets of Langerhans. It binds to receptors on glucagon-secreting α cells in the mantle region, and to receptors on insulin-secreting β cells in the central region of the islets. Paracrine secretion is the release of locally acting hormones from endocrine cells into the intercellular space to act on nearby cells. Release of hormones to capillaries for transport to a distant site is an endocrine function. Apocrine, holocrine, and merocrine refer to a classification of exocrine glands based on mechanism of secretion.

139. The answer is A [Chapter 11 VIII E]. The point of origin of the channel and its diameter indicate that this is a perforating (Volkmann) canal. A perforating canal and an osteonal (Haversian) canal may be of similar diameter and both contain blood vessels, but a perforating canal always opens onto the periosteal or endosteal surfaces of the bone, and an osteonal canal is always surrounded by concentric lamellae of bone. Osteocytic canaliculi are much narrower than the described channel and contain processes of osteocytes. Howship lacunae are broad depressions on the surface of a bone and contain osteoclasts.

140. The answer is E [Chapter 28 VIII B 2 a]. The lining of a pulmonary alveolus is formed mainly by squamous epithelial type I cells. The other cellular component of the alveolar surface lining is the cuboidal, surfactant secreting type II cell. Dust cells (alveolar macrophages) are cells that pass back and forth across the alveolar lining and may rest temporarily in the cellular lining of the alveolus. Endothelial cells line the capillaries in the interalveolar septum and Clara cells are found in the epithelium of bronchioles.

141. The answer is C [Chapter 5 V C 2 a]. The connexon is a subunit of a gap junction. The connexon is a hexamer of six protein molecules, which are symmetrically arranged around a central channel 2 nm in diameter. The functional unit of a gap junction is formed by two connexons joined end to end. The central channel of the connexon pair provides a continuous aqueous pathway from the cytoplasm of one cell to the cytoplasm of an adjacent cell.

142. The answer is D [Chapter 38 III C]. The auditory tube, connecting the pharynx and middle ear, enables air pressure to equilibrate between the middle ear (an air-filled space) and the atmosphere. The tube normally is closed, but opens briefly during swallowing to allow pressure equilibration. Microorganisms from the pharynx may enter the middle ear through the auditory tube, causing a middle ear infection.

143. The answer is D [Chapter 1 II C 1; Figure 1-1]. Phospholipids provide a continuum throughout a biological membrane. The phospholipid molecules form a bilayer with their hydrophobic chains oriented toward the inside and their hydrophilic regions oriented outward toward the aqueous cytoplasmic compartment or the extracellular space. Cholesterol, glycolipids (including gangliosides), and glycoproteins are important components of membranes but they occur as isolated molecules or groups of molecules, not as a continuum.

144. The answer is C [Chapter 26 IX B 1]. The concentration of bile is driven by the active transport of Na^+ and Cl^- and HCO_3^- from the cell into the intercellular compartment by a transport ATPase located in the lateral plasma membrane. Water follows passively down its concentration gradient. The removal of electrolytes and water from the bile concentrates the bile acids. Transport of H^+ and Cl^- is associated with acid secretion by the oxyntic cells of the gastric mucosa.

145. The answer is C [Chapters 8 IV A 3 b; Chapter 12 V B 2]. Heparin is found in the granules of mast cells but not in the granules of basophils. Both cells, however, contain histamine. While basophils lack heparin, they do contain heparan sulfate, a closely related glycosaminoglycan. Neither cell has a basal lamina. Both cells contain cytoplasmic granules.

146. The answer is C [Chapter 6 V D 2,3]. Saltatory conduction refers to conduction of a nerve impulse in a myelinated axon. The nerve impulse "jumps" from node of Ranvier to node of Ranvier. If nodes are absent, as they are in unmyelinated nerves, then saltatory conduction cannot occur.

147. The answer is B [Chapter 25 II B 2 b]. The stem cell population in the colon is located in the base of the crypt. The replicating cell population extends through the lowest one-third of the crypt, where newly formed cells may divide 2 to 3 more times while beginning to differentiate into goblet cells, absorptive cells, and enteroendocrine cells. The replicating cell population in the small intestine is also located in the crypt, but usually extends through the lower one-half of the crypt. The esophagus is lined with a stratified squamous epithelium and, as such, has a stem cell population in the deepest layer of the epithelium, adjacent to the lamina propria. The replicative zone in the stomach is located in the gastric neck, from which cells migrate both to the free surface and into the depth of the gastric (fundic) gland.

148. The answer is C [Chapter 12 III D 4]. The accumulation of neutrophils in connective tissue, close to an epithelium, is evidence of the acute phase of inflammation. This is commonly seen in areas of the respiratory system and in the alimentary canal where epithelial surfaces are normally exposed to a rich bacterial flora. Penetration of the epithelial barrier by microorganisms may provoke an acute inflammatory response.

149. The answer is D [Chapter 35 XI C 1]. Placental villi develop from the trophoblast of the embryo. A single villus is formed by the syncytial and cellular trophoblast layers and a core of vascularized connective tissue. The

villi are the major contribution of the embryo (and fetus) to the placenta.

150. The answer is B [Chapter 20 IV B, C]. Several hair follicles in transverse section are visible in this light micrograph. The hair shaft is darkly stained. The external and internal root sheaths are not sharply differentiated from each other at this level of the follicle. Dermal connective tissue, formed primarily by adipose tissue, surrounds the follicles.

151. The answer is D [Chapter 35 VIII B 2 b]. Straight endometrial glands are characteristic of the proliferative phase of the cycle. Late in the proliferative phase or early in the secretory phase, the glands acquire a distinctive coiled structure. Later in the secretory phase, the glands become sacculated as secretions accumulate in the tubule lumen.

152. The answer is E [Chapter 15 VI A 1]. Reticular cells have the structural characteristics of fibroblasts and they synthesize the collagen fibrils and proteoglycans that form the fibrous reticulum. Reticular cells were once thought to be phagocytic and to have an endothelial function, but these have been shown to be incorrect conclusions that were based on the limitations of the light microscope.

153. The answer is E [Chapter 12 III C 1 b]. The azurophilic granules of a neutrophil contain hydrolytic enzymes that function optimally at a low pH. This indicates that the azurophilic granules are lysosomes. Lysosomal enzymes, like other proteins, are packaged into granules in the Golgi apparatus. Phagosomes are membrane-limited vacuoles that contain exogenous or endogenous materials that later will fuse with lysosomes. Residual bodies are the endpoint of the catabolic processes involving phagosomes, specific granules, and azurophilic granules. Although they contain peroxidase, azurophilic granules are not peroxisomes.

154. The answer is B [Chapter 36 IV B, C 4]. Complex Sertoli–Sertoli cell junctions that include a well-developed tight junction component are the morphologic basis of the blood–testis barrier. Cytoplasmic bridges between spermatocytes and their derivatives allow synchronous development of the clone of cells derived from each type B spermatogonium that becomes committed to develop. There are no gap junctions between spermatogonia.

155. The answer is D [Chapter 7 IV D 7 a].
Each titin molecule spans approximately half the length of a sarcomere as it joins Z disk to M line. Titin is the largest protein known. It is a filamentous molecule greater than 1 μm in length, with a molecular weight of about 3 million (3000 kD). The spring-like nature of this molecule may aid in maintaining the precise geometric structure of the sarcomere and restoring actin–myosin relationships after contraction.

156. The answer is C (Chapter 17 V A 1].
The connective tissue capsule covering the broad convex surface of a lymph node is penetrated at several points by afferent lymphatic vessels. The lymph in the afferent vessel arrives at the node from another more distal node or from a connective tissue space. The lumen of the afferent vessel is directly continuous with the lumen of the subcapsular sinus. The efferent lymphatic vessels and the blood vessels that supply and drain the node are all found at the hilum.

157. The answer is C [Chapter 36 III D 3].
Capacitation involves the removal or modification of some sperm surface oligosaccharides in the female reproductive tract.

158. The answer is B [Chapter 12 II D 2 b].
Red blood cells (RBCs) in a hypertonic solution become crenated. Water moves out of the cell by osmosis, producing the characteristically spiny surface of a crenated cell.

159. The answer is D [Chapter 27 II; IV A, D 1]. The characteristics listed are those of the exocrine pancreas. The intercalated ducts of the exocrine pancreas actually begin in the lumen of the acini as centroacinar cells. The interlobular ducts form a herringbone pattern as they enter the main duct that runs the length of the organ. The sublingual gland and the submandibular gland are both mixed serous and mucus glands. The parotid gland, although exclusively serous, does not have centroacinar cells in its secretory units.

160. The answer is C [Chapter 28 VIII B 2 a, b]. The alveolar epithelial surface is formed by squamous (type I) cells and cuboidal (type II) cells that are joined by tight junctions. Alveolar macrophages (dust cells) may be seen beneath, crossing, or on top of the alveolar epithelium, but such macrophages do not form junctions with either type I or type II cells.

161. The answer is D [Chapter 11 VII F 6]. A mixed spicule has a core of calcified cartilage that is covered by a layer of new bone. The calcified cartilage is a surviving remnant of the hyaline cartilage of the growth plate. The zone of mixed spicules is the part of the growth plate that is closest to the center of the developing bone and is contained within the metaphysis. The zone of mixed spicules, which forms a three-dimensional skeletal meshwork, is a temporary structure that gives structural stability to the growing bone.

162. The answer is C [Chapter 14 VII]. A portal system of blood circulation is defined as two capillary beds that are joined by an arterial or venous blood vessel. An example is the portal vein connecting the mucosal capillaries of the small intestine to the sinusoids (i.e., capillaries) of the liver. While capillary beds may connect parts of an organ (e.g., adrenal cortex, pancreatic islet), capillaries do not extend between organs.

163. The answer is D [Chapter 4 IX B 1 b]. Crossing over is the exchange of genetic material between non-sister chromatids in a tetrad during the first prophase of meiosis. Synapsis of homologous chromosomes must be completed in order for crossing over to occur. Crossing over introduces genetic diversity into the gene pool.

164. The answer is C [Chapter 13 I C 3 a]. The indicated myeloid cell contains many cytoplasmic granules. This characteristic immediately assigns it to the granulopoietic line of hematopoiesis. Granules are not found in those cells leading to the formation of erythrocytes, megakaryocytes, or monocytes.

165. The answer is D [Chapter 12 III A 1, B 1]. The indicated cell is a neutrophilic leukocyte. Mature neutrophils are found both in marrow smears and in peripheral blood smears. In fact, many more neutrophils are found stored in the marrow than are found in circulation. Identifying characteristics of this cell are its size, which is larger than an erythrocyte, and its lobulated nucleus, which gives the cell another of its names—polymorphonuclear leukocyte (PMN). Cytoplasmic granules are indistinct in the granulocyte because of their poor affinity for any of the dyes used in the staining mixture (i.e., the granules are *neutrophilic*).

A reticulocyte is an anucleate cell; possibly some of the nearby erythrocytes (after brilliant cresyl blue staining) could be shown to be reticulocytes. A neutrophilic myelocyte has a nucleus that is only slightly indented, not lobulated. A polychromatophilic erythroblast has a spheroidal nucleus. A band cell is a precursor of a neutrophil, but its horseshoe-shaped nucleus is not yet lobulated.

166. The answer is D [Chapter 13 IV B 1]. The cell labeled *Y* is an example of a promyelocyte. Identifying characteristics of a promyelocyte include its large size (2 to 3 times the diameter of an erythrocyte), presence of cytoplasmic granules (shown are azurophilic granules), and an essentially spheroidal nucleus. (The nucleus will undergo dramatic morphologic changes and, after several generations, may form a nucleus similar to that seen in cell *X*.)

An erythroblast, at any stage of development, does not contain granules. A myelocyte, whether neutrophilic, eosinophilic, or basophilic, is closely related to cell *Y* but it has an indented nucleus and shows evidence of specific granule accumulation. A normoblast is a cell with an agranular cytoplasm and a pyknotic nucleus, characteristics very different from the granule-filled cytoplasm and large euchromatic nucleus seen in this cell.

167. The answer is A [Chapter 28 II C 1 a]. Bipolar neurons are found in the olfactory mucosa of the nasal cavity, where they function as the sensory cells in olfaction. The dendritic pole of the neuron develops extremely long cilia that extend into the nasal cavity and probably contain olfactory receptors in their cell membranes. The axonal pole of the neuron forms a slender process that leaves the olfactory epithelium and, together with a large number of similar processes of nearby neurons, forms the olfactory nerve (cranial nerve I).

168. The answer is B [Chapter 14 IV B 1, 3]. A blood vessel of this size with a distinct tunica media and internal elastic lamina is a muscular artery. An elastic artery lacks a distinct internal elastic lamina. Arterioles are considerably smaller in diameter than 2 mm. A pericytic venule and a small vein each lack both an internal elastic lamina and a prominent tunica media.

169. The answer is D [Chapter 13 III D 2]. The nucleus is lost from the developing red blood cell (RBC) during the normoblast stage.

The cell identified as a reticulocyte is anuclear. All cells preceding the reticulocyte have a nucleus. The nucleus progresses from a large euchromatic structure in the proerythroblast, to a smaller structure with a checkerboard chromatin pattern in the polychromatophilic erythroblast, to a small pyknotic structure in the normoblast, from which it is ultimately expelled.

170. The answer is B [Chapter 17 III A 2 b, c]. The thymus-dependent region of a lymph node is the deep cortex, which is bounded on one side by the nodular cortex and on the other side by the medulla. The deep cortex does not contain nodules. The thymus-dependent region has large numbers of T cells and postcapillary venules with cuboidal or columnar endothelium.

171. The answer is D [Chapter 3 II B]. Polymerization of G-actin subunits to form filamentous F-actin is a cytoplasmic event. Actin filaments form one of the three filamentous elements of the cytoskeleton; the other two are microtubules and intermediate filaments. Proline and lysine are hydroxylated cotranslationally in the rough endoplasmic reticulum (rER), proteins are glycosylated in the rER and Golgi apparatus, and β-oxidation of fatty acids occurs in mitochondria and in peroxisomes.

172. The answer is C [Chapter 2 II B 3; IV]. The mitochondrion is the site of synthesis of adenosine triphosphate (ATP), the principal carrier of chemical energy in cells. The other molecules listed are synthesized in the rough endoplasmic reticulum (rER).

173. The answer is C [Chapter 9 I A; II A]. The primary function of adipose tissue is to store neutral fats that can be metabolized to fatty acids, which are subsequently broken down to two-carbon fragments that enter the general metabolic pool. Glycogen is a stored form of glucose that is found in other tissues (e.g., muscle, liver) and in developing lipoblasts as a source of two-carbon fragments for neutral fat synthesis. However, it is not stored in mature adipose cells.

174. The answer is B [Chapter 15 VIII B 4]. The one cell that is not found in germinal centers is the killer cell. Germinal centers are evidence of B-lymphocyte function and the humoral immune response. Killer cells are the cytotoxic effector cells of the cell-mediated immune response, which is a T-lymphocyte function.

175. The answer is C [Chapter 25 I B 4 c]. The pericryptal fibroblasts are components of the intestinal mucosa but not of the epithelium. They are located in the lamina propria immediately beneath the basal lamina of the epithelium. They secrete the small collagen fibers of the reticular layer of the basement membrane and, in the colon, also secrete the collagen table that lies beneath the absorptive surface. The other four cell types are all components of the small intestinal epithelium and are derived from the same stem cell population located at the base of the crypt of Lieberkühn.

176. The answer is E [Chapter 28 IX]. The air–blood barrier does not include smooth muscle. Gases must move across squamous alveolar cells, across endothelial cells, across the basal laminae of those epithelial cells, and across intervening connective tissue, if present. The makeup of the air–blood barrier varies with the cells and cell products that occur between the alveolar lumen and the capillary lumen. Smooth muscle extends distally in the system only as far as the nonalveolar portion of the wall of alveolar ducts.

177. The answer is E [Chapter 2 II A 2]. The major function of the smooth endoplasmic reticulum (sER) is the synthesis of phospholipids. Although the membranes of the sER and the rough endoplasmic reticulum (rER) are continuous, proteins that are synthesized on the rER are not post-translationally modified in the sER. Post-translational modification of rER-synthesized proteins can occur in the rest of the cytoplasmic structures listed, including the rER itself.

178. The answer is C [Chapter 8 I; IV A 1 a (2) (b)]. Fibroblasts do not form junctions with other fibroblasts in adult tissue. The primary characteristic of connective tissue is that its cells exist as individual cells surrounded by an extracellular matrix secreted by the fibroblasts. In nearly all connective tissues, the volume of the extracellular compartment is significantly greater than that of the cellular compartment. Connective tissue is usually separated from the other basic tissues by a basal lamina or external lamina secreted by the epithelium, muscle, or nerve tissue.

179. The answer is C [Chapter 25 I B 1,2,3; I C 1 d]. Intracellular canaliculi increase the surface area of membrane available for secretion of electrolytes, as in the parietal cells of the gastric glands. Plicae circulares are permanent transverse folds that involve the mucosa and submucosa of the small intestine. Villi are expansions of the lamina propria that extend the intestinal mucosal surface. Microvilli are microscopic, finger-like projections of the apical plasma membrane of intestinal epithelial cells. The glycocalyx extends into the lumen from the microvilli and contains hydrolytic enzymes for dipeptides and oligosaccharides.

180. The answer is B [Chapter 2 III A 2, C 3; Chapter 27 III A]. Newly formed vacuoles that will become storage granules pinch off of the *trans* Golgi network as condensing vacuoles. They then undergo maturation to become storage granules (i.e., secretory granules). Vesicles clustered near the *cis* face of the Golgi apparatus function in the transport of molecules from the rough endoplasmic reticulum (rER) to the Golgi apparatus.

181. The answer is E [Chapter 22 III; Chapter 19 VIII A]. The thymus, not the tongue, is the site of differentiation of T lymphocytes. While the tongue does contain diffuse lymphatic tissue and lymphatic nodules, namely the lingual tonsils, which are part of the immune barrier at the entrance of the oropharynx, it is not primarily a lymphatic organ. Its important functions are in swallowing and speech, and in the reception of simple taste sensations.

182. The answer is D [Chapter 8 IV B 2; Chapter 26 V B 1 a, 2]. Synthesis and secretion of immuoglobulins are the role of plasma cells in the connective tissue, not of hepatocytes. Immunoglobulin A (IgA), however, may be transported in vesicles across the hepatocyte from the perisinusoidal space to the bile canaliculus. Hepatocytes synthesize and secrete nonimmune globulins, albumin, and other proteins and lipoproteins found in the blood. Hepatocytes are a major storage site for energy in the form of glycogen synthesized from glucose that is taken up by the hepatocytes, along with chylomicrons and other nutrients that come to the liver in the portal blood. Degradation and conjugation of toxins and drugs are a major function of the smooth endoplasmic reticulum of the hepatocyte. Bile, with its contained bile acids, cholesterol, lecithin, and electrolytes, is the principal exocrine secretion of the hepatocyte.

183. The answer is B [Chapter 4 IX A]. Meiosis and mitosis share some similarities but differ significantly. Meiosis results in the production of haploid gametes whose genetic compositions are different from one another because of crossing over and random segregation of homologous chromosomes. Mitosis results in the production of two identical daughter cells.

184. The answer is D [Chapter 25 I C 1 a, d (1), (3) e]. Epithelial cells with basal infoldings associated with mitochondria are characteristically found in the kidney tubules and the striated ducts of the salivary glands, not in intestinal absorptive cells. Microvilli, lateral plications, and an apical concentration of mitochondria are specializations associated with the transport of metabolites, electrolytes, and water across all transporting and absorptive epithelia. Tight junctions seal the intercellular space from the intestinal lumen and serve as an intramembrane barrier that restricts terminal digestive enzymes to the apical surface, and transport enzymes (e.g., Na^+,K^+-ATPase) to the lateral surface.

185. The answer is E [Chapter 36 I A 1; IV C]. Testosterone is secreted by the interstitial cells (Leydig cells) of the testis. All of the other functions are among those of the Sertoli cells, which support and isolate the developing sperm in the seminiferous tubules.

186. The answer is E [Chapter 3 I A; IV A 1, 2; Chapter 37 VII C 1 a (2)]. Zonular fibers are the suspensory ligaments of the lens of the eye. They are extracellular components of connective tissue origin. Vimentin, keratin, actin, and microtubules are all part of the intracellular cytoskeleton.

187. The answer is C [Chapter 21 III A 1 b, 2]. Epithelial junctional complexes are components of the physiologic exclusion barrier in the gastrointestinal tract and have an important function in the regulated active transport of metabolites, electrolytes, and water across the absorptive epithelium. All of the cells and cell aggregates listed are components of the gut-associated lymphatic tissue (GALT) and, thus, are part of the mucosal immunologic barrier.

188. The answer is D [Table 8-4]. Connective tissue is one of four basic types of tissue; the other three are nerve, muscle, and epithelia. The capillary endothelium is a simple squamous epithelium that separates two connective tissues: the blood within the capillary and the loose connective tissue in which the capillary travels. Some connective tissues have structural roles (e.g., bone and cartilage), others store energy (e.g., adipose tissue), and others are part of the immune system (e.g., lymphatic tissue). All, however, are characterized by a relatively small number of cells and a relatively large amount of extracellular material, usually secreted by the cells.

189. The answer is D [Chapter 29 X C; Chapter 36 VI]. The ureters convey urine from the pelvis of the kidney to the urinary bladder. The other structures are all part of the excurrent duct system of the male genital system.

190. The answer is D [Chapter 26 III A 3 b]. The terminal hepatic venule, or central vein, is the one structure listed that is not part of a portal triad. It is located in the center of the hexagonal classic lobule; the portal triads form the corners of the periphery of the lobule. The triad contains portal vein branches and hepatic arterioles that bring blood to the liver parenchyma, and bile ducts and lymphatic vessels that carry bile and lymph away from the liver parenchyma. The term *triad* is a misnomer because it usually contains these four structures, and often contains multiple examples of each of them.

191. The answer is D [Chapter 23 I B, C]. The pancreas is an extramural digestive gland that secretes enzyme precursors into the proximal portion of the duodenum. The exocrine secretory portion of the pancreas is purely serous. The parotid, sublingual, and submandibular glands are the major paired salivary glands that secrete into the oral cavity. The buccal glands are among the many minor salivary glands that also secrete into the oral cavity.

192. The answer is A [Chapter 4 II A]. The double-stranded DNA in the nucleus of eukaryotic cells is packaged into linearly arranged units called chromosomes that are always present in the nucleus. Chromosomes are most obvious in dividing cells because the DNA is in a highly condensed form. During interphase, chromosomal DNA is amorphous in appearance.

193. The answer is E [Chapter 26 III B 3]. The absence of a continuous basal lamina underlying either the sinusoidal endothelium or the hepatocytes is an important characteristic of liver structure and function. There is only a very porous cellular barrier between the blood in the sinusoid and the hepatocyte plasma membrane. Soluble and particulate materials in the blood pass freely between the sinusoid and the perisinusoidal space; only blood cells are retarded by the fenestrated, separated endothelial cells and the Kupffer cells that line the sinusoid.

194. The answer is B [Chapter 8 II A; Chapter 3 I A]. Collagen is the principal extracellular fibrous component of connective tissue. The cytoskeleton is an intracellular structure that includes microfilaments (actin), microtubules (tubulin), and intermediate filaments; collagen is never found as part of the cytoskeleton. Collagen is synthesized primarily by fibroblasts, the stereotypic cells of connective tissue, and by chondroblasts and osteoblasts, of cartilage and bone, respectively. Cells of each of the other three basic tissues synthesize collagen, as well. All epithelial cells secrete type IV and type VII collagen as components of the basal lamina. Some developing epithelial cells even secrete fibrillar collagen. Schwann cells of the nervous system and smooth muscle cells secrete external lamina collagens. In addition, Schwann cells secrete fibrillar collagen as a component of the endoneurium, and smooth muscle cells secrete fibrillar collagen as a component of the tunica media of blood vessels.

195. The answer is B [Chapter 27 IV B]. Unlike the parotid and submandibular salivary glands, the pancreas does not contain striated ducts. Modification of the pancreatic acinar secretion is accomplished by the cells of the intercalated and intralobular ducts, which add fluid and bicarbonate ion to the secretion. Centroacinar cells are the cells at the beginning of the intercalated duct, located within the acinar lumen.

196. The answer is D [Chapter 14 II A 2]. The entry of the pulmonary veins into the left atrium is not guarded by valves. Semilunar valves guard against backflow of blood from the pulmonary trunk into the right ventricle, and from the aorta into the left ventricle. The tricuspid valve prevents backflow of blood from the right ventricle to the right atrium.

197. The answer is B [Chapter 9 II B]. Adipocytes—like connective tissue cells—ultimately derive from undifferentiated mesenchymal cells. The first stage of differentiation of such cells is a cell that is morphologically indistinguishable from a fibroblast. The first changes that begin to identify a cell that will develop into an adipocyte are the secretion of an external (basal) lamina and the accumulation of small lipid droplets. Cells that have these characteristics are called lipoblasts (to distinguish them from "typical" fibroblasts) or preadipocytes. Monocytes are of hemopoietic origin and give rise to connective tissue macrophages and other cells of the mononuclear phagocytic system, not to adipocytes.

198. The answer is D [Chapter 28 VII A 3]. Cartilage is found in the walls of the larynx, trachea, and all bronchi, but not in narrower diameter tubules of the respiratory system such as bronchioles. In histologic sections, small bronchi can be distinguished from large bronchioles by the presence of cartilage in the wall of the bronchi.

199. The answer is D [Chapter 4 IV; Chapter 2 II B 2]. The proteins that form elements of the nuclear matrix are synthesized on polysomes that are free in the cytoplasm. The proteins are then transported into the nuclear compartment via nuclear pores. Although the membranes of the nuclear envelope are continuous with those of the rough endoplasmic reticulum (rER), proteins that are made on the nuclear envelope enter the intracellular pathway for secretion and do not enter the nucleus.

200. The answer is D [Chapter 8 II A 2 c]. Collagen contains few, if any, sulfur-containing amino acids in its fibrillar form. Sulfur-containing amino acids in procollagen are restricted to the globular (nonhelical) portions of the molecule that are largely cleaved at the time of secretion from the fibroblast. Cross-linking in the triple-helical portion of the molecule is accomplished through hydrogen bonds between the α chains that involve the hydroxyl groups of hydroxyproline and hydroxylysine.

201. The answer is D [Chapter 36 II C 1 a, b]. Sertoli cells are the columnar epithelial cells of the seminiferous tubules. Leydig cells are located in the connective tissue between seminiferous tubules. Cells in all of the stages of spermatogenesis are partially enclosed by surface invaginations of the Sertoli cells. The seminiferous epithelium is populated by the stem cells of the male germ cells in early embryonic life.

202. The answer is D [Chapter 22 IV A 3]. Mature enamel is acellular and nonreplaceable. It is produced during tooth development by secretory ameloblasts. These cells secrete the organic matrix onto which calcium and phosphate, transported by maturation ameloblasts, are deposited as hydroxyapatite.

203. The answer is B [Chapter 9 II C 2]. Plasma cells, which are part of the immune system, are not usually found in adipose tissue. They are commonly present in loose connective tissue that subtends body surfaces, as in the lamina propria of the alimentary canal, the respiratory tract, and the urinary tract. They are also found in lymph nodes, where they differentiate from transformed B lymphocytes.

204. The answer is E [Chapter 27 III A 1; Chapter 25 I C 1 d (2) (b) (ii)]. Enterokinase is a membrane-associated enzyme in the glycocalyx of intestinal absorptive cells that converts the proenzyme trypsinogen, secreted by the exocrine pancreas, to its active form, trypsin. All of the other enzymes are secreted as proenzymes by pancreatic acinar cells.

205. The answer is D [Chapter 25 I B 4 c; II B 3 c]. The replicative zone of the pericryptal fibroblasts is restricted to the immediately subepithelial lamina propria underlying the base of the intestinal crypt. From here, the fibroblasts migrate up the outside of the crypt, differentiating and secreting collagen, glycosaminoglycans (GAGs), and proteoglycans (PGs) of the pericryptal sheath and, in the colon, of the collagen table.

206. The answer is E [Chapter 9 II D 2]. Parathormone, secreted by the parathyroid glands, is a regulator of calcium metabolism, not of lipid metabolism. Its primary role is in regulating the storage and release of calcium and phosphate from bony tissue. All of the other hormones listed have either direct or indirect effects on important steps in lipid metabolism and in the relationship between glucose metabolism and lipid metabolism.

207. The answer is E [Chapter 37 VI B; VIII A]. The aqueous humor of the eye is a fluid secretion, not a connective tissue gel. Vitre-

ous humor is connective tissue gel that fills the space between the lens and the retina. It does not circulate or interact with the lens or cornea. It is secreted by hyalocytes, not by the ciliary epithelium.

208. The answer is D [Chapter 7 V A 5 c]. Triads are formed by two terminal cisternae of the sarcoplasmic reticulum and a transverse tubule. They function in excitation–contraction coupling in skeletal muscle and are not found in cardiac muscle. The comparable structure in cardiac muscle is the dyad, which is formed by one terminal cisterna and a transverse tubule.

209–211. The answers are: 209-E [Chapter 1 IV C], **210-D** [Chapter 1 IV B 1 b], **211-B** [Chapter 1 III A 3 c (2)]. In phagocytosis, regions of the plasma membrane extend around and engulf large particles (e.g., bacteria, cell debris), internalizing the material in large cytoplasmic vacuoles.

The uptake of ligands into cells by receptor-mediated endocytosis requires that ligand-receptor complexes be located in clathrin-coated regions of the plasma membrane, which then become coated pits. The coated pits become clathrin-coated vesicles as they are pinched off into the cytoplasm.

The inositol trisphosphate (IP$_3$) signaling pathway is activated by one class of G protein–linked receptors. The IP$_3$ that is produced binds to vesicles of the smooth endoplasmic reticulum and induces the release of stored calcium into the cytoplasm.

212–218. The answers are: 212-C [Chapter 7 IV D 5], **213-A** [Chapter 7 V A 1], **214-C** [Chapter 7 IV D 5], **215-D** [Chapter 8 IV A 1 e], **216-A** [Chapter 7 V A 2], **217-E** [Chapter 7 VI A], **218-B** [Chapter 23 II B]. Transverse tubules are invaginations of the plasma membrane that penetrate deeply into striated muscle fibers. The transverse tubules are located at the A–I band junction in mammalian skeletal muscle and at the Z disk in mammalian cardiac muscle.

Cardiac muscle tissue consists of single cells organized into long fibers. The cells are joined to each other by specialized intercellular junctions called intercalated disks. Components of the intercalated disks include adherens junctions and gap junctions, which provide cell–cell attachment and cell–cell communication.

In skeletal muscle cells, transverse tubules are located between adjacent terminal cisternae of the sarcoplasmic reticulum to form an association called the triad.

The myofibroblast is an elongated, spindle-shaped cell that displays physiologic and morphologic characteristics of both fibroblasts and smooth muscle cells. The myofibroblast is implicated in wound contraction, a natural process that closes a wound in which tissue loss has occurred.

Cardiac muscle cells are organized into long, branching fibers. The nucleus of a single cardiac muscle cell is located in the center of the cell.

Smooth muscle cells are elongate fusiform (spindle-shaped) cells. They synthesize and secrete several components of the extracellular matrix that surrounds them, including reticular (type III) collagen.

Myoepithelial cells are contractile cells that lie between the basal plasma membrane of acinar cells and the basal lamina in exocrine glands. Their contraction plays an important role in moving the secretory products of an exocrine gland toward its secretory duct.

219–224. The answers are: 219-B [Chapter 11 II D 1], **220-D** [Chapter 13 I A 1], **221-A** [Chapter 11 II C 2], **222-E** [Chapter 11 III C], **223-F** [Chapter 11 III C 1], **224-C** [Chapter 13 V C 1]. This micrograph depicts a section of a spicule of bone in the metaphysis of a growing long bone. An osteoclast (B) is visible on the surface of the spicule. Note its very large size and its several nuclei. At least two additional osteoclasts are also visible at other points on the surface of the bony spicule.

Several hematopoietic, myeloid cells are shown enclosed by a circle (D). This is bone marrow. Structural details of these blood-forming cells are not clear in this relatively low magnification micrograph of sectioned material.

Cells in bone tissue that are found in lacunae are osteocytes (A). Several unlabeled osteocytes are also visible in this spicule of bone. Not visible in this example of decalcified bone are the many canaliculi that radiate from each lacuna.

In a region of active bone formation, osteoblasts (E) form a compact, epithelial-like layer on the surface of the bone. The newest bony matrix formed by an osteoblast is osteoid.

The junction between osteoid and calcified bony matrix (F) is visible in histologic sections of rapidly growing bone such as this. The growing region of the spicule is covered by osteoblasts. Osteoclasts are associated with the older, calcified region of the spicule.

A megakaryocyte (C) is much larger than other hematopoietic cells. Megakaryocytes and osteoclasts may be of similar size and may be in close proximity to one another. Megakaryocytes, however, have a single polyploid nucleus, whereas osteoclasts have many diploid nuclei.

225–229. The answers are: 225-D [Chapter 6 VIII A 1 a (2)], **226-C** [Chapter 2 III B 2], **227-E** [Chapter 7 IV E 1], **228-B** [Chapter 2 IV B], **229-A** [Chapter 8 III A 2, 4]. This electron micrograph depicts a fibroblast of the endomysium together with a portion of a skeletal muscle fiber and an unmyelinated axon. The unmyelinated axon, with two mitochondria, is visible partially enveloped by a process of a Schwann cell. The small size of the axon–Schwann cell complex suggests that this nerve process is close to its point of termination. Part of the surface of the axon is exposed, and it is separated from the extracellular matrix only by the basal lamina.

The Golgi apparatus is a site of glycosylation of cellular secretions. A particularly clear example of the organelle is visible in this fibroblast. Numerous small vesicles, some possibly containing recently glycosylated secretions, are visible close to the Golgi apparatus.

Overlap of actin and myosin occurs in the myofibrils of striated muscle cells. The region of overlap occurs in the A band of the sarcomere. One sarcomere is defined as the expanse of a myofibril enclosed by two successive Z lines.

Oxidative phosphorylation and adenosine triphosphate (ATP) synthesis occur in mitochondria. The mitochondria of the muscle cell are branched and relatively dark in appearance, whereas the mitochondria of the fibroblast are unbranched and lighter in appearance. The significance of this variation in appearance is not known.

Proteoglycans, collagen, and fibronectin are components of the extracellular matrix. They contribute to the delicate filaments and amorphous substances in this region of the matrix shown in this micrograph between a fibroblast and an unmyelinated axon. Note also the distinct basal lamina of the skeletal muscle cell and the basal lamina–free surface of the adjacent fibroblast.

230–236. The answers are: 230-D [Chapter 17 III A 1 b], **231-F** [Chapter 17 III B 2 a (2)], **232-E** [Chapter 17 III A 2 b (2)], **233-C** [Chapter 17 V B], **234-D** [Chapter 15 VIII B 2 a], **235-G** [Chapter 17 V E], **236-D** [Chapter 15

VIII B 1]. This light micrograph depicts a section of a lymph node. B lymphocytes are concentrated in nodules, and the germinal center of the nodule is a site of B lymphocyte blastic transformation, one indication of which is the presence of lymphoblasts. The deep, non-nodular cortex (paracortex) contains more T lymphocytes than B lymphocytes, and is the thymus-dependent subcompartment of the node. The subcapsular (marginal) sinus lies between the capsule and the nodular cortex. Antibody-secreting plasma cells are numerous in the cords of the dense lymphatic tissue of the medulla. Medullary sinuses are continuous with the lumen of the efferent lymphatic vessel.

237–241. The answers are: 237-D [Chapter 24 II C 1 a], **238-C** [Chapter 24 III A 3], **239-A** [Chapter 24 III A 2], **240-A** [Chapter 24 III A 2], **241-B** [Chapter 24 III A 4 d]. Surface mucous cells and mucus-secreting cells of the gastric pit secrete a thick, basic mucus that protects the gastric epithelium from both the abrasive action of chyme and the acid environment of the stomach lumen.

The chief cells of the gastric gland secrete pepsinogen and other enzyme precursors into the stomach. They are converted to active enzymes by hydrochloric acid secreted by the parietal cells.

In humans, intrinsic factor, a glycoprotein essential for the absorption of vitamin B_{12} by the ileum, is secreted by the parietal cells along with 0.16N hydrochloric acid.

Parietal (oxyntic) cells of the gastric glands secrete 0.16N hydrochloric acid, which passes from the lumen of the gland to establish an acidic environment in the lumen of the stomach. The peptidases and other enzymes secreted by the chief cells have optimum enzymatic activity at an acid pH.

Gastrin is one of the more than 20 polypeptide hormones secreted by enteroendocrine cells of the gastrointestinal epithelium. Gastrin is secreted in response to filling of the stomach and promotes the secretion of acid by the parietal cells of the gastric glands. Enteroendocrine cells secrete across the basal lamina, where their hormones may act locally on other epithelial cells (i.e., paracrine function) or may enter the blood circulation and be carried to other sites of action (i.e., endocrine function).

242–244. The answers are: 242-E [Chapter 29 V A 1 b], **243-C** [Chapter 29 V G 1 b, 2 a], **244-A** [Chapter 29 V G 2 a]. The diagram depicts a renal corpuscle. The visceral epithelial cell of the renal capsule is also called a podocyte (E). Processes of this cell are the pedicels, or foot processes, that are aligned along the glomerular basement membrane. Spaces between the foot processes are the filtration slits that are a component of the filtration barrier.

Juxtaglomerular (JG) cells (C) are modified smooth muscle cells that secrete renin, a proteolytic enzyme that converts angiotensinogen to angiotensin I. They are found in the wall of the afferent arteriole to the glomerulus.

The cells of the macula densa of the distal convoluted tubule (A) monitor blood sodium concentration and blood volume. Decreases in either cause the macula densa cells to release a factor that stimulates the JG cells of the afferent arteriole to release renin.

245–251. The answers are: 245-A [Chapter 17 III B 2 a], **246-A** [Chapter 17 V B], **247-B** [Chapter 16 III B 2 b], **248-A** [Chapter 17 II B 1], **249-C** [Chapter 18 III A], **250-D** [Chapter 19 VIII A] **, 251-E** [Chapter 16 II B 2–4]. Plasma cells are a prominent component of the dense lymphatic tissue that forms the medullary cords of lymph nodes. Plasma cells are also found in Peyer patches, spleen, and tonsils, but not in the concentrations noted in medullary cords of nodes. Plasma cells are not usually found in the thymus gland. The subcapsular sinus is the lymph space that is fed by the afferent lymphatic vessels and drained by the cortical sinuses. It is present in lymph nodes but not in any of the other lymphatic tissues listed.

Peyer patches are masses of lymphatic nodules in the distal small intestine (i.e., the ileum). The development of this lymphatic tissue presumably is in response to antigens produced by the abundant microbial flora of the gut. Peyer patches develop initially from the gut-associated lymphatic tissue (GALT) of the mucosa of the ileum. The nodules enlarge beyond the limited space of the mucosa, pushing through the muscularis mucosae into the submucosa. In a fully developed nodule of a Peyer patch, a greater portion of the nodule is found in the submucosa than in the mucosa.

Lymph nodes are situated in the flow of lymph. The afferent lymphatic vessels transport lymph into the node. Many afferent vessels enter a node along its convex surface. Valves are often present in these lymphatic vessels. None of the other listed lymphatic tissues has as numerous and distinct afferent lymphatic vessels.

The white pulp of the spleen forms the periarteriolar lymphatic sheath (PALS), a continuous sleeve of lymphatic tissue that surrounds the small arteries and arterioles of the organ. Other lymphatic organs are vascularized and contain dense lymphatic tissue but not in the unique relationship that is characteristic of the spleen.

The thymus gland is the site of maturation of T-lymphocytes, which are the cells responsible for cell-mediated immunity. The thymus gland provides a protected environment for the development of these cells; T-lymphocytes that might react against self (i.e., produce an autoimmune reaction) are recognized and prevented from entering the circulation.

Tonsils contain nodules with germinal centers and they are close to a mucosal surface. Villi are not present on the mucosal surface of tonsils. This surface is formed by a stratified squamous epithelium or by a pseudostratified epithelium, neither of which forms villi.

252–256. The answers are: 252-D [Chapter 8 I], **253-B** [Chapter 7 IV D 5 a], **254-D** [Chapter 5 VII B 2], **255-A** [Chapter 5 V A, D], **256-C** [Chapter 6 V]. A characteristic of connective tissue, in general, is the wide dispersal of its component cells (e.g., fibroblasts and macrophages). Most of the mass of a connective tissue sample consists of extracellular matrix secreted by the widely dispersed cells.

An intimate association between the plasma membrane and the smooth endoplasmic reticulum is seen in the triads of skeletal muscle. A triad is formed by an invagination of the cell membrane located between two cisternae of the sarcoplasmic reticulum. Thousands of triads exist in a typical skeletal muscle fiber and they have an important role in the coupling of excitation and contraction.

Connective tissue cells do not have a basal or external lamina. Basal and external laminae are regularly found at the junction of connective tissue with other basic tissues (i.e., epithelium, muscle, and nerve). Neither lamina is found at the interface between a connective tissue cell and connective tissue matrix.

Tight junctions and desmosomes are characteristics of epithelia. Such junctions are found only rarely in skeletal muscle and peripheral nerve. They are virtually absent from connective tissue.

Myelin is the plasma membrane of a Schwann cell. In the fully developed myelin sheath of a peripheral nerve, the layers of membrane that form the myelin are tightly laminated to each other.

257–261. The answers are: 257-E [Chapter 32 IV A 1], **258-B** [Chapter 32 III B 2], **259-C**

[Chapter 32 IV C 2], **260-C** [Chapter 32 III C], **261-E** [Chapter 32 IV B 1]. The adrenal medulla is derived from presumptive sympathetic ganglion tissue, a neural crest derivative. The principal cells in this region of the adrenal gland secrete epinephrine and norepinephrine, which are catecholamines.

The zona glomerulosa of the adrenal cortex synthesizes and secretes mineralocorticoids under the control of the renin–angiotensin system.

Glucocorticoids are synthesized and secreted by cells in the zona fasciculata of the adrenal cortex. Glucocorticoids secreted by the zona fasciculata stimulate cells in the adrenal medulla to synthesize the enzyme phenylethanolamine N-methyltransferase (PNMT), which converts norepinephrine to epinephrine.

Adrenal medullary cells synthesize and secrete catecholamines. In the chromaffin reaction, catecholamines are oxidized by chromium salts to dark brown, insoluble pigments, staining the cells brown.

262–266. The answers are: 262-F [Chapter 20 II D 2], **263-B** [Chapter 20 V C 1], **264-C** [Chapter 20 IV D], **265-D** [Chapter 20 VI B 2], **266-G** [Chapter 20 IV C]. The epidermis is indicated by F. Keratin intermediate filaments are aggregated by filaggrin in the epidermis. The aggregation process begins in the stratum granulosum and is completed by the time the cell takes its place in the stratum corneum.

A portion of a sebaceous gland is shown at B. Sebaceous glands have ducts, and are therefore exocrine glands. They are holocrine glands because cells die in the secretory process, contributing their remains to the secretory product.

An arrector pili muscle is indicated by C. This is a bundle of smooth muscle that extends between the wall of the hair follicle and the superficial dermis. The follicular end of the muscle is not visible in this micrograph. Contraction of the muscle causes the mobile hair follicle to move in the dermis, causing the hair shaft to project at nearly a right angle from the skin surface (i.e., causing the hair to "stand on end").

The straight portion of the duct of an eccrine sweat gland is shown at D. Because of the plane of section, continuity of this portion of the duct is not evident either with its deeper coiled portion or with its orifice on the surface of the epidermis.

Part of a hair follicle is shown at G. The epithelial wall of the follicle is continuous with the epithelium forming the epidermis. A fully keratinized, unstained hair shaft is visible inside the follicle. This is an example of a large hair follicle that has produced a terminal hair.

A blood vessel is indicated by A, and dense irregular connective tissue of the dermis is indicated by E.

267–276. The answers are: 267-C [Chapter 37 VII B], **268-E** [Chapter 37 II A 2], **269-B** [Chapter 37 I C; II A; IV A], **270-I** [Chapter 37 IX B], **271-F** [Chapter 37 VII C 3], **272-E** [Chapter 37 VII D 2 b], **273-H** [Chapter 37 VIII B 2], **274-D** [Chapter 37 III A 2], **275-B** [Chapter 37 IV B 3], **276-G** [Chapter 37 VII C 2 a, 3]. The pupil (C) is the circular opening surrounded by the medial edge of the iris. Muscles in the iris change the diameter of the pupil, regulating the amount of light entering the eye.

The lens (E) becomes more rounded with contraction of the ciliary muscles, focusing near objects on the retina. This process is accommodation.

The transparent cornea (B), the most anterior portion of the eye, is the primary image-forming element (dioptric) of the eye.

The axons of the ganglion cells of the neural retina leave the eye at the optic disc and pass directly to the brain as the optic nerve (cranial nerve II) (I).

From the basal lamina of the nonpigmented epithelium of the ciliary body (F) to the lens capsule, zonular fibers (G) form the suspensory ligament of the lens. The nonpigmented epithelial cells of the ciliary body secrete zonular fibers and the aqueous humor.

The anterior lens epithelium continues to divide throughout life and the newly formed cells migrate to the equator of the lens (E), where they turn in on themselves to form lens fibers. Increased cross-linking of proteins (crystallins) that accumulate in the lens fibers likely produces the gradual loss of elasticity of the lens with age.

Drying and shrinkage of the vitreous humor (H) with age can cause it to pull away from the retina. The resulting loss of pressure on the neural retina or tension on the retina can lead to separation of the neural retina from the pigmented retina.

The medial border of the iris (D) forms the pupil. The iris develops from the two layers of the optic cup. It separates the anterior and posterior chambers and, with the lens, forms a ball valve that prevents reflux of aqueous humor from the anterior to the posterior chamber.

Close to 90% of the cornea (B) is corneal stroma composed of fine collagen fibrils arranged in about 60 lamellae parallel to the corneal surface. This orthogonal array, and the regular size and spacing of the fibrils, likely underlie the transparency of the cornea.

Zonular fibers (G), also known as the suspensory ligament of the lens, are normally under tension and hold and shape the lens. Contraction of the ciliary muscle relaxes this tension and allows the lens to become more rounded, thus becoming a stronger dioptric element.

277–280. The answers are: 277-B [Chapter 22 I B 2], **278-A** [Chapter 22 I B 3; Chapter 23 VI], **279-D** [Chapter 22 I B 4; Chapter 16 II], **280-C** [Chapter 22 I B 1]. The teeth grind and tear food during chewing so that a macerated mass can be passed on to the esophagus in swallowing.

Salivary glands secrete mucins to lubricate the oral cavity and mix with the chewed food. They also secrete enzymes, notably amylase, that begin digestion of the chewed food.

Diffuse lymphatic tissue and lymphatic nodules, organized as the lingual, palatine, and pharyngeal tonsils, form an immunoprotective ring at the junction of the oral cavity and the pharynx.

The tongue is a muscular organ projecting from the floor of the mouth; it moves food around the oral cavity during chewing and swallowing. It also serves an essential role in speech and in gathering information about the mouth and its contents.

281–286. The answers are: 281-I [Chapter 31 II C 1 a], **282-D** [Chapter 30 IV A 1], **283-H** [Chapter 35 XI], **284-F** [Chapter 31 III], **285-G** [Chapter 34 III], **286-B** [Chapter 32 II B 1, C 1]. Thyroid gland follicular cells secrete the large glycoprotein precursor thyroglobulin into the lumen of the follicle, where it is temporarily stored. Thyroglobulin is taken up from the lumen by endocytosis and digested in lysosomes to produce thyroid hormones.

The neurohypophysis is the site of storage of peptide hormones oxytocin and antidiuretic hormone (ADH). The hormones are synthesized and packaged into secretory granules in the cell bodies of neurosecretory cells of the hypothalamus. The axons of these neurons end in the neurohypophysis. Secretory granules move down the axon by axonal transport to the axonal ending, where they are stored and, eventually, released by exocytosis following appropriate stimulation.

The placenta is a major endocrine organ and is also the point of exchange of metabolites, gases, and waste products between the fetus and mother. Hormones synthesized by the trophoblast affect both the fetus and the mother.

Total removal of the parathyroid gland results in a drop in serum calcium levels that produces tetanic convulsions and death.

The pineal gland mediates the responses of the reproductive system of seasonally breeding animals to changes in day length.

The zona fasciculata of the adrenal cortex secretes hydrocortisone, a glucocorticoid that acts on many different cells and tissues to increase the availability of glucose and fatty acids. The zona glomerulosa secretes aldosterone, a mineralocorticoid that acts on the collecting ducts of the kidney to increase Na⁺ retention.

287–292. The answers are: 287-D [Chapter 20 II F 2], **288-B** [Chapter 20 II E 4 a], **289-E** [Chapter 20 V B, C], **290-F** [Chapter 20 III C], **291-B** [Chapter 20 II E 4 a (2), 5], **292-C** [Chapter 20 II F 1]. The antigen-presenting cells found in the epidermis are the Langerhans cells. Once thought to be worn-out melanocytes, it is now generally accepted that Langerhans cells function in skin-associated immune responses.

The interfilamentous matrix of the anucleate, squamous keratinized cell is filaggrin.

A sebaceous cell synthesizes lipid; its final act is to die in the holocrine mechanism of secretion.

The dermal fibroblast is a synthetically active connective tissue cell that lies in the dermis, not the epidermis. It synthesizes collagen, elastin, and other components of the extracellular matrix.

The layer of dead, desiccated, squamous keratinized cells of the stratum corneum is an important component of the water diffusion barrier of the epidermis. Removal of the stratum corneum results in loss of the barrier.

The melanocyte oxidizes tyrosine in melanogenesis. Melanin-secreting cells in the skin, neural ganglia, and the iris are derived from the neural crest of the embryo.

293–298. The answers are: 293-A [Chapter 21 IV B 4], **294-D** [Chapter 21 IV A 2 c (1); Chapter 24 III A 2], **295-A** [Chapter 21 IV B 2], **296-D** [Chapter 21 IV A 4], **297-A** [Chapter 21 IV B 3], **298-B** [Chapter 21 II C 5 c]. Microvilli increase the surface area of intestinal absorptive cells up to 600 times, provid-

ing more surface across which metabolites may be absorbed. Microvilli are also covered with a glycocalyx containing membrane-associated glycoprotein enzymes, particularly dipeptidases and disaccharidases that produce amino acids and sugars for absorption.

Intracellular canaliculi in the acid-secreting cells (parietal cells) of the gastric glands increase the apical surface area across which hydrochloric acid is secreted. Hydrochloric acid begins the breakdown of ingested proteins by acidifying the macerated bolus of food in the stomach. The acid environment also stimulates the conversion of pepsinogen to pepsin, a potent proteolytic enzyme.

Plicae circulares are permanent submucosal circumferential folds in the small intestine that increase the luminal surface area of this organ. Covering the plicae and the interplical surface are villi, mucosal folds that further increase the surface area. Villi, in turn, are covered with absorptive epithelial cells with apical microvilli.

The extramural glands of the digestive system are the pancreas and liver. They secrete digestive enzymes and bile, respectively, that are delivered to the proximal portion of the small intestine (duodenum), where they act on the partially digested chyme. The liver is the largest gland in the body. Like the pancreas, it is both an exocrine and an endocrine gland.

Villi are finger-like and leaf-like mucosal projections on the wall of the small intestine. They are covered with absorptive epithelial cells. Fenestrated absorptive capillaries lie in the lamina propria immediately beneath the epithelium, and a blind-ending lymphatic capillary, the lacteal, is located in the core of the lamina propria. Most substances absorbed across the epithelium enter the fenestrated blood capillaries to be carried to the liver and then to the rest of the body. Molecules too large to enter the capillaries diffuse to the lacteal and reach the general circulation via the lymphatic circulation.

The teniae coli are thickened bands of the outer (longitudinal) layer of the muscularis externa. Their contraction provides the propulsive force for defecation.

299–304. The answers are: 299-D [Chapter 38 IV F 1 b], **300-C** [Chapter 38 III B 1; V C 3 b (1)], **301-E** [Chapter 38 V C 3 d (2)], **302-B** [Chapter 38 V C 3 c (1)], **303-C** [Chapter 38 III B 1; IV C], **304-A** [Chapter 38 III B 1; V C 3 a]. The stria vascularis of the cochlear duct is a thick, pseudostratified epithelium that is richly vascularized, as is implied by its name. It is thought to synthesize and secrete endolymph. The stria vascularis extends the entire length of the scala media, from base to apex of the cochlea.

The oval window is an aperture in the bony wall that separates the middle ear from the inner ear. The footplate of the stapes fits into the oval window and transmits vibrations from the chain of ossicles to the inner ear.

The tectorial membrane overlies the organ of Corti and the stereocilia of the hair cells of the organ are attached to it. One effect of sound vibrations on the inner ear is production of a shearing force between the hair cells and the tectorial membrane. The stereocilia are affected by this shearing effect.

The traveling wave that forms in the cochlea during sound perception is in the basilar membrane. This membrane forms the floor of the scala media and is the supporting substratum of the organ of Corti.

The oval window is one of two openings in the wall between the middle and inner ears (the other opening is the round window). The middle ear is an air-filled space and the inner ear is a fluid-filled space.

The auditory ossicles are three small bones that connect the tympanic membrane to the oval window. The ossicles thus establish communication between the tympanic membrane of the outer ear and the oval window, which is the main portal by which sound energy is transmitted to the inner ear.

305. The answer is C [Chapter 11 II C 2 b]. Canalicular channels (canaliculi) are narrow-diameter channels that permeate lamellar bone. Canaliculi extend out from lacunae and contain processes of osteocytes. Canaliculi should not be confused with osteonal (Haversian) canals or with perforating (Volkmann) canals.

306. The answers are: C [Chapter 11 II C 2 a], **A, E, G** [Chapter 10 II C 2]. Lacunae are characteristic of cartilage and bone. Lacunae are microscopic-sized compartments, surrounded by matrix, that are occupied by chondrocytes or osteocytes.

307. The answers are: B, D [Chapter 8 II C 1), **G** [Chapter 10 IV B 1). Elastic fibers are found in many, but not in all, types of connec-

tive tissue, and are especially numerous in elastic cartilage. Elastic fibers are present in loose irregular (i.e., areolar) and dense irregular connective tissues as a fibrous component of the extracellular matrix.

308. The answer are: A, E, G [Chapter 10 III C 1]. The territorial matrix is a characteristic of cartilage and is the matrix adjacent to chondrocytes (i.e., the territory of the cells). The territorial matrix stains differently from the interterritorial matrix, which is some distance removed from chondrocytes. This is because of the greater concentration of stainable, highly charged macromolecules present in the matrix close to chondrocytes.

309. The answers are: C [Chapter 11 III A 2], **A** [Chapter 11 VII F 4]. Hydroxyapatite crystals (calcium phosphate) are characteristic of bone. In fully mineralized bone, hydroxyapatite accounts for about 75% of dry weight. During endochondral ossification, hydroxyapatite crystals are deposited in hyaline cartilage in one zone of the growth plate.

310. The answers are: C [Chapter 11 III E], **A, E, G** [Chapter 10 VI A]. Appositional growth is characteristic of both bone and cartilage. The term refers to the deposition of new matrix on the surface of pre-existing bone or cartilage, and the resulting growth of the original bone or cartilage. Appositional growth is the sole growth process in bone; cartilage, however, grows by both appositional and interstitial processes.

311. The answer is C [Chapter 11 VIII F]. Cement lines are characteristic of lamellar bone, particularly bone in which extensive remodeling has occurred. Cement lines mark the boundaries between newly deposited bone and older, partially eroded bone.

312. The answers are: C [Chapter 11 VIII A 2], **B, D, F** [Chapter 8]. All of the connective tissues listed have blood vessels that permeate their matrices except for the three types of cartilage. Chondrocytes exist in an avascular environment. Their survival depends upon the diffusion of nutrients through the surrounding matrix from the blood vessels of the perichondrium.

Index

Italic page numbers indicate figures; page numbers with t indicate tables.

A

A bands, 85
A bundle, 171
Absorption, 468Q, 497E
Absorptive cells, 237, 276, 285–286
Accessory glands, 391
Accessory pancreatic duct, 309
Accessory proteins, 25
Accessory sex glands, 391, 404
Accommodation, 409
Acetylcholine, 92, 272
Acid hydrolases, processing, 17, 19
Acid secretion, mechanism and regulation, 272
Acidic protein, 348
Acidophils, 344
Acne, 232
Acquired pellicle, 261
Acrosome, 398
Actin, 25, 81, 94, 461Q, 493E
  binding proteins, 25, 26–27
  disruptive toxins, 27–28
  interaction between myosin and, during contraction, 88–89, 90, 91
  polymerization, 26
  types, 25–26
Actin microfilaments, 107, 278
Actin-disruptive toxins, 27–28
α-Actinin, 88, 94
Activated lymphocytes, 185
Acute inflammation, 454Q, 486E
Adenohypophysis, 342, 344–346, 345t, 346, 347, 467Q, 496–497E
Adenoids, 195
Adenosine triphosphate (ATP)
  hydrolysis, 26
  production, 20–21
  synthesis, 463Q, 493E
Adenosine triphosphate (ATP)-dependent process, 39
Adhesion belts, 56, 451Q, 483E
Adipocytes, 356, 459Q, 491E
Adipose cells
  histologic characteristics, 110–111
  of Ito, 298–299
  origin, 110
Adipose tissue, 111, 171, 457Q, 488E
  definition, 115, 116
  metabolic function, 115
  regulation, 119, 460Q, 492E
  types, 115, 116, 117
  brown, 116–117
  white, 115–119, 117
Adrenal androgens, 362
Adrenal cortex, 467Q, 496–497E
Adrenal gland, 323, 359–365
  cortex, 359
    androgens, 362
    glucocorticoids, 361–362
    histologic organization, 360, 360
    mechanisms of steroid activity, 362
    mineralocorticoids, 360–361
  development, 359

fetal, 364–365
medulla, 467Q, 496–497E
  development, 362
  effects of catecholamines, 364
  histologic characteristics, 362–363, 363
  synthesis of catecholamines, 363–364
  structure, 359
Adrenalin, 362
Adrenocorticotropic hormone (ACTH), 345, 361
  specificity, 361–362
Adult thymectomy, 220
Adventitia, 284, 288
  in alimentary canal, 240
  in gallbladder, 303
Afferent arterioles, 335, 336
Afferent lymphatic vessels, 201, 455Q, 487E
Afferent receptors, 78–79
Air-blood barrier, 320, 320–321, 321
Air-phospholipid interface, 321
Aldosterone, 262, 333, 334, 361
Alimentary canal, 435Q, 470E
  basic plan for wall, 237, 238
    adventitia, 240
    mucosa, 237, 239
    muscularis externa (muscularis propria), 239–240
    serosa, 240
    submucosa, 239
  functional specializations in wall, 243–244
Alimentary mucosa, functions, 240, 241, 242–243
Alimentary tract, 237–244, 458Q, 490E
  components, 237
  phylogenetic and general functional considerations, 237
Alpha granules, 151
Alveolar air-blood barrier, 457Q, 489E
Alveolar bone, 252
Alveolar macrophages, 319
Alveolar processes, 252
Alveoli, 318–320, 319
  collateral air circulation, 320
  histologic characteristics, 318–320, 319
  interalveolar septum, 319–320
  structural organization, 318
Alveolus, 448Q, 480–481E
Ameloblasts, 250–251
Amelogenesis, 248, 250
Amino acids, 405
  analog and derivatives, 341
Ampulla, 380, 427
  of oviduct, 444Q, 478E
Anabolic effects, 361
Anagen, 230
Anal canal, 285
Anal sinuses, 285

Anaphase, 42, 396–397
Anaphase I, 45
Anaphase II, 45
Anchoring filaments, 59
Androgen-binding protein, 391, 401
Androgens, 391
Androstenedione, 362
Angiotensin I, 334, 361
Angiotensin II, 334, 361
Angiotensin-converting enzyme (ACE), 361
Angiotensinogen, 334, 361
Annulate lamellae, 400
Annuli fibrosi, 171
Anterior chamber and associated structures, 415–416, 416
Anterograde degeneration, 77
Antibody-secreting cells, 463Q, 493–494E
Antidiuretic hormone (ADH), 335, 347, 440Q, 474E
Antigen, recognition of, by B cells, 186
Antigen presentation, 109
Antigenic stimulation, 192
Antigen-presenting cells, 190–191
Antral (tertiary) follicles, 375, 375–376
Antrum, 375, 376, 435Q, 470E
Anus, 285
Aortic valve, 169
Apical domain, 278
Apical foramen, 252
Apical processes, 252
Apocrine glands
  distribution, 234
  function, 234
  structure, 234
Apocrine secretion, 259
  of lipids, 388
Apoptosis, 232, 376–377, 377
Appendix, 197, 284–285
  function, 198
  histologic characteristics, 198, 198
Appositional growth, 126, 130
Aqueous humor, 409, 416, 460Q, 492E
Arcuate arteries, 335
Area cribrosa, 334
Areolar tissue, 112
Argentaffin cells, 271
Arginine vasotocin, 372
Argyrophil cells, 271
Arterial capillaries, 213
Arterial vessels, 174–176, 175, 176
Arteries
  central, 213
  splenic, 213
  trabecular, 213
Arteriolae rectae, 336, 337
Arterioles, 175–176, 176, 213
  penicillar, 213
  sheathed, 213
Arteriovenous anastomosis (AVA), 182
Ascorbic acid, 405

Associated proteins, 25
Astrocytes, 69–70
Atresia, 376, 449Q, 481E
  histologic indications, 376–377
Atrial granules, 93
Atrial muscle cells, 170
Atrial natriuretic factor (ANF), 170
Atrioventricular (AV) node, 171
Atrioventricular (AV) valve, 169
Attachment epithelium, 253
Attachment plaques, 52
Attenuation reflex, 426
Auditory ossicles, 425, 426, 468Q,
  497–498E
Auditory tubes, 314, 425–426, 453Q,
  485E
Auerbach plexus, 240, 452Q, 484E
Auricle, 425
Autonomic nervous system, 61
Autonomic sensory receptors, 172
Autophagocytosis, 22
Avascular tissue, 125
Axon terminal, 92
Axonal process, 311
Axonemal complex, 397
Axons, 311
  cytologic characteristics, 65
  hillock, 65
  initial segment, 65
  length, 65
  transport, 65–66
Axoplasmic flow, 66
Axoplasmic transport, 66
Azurophilic granules, 146, 151, 454Q,
  486E

B
B memory cells, 188–189
Bacteria, phagocytosis of, 146
Band cell, 163–164, 443Q, 477E
Barr body, 35, 146, 452Q, 484E
Basal bodies, 30
Basal cells, 222–223, 312–313, 314,
  404
Basal cytoplasm, 307
Basal infoldings, 458Q, 490E
Basal infoldings and striations, 12
Basal interdigitations, 332
Basal lamina, 58, 59, 59–60, 226,
  446Q, 459Q, 479E, 490–491E
  comparison of basement membrane
    and, 60
  functions, 60
  and hemidesmosomes, 53–54
Basal layer, 451Q, 452Q, 483–484E,
  484E
Basement membrane, 58
  and comparison of basal lamina, 60
Basilar membrane, 431, 468Q,
  497–498E
Basolateral domain, 278
Basophilic erythroblast, 158, 456Q,
  488E
Basophils, 111, 148, 344, 345, 450Q,
  483E
Bicuspid valve, 437Q, 471E
Bile, 453Q, 485–486E
  secretion, 300–302, 301t
Bile acids, 301
Bile canaliculi, 299, 299–300, 438Q,
  472E
Biliary system, 299, 299–300
Bilirubin glucuronide, 301
Biochemical activity of nerve cells, 64
Biological membranes
  organization, 1–4, 2
  structure, 437Q, 471E

Biosynthesis, location, 14
Biosynthetic pathways, 13
Bipolar neurons, 64
Bladder, urinary, 339–340
Blastic transformation, 109, 186
  products, 187
  of T cells, 189
Blastocyst, 388
  implantation of, in uterine wall, 388
Blind spot, 421
Blood, 143–153, 144t
  basophils in, 148
  definition, 143
  eosinophils in, 145, 147–148
  erythrocytes in, 143–144
  lymphocytes in, 149, 149–150, 150
  monocytes in, 149, 150–151
  neutrophils in, 145, 145–146
  pathway through lymph nodes,
    205–206
  platelets in, 151–153, 152
Blood cells
  morphologic criteria, 155, 157
  types, 450Q, 483E
Blood pressure, 464Q, 494E
Blood sodium concentration, 464Q,
  494E
Blood vessels, 449Q, 482E
  general structure, 173, 173–174
  portal, 181–182
  of spleen, 213
Blood-brain barrier, 77
Blood-ocular barrier, 421–422
Blood-retinal barrier, 419
Blood-testis barrier, 401–402, 454Q,
  486E
Blood-thymus barrier, 217–218
B-lymphocytes, 149, 440Q, 441Q,
  443Q, 463Q, 473E, 474–475E,
  476E, 493–494E
  blastic transformation, 186
  in germinal centers, 193
  and humoral immunity, 186–189
Bone, 127–141
  cells, 127–129, 128
  definition, 127
  fracture repair, 140
  function, 127
  growth and remodeling of flat,
    139–140
  growth and remodeling of long, 139
  and hormonal control of calcium,
    140–141
  lamellar, 136–139, 137, 138
  matrix, 129–130
  osteogenesis
    endochondral ossification, 133–136
    intramembranous ossification,
      132–133
  types, 130, 130–131, 132
Bone marrow, numbers of neutrophils
  and erythropoietic cells in, 164,
  165t
Bone resorption, 461Q, 493E
Bone-associated fibrous connective
  tissue, 131
Bony labyrinth, 427
Bound ribosomes, 24
Boutons, 66–67
Bowman membrane, 413
Bowman's glands, 313
Brain sand, 371
Bronchi, 315–317, 316
  extrapulmonary, 316
  histologic characteristics, 316–317
  intrapulmonary, 316, 316
Bronchioles, 317, 317–318, 459Q,
  491E

  histologic characteristics, 317–318
Bronchus, 452Q, 484E
Brown adipose tissue
  histogenesis, 120
  histologic characteristics, 119–120
  physiologic function, 119
Bruch membrane, 419
Brunner glands, 273, 283–284
Brush border, 8, 278
Bulbar conjunctiva, 411
Bulbourethral glands, 406
Bundle of His, 171

C
Cadherin transmembrane linker
  proteins, 56
Calcification, zone of, 134
Calcified bone matrix, 461Q, 493E
Calcified cartilage, 455Q, 487E
Calcitonin, 354, 435Q, 470E
  physiologic roles, 357
Calcium
  homeostasis, 356–357
  hormonal control, 140–141
  regulation, 91–92
  release, 92
Callus, 140
Calmodulin, 27
Calmodulin-dependent myosin light
  chain kinase, 95
Calyces, 338–339
Canal of Schlemm, 415
Canaliculi, 128, 136
Cancellous bone, 130–131
Capacitation, 399
Capillaries, 119, 176–180, 178, 435Q,
  470E
  arterial, 213
  classification, 179–180
  lymphatic, 182–183
Capillary endothelium, 458Q, 490E
Capillary wall, components of,
  178–179
Capsule, 209
  connective tissue, 201
Carbon dioxide, transport of, in blood,
  143
Cardia, 265
Cardiac glands, 267
Cardiac muscle, 83, 93–94, 460Q,
  461Q, 492E, 492–493E
  morphologic characteristics, 93–94
  repair and renewal of cells, 96
Cardiac skeleton, 171
Cardiac structures, 459Q, 491E
Cardiac valves, 169
Cardiovascular system, 169–183,
  450Q, 482E
  arterial vessels, 174–176, 175, 176
  arteriovenous anastomosis, 182
  capillaries, 176–180, 178
  function, 169
  general structure of blood vessels,
    173, 173–174
  heart
    anatomy, 169, 170
    cardiac tissues, 169–171
    impulse-generation and impulse-
      conduction system, 171–172, 172
    lymphatic vessels, 182–183
    portal blood vessels, 181–182
    venous vessels, 180–181
Carotid body, 172–173
Carotid sinus, 172
Cartilage, 121–126, 459Q, 491E
  functions, 121
  growth, 126

organization, 121
types, 121, 124–125
zone of breakdown, 134–135
Cartilage cells
chondroblasts, 121
chondrocytes, 121, *122, 123*
perichondrial, 121
Cartilage matrix, 122–124
ground substance component, 123
Catabolic effects, 361
Catagen, 230
Catalase, 22
Catalytic receptors, 5
Catecholamines, 67
Caveolated cells, 286
Cecum, 284–285
Cell cortex, 25, 27
Cell cycle, 450Q, 482E
division, 43
interphase, 40–41, *41*
mitosis, 41–42, *42*
Cell-cell communication, 66
Cell-mediated immunity, 189–190,
465Q, 495E
Cells
classification, 1
plasma membrane functions in
regulation and signaling, 4–5
renewal, 450Q, 483E
α-Cells, 367
β-Cells, 367
σ-Cells, 367
Cellular junctions, 440Q, 473E
Cellular membranes, microscopy of, 4
Cellular reticulum, 191, 216
Cellular reticulum-fibrous reticulum
relationships, 191
Cellular similarity, 190
Cellular trophoblast, 388
Cement lines, 139, 448Q, 480–481E
Cementoblasts, 251
Cementum, 251
Central arteries, 213
Central nervous system (CNS), 61
myelin sheath, 74–75
nodes of Ranvier, 75
regeneration, 78
unmyelinated nerves, 76
Central vein, 441Q, 475E
Centrioles, 30
Centroacinar cells, 308, *308*
Centromere, 41
Centrosome, 25, 30
Ceruminous glands, 425
Cervical canal, 383
Cervical epithelium, 383
Cervical-vaginal junction, 383
Cervix, 381, 383
Chemical synapses, 66–69
functions, 68–69
Chemiosmotic coupling, 21
Chemoreceptors, 312
Chief cells, 355, 464Q, 494E
Choana, 311
Cholecystokinin (CCK), 272, 281, 309,
446Q, 479E
Cholesterol, 3
Chonchae, 311
Chondroblasts, 121
formation, 126
Chondroclasts, 122
Chondrocyte hypertrophy, 133
Chondrocytes, 121, *122, 123*
formation, 126
supply of nutrients to, 125–126
Choriocapillaris, 422
Choroid, 422
Chromaffin cells, 362

Chromaffin granules, 362
Chromaffin reaction, 465Q, 495E
Chromatids, 396, 455Q, 487E
Chromatolysis, 77–78
Chromophores, 344, 345
Chromosomes, 396, 459Q, 490F
chromatin, 35–37, *36*
general appearance, 35
number, 35
types, 36–37, *37*
Chronic inflammation, 191–192
Cilia, 9–10, *10, 11,* 12, 30
beating, 445Q, 478E
olfactory, 312
Ciliary body, 417–418
Ciliated columnar cells, 314
Ciliated pseudostratified, 449Q, 482E
Ciliated pseudostratified columnar
epithelium, 311, 314
Circumanal glands, 285
Circumferential lamellae, 138
Circumferential microtubule band, 151
Circumvallate papillae, 247, 248
Cis Golgi, 17
Cisternal compartment, 2
Clathrin, 6, 19
Clear cells, 355
Cleavage, 43
Clonal selection theory, 186
Clot formation, 153
Coated pit, 7
Coated vesicles, 6, 7
Cochlea, 427
Cochlear canal, 428–429, *429*
Cochlear duct, 427, 428
Colchicine, 30, 444Q, 477E
Collagen, 97–100, *99, 100,* 101–102t,
441Q, 459Q, 460Q, 463Q, 474E,
490–491E, 491E, 493E
in bone matrix, 129
composition and structure, 97–98, *99*
distribution, 97
synthesis, 98–99, *100*
types, 99–100, 101–102t
Collagen fibrils, 419, 438Q, 466Q,
472E, 496E
assembly, 99
Collagen table, 288
Collecting ducts, 324
Collecting venules, 180
Colloid, 351, 353
Colon, 237, *284,* 284–288
Colony-forming cells (CFCs), 155
numbers, 158
structure, 158
types, 158
Colony-forming units (CFUs), 155
Colostrum, 387
Columnar epithelial cell, 48
Committed progenitor cells, 158
Compact bone, 130, *130,* 131
transformation of spongy bone to,
133
Complex intercellular junctions, 457Q,
489E
Concurrent immune responses, 190
Condensation, 19
Condensing vacuoles, 19
Cones, 409–410, 419
Coni vasculosi, 402
Conjunctiva, 411
Connective tissue capsule, 201
Connective tissue sheaths of peripheral
nerve, *76,* 76–77
Connective tissue-epithelium interface,
446Q, 479E
Connective tissues, 97–114, *98,* 457Q,
458Q, 489E, 490F

associated with skeletal muscle, 84
bone-associated fibrous, 131
cells, 106–111, 107t
classification, 111–112, 112t
dense, 112–113, *113*
elastic, 113
loose, 112
reticular, 113
specialized, 113
dermis as, 221
fibers, 97
collagen, 97–100, *99, 100,*
101–102t
elastic, 102–103
reticular, 100, 102–103
ground substance, 103
fluid, 106
histologic characteristics, 105–106
macromolecules, 104, *104,* 105t
organization, 105
histogenesis, 113–114
histologic section, 435Q, 470E
Connexin molecules, 54
Connexons, 54, 453Q, 485E
Constituent cells, 465Q, 495E
Constitutive secretion, 19
Continuous capillaries, 179
Contractile proteins, 81
Contraction
initiation, 92
interaction between myosin and actin
filaments during, 88–89, *90,* 91
regulation, 91–92
Cornea, 409, 413
characteristics, 413
layers, 413–415, *414*
Corneal endothelium, 413, 414–415,
415
Corneal epithelium, 411, 413
Corneal stroma, 413–414
Corneosclera, 411
Corneoscleral layer, 409
Corneoscleral margin, 413
Cornified cells, characteristics, 225
Corona radiata, 376
Corpora albicans, 376
Corpora amylacea, 406
Corpora arenacea, 371
Corpora cavernosa, 406
Corpus luteum, 378–379
function, 379
of pregnancy, 379
regression, 379
Corpus spongiosum, 340, 406
Cortex
of kidney, 323–324
of lymph node, 201–203, *202*
of thymus, 216
Cortical actin network, 25
Cortical arterioles, 359
Cortical capillaries, 359
Cortical cells, 229
Cortical labyrinth, 330–332
Cortical sinuses, 205
Corticotropes, 345
Corticotropin-releasing hormone, 361
Cortilymph, 428
Cortilymphatic space, 428
Cortisol, 361
Cotranslational modifications, 16
Countercurrent exchange, 337–338
Crenated red blood cells, 455Q, 487E
Crevicular epithelium, 253
Crista, 20, 429
of semicircular canals, 428
Crossing-over, 45, 396, 455Q, 487E
Cross-striations, 84–85
ultrastructure, 85, *86*

Crypt of Lieberkühn, 450Q, 483E
Cryptorchidism, 391
Crypts of Lieberkühn, 275, *277*
Crypt-villus junction, 460Q, 492E
Crypt-villus relationship, 275, *277*
Crystallins, 418
Crystals of Reinke, 395
Cuboidal epithelial cell, 48
Cumulus oophorus, 376
Cupula, 429–430, 444Q, 477E
CURL, 7, 19
Cuticle, 235
Cuticle cells, 229
Cytochalasin, 27–28
Cytokinesis, 43
Cytoplasm, organization, 25
Cytoplasmic basophilia, 187, 188
  significance, 158
Cytoplasmic Ca^{2+} concentration,
    443Q, 477E
Cytoplasmic components, 13, 62, *64*
Cytoplasmic dynein, 66
Cytoplasmic events, 43–44
Cytoplasmic granules, 146, 155
Cytoplasmic organelles, 93, 94, 457Q,
    488E
Cytoplasmic polychromatophilia, 159
Cytoplasmic scaffold, 25
Cytoplasmic space
  integration, 33
  integrators, 25
Cytoskeleton, 25–34, 458Q, 459Q,
    490E, 491E
  actin, 25
    binding proteins, 26–27
    disruptive toxins, 27–28
    polymerization, 26
    types, 25–26
  intermediate filaments, 30–31
    assembly, 33
    functions, 33–34
    types, *31*, 31*t*, 31–33
    ultrastructure, 33
  microtubules, 28, *28*
    composition, 28
    polymerization of tubulin, 28–29
Cytotoxic T cells, 189–190
  as effector cells, 189–190

D
Dawn of neutrophilia, 162
Deep cortex, 456Q, 488E
Dehydroepiandrosterone, 362
Deiodination of thyroxine (T$_4$), 295
Dendrites, 64–65, 311
  cytologic characteristics, 65
Dendritic process, 311
Dense bodies, 94, 107
Dense granules, 151
Dense irregular connective tissue,
    465Q, 469Q, 495E, 498E
Dense regular connective tissue,
    469Q, 498E
Dental caries, 248, 466Q, 496E
Dentin, 251–252
Dentinal tubules, 252
Deoxyribonuclease, 305
Dephosphorylation, 95
Depolarization, 92
  propagation, 92
Dermal fibroblast, 468Q, 497E
Dermal papilla, 228
Dermal repair, 236
Dermatoglyphics, 227–228
Dermis
  components, 226–227
  dermoepidermal junction, 227–228

fibroblasts, 227
general characteristics, 226
hypodermis, 228
Langer lines, 227
Descemet membrane, 414
Desmin, 32, 88, 94
Desmosine, 103
Desmosomal plaques, 25
Desmosomes, 50–53, *53*, 93, 223,
    465Q, 495E
  and hemidesmosomes, 54
Diad, 94
Diaphysis, 134, 139
Diencephalon, evagination of, 412
Diffuse lymphatic tissue, 191–192,
    192
Diiodotyrosine (DIT), 353
Dilator pupillae, 417
Dimer formation, 33
Diplotene, 396
Discontinuous capillaries, 179
Distal tubule, 438Q, 472E
  convoluted, 333
  straight, 333
DNA, 448Q, 480–481E
  linker, 36
  nuclear, 447Q, 480E
Dopa, 363
Dopamine β-hydroxylase, 363
Duct of Santorini, 309
Duct of Wirsung, 309
Duct system, 307–309, 459Q, 491E
Ductus deferens, 404
Ductus epididymis, 399, 402, 403
Duodenal enteroendocrine cells,
    446Q, 479E
Duodenum, 273, 441Q, 474E
Dynein, 29

E
Ear, 425–431
  external
    auditory canal, 425
    auricle, 425
  inner, 426
    bony labyrinth, 427
    cochlear canal, 428–429, *429*
    functions, 429–431
    hair cells, 428
    membranous labyrinth, 427
    perilymphatic space, 427–428
    sensory areas, 428
  middle, 453Q, 485E
    auditory (eustachian) tube, 425–426
    auditory ossicles, 425, *426*
    muscles of, and attenuation reflex,
      426
    tympanic membrane, 425
Eccrine sweat glands
  distribution, 232–233
  function, 233–234
  structure, 233, *233*
Ectoderm, 47
Ectomesenchyme, 114
Ectomesoderm, 114
E-face, 4
Effector cells, cytotoxic T cells as,
    189–190
Efferent arterioles, 335
Efferent lymphatic vessels, 201, 463Q,
    493–494E
Efficient packing, 35
Ejaculatory duct, 404
Elastic cartilage, 124, *124,* 469Q,
    498E
Elastic fibers, 102–103

composition, 103
distribution, 102
structure, 102–103
synthesis, 103
system, 103
Elastic tissue, 113
Elastin, 103
Elaunin fibers, 103
Electric coupling, 55
Electrical synapses, 69
Electronic conduction, 95
Elementary particles, 21
Emotional sweating, 234
Enamel, 460Q, 492E
Endocardium, 169
Endochondral ossification, 455Q, 487E
Endocrine glands, 48, 341
  blood supply, 341
Endocrine pancreas, 305
Endocrine system, 341
Endocytosis, 5, 19, 22, 68
  receptor-mediated, 6–7
  and release of thyroid hormone, 353
Endocytotic vesicles, 7
Endoderm, 47
Endolymph, 428
Endolymphatic space, 428
Endometrial glands, 384
Endometrium, 107, 382–383, 454Q,
    486E
Endomysium, 84
Endoneurium, 76, 438Q, 472E
Endoplasmic reticulum
  rough, *15*, 15–17
  smooth, 13–15, *14*
Endosteum, 131
Endothelial cells, 178
Endothelial fenestrations, 437Q, 471E
Endothelium, 169, 173–174
Enterochromaffin cells, 271
Enteroendocrine cells, 239, 243, 265,
    271–272, 281, *281*, 283, 464Q,
    494E
Enteroeptors, 78
Enteroglucagon, 282
Enterokinase, 460Q, 492E
Enzymatic receptors, 5
Enzymes and bicarbonate ions, 448Q,
    481E
Eosinophilic chemotactic factor of
    anaphylaxis (ECF-A), 110
Eosinophils, 111, *145*, 147–148,
    450Q, 483E
Ependymal cells, 70
Epicardium, 170–171
Epidermal appendages, 221
Epidermal germinative cell, 443Q,
    477E
Epidermal-melanin unit, 226
Epidermis, 451Q, 483–484E
  basal cells, 222–223
  general characteristics, 221–222, *223*
  granular cells, 224
  keratinized cells, 224–225
  nonkeratinocytes, 225–226
  spinous cells, 223–224
Epimysium, 84
Epinephrine, 362
  hormonal control of synthesis,
    363–364
Epinephrine-secreting cells, 363
Epineurium, 77
Epiphyses, 139
  closure, 136
Epiphysis, 134
Epithelia-connective tissue interface,
    58–60

Epithelial cells, 98, 441Q, 451Q, 475E, 483E
  intercellular junctions, 50–58, 51, 52t, 53
  mitosis and tissue renewal, 58
  renewal, 266–267, 283, 286–287
Epithelial destruction, 235–236
Epithelial repair, 235
Epithelial structure, 466Q, 496E
Epithelium, 47–60, 415
  in alimentary canal, 237, 239
  classification, 48, 49, 50, 50t
  in esophagus, 263
  functions, 48
  general characteristics, 47–48
  in oral cavity, 245
Eponychium, 235
ER cisternae, 13
Erythroblasts, 167, 456Q, 488E
Erythrocytes, 143–144, 435Q, 452Q, 470E, 484E
  distribution, 160
  life-span of mature, 160
Erythropoiesis, 456Q, 488E
  basophilic erythroblast, 158
  duration, 160
  kinetics of red blood cell development, 160
  mitotic phase, 160
  normoblast (orthochromatic erythroblast), 159
  polychromatophilic erythroblast, 158–159, 159
  postmitotic phase, 160
  proerythroblast, 158
  reticulocyte, 160
Erythropoietin, 323, 335
Esophageal cardiac glands, 263
Esophageal glands, 263, 265
Esophageal wall layers, 263, 264, 265
Esophagogastric, 435Q, 470E
Esophagus, 237, 240, 448Q, 450Q, 480–481E, 482E
Esterases, 444Q, 478E
Euchromatin, 36–37
Eukaryotic cells, 1
  membranous compartments, 1
Eumelanin, 226
Eustachian tubes, 314, 425–426
Exchange vessels, 177
Excitatory synapses, 68
Excretory ducts, 259
Exocrine glands, 48, 255–262, 441Q, 447Q, 453Q, 465Q, 475E, 480E, 485E, 495–496E
  duct system, 256–257, 258, 259
  general characteristics, 255–257, 256, 257, 258, 259
  major, 255
  minor, 255
  parotid, 259–260
  saliva, 261–262
  sublingual, 260–261
  submandibular, 260
Exocrine pancreas, 237, 305–310, 306, 447Q, 455Q, 460Q, 479E, 487E, 492E
  control of secretion, 309–310
  duct system, 307–309
  histologic characteristics, 305, 306
  serous acinar cells, 305, 307, 307
Exocytosis, 68, 307, 437Q, 445Q, 471E, 478E
Exocytotic release, 67
Exocytotic secretion of proteins, 388
Extended tongue model, 72–73
External auditory canal, 425

External laminae, 447Q, 479–480E
Exteroceptors, 78
Extracellular space, 11
Extraglomerular mesangial cells, 330, 333
Extrahepatic bile ducts, 300
Extramural digestive glands, 244
Extraocular muscles, 423
Extraosteonal lamellae, 138
Extratesticular genital ducts, 403–404
Eye, 409–423, 466Q, 496E
  anterior chamber and associated structures, 415–416, 416
  blood-ocular barrier, 421–422
  choroid, 422
  concentric layers, 409, 410
  cornea
    characteristics, 413
    layers, 413–415, 414
  embryonic development, 411–413, 412, 412t
  extraocular muscles, 423
  eyelids, 422–423
  function, 409
  lacrimal apparatus, 423
  location, 409
  posterior chamber and associated structures, 416–418
  retina, 419–421, 420
  sclera, 415
  size and suspension, 409
  specific functions of ocular tissues, 409–411, 411
  vitreous body, 418–419
Eyelashes, 423
Eyelids, 422–423

F
F-actin, 81
Fallopian tubes, 380, 449Q, 482E
Fasciae adherentes, 93
Fascicles, 83, 84
Fast twitch fibers, 84
Fat, 449Q, 481E
Fatty acids, β-oxidation of, 22
Female reproductive system, 373–389, 374
  fertilization, 381
  luteinization of ovarian follicle, 378, 378–379
  mammary gland, 386, 386–388, 387
  menstrual cycle, 384–385
  mitosis and meiosis of female germ cell
    oogonia, 379
    ova, 379–380
    primary oocytes, 379
    secondary oocytes, 379
  ovaries, oocytes, and ovarian follicles and age of female, 376
    atresia of, 376–377, 377
    female germ cells, oogonia and oocytes, 373
    gross aspects, 373
    ovarian, 373–376, 375
  oviducts
    histologic structure of, 380
    regions, 380
  ovulation, 377–378
  placenta, 388–389
  uterus, 381, 382
    cervix, 383
    endometrium, 382–383
    myometrium, 382, 383
    perimetrium, 382
    regions, 381
  vagina, 385–386

Fenestrae and gaps, 291
Fenestrated capillaries, 179
Fertilization, 381, 444Q, 478E
Fetal adrenal gland, 364–365
Fetal-placental unit, 365
Fibril assembly, 97
Fibrillar collagen, 446Q, 479E
Fibrillar regions, 37
Fibrinolysin, 405
Fibroblasts, 98, 102, 454Q, 486E
  function, 106
  histologic characteristics, 106
  morphologic heterogeneity, 107
  replication and renewal, 106–107
Fibrocartilage, 125, 125, 469Q, 498E
Fibroelastic tissue, 169
Fibronectin, 463Q, 493E
Fibrous proteins, 33
Fibrous reticulum, 191
Fight-or-flight response, 364
Filaggrin, 224, 465Q, 495–496E
Filament ratio, 94–95
Filamentous actin, 25–26
Filamentous mitochondria, 118
Filaments, intermediate, 30–31
Filiform papillae, 247
Fimbriae, 380
Fimbrin, 27
Flagella, 9–10, 10, 11, 12, 30, 398, 445Q, 478E
Flat bones, 132
Flippases, 14
Fluid-phase endocytosis, 461Q, 492E
Fluid-phase pinocytosis, 6, 6
Foliate papillae, 247, 248
Follicle bulb, 228
Follicle epithelium, 351
Follicle matrix, 228
Follicle-stimulating hormone (FSH), 345
Follicular mantle, 193
Foramen cecum, 246
Foreign antigens carried in blood, 445Q, 478E
Fovea, 421
Fovea centralis, 421
Foveolae, 266
Fracture repair, 140
Free ribosomes, 24
Freeze-fracture, 54, 56
  of membranes, 438Q, 472E
Freeze-fracture electron microscopy, 4
Fructose, 405
Functional syncytium, 93
Fundus, 265, 381
Fungiform papillae, 247

G
G₁ phase, 40
G₂ phase, 41, 443Q, 477E
G-actin, 81
Gallbladder, 237, 289, 453Q, 485–486E
  mechanism of bile concentration, 303–304, 304
  structure, 302, 302–303
Ganglia, 61, 427
Ganglion cells, 409
Gap junctions, 4, 54–55, 93, 95, 441Q, 453Q, 475E, 485E
Gastric emptying, 269
Gastric epithelium, 449Q, 481–482E
Gastric glands, 242, 267, 268
  cells of, 269–272, 270, 271
Gastric inhibitory peptide, 281
Gastric mucosa, 266, 266–267, 268, 269

Gastric pits, 265–266
Gastrin, 265, 272, 310, 464Q, 494E
Gastroduodenal (pyloric) sphincter, 265
Gastroenteropancreatic endocrine system, 272, 281, *281*
Gastrointestinal epithelial cells, 453Q, 486E
Genetic diversity, 45
Genital ducts, 391
Genome, 35
Germinal centers, 192–193, 195, 209, *210*, 443Q, 457Q, 476E, 488–489E
Germinative cells, 223
Ghost, 144
Gingiva, 253
Gingival sulcus, 253
G-labeled structures, 466Q, 496E
Glial cells, 61
Glial fibrillary, 348
Glial fibrillary acidic protein (GFAP), 32, 69
Glisson capsule in liver, 289
Glomerular basement membrane, 329–330, 330
Glomerular capillary endothelium, 330
Glomerular endothelium, 329
Glomerular filtrate, 325, 330, 440Q, 473E
Glomerular filtration, 330
Glomerular filtration barrier, 464Q, 494E
Glomerular mesangial cells, 330
Glomerulus, 325, 328–329
Glomerulus-cortical tubule portal system, 181
Glucagon, 367
 control of release, 369–370
Glucocorticoids, 359, 361–362
 synthesis, 465Q, 495E
Gluconeogenesis, 361
Glucuronic acid, 301
Glycine, 446Q, 479E
Glycocalyx, 8, *9*, 244, 278–279, 286
Glycogen, 24, 297
Glycogen granules, 88
Glycogenesis, 361
Glycolipids, 3
Glycoproteins, 97, 104, 341, 440Q, 474E
 membrane, 3
Glycosaminoglycans, 104
Glycosphingolipids, 3
Glycosyltransferases, 17
Goblet cells, 243, 280–281, 286, *287*, 314–315
Goiter, 354
Golgi apparatus, 13, 63–64, 188, 296–297, 307, 458Q, 489E
 function, 17, 19
 morphology, 17, *18*
 in secretion, 19
Golgi complex, 88
Golgi method, 66
Golgi phase, 397
Golgi tendon organs, 79
Gonadotropes, 345
Gonadotropin-releasing factor, 372
Graafian follicles, 376
Graft rejection, 189
Granular cells, 224
Granular regions, 38
Granules, 452Q, 484E
Granulocytes, 146
Granulomere, 151
Granulopoiesis, 437Q, 456Q, 472E, 487E

band cell, 163–164
 metamyelocyte, 163
 myeloblast, 160–161
 myelocyte, 161–162, 161–163
 promyelocyte, 161, *161*
Granulosa cells, 376
Granulosa lutein cells, 378
Grave disease, 354, 447Q, 479E
Gray matter, 61
Ground substance
 in bone matrix, 123, 129
 in connective tissue, 103
  fluid, 106
  histologic characteristics, 105–106
  macromolecules, 104, *104*, 105t
 organization, 105
Growth plates, 134–136, *135*
 cartilage model growth and formation, 134
Gum, 253
Gut-associated lymphatic tissue (GALT), 195, 242, 274, 283, 287

H
H zone, 85
Hair cells, 428, 431
 function, 444Q, 477E
Hair follicles, 228, *229*, 454Q, 465Q, 486E, 495–496E
 arrector pili muscles, 230
 baldness, 230
 differentiating region, 228–229
 germinative region, 228
 growth cycle, 230
 sebaceous glands, 230
 size, 228
Halo cells, 404
Haploid cells, 35
Hassall corpuscles, 443Q, 477E
Haustra, 288
Haversian canal, 136
Heart
 anatomy, 169
 cardiac tissue, 169–171
 impulse-generation and impulse-conduction system, 171–172, *172*
 regulation of, by nervous system, 172–173
Helper T cells, 187, 190
Hematocrit, 144
Hematopoiesis, 155–167
 definition, 155, *156*
 morphologic criteria of blood cell development, 155, *157*
 site, 155
 tissue characterization, 155
Hematopoietic stem cells, 155, 157–158, 443Q, 477E
 and erythropoiesis, 158–160, *159*
 and granulopoiesis, 160–164, *161*, *162*, *163*, 165t
 and megakaryocytopoiesis, 164–165, *166*
 and microscopic anatomy of marrow compartment, 166–167
 and monocytopoiesis, 166
Hematoxylin-eosin-stained section, 448Q, 480–481E
Hemidesmosomes, 53–54
 and basal laminae, 53–54
 and desmosomes, 54
Hemoglobin, 143, 155, 159
Hemolysis, 144
Hemostasis, platelets in, 152–153
Henle layer, 229
Heparan sulfate, 148, 329

Heparin, 110, 453Q, 486E
Hepatic artery, 289–290
Hepatic portal triad, 459Q, 490E
Hepatic portal vein, 181, 289, 443Q, 477E
Hepatic sinusoids, 179
Hepatocytes, 14, 293–298, *294*, *296*, 458Q, 489E
 in liver, 289
 recycling by, 301
Herring bodies, 347
Heterochromatin, 36
Hilum, 323
Histamine, 109, 148, 272
Histogenesis of connective tissue, 113–114
Histones, 35
Holocrine, 452Q, 465Q, 484E, 495–496E
Holocrine secretion, 232, 259
Homeostasis, 289
Homeostatic activity, 357
Homologous chromosomes, 43
Hormones, 341
 classes, 341
 control of calcium, 140–141
Howship lacuna, 129
Humoral immunity, 186–189
Huxley layer, 229
Hyaline cartilage, 124, 469Q, 498E
Hyaline membrane disease, 321
Hyalocytes, 419
Hyalomere, 151
Hyaluronic acid, 104
Hydrochloric acid, 265, 464Q, 494E
Hydrocortisone, 361
Hydrogen peroxide degradation, 22
Hydrophilic polar head groups, 1
Hydrophilic portion, 3
Hydrophobic hydrocarbon tails, 1
Hydrophobic portion, 3
Hydroxyapatite, 130, 248
Hydroxylation, 16
Hydroxylysine, 97
Hydroxyproline, 97
Hypercalcemia, 354, 356
Hyperglycemia, 369
Hyperpolarization, 420
Hyperthyroidism, 354
Hypertonic urine, 442Q, 476E
Hypertrophy, zone of, 134
Hypocalcemia, 356
Hypoglycemia, 369
Hyponychium, 235
Hypophyseal portal system, 342–343, *344*
Hypophysis, 341
 hypothalamic regulation, 348t, 348–349
Hypophysis-initiated feedback loop, 348–349
Hypothalamic regulation of hypophysis, 348t, 348–349
Hypothalamic-hypophyseal portal system, 181
Hypothalamic-hypophyseal tract, 348
Hypothalamus, 341
Hypothalamus-pituitary-adrenal interactions, 361–362
Hypothyroidism, 354

I
I bands, 85
Ileocecal valve, 240
Ileum, 273, 437Q, 471E
Immune exclusion, 242, 283

Immune reactions
  basophils in, 148
  eosinophils in, 148
  lymphocytes in, 149–150
  specificity, 186
Immune responses
  concurrent, 190
  features of humoral and cell-
    mediated, 190–191
  sites, 207
  thymus in, *219, 220*
Immune surveillance, 206
Immune system
  macrophages in, 109
  role of, 272
Immunity
  cell-mediated, 189–190
  humoral, 186–189
Immunoglobulin A (IgA), 261, 301
Immunoglobulins, 458Q, 489E
  production, 283
Immunoregulation, 109
Immunosurveillance, 111
Impulse-conduction system, 448Q,
    481E
Impulse-generation, 448Q, 481E
Incus, 425
Inflammation, 146
Infundibulum, 341, 380
Inhibin, 391
Inhibitory synapses, 68–69
Initial immune reactions, 211
Inner leaflet, 2
Inositol triphosphate, 461Q, 492E
Inositol triphosphate signaling
    pathway, 5
Insulin, 119, 441Q, 475E
  control of release, 369–370
Integral membrane proteins, 3
Intercalated disks, 93
Intercalated ducts, 308, *308*
Intercellular junctions of epithelial
    cells, 50–58, *51, 52t, 53*
Intercellular material, 224
Intercellular space, dilation of, 435Q,
    470E
Interdigitations, *11,* 12
Interlobular arteries, 335, 437Q, 471E
Interlobular ducts, 309
Intermediate cells, 282
Intermediate filaments, 30–31
  assembly, 33
  functions, 33–34
  types, *31,* 31*t,* 31–33
  ultrastructure, 33
Intermembrane space, 20
Internal anal sphincter, 240
Interphase, 40–41, *41*
Interphase cells, 35
Interstitial cells, 371
Interstitial cell-stimulating hormone,
    395
Interstitial growth, 126
Interstitial lamellae, 138
Interstitial tissue, 395
Interterritorial matrix, 124
Interventricular septum, 451Q, 483E
Intestinal absorptive cells, 458Q, 490E
Intestinal epithelial cells, 276,
    278–283, *279, 280, 281*
Intracellular calcium concentration,
    461Q, 492E
Intracellular canaliculi, 243, 457Q,
    489E
Intraepithelial barrier, 283
Intraepithelial bipolar neurons, 456Q,
    488E

Intraepithelial gaskets, 56
Intraepithelial glands, 243
Intrahepatic bile ducts, 300
Intralobular collecting ducts, 308–309
Intraorbital fat, 411
Intratesticular genital ducts, *402,*
    402–403
Intrinsic factor, 265, 464Q, 494E
Iodination, 353
Iodine-deficiency goiter, 354
Iodopsins, 419
Iridial epithelium, 417
Iridial pigment, 417
Iris, 416–417
Islet β cell, 441Q, 475E
Islets of Langerhans, 305, 367–370
  control of release of insulin and
    glucagon, 369–370
  structure and development,
    367–369, *368, 369t*
Isodesmosine, 103

J

Jaundice, 301
Jejunum, 273, 441Q, 475E
Junctional complexes, 56–58, 307,
    438Q, 472E
Junctional epithelium, 253
Juxtaglomerular apparatus, 96,
    333–334
Juxtamedullary nephrons, 325

K

Karyokinesis, 43, 440Q, 473E
Karyosomes, 400
Keratin filaments, *31,* 31–32
Keratinized cells, 222, 224–225
  transformation to, 225
Keratinized cells, characteristics of,
    225
Keratinized epithelium, 245
Keratinocytes, 221
  differentiation, 222, *223*
  keratinized, 468Q, 497E
  nonkeratinized, 468Q, 497E
  postmitotic, 223
Keratohyalin granules, 224
Kidneys
  duct system, 334–335
  general characteristics, 323
  histophysiology, 337–338
  interstitium, 325
  nephron, 325, *326, 327,* 327–334,
    328, 329, 331
  organization of parenchyma,
    323–325
  renal circulation, 335–337, *336*
Killer cells, 457Q, 488–489E
Kinesin, 29, 66
Kinetics of red blood cell
    development, 160
Kinetochore, 41
Kinetochore microtubules, 42
Kupffer cells, 291

L

Lacrimal apparatus, 423
Lacrimal ducts, 423
Lacrimal glands, 255, 411, 423
Lacrimal sac, 423
Lacteal, 274
Lacuna, 461Q, 493E
Lacunae, 121, 128, 136
Lamellae

circumferential, 138
extraosteonal, 138
formation, 71–72
interstitial, 138
Lamellar bone, 129, 131, *132,*
    136–139, *137, 138,* 441Q, 469Q,
    474E, 498E
Lamellipodia, 27
Lamina densa, 330
Lamina propria, 239, 245, 267,
    287–288, 303, 338, 380
  in esophagus, 263
  in oral cavity, 246
Lamina rara externa, 330
Lamina rara interna, 329
Laminated plasma membrane, 465Q,
    495E
Langerhans cells, 226, 468Q, 497E
Lanthanum staining, 54
Large intestine, 242
Larynx, 314
Late endosome, 19
Lateral plications, 279–280, *280*
Left atrium, 169
Left atrium-pulmonary veins, 459Q,
    491E
Left ventricle, 169
Lens, 409, 413, 418
  focusing role of, 409
Leptotene, 396
Leydig cells, 395, 437Q, 444Q, 471E,
    478E
Lids, 411
Ligaments, 131
Ligand, 461Q, 492E
Ligand-gated receptor, 5
Limbus, 413
Lingual papillae, 246, 247
Lingual tonsillar crypts, 196
Lingual tonsils, 195, 246
Linker DNA, 36
Lipase, 119, 271, 305
Lipid bilayer, 1–2
Lipid droplets, 24, 297
Lipids
  apocrine secretion, 388
  membrane, 2–3
Lipoblasts, 118
Lipofuscin, 23
Lipolysis, 361
Lipotropes, 345
Liver, 237, 242, 244, 289, 443Q,
    444Q, 477E, 478E
  endocrine function, 443Q, 476E
  enzymes from, 273
  general structure
    perisinusoidal space, 289
    sinusoids, 289
  hepatic circulation, 289–292, *290*
  hepatocytes, 293–298, *294, 296*
  parenchyma, 289
    organization, *292,* 292–293
    stroma, 289
  perisinusoidal space, *298,* 298–299
  secretion of bile, 300–302, 301*t*
  sinusoids of, 459Q, 490–491E
Liver acinus, 293
Liver lobule, 441Q, 475E
Lobar bronchus, 449Q, 482E
Lobes of kidney, 325
Lobules of kidney, 325
Long bones, 133
  regions of developing, 134
Loop of Henle, 324, 332, 443Q, 476E
Loose irregular connective tissue,
    469Q, 498E
Lumen, 427

Lunula, 235
Luteinization of ovarian follicle, *378,* 378–379
Luteinizing hormone (LH), 345, 395, 437Q, 471E
Lymph circulation, 291–292
Lymph nodes, 201–207, 438Q, 464Q, 473E, 494–495E
  blood pathway through, 205–206
  blood to, 438Q, 473E
  cellular filters, 207
  compartments
    cortex, 201–203, *202*
    medulla, *203,* 203–204
    medullar sinuses, 204
    medullary cords, 204, *204*
  distribution, 201
  and drainage, 201
  filtering, 201
  flow of, 438Q, 473E
  functions, 206–207
  lymph pathway through, 205, *206*
  mechanical filters, 206–207
  pathway through, 205, *206*
  surface landmarks, 201, *202*
  transport, 183
Lymph pathway through lymph node, 205, *206*
Lymphatic capillaries, 182–183
Lymphatic cells and tissues, 185–193
  B lymphocytes and humoral immunity, 186–189
  components, 185
  function, 185
  nodules, 192, *193*
  T lymphocytes and cell-mediated immunity, 189–190
Lymphatic nodule-germinal center complex, 193
Lymphatic nodules, 192, *193,* 209, 452Q, 464Q, 465Q, 484–485E, 494–495E
Lymphatic sinuses, *203,* 204–205
Lymphatic tissues, 242
  diffuse, 191–192, *192*
  structural framework, 191
Lymphatic vessels, 182–183, 201, 464Q, 494–495E
  functions, 182
  renal, 336–337
Lymphoblasts, 185, 186, 463Q, 493–494E
Lymphocyte packing, 217
Lymphocytes, 111, *149,* 149–150, *150,* 185–186, *186,* 203, 404, 450Q, 483E
  differentiation, 220
  in immune reactions, 149–150
  significance of recirculation, 206
  structural characteristics, 149
Lysosomal storage diseases, 23
Lysosomes, 7, 146, 151, 297, 437Q, 454Q, 471E, 486E
  function, 23
  morphology, 22–23, *23*
  primary, 22
  secondary, 22
  tertiary, 23
Lysozyme, 423

M
M cells, 198, 282
  location, 198–199
  significance, 199
  structure, 198–199
M line, 85

Macrocytes, 143
Macromolecules of ground substance, 104, *104,* 105t
Macrophage activation, 109
Macrophages, 27, 107, 107t, 167, 444Q, 478E
  histologic characteristics, 107–108
  in immune system, 109
  origin, 107
  protective activities, 108
  secretory activities, 108–109
  in wound healing, 109
Macula densa, 333, 438Q, 472E
Macula lutea, 421
Maculae, 430
Maculae adherentes, 50–53, *53*
Maculae of vestibule, 428
Male genital system, 458Q, 490E
Male reproductive system, 391–407, *392*
  accessory sex glands, 404
    prostate gland, *405,* 405–406
    seminal vesicles, 405
  extratesticular genital ducts, 403–404
  functions, 401–402
  intratesticular ducts, 402–403
  penis, *406,* 406–407
  Sertoli cells, 400
    structure, 400
    unique junctions, 400–401
  spermatogenesis, 395–400, *399*
  testes, 391, *393,* 393–395
Malleus, 425
Malpighian layer, 221
Mammary gland, *386,* 386–388, *387,* 435Q, 448Q, 470E, 480–481E
Manchette, 398
Mannose-6-phosphate, 17
Marginal zone, 211
Marrow compartment, microscopic anatomy of, 166–167
Mast cells, 435Q, 470E
  contents of granules, 109–110
  degranulation, 110
  histologic characteristics of, 109
  longevity, 110
  origin, 110
Matrix, 20
  interterritorial, 124
  subcompartments, 123–124
Matrix calcification, 133
Matrix enzymes, 21
Matrix erosion, 133
Maturation ameloblasts, 250
Mechanisms of steroid activity, 362
Medial Golgi stacks, 17
Mediastinum, 393
Medulla, 464Q, 494–495E
  of kidney, 324
  of lymph node, *203,* 203–204
  of thymus, 217, *217*
Medullary capillaries, 336, 359
Medullary cells, 229
Medullary collecting ducts, 440Q, 474E
Medullary cords of lymph node, 204, *204*
Medullary osmotic gradient, 337
Medullary pyramids, 324
Medullary rays, 441Q, 475E
  of kidney, 324–325
Medullary sinuses, 205, 438Q, 473E
  of lymph node, 204
Medullary vein, 359
Medullipin I, 323, 325
Medullipin II, 325
Megakaryoblast, 164

Megakaryoblast-megakaryocyte transition, 164–165
Megakaryocytes, 164, 165, *166,* 167, 447Q, 480E
Megakaryocytopoiesis, 164–165
Meibomian glands, 422–423
Meiosis, 43–44, *44,* 373, 446Q, 458Q, 479E, 490E
  anaphase I, 45
  anaphase II, 45
  crossing over, 45
  metaphase I, 45
  metaphase II, 45
  prophase I, 44–45
  prophase II, 45
  synapsis, 45
  telophase I, 45
Meissner plexus, 239
Meissner's corpuscles, 79
Melanin, 226
Melanocytes, 226, 468Q, 497E
Melanosomes, 226
Melanotropes, 346
Melanotropins, 346
Melatonin, 372
Membrane components, mobility of, 4
Membrane enzymes, 21
Membrane glycoproteins, 3
Membrane lipid asymmetry, 14
Membrane lipids, 2–3
Membrane phospholipid biosynthetic pathway, 13
Membrane proteins, 3, 16
  topographic distribution, 5
Membranous cochlea, 427
Membranous labyrinth, 427
Membranous semicircular canals, 427
Membranous triads, 460Q, 492E
Membranous urethra, 340
Menstrual cycle, 384–385
Merkel cells, 226, 468Q, 497E
Merkel's corpuscles, 78, 226
Merocrine secretion, 259
Mesangial cells, 452Q, 484E
  functions, 330
Mesangium, 330
Mesaxons, 71, 75
Mesenchymal cells, undifferentiated, 111
Mesenchyme, 113–114
Mesoderm, 47, 113–114
Mesothelium
  in alimentary canal, 240
  in gallbladder, 303
Metabolic coupling, 55
Metamyelocyte, 163
Metaphase, 42, 396–397
Metaphase I, 45
Metaphase II, 45
Metaphase plate, 42
Metaphyses, 139
Metaphysis, 134
Metarterioles, 176, *177*
Microcytes, 143
Microfibrils, 103
Microfold cells, 282
Microglia, 69–70
Microtubule organizing centers, 29–30
Microtubule-associated proteins (MAPs), 29
Microtubule-disruptive toxins, 30
Microtubules, 28, *28*
  composition, 28
  dynamic instability, 29
  polymerization of tubulin, 28–29
Microvillar (brush) cells, 313, 315

Microvillar surface enzymes, 8
Microvilli, 8, *9,* 27, 244, 275, 278
Micturition reflex, 340
Middle ear, 453Q, 485E
Milk letdown reflex, 387–388
Mineralocorticoids, 359, 360–361
Minimal extracellular space, 47
Mitochondria, 19–20, *20,* 88, 93–94, 297, 398
  division, 21
  filamentous, 118
  function, 20–21
  genome, 21
  growth, 21
  morphology, 20
  origins, 21
Mitochondrial enzymes, 21
Mitochondrial genome, 21
Mitochondrial growth and division, 21
Mitosis, 41–42, *42,* 373, 458Q, 490E
  intraepithelial site, 58
Mitosis and meiosis of female germ cell
  oogonia, 379
  ova, 379–380
  primary oocytes, 379
  secondary oocytes, 379
Mitotic cells, 35
Mitotic compartment, 58
Mitotic spindles, 41
  of dividing cells, 444Q, 478E
Mitral valve, 169
Mixed spicule, 455Q, 487E
Modified fluid-mosaic model, 1, *2*
Modified vascular smooth muscle cells, 445Q, 478E
Monoblasts, 166
Monocytes, 107, 111, *149,* 150–151, 450Q, 452Q, 459Q, 483E, 484E, 491E
  in mononuclear phagocyte system, 151
  structural characteristics, 151
Monocytopoiesis, 166
Monoiodotyrosine, 353
Monomeric actin, 26
Mononuclear phagocyte system, 70
  monocytes in, 151
Mononuclear phagocytic cells, 166
Mononuclear phagocytic system, 129
Morula, 388
Motilin, 282
Motor proteins, 25
Motor unit, 92–93
Mouth, 245
Mucosa, 405
  aggregation of lymphatic nodules in, 437Q, 471E
  of alimentary canal, 237, 239
  of colon, 285–286, *286*
Mucosal glands, 243–244, 263
Mucosal invaginations, 195
Mucous cells, 255–256, *257*
Mucous secretory cells, 237
Müller cells, 410
Multilamellar bodies, 319
Multilaminar follicles, 374
Multipolar neurons, 64
Mumps, 260
Muscle
  cardiac, 93–94
    morphologic characteristics, 93–94
  classification, *82,* 83
  skeletal, 82–93
    connective tissue associate with, 84
    general characteristics, 82
    histologic characteristics, 84–85, *86, 87,* 88

types, 84
smooth
  contraction, 95
  morphologic characteristics, 94–95
  noncontractile functions, 95–96
Muscle spindles, 79
Muscle tissue
  contractile proteins, 81
  repair and renewal in, 96
Muscle triad, 88
Muscular artery, 456Q, 488E
Muscular venules, 180
Muscularis externa, 269, 284, 450Q, 452Q, 482–483E, 484E
  in alimentary canal, 239–240
  in esophagus, 263
  in gallbladder, 303
  in large intestine, 288
Muscularis mucosae, 239, 266, 269
  in esophagus, 263
Myelin
  comparison of peripheral myelin and central, 75
  mechanisms of formation, 72–73
Myelin sheath
  of central nervous system, 74–75
  of peripheral nervous system, 70–74
  ultrastructure, 71
Myelinated peripheral nerve, 465Q, 495E
Myeloblast, 160–161
Myelocytes, 161–163, 167, 437Q, 472E
Myeloid differentiation, 456Q, 487E
Myeloid tissue, 461Q, 493E
Myenteric plexus, 240, 452Q, 484E
Myoblasts, 83
Myocardial fibers, 448Q, 481E
Myocardium, 170
Myoepithelial cells, 256, 461Q, 492–493E
Myofibril, 83
Myofibroblastic cells, 461Q, 492–493E
Myofibroblasts, 107
Myofilaments
  overlapping of, 88
  three-dimensional organization of, 85
Myoglobin, 84
Myoid cells, 394
Myomesin, 85, 88
Myometrium, 382, *383*
Myosin, 81, 94, 461Q, 493E
  interaction between actin and, during contraction, 88–89, *90,* 91
Myosin I, 27
Myosin-binding site, 81
Myotendon junction, 84
Myotube formation, 96

N
Nail
  growth, 235
  structure, 235
Nail bed, 235
Nail matrix, 235
Nail plate, 235
Nail root, 235
Na^+,K^+-ATPase, 278, 286, 461Q, 492E
Nares, 311
Nasal cavity, 311, 449Q, 456Q, 481F, 488E
  anatomy, 311

functions of mucosa, 311
  olfactory mucosa, 311–313, *313*
Nasal septum, 311
Nasolacrimal duct, 423
Nasopharynx, 314
Natural killer (NK) cells, 149
Nebulin, 88
Neonatal thymectomy, 220
Nephron, 325, *326, 327,* 327–334, *328, 329, 331,* 443Q, 476E
Nerve cell processes, 64–66
Nerve cells
  biochemical activity, 64
  classification, 64–66
Nerve supply, renal, 338
Nervous system
  components, 61
  degeneration and regeneration, 77–78
  functions, 61
  regulation of heart, 172–173
  supporting cells, 69
    astrocytes, 69–70
    oligodendrocytes, 69
Neurofilaments, 32, *32*
Neurohypophysis, 342, 346–348, 347t, 467Q, 496–497E
Neuromuscular junction, 92
  structure, 92
Neurons, 61, *62, 63,* 450Q, 483E
  cell body, 61–62
  Golgi apparatus, 63–64
  Nissl bodies, 62–63
Neurotransmitter binding, 92
Neurotransmitter breakdown, 92
Neurotransmitter release, 92, 448Q, 481E
Neutrophilic leukocyte, 456Q, 487–488E
Neutrophils, 23, 111, *145,* 145–146, 160, 450Q, 452Q, 483E, 484E
  functions, 146
  kinetics of development, 164
Nissl bodies, 62–63
Nissl substance, 16
N-linked glycosylation, 16
N-linked oligosaccharide chains, processing of, 17
Nodes of Ranvier, 453Q, 486E
  in central nervous system, 75
  in peripheral nervous system, 73–74
Nodular mantle, 193
Nodules with germinal centers, 445Q, 478E
Noncoated pinocytotic vesicles, 6
Nonhistone proteins, 35
Nonkeratinized cells, 221
Nonkeratinized stratified squamous epithelium, 448Q, 450Q, 480–481E, 482E
  in esophagus, 263
Noradrenalin, 119, 362
Norepinephrine, 119, 362
Norepinephrine-secreting cells, 363
Normoblasts, 159, 167
Nuclear chromatin, 442Q, 476E
Nuclear DNA, 447Q, 480E
Nuclear envelope, *38,* 38–39, 459Q, 491E
Nuclear events, 43
Nuclear lamina, 39–40
Nuclear lamins, 32–33, 449Q, 481E
  dynamic function, 34
Nuclear location sequences, 39
Nuclear matrix, 40, 459Q, 491E
Nuclear pore complex, 39

Nuclear pores, 39
Nucleating structure, 26
Nuclei, 88
Nucleolus, 440Q, 449Q, 473E, 481E
  functional regions, 37–38
  morphology, 37
Nucleosomal histones, 35
Nucleosomes, 36, 442Q, 476E
Nucleotide-binding site, 81
Nucleus, 1, 35–45, 62, 94
  cell cycle
    division, 43
    interphase, 40–41, *41*
    mitosis, 41–42, *42*
  chromosomes
    chromatin, 35–37, *36*
    general appearance, 35
    number, 35
    types of, 36–37, *37*
  meiosis, 43–44, *44*
    anaphase I, 45
    anaphase II, 45
    crossing over, 45
    metaphase I, 45
    metaphase II, 45
    prophase I, 44–45
    prophase II, 45
    synapsis, 45
    telophase I, 45
  nuclear envelope, *38*, 38–39
  nuclear lamina, 39–40
  nuclear matrix, 40
  nuclear pores, 39
  nucleolus
    functional regions, 37–38
    morphology, 37
Nutrients, supply of, to chondrocytes,
    125–126

O

Odontoblast processes, 252
Odontoblasts, 251
Olfactory cilia, 312
Olfactory mucosa, 311–313, *313*
Oligodendrocytes, 69, 75, 440Q, 474E
O-linked glycoproteins, synthesis of,
  17
Oocyte-containing ovarian follicles,
  373
Oocyte-granulosa cell gap junctions,
  440Q, 474E
Oocytes, 44, 449Q, 451Q, 481E, 483E
Oogonia, 379
Opsonins, 8
Opsonization, 8
Optic cup, 412, 438Q, 466Q, 472E,
  496E
Optic nerve, 409, 421
Oral cavity, 245–253
  mucosa, 245–246
  teeth, 248, *250*
    cementum, 251
    dentin, 251–252
    enamel, 248, 250–251
    pulp cavity, 252
    supporting tissues of, 252–253
  tongue, 246
    gross appearance of dorsal surface,
      246, *247*
    lingual papillae, 247
    muscles, 246
    taste buds, 247–248, *249*
Organ of Corti, 428, 430–431, 442Q,
  476E
Organelles, 1
Orthochromatic erythroblast, 159, 167

Ossification
  secondary centers of, 136
  zone, 135
Osteoblasts, 127, *128*, 435Q, 470E
Osteoclasia, 128–129
Osteoclasts, 23, *128*, 128–129, 440Q,
  442Q, 473E, 475–476E
Osteocytes, 127–128, *128*
  maintaining and maintenance of
    bone matrix, 129
Osteocytic osteolysis, 128
Osteogenesis
  endochondral ossification, 133–136
  intramembranous ossification,
    132–133
Osteoid, 435Q, 461Q, 470E, 493E
  maintaining and maintenance of
    bone matrix, 129–130
Osteonal canal, 136
Osteons
  development, 137
  relationship of, to ossification
    processes, 137–138
Osteoprogenitor cells, 127
  modulation, 133
Otitis media, 426
Otoliths, 430
Outer leaflet, 2
Ova, 379–380
Oval window, 468Q, 497–498E
Ovarian follicles, 435Q, 470E
  and age of female, 376
Ovarian stroma, 373, 374
Ovaries
  and age of female, 376
  atresia of, 376–377, *377*
  cortical compartment, 373
  female germ cells, oogonia and
    oocytes, 373
  gross aspects, 373
  medullary compartment, 373
  ovarian, 373–376, *375*
Oviducts
  histologic structure, 380
  regions, 380
Ovulation, 377–378, 440Q, 474E
Oxidative phosphorylation, 463Q,
  493E
Oxygen, transport of, in blood, 143
Oxyntic cells, 270
Oxyphil cells, 355, *356*
Oxytalin fibers, 103, 253
Oxytocin, 347, 388

P

Pachytene, 396
Pacinian corpuscles, 79
Palatine tonsillar crypts, 196
Palatine tonsils, 195, 246, 444Q,
  452Q, 477E, 484–485E
Pale-staining regions, 38
Palpebral conjunctiva, 411
Pancreas, 242–243, 244, 255, 459Q,
  490E
  enzymes from, 273
Pancreatic exocrine secretion, 446Q,
  479E
Pancreatic islet, 467Q, 496–497E
Pancreatic polypeptide, 282, 310
Pancreozymin, 309
Paneth cells, 282, 283, 450Q, 483E
Panniculus adiposus, 115, 228
Panniculus carnosus, 228
Papillae, lingual, 247
Papillary lamina propria in oral cavity,
  246

Paracortex, 202
Paracrine, 453Q, 485E
Paracrine effects, 370
Parafollicular cells, 141, 351
Parakeratinized epithelium, 245
Paranasal sinuses, 313
Parasympathetic fibers, 310
Parasympathetic stimulation, 262
Parathormone, 460Q, 492E
Parathyroid glands, 140–141,
  354–357, 446Q, 467Q, 479E,
  496–497E
  calcium homeostasis, 356–357
  histologic characteristics, 355–356,
    356
  structure and development, 355
Parathyroid hormone, 356
  physiologic roles, 356–357
Parenchyma in liver, 289
Parietal bone, 442Q, 475–476E
Parietal cells, 270, 449Q, 464Q, 482E,
  494E
Parietal eye, 372
Parotid glands, 259–260
Pars distalis, 342, 344
Pars intermedia, 342, 346
Pars nervosa, 346–347
Pars plana, 417
Pars plicata, 417
Pars tuberalis, 344
Pedicels, 327–328
Peg cells, 380
Penicillar arterioles, 213
Penile urethra, 340
Penis, 391, *406*, 406–407
Pepsinogens, 265, 270–271, 464Q,
  494E
Pepsins, 270–271
Peptidase proenzymes, 305
Peptides, 341
Perforating canals, 138, 453Q, 485E
Periarteriolar lymphatic sheath, 209
Pericardium, 170
Perichondrial cells, 121
Perichondrium, 121
Pericryptal fibroblast sheath, 275,
  287–288
Pericryptal fibroblasts, 457Q, 460Q,
  489E, 492E
Pericytes, 96, 178–179, 437Q, 471E
Perilymph, 428
Perilymphatic space, 427
Perimetrium, 382
Perimysium, 84
Perineurium, 77
Perinuclear space, 38
Periodic acid-Schiff (PAS) reaction,
  102, 191
Periodontal ligament, 252–253
Periodontium, 253
Periosteum, 127, 131
Peripheral blood, 444Q, 478E
Peripheral membrane proteins, 3
Peripheral myelin sheath, development
  of, 71–73, *72*, *73*
Peripheral nerve, connective tissue
  sheaths of, *76*, 76–77
Peripheral nervous system (PNS), 61
  myelin sheath, 70–74
  nodes of Ranvier, 73–74
  regeneration, 78
  unmyelinated nerves, 75–76
Perirenal adipose tissue, 323
Perisinusoidal space, *298*, 298–299,
  443Q, 476E
  in liver, 289
Peristalsis, 269, 284

Peritoneal covering, 373
Peritonsillar tissues, 196
Peritubular capillaries, 335
  network, 329
Peritubular tissue, 394
Peroxisomes, 297
  biogenesis, 22
  functions, 22
  morphology, 22
Peyer patches, 195, 273, 464Q,
    494–495E
  function, 197
  histologic characteristics, 197, 197
  location, 196–197
P-face, 4
PG, 463Q, 493E
Phagocytic cells, 401
Phagocytic vacuoles, fate of, 8
Phagocytosis, 5, 7–8, 22, 461Q, 492E
  and sinuses, 205
Phagosomes, 7–8, 146
  formation, 7–8
Phalangeal cells, 430
Phalloidin, 27, 28
Pharyngeal tonsil, 195, 314
Pharyngoesophageal sphincter, 240
Pharynx, 453Q, 485E
Phenylethanolamine N-
    methyltransferase, 363
Pheomelanin, 226
Pheromones, 234
Phosphatases, 444Q, 478E
Phosphatidylcholine, 3
Phosphatidylethanolamine, 3
Phosphatidylinositol, 3
Phosphatidylserine, 3
Phospholipid exchange proteins, 13
Phospholipid translocation, 14
Phospholipids, 3, 453Q, 485E
Phosphorylation, 95
Photoreception, 372, 409–410
Photoreceptor cell, 419–420
Photosensitive layer, 409
Pigment cells, 422
Pigmentation, 410
Pilosebaceous canal, 230
Pineal antigonadotropin, 372
Pineal gland, 371–372, 467Q,
    496–497E
  functions, 371–372
  parenchymal cells, 371
  role, 444Q, 477E
Pinealocytes, 371
Pinocytosis, 5
  fluid-phase, 6, 6
Pituicytes, 348
Pituitary gland, 341–343, 342, 343,
    344
Placenta, 388–389, 467Q, 496–497E
  blood circulation through, 389
  functions, 389
Placental barrier, 389
Placental villi, 454Q, 486E
  formation, 389
Plasma cells, 111, 460Q, 492E
  as effector cells, 187
  in germinal centers, 193
  structural characteristics, 187,
    187–188, 188
Plasma membrane, 1
  functions in cell regulation and
    signaling, 4–5
  specializations, 8–10
  surface structures, 8–10, 9, 12
Plasma membrane proteins, classes of,
    4–5
Platelets, 151–153, 152, 444Q, 461Q,
    478E, 493E

aggregation, 152
  in hemostasis, 152–153
  quantity, 151
  shape, 151
  size, 151
  structural characteristics, 151–152
Plicae circulares, 244, 273
Pluripotential stem cell, 158
Podocytes, 327–328
Polar bodies, 44
Polychromatophilic erythroblast,
    158–159, 159, 456Q, 488E
Polymerization, regulation of, 26
Polymerization of tubulin, 28–29
Polymorphonuclear leukocyte (PMN),
    145, 164
Polypeptide chains, 98
Polyribosomes, 98–99, 159
Polysaccharides, 448Q, 481E
Polysomes, 24
Porta hepatis, 290
Portal blood vessels, 181–182
Portal lobule, 293
Portal system of blood vessels, 455Q,
    487F
Portal triads, 290
Postcapillary venules, 180
Postmitotic compartment, 58
Postmitotic keratinocytes, 223
Postsynaptic component, 66
Post-translational modifications, 16–17
Postvenule veins, general
    characteristics of, 180
Power stroke, 12, 89
Preadipocytes, 118
Precursor cell, 452Q, 484E
Predentin, 251
Pregnancy, corpus luteum of, 379
Preproparathyroid hormone, 356
Prepuce, 407
Presynaptic component, 66
Presynaptic plasma membrane, 448Q,
    481E
Primary follicles, 374
Primary lysosomes, 22
Primary nodule, 193
Primary oocytes, 379
Primordial follicles, 374
Proacrosomal granules, 397
Procollagen, synthesis of, 98–99
Procollagen peptidase, 99
Proenzymes, release of, 445Q, 478E
Proerythroblast, 158
Profilin, 26
Prokaryotic cells, 1
Proliferation, zone of, 134
Proliferative, 454Q, 486E
Proline, 97, 446Q, 479E
Prometaphase, 42
Promonocytes, 166
Promyelocyte, 161, 161, 443Q, 456Q,
    476E, 488E
Pro-opiomelanocortin, 345–346
Prophase, 41, 397
Prophase I, 44–45, 446Q, 479E
Prophase II, 45
Proprioceptors, 78
Propulsion, 468Q, 497E
Prostaglandins, 405
Prostate gland, 391, 405, 405–406
Prostatic urethra, 340
Prostatic utricle, 404
Proteases, 444Q, 478E
Protection, 468Q, 497E
Protein biosynthesis, 16
Protein biosynthetic pathway, 13

Protein synthesis
  capacity, 63
  location, 16
Proteins, 341, 438Q, 472F
  exocytotic secretion, 388
  membrane, 3, 16
  nonhistone, 35
  sulfation, 19
  translocation, 16
Protein-secreting cells, 270
Proteoglycans, 104, 414, 448Q, 461Q,
    481E, 493E
  sulfation of sugars in, 435Q, 470E
Protofilaments, 28
Proton gradients, 21
Proton motive force, 21
Proximal convoluted tubule, 330–332,
    438Q, 440Q, 472F, 473F
Proximal straight tubule, 332
Pseudostratified epithelium, 403–404,
    404
Puberty, 391, 443Q, 477E
Pulmonary alveolus, 453Q, 485E
Pulmonary surfactant, 450Q, 482E
Pulmonary valve, 169
Pulp cavity, 252
Pulp veins, 213
Pumps, 278
Pupil, 416
Purkinje fibers, 171–172, 172, 451Q,
    483E
Pyloric glands, 267
Pyloric sphincter, 240
Pylorus, 265

Q
Quarter-molecule stagger, 97

R
Rathke pouch, 342
Receptor down-regulation, 7
Receptor proteins, 5
Receptor-ligand interactions, 7
Receptor-mediated endocytosis, 6–7,
    461Q, 492E
Receptor-mediated process, 39
Recovery stroke, 12
Rectal glands, 285
Rectum, 237, 285
Red blood cells (RBCs), 447Q, 450Q,
    455Q, 480E, 483E, 487E
  alteration of shape, 144–145
  kinetics of development, 160
Red bone marrow, 443Q, 476E
  cell associations in, 167
Red fibers, 84
Red pulp, 209, 211, 211–213
  blood circulation through, 214, 214
  functions, 213
  of spleen, 447Q, 480E
  venous drainage, 213
Refractive index, 409
Regeneration, 78
Regulated secretion, 19, 27
Reissner membrane, 428
Renal capsule, 325, 327–328
Renal circulation, 335–337, 336
Renal columns of kidney, 324
Renal corpuscles, 324, 325
Renal glomerular capillary, 452Q,
    484E
Renal lobule, 441Q, 475F
Renal lymphatic vessels, 336–337
Renal nerve supply, 338
Renal pelvis, 339
Renal sinus, 323

Renal vessels, 437Q, 471E
Renin, 96, 323, 333, 361
  secreted, 445Q, 478E
Renin-angiotensin, 465Q, 495E
Renin-angiotensin system, 361
Replicative zone, 275
Reproductive system. (*See* Female
  reproductive system; Male
  reproductive system.)
Residual bodies, 23
Resorption, zone of, 135–136
Respiratory bronchioles, 318
Respiratory epithelium, 311
Respiratory system, 311–321, *312*
  air-blood barrier, *320,* 320–321, *321*
  alveoli, 318–320, *319*
    collateral air circulation, 320
    histologic characteristics, 318–320,
      319
    interalveolar septum, 319–320
    structural organization, 318
  bronchi, 315–317, *316*
    extrapulmonary, 316
    histologic characteristics, 316–317
    intrapulmonary, 316, *316*
  bronchioles, *317,* 317–318
    histologic characteristics, 317–318
  larynx, 314
  nasal cavity, 311
    anatomy, 311
    functions of mucosa, 311
    olfactory mucosa, 311–313, *313*
  nasopharynx, 314
  paranasal sinuses, 313
  surfactant, 321
  trachea, 314–315, *315*
    anatomy, 314
    histologic characteristics, 314–315
Resting cartilage, zone of, 134
Rete testis, 402
Reticular cells, 102
  of lymph node, 454Q, 486E
Reticular fibers, 100, 102–103, 119
  composition and structure, 102
  distribution, 100, 102
  synthesis, 102
Reticular lamina, 58
Reticular membrane, 430
Reticular tissue, 113
Reticulocytes, 143, 160
Retina, 419–421, *420,* 466Q, 496E
Retinal detachment, 438Q, 466Q,
  472E, 496E
Retinal layer, 409
Retinal pigment epithelium (RPE), 419
Retrograde degeneration, 77
Rhodopsin, 419
Ribonuclease, 305
Ribosomal RNA, 37
Ribosomal subunits, 440Q, 473E
Ribosomes, 24
  bound, 24
  free, 24
Right atrium, 169
Right ventricle, 169
  and left ventricle, 437Q, 471E
Rigor mortis, 89
Rods, 409–410, 419
Rokitansky-Aschoff sinuses in
  gallbladder, 303
Rotating cell model, 72
Rough endoplasmic reticulum, 13, *15,*
  15–17, 88, 187, 295, 440Q,
  457Q, 474E, 488E
Rouleaux, 143
Ruffini's corpuscles, 79
Ruffled border, 129
Rugae, 244, 265

S
S phase, 40–41
Sacculations, 288
Saccule, 427, 430
Saliva, 261–262
Salivary glands, 237, 245, 255–262,
  448Q, 459Q, 467Q, 481E, 490E,
  496E
  general characteristics of, 255–257,
    256, 257, 258, 259
  major, 255
  minor, 255
  parotid, 259–260
  saliva, 261–262
  sublingual, 260–261
  submandibular, 260
Salivation, control of, 261–262
Saltatory conduction, 73–74, 453Q,
  486E
Sarcolemma, 83
Sarcomere, 85, 455Q, 487E
  supporting proteins of, 88
Sarcomeres, 93
Sarcoplasm, 83
Sarcoplasmic reticulum, 14, 83, 85,
  87, 94
Satellite cells, 61, 70, 96
Saw-toothed epithelium, 402–403
Scala media, 428
Scala tympani, 429
Scala vestibuli, 429
Scar formation, 78
Schmidt-Lantermann, incisures of, 74
Schwann cells, 61, 70, 75–76, 98, 102
Schwann sheath, 71
Schwann tubes, 78
Sclera, 415
Scurvy, 99
Sebaceous cell, 468Q, 497E
Sebaceous glands, 230, *231, 232,* 423
  function of sebum, 232
  secretion, 232
  structure, 230–231
  transformation, 231
Sebum, 232, 452Q, 484E
Secondary lysosomes, 22
Secondary nodule, 193
Secondary oocytes, 379, 449Q, 482E
Secretin, 272, 281, 309, 446Q, 479E
Secretion, 468Q, 497E
  constitutive, 19
  regulated, 19
  role of Golgi apparatus in, 19
  stimulation, 272
Secretory acini and tubules, 255–256,
  256
Secretory ameloblasts, 250
Secretory cells, 401
Secretory IgA (sIgA), 242, 261
Secretory proteins, 16, 457Q, 489E
Segmentation, 284
Selective aggregation, 19
Sella turcica, 341
Semen, 406
Semicircular canals, 427, 429–430
Seminal vesicles, 391, 405
Seminiferous epithelium, 394, 441Q,
  475E
  cycles of, 399–400
Seminiferous tubules, 393–394, 460Q,
  491–492E
Sensory areas, 428
Serosa, 284, 380
  in alimentary canal, 240
  in gallbladder, 303
  in large intestine, 288
Serous acinar cells, 305, 307, *307*

Serous acini, 305
Serous cells, 255, 256
Serous demilune, 256
Sertoli cells, 391, 394, 454Q, 458Q,
  460Q, 486Q, 490E, 491–492E
  functions, 401–402
  structure, 400
  unique junctions, 400–401
Sertoli-Sertoli junctions, 400–401
Sertoli-spermatid junctions, 401
Sex chromatin, 146
Sharpey's fibers, 131
Shearing effect, 431
Sheathed arterioles, 213
Sialoglycoproteins, 330
Signal peptidase, 16
Signal recognition particle (SRP), 16
Signal sequence, 16
Simple columnar epithelium, 465Q,
  495E
Simple squamous epithelium, 450Q,
  482E
Sinoatrial (SA) node, 171
Sinuses
  anal, 285
  cortical, 205
  lymphatic, *203,* 204–205
  medullary, 204, 205
  paranasal, 313
  in red pulp, 211–212
  renal, 323
  Rokitansky-Aschoff, 303
  subcapsular (marginal), 205
Sinusoidal circulation, 290–291
Sinusoidal endothelium, 291
Sinusoidal wall, 167
Sinusoids, 179, 290
  in liver, 289
Sister chromatids, 41
Skeletal muscle, 83, 461Q, 492–493E
  connective tissue associate with, 84
  general characteristics, 83
  histologic characteristics, 84–85, *86,*
    87, 88
  repair and renewal of cells, 96
  types of fibers, 84
Skin, 221–236
  apocrine glands, 234
    distribution, 234
    function, 234
    structure, 234
  components, 221, *222*
  dermis, 226
    components, 226–227
    dermoepidermal junction, 227–228
    fibroblasts, 227
    general characteristics, 226
    hypodermis, 228
    Langer lines, 227
  eccrine sweat glands
    distribution, 232–233
    function, 233–234
    structure, 233, *233*
  epidermal appendages, 221
  epidermis, 221
    basal cells, 222–223
    general characteristics, 221–222,
      223
    granular cells, 224
    keratinized cells, 224–225
    nonkeratinocytes, 225–226
    spinous cells, 223–224
  functions, 221
  hair follicles, 228, *229*
    arrector pili muscles, 230
    baldness, 230
    differentiating region, 228–229